D1557847

ANAC's
Core Curriculum for
HIV/AIDS Nursing

Kathleen McMahon Casey, MEd, MA, RN
Felissa Cohen, PhD, RN, FAAN
Anne M. Hughes, MN, RN, FNP, OCN

Editors

Association of Nurses in AIDS Care

ANAC's
Core Curriculum for
HIV/AIDS Nursing

Published by: Nursecom, Inc.
1211 Locust St.
Philadelphia, PA 19107

For: The Association of Nurses in AIDS Care

Printed in the United States of America
10 9 8 7 6 5 4 3 2 1

ISBN: 0-963702-2-2

Library of Congress Catalog Card Number: 96-69700

A Nursecom Book

To all nurses who care for or have cared for people whose lives have been affected by HIV/AIDS

Kathleen McMahon Casey, Felissa Lashley Cohen,
and Anne M. Hughes

Contents

Appendices

References

Bibliography

Index

Figures

Tables

Preface

The epidemic associated with HIV infection, first recognized 15 years ago, began almost unnoticed with the suffering and deaths of a few people—gay men, people with hemophilia, people who had received blood transfusions, injecting drug users, and their sexual partners (and in some cases their children). Lost human lives marked what would become known as the global public health tragedy of the 20th century. While the etiology of the rare illness frightened many and led to abandonment and stigmatization, some nurses responded with uncommon courage, commitment, and compassion.

Little was known about the phenomenon. An infectious agent was hypothesized and in 1983 a human retrovirus was identified as the probable cause. In the years since the human immunodeficiency virus was classified and the natural history of HIV infection described, nurses have studied medical sciences such as epidemiology, virology, infectious diseases, oncology, neurology, and psychiatry. They have been required to learn, or relearn in some instances, about health psychology, adult education theory, legal-ethical issues, infection-control practices, and communities and cultures different from their own in order to provide competent care.

In fall 1987 and through spring 1988, a small group of nursing visionaries met to form what is now known as the Association of Nurses in AIDS Care (ANAC). ANAC is a nursing specialty organization with more than 2,500 members from around the United States and the world. ANAC has 42 local chapters in the United States. In what would be an historic effort, nurses—the unsung heroes in providing care to individuals, families, and communities affected by HIV/AIDS—began an organization that continues to provide leadership in this nursing-intensive, chronic illness.

The vision for a core curriculum and its initial planning (i.e., soliciting ANAC Board support and coordinating the two-round Delphi survey) was most ably done by James Halloran, president of ANAC from 1991 to 1992. Its form and substance, however, are the gift of more than 90 volunteer contributors and editors who together donated thousands of hours fine tuning this curriculum into a scientifically based work of nursing art.

In the years since the epidemic was first noticed, nurses have amassed a sizeable body of knowledge, which is included in this core curriculum. A two-round Delphi survey method was used to validate the content; the first round was conducted in fall 1993 and the second in winter 1994. Each respondent was asked to rate the relative importance of a topic on a scale of 0 to 4 (0 = not at all important, 4 = essential knowledge for HIV/AIDS nursing practice). None of the 27 ANAC leaders who responded rated any item as unimportant or not necessarily essential information for the HIV/AIDS nurse. Listed here are selected items and their mean scores from the first round of surveys:

Topic	Mean Score
Clinical manifestations of HIV infection	4.0
Nursing management of HIV disease	4.0
Risk behaviors for transmission of HIV	3.96
End-of-life decisions	3.93
Pathophysiology of HIV disease	3.81
Occupational safety for healthcare workers	3.7
Impact of HIV infection on the family	3.69
Meaning of HIV infection in various cultures	3.44
Medical management of HIV disease	3.33
Prevention/education issues among gay men	3.11
Prevention/education among women	3.11
Quackery/fraud	2.52
Harm reduction model	2.17

In the second round, ANAC leaders were also to describe key content to be included in the topic areas previously identified. These key concepts were used to develop the breadth of the core curriculum.

Nurse clinicians, nurse researchers, nurse educators, nurse administrators, and some other colleagues collaborated to develop this core curriculum. Some of the contributors have spent their professional careers studying the work they have presented and have published extensively; others are clinical experts with possibly less publishing experience. Proudly we acknowledge, thank, and list our contributors along with the titles of their work, starting on page xvii. Please read this list to appreciate the experts who have developed this curriculum.

The core curriculum supports the mission of ANAC. As the ANAC Bylaws state:

The mission of the Association is to promote the individual and collective professional development of nurses involved in the delivery of health care to persons infected or affected by the Human Immunodeficiency Virus (HIV) and to promote the health and welfare of infected persons by

- Creating an effective network among nurses in AIDS care;
- Studying, researching, and exchanging information, experience, and ideas leading to improved care for persons with AIDS/HIV infection;
- Advocating by HIV-infected persons; and
- Promoting social awareness concerning issues related to HIV/AIDS.

Inherent in these goals is the abiding commitment to the prevention of further HIV infection.

The core curriculum helps document not only the history of ANAC but also the development of HIV as a nursing specialty that crosses practice settings, roles, research interests and other professional nursing identities. HIV/AIDS nurses (like our contributors) are adult health nurses, pediatric nurses, psychiatric nurses, community health nurses, acute care nurses, nurse scientists, nurse practitioners, nurse midwives, nurse managers, nurse educators, and case managers. For some of our contributors, HIV was the reason for becoming a nurse; for others, HIV is a natural extension of the value accorded professional and social responsibility.

Finally, the core curriculum is a key first step in developing a certification process to assure competency in HIV/AIDS nursing practice. The editors have made every possible effort to ensure that the content in this book is accurate, scientifically based, and current at the time of publication. One of the challenges of this age is keeping current in a specialty that is always advancing. ANAC and the editors of this book (who are listed alphabetically, and not in order of contribution) would like your feedback, ideas, and comments.

Kathleen McMahon Casey
Felissa Lashley Cohen
Anne M. Hughes

Acknowledgments

Several people made important contributions to the project and supported me through the process. I am indebted to James M. Casey for editorial critiques, administrative support, and his belief in the importance of the book; to Jim Halloran for asking me to be an editor; to Mária Cipriani for word processing support; to my family (Eileen and sisters Eileen [and family], Mary Ellen [and family], Patricia, and Rosemary) for sharing in my delight; and to my Helix Community for their encouragement and care. I also feel gratitude toward ANAC for allowing me to make this contribution to HIV/AIDS nursing and to the 44 contributing authors with whom I worked for making the process so smooth.

K.M.C.

With love and thanks to my children who are so special to me: Pete and Julie, Heather, and Neal and Anne. With special recognition to my parents, Ruth and Jack Lashley, and to Tony O. I also want to thank all those who helped on this project, including Mary Allen for reviewing selected parts of the manuscript, the library staff at Southern Illinois University at Edwardsville (especially Kathy Behm) and at Southern Illinois University School of Medicine at Springfield, and to all my friends who listened to me moan and are still my friends. Especially I want to pay tribute to all the nurses, families, and others that I have worked with who are so committed to those affected by HIV/AIDS. Finally, to all the contributors to the sections I edited, thank you for all your hard work, commitment, and cooperation; it is due to you that this book exists.

F.L.C.

Many wonderful people supported me during the development of this book. My partner Marylin provided unfailing support, belief in the importance of the project, and understanding why I always seemed too busy. My co-editors have become cherished colleagues and good friends over the past several years. Felissa's wisdom, practicality, and tolerance was so appreciated, as was Kathleen's drive, creativity, and her sense of humor. Margo Neal, our publisher, provided mentorship, and her optimism made me believe we would complete the project. My family, friends, and co-workers gave their love and support in all kinds of ways, listening when I needed to talk and letting me be quiet at other times. Ann Kurth provided critical leadership at a critical part of this project; other ANAC board members and ANAC friends offered hope and belief in the importance of this work. Rita Fahrner generously agreed to be an external reviewer for a portion of the book. Lastly, I would like to thank the wonderful contributors I had the privilege of working with; their work has made this book a work of art and of science.

A.M.H.

Introduction

The goals of *ANAC's Core Curriculum for HIV/AIDS Nursing* are

- To identify the essential information required by nurses to care for people with HIV/AIDS regardless of practice setting or role responsibilities
- To serve as foundation for the ANAC certification process for HIV/AIDS specialty nurses/nursing, and
- To provide a framework for core curriculum content that may be used in undergraduate, staff development, and continuing education programs related to HIV/AIDS nursing care.

We intend the book to be used by novice HIV nurses as a reference text, to assist in planning of care, and to stimulate discussion. For the more expert nurse, we expect this text may guide staff/patient educational efforts and quality-improvement activities, and support the demands of expert clinical practice.

We have used the standardized, outline format to enable the reader to scan headings and subheadings rapidly to find topics of interest. There are more than 90 contributors to this book. Read the *Contributors* list to identify the authors of specific content in the text. In some instances, contributing authors' text is divided among two or more sections of the book.

Contributing Authors

Joyce K. Anastasi, PhD, RN
Assistant Professor; Director, AIDS Program;
Co-director, Center for AIDS Research
Columbia University School of Nursing
New York, NY
  *Condylomata acuminata, pelvic inflammatory
  disease*

Heather Anderson, MN, RN
Faculty Member, University of Washington
Schools of Social Work & Nursing
Nursing Consultant, Human Source,
Seattle, WA
  Humor

Douglas Arditti, MN, FNP
University of Washington AIDS Education &
  Training Center and School of Nursing
Seattle, WA
Medford Clinic, Medford, OR
  *Cytomegalovirus, herpes simplex virus, varicella
  zoster virus*

Mary C. Angerame, MS, RN, CS, OCN
Adult Nurse Practitioner
Community Health Network, Inc.
Rochester, NY
  All parasitic infections; sinusitis

Linda Augustyniak, RN, BSN
Nurse Consultant
The National Hemophilia Foundation
New York, NY
  People with hemophilia

John Barfield, MSW, RN, CS
Clincial Nurse Specialist
San Diego County Department of Health
  Services
San Diego, CA
  The incarcerated

Cynthia Reno Balkstra, MS, RNC
Pulmonary CNS
Candler Hospital
Candler, GA
  Cough, dyspnea

Bill Barrick
Head Nurse
HIV Research Clinic
National Institutes of Health
Bethesda, MD
  Natural history

Crystal C. Bennett, RN, DNSc
Administrative Nurse IV
School of Nursing, UCLA
Los Angeles, CA
  Social support

Barbara E. Berger, PhD, RN
University of Illinois at Chicago
Chicago, IL
  Stigma

Christine M. Boenning, MSN, RN
Nurse Specialist/Study Coordinator
NIAID, Nation Institutes of Health
Bethesda, MD
  *Immune system enhancement or restoration:
  Gene therapy*

Julia A. Bucher, PhD, RN
Assistant Professor,
Bloomsburg University
Bloomsburg, PA
  Rural communities

Cynthia Brogdon, MSN, RN
Clinical Support Specialist
Amgen
Thousand Oaks, CA
  *Potential for infection: neutropenia, potential for
  bleeding: thrombocytopenia*

Gerald A. Burns, MSN, RN
Infectious Diseases Clinical Nurse Specialist
Harper Hospital
Detroit, MI
  *High risk for ineffective management of
  therapeutic regimen*

Carolyn Keith Burr, MS, RN
Associate Director
National Pediatric & Family HIV Resource
  Center
Newark, NJ
  Clinical management of pediatric patients

Kathleen McMahon Casey, MEd, MA, RN
Nursing Consultant, AIDS and Oncology
Associate, Columbia University School of
    Nursing
New York, NY
    Immune system enhancement or restoration
    (through vaccine development), pelvic
    inflammatory disease, meditation

Mária I. Cipriani, MA
Psychospiritual Counselor, Private Practice
Brooklyn, NY
    Meditation

Cecily D. Cosby, MSN, FNP
NP III, UCSF, HIV Practice
San Francisco, CA
    All dermatologic complications, aphthous ulcers,
    syphilis

Noreen Coyne, MSN, RN, OCN, CRNI
National Director, Infusion Therapy
Staff Builders' Home Health Care
Lake Success, NY
    Hearing loss, hiccups, idiopathic thrombocy-
    topenic purpura

Donna Davage (Amrita), MS
Certified Kundalini Yoga Teacher
New York, NY
    Yoga

Ann S. Dellaira, PhD, RN(C)
Assistant Professor & Coordinator, HIV
    Subspecialization MSN Tract
Department of Nursing
Rutgers University
Camden, NJ
    All endocrine complications

Alice S. Demi, DNS, RN, FAAN
Professor, School of Nursing,
Georgia State University
Atlanta, GA
    Grief & loss

Pamela J. Dole, DEd, FNP, RN
Nurse Researcher/Colpo-scopist, Department
    of OB/GYN Pathology and Clinical
    Instructor, School of Nursing,
Columbia University
New York, NY
    Menstrual irregularities

Julie C. Funesti Esch, BSN, RN, CCM
Clinical Research Nurse
AIDS Supportive Care Clinic
Memorial Sloan Kettering Cancer Center
New York, NY
    Appendix: Drug development

David Feldt, RN
Manager, AIDS Program & Special Projects
Visiting Nurse Association of Cleveland
Cleveland, OH
    HIV-positive nurses

Richard S. Ferri, RN, PhD, ANP
HIV/AIDS Nurse Practitioner
MediCenter
Harwich, MA
    Sexual transmission

Stuart N. Fisk, RN, PHN
Nurse Case Manager
Visiting Nurses & Hospice of San Francisco
San Francisco, CA
    Sex industry workers, substance users

Kathryn J. Foley, MS, RN
Nurse Practitioner
Community Medical Alliance
Boston, MA
    Mycobacterium tuberculosis

Paul N. Franquist, MSN, RN
Clinical Nurse Specialist,
Medical-Surgical/ Immunodeficiency
Desert Samaritan Medical Center
Mesa, AZ
    Anorectal signs & symptoms, body image
    disturbance

Vivian Gaits, MSN, RN, CS, OCN
Instructor, Englewood Hospital & Medical
    Center
School of Nursing
Englewood, NJ
    All hematologic system complications

Donna M. Gallagher, MS, RN-C, ANP
Director, New England AIDS Education &
    Training Center
Univ. of MA. Medical Center
Worcester, MA
Senior Nurse Practitioner
Community Medical Alliance
Boston, MA
    HIV testing & counseling

Christine Grady, PhD, RN
Acting Clinical Director
National Institute of Nursing Research, NIH
Bethesda, MD
Vaccine development

Patricia Harrington, EdD, RN, CS
Chairperson, Department of Nursing
University of Scranton
Scranton, PA
All hematologic complications

Hilarie S. Harris, MS, RN,
Director, AIDS Dementia Unit
St. Mary's Hospital & Medical Center
San Francisco, CA
AIDS dementia complex

Betsey R. Herpin, MSN, RN
Research Study Coordinator, HIV/AIDS Clinical
     Trials
NIAID, National Institutes of Health
Bethesda, MD
*The use of surrogate markers to evaluate HIV
treatment & efficacy*

Susan Holman, MS, RN
Project Director, Women's Interagency HIV
     Study
SUNY Health Science Center at Brooklyn
Brooklyn, NY
Women

Barbara J. Holtzclaw, PhD, RN, FAAN
Professor, Director of Nursing Research
School of Nursing
University of Texas Science
Center at San Antonio
San Antonio, TX
Fever & night sweats

Joseph T. Horan, LMT
Director, Reflexology Seminars of New York
New York, NY
Reflexology

Mary Jo Hoyt, MSN, RN, FNP
Director, Women's Program
AIDS Center, St Vincent's Hospital
New York, NY
Lab values

Anne Hughes, MN, RN
Clinical Nurse Specialist, HIV Disease
San Francisco General Hospital
San Francisco, CA
Potential for injury: falls

Valery Hughes, BSN, RN
HIV Clinician, Retroviral Disease Clinic AIDS
     Center Program
Lenox Hill Hospital
New York, NY
Periodontal disease

Barbara E. Joël, LMT
Private Practice, Massage Therapy
New York, NY
Massage

Ernestine King-McCoy, RN, CS
HIV Program Administrator
Greater Baltimore Medical Center Community
     Health Center
Baltimore, MD
African-American community

Vi Kunkle, MS, RN
Assistant Professor
West Suburban College of Nursing
Oak Park, IL
Epstein-Barr virus

Ann Kurth, MPH, MSN, CNM
Indiana State Dept. of Health
Indianapolis, IN
Vertical transmission

Frank P. Lamendola, PhD(C), CS, CRNH
Consultant & Educator
Journeywell
Minneapolis, MN
HIV-positive nurses; spiritual distress

Jennifer Lang-Kummer, MN, RN, CS
Director, Case Management Services
Pitt County Memorial Hospital
Washington, NC
Impaired/risk for impaired skin integrity

Suzanne Lego, PhD, RN, CS, FAAN
Private Practice
Pittsburgh, PA & Kent, OH
Individual psychotherapy, support groups

Wende Levy, BS, RN
Clinical Trials Specialist
Social and Scientific Systems
Rockville, MD
All renal complications

Gene London, LAc, Dipl. AC
Acupuncturist/Herbalist
Immune Enhancement Project
San Francisco, CA
*Acupuncture, Chinese herbal medicine, qi gong,
traditional Chinese medicine*

Edward Lor, Pharm.D
Assistant Clinical Professor
San Francisco General Hospital,
School of Pharmacy, UCSF
San Francisco, CA
*Appendix: Common medications used in treating
the patient with HIV/AIDS*

R. Kevin Mallinson, BSN, RN
Nurse Educator,
Maryland AIDS Professional Education Center
University of Maryland Medical System
Baltimore, MD
Deaf community, gay male community

Mary McCarthy, RN, NP
Research Nurse Practitioner
HIV Neurobehavioral Research Center, UCSD
San Diego, CA
Altered mental status: delirium

Denise McDermott, MSN, RN, CCRN
AIDS Clinical Nurse Specialist
Rivington House Adult Day Health Care
Program
New York, NY
Peripheral neuropathy

N. Holly Melroe, MS, RN
HIV Nurse Specialist
St. Paul Ramsey Medical Center
St. Paul, MN
*Infection control: preventing the transmission of
HIV in the patient care setting*

Howard H. Moffet, MS, LAc, FNAAOM
HIV Clinic Coordinator
American College of Traditional Chinese
Medicine
Executive Director, AIDS & Chinese Medicine
Institute
San Francisco, CA
*Acupuncture, Chinese herbal medicine, qi gong,
traditional Chinese medicine*

Theresa A. Moran, MS, RN-C
AIDS/Oncology Clinical Nurse Specialist and
Family Nurse Practitioner
Assistant Clinical Professor
University of California, San Francisco
San Francisco General Hospital
San Francisco, CA
Malignancies

Janet Muff, MSN, RN, CS
Private Practice
South Pasadena, CA
Dreamwork

B. Anna Mullen, RN
Clinical Research Nurse
Infectious Disease Program, Department of
Epidemiology
School of Hygiene and Public Health
Johns Hopkins University
Baltimore, MD
African-American community

Gayle Newshan, PhD, RN, CS
Adult Nurse Practitioner
AIDS Center, St. Vincent's Hospital
New York, NY
Pain

Pat Nishimoto, DNS, RN
Pediatric HIV Clinical Nurse Specialist
& Adult Oncology Clinical Nurse Specialist
Tripler Army Medical Center
Honolulu, HI
Sexual transmission

Kathleen M. Nokes, PhD, RN, FAAN
Associate Professor & Project Director,
Nursing of Persons With HIV/AIDS,
Hunter College, CUNY Hunter Bellevue School
of Nursing
New York, NY
*Appendix: HIV assessment tool, vaginal
symptoms*

Adeline M. Nyamathi, PhD, RN, FAAN
Associate Professor
School of Nursing, UCLA
Los Angeles, CA
Social support

Mary Jo O'Hara, MSN, RN, CPNP
PNP/Clinical Educator
National Pediatric & Family HIV Resource
    Center
Newark, NJ
Clinical management of pediatric patients

Charles Owen, MEd, RN
Research Study Coordinator
National Institutes of Health
Bethesda, MD
Protease inhibitors

**Kristin Kane Ownby, MPH, MSN, RN, CS,
    OCN**
Doctoral Student
Texas Woman's University
Houston, TX
Transmission, cofactors, risk factors

Joan Piemme, MNEd, RN, FAAN
HIV Coordinator
VA Medical Center
Martinsburg, WV
Adolescents

Gail M. Powell-Cope, PhD, RN
Assistant Professor, College of Nursing
University of South Florida
Tampa, FL
*Alteration in family functioning, family
caregiver burden/strain*

Carmen J. Portillo, PhD, RN
Assistant Professor & Education Coordinator
International Center for HIV/AIDS Research
    and
Clinical Training in Nursing
School of Nursing, UCSF
San Francisco, CA
Hispanic community

David Rabinowitsch, MS, RN
Adjunct Clinical Instructor
Orange County Community College
Private Practice, Holistic Nursing
Per diem nurse, Hospice at Orange and Sullivan
    County
*Therapeutic touch, healing touch, & other energy
modalities*

Tracy A. Riley, MSN, RN, CS
Instructor, University of Akron;
Clinical Nurse Specialist,
Akron General Medical Center
Akron, OH
Fatigue, impaired mobility, visual loss

Mary E. Ropka, PhD, RN, FAAN
Associate Professor & Chairman,
Adult Health UCU School of Nursing
Richmond, VA
Epidemiology

Albert A. Rundio, Jr., PhD, RN, CS, CNAA
VP for Nursing & Clinical Nurse Specialist,
    HIV/AIDS
Shore Memorial Hospital
Somers Point, NJ
Suppression of HIV disease

Barbara Russell, MPH, RN, CIC
Director, Infection Control Services
Baptist Hospital of Miami
Miami, FL
Infection control

Patricia Sanders, MSN, NP, LAc
HIV NP, Kaiser Permanente Medical Center
San Francisco, CA
*Acupuncture, Chinese herbal medicine, qi gong,
traditional Chinese medicine*

Judith M. Saunders, DNSc, RN, FAAN
Assistant Professor
University of Southern California
Los Angeles, CA
*Guilt, hopelessness, powerlessness, social
isolation*

Deanne P. Sayles, MN, RN, OCNS
Oncology Clinical Nurse Specialist
Bone Marrow Transplant Unit
Lutheran General Hospital
Park Ridge, IL
Nausea & vomiting, stomatitis

Helen Schietinger, MA, RN
HIV/AIDS Consultant
Washington, DC
Context & setting of epidemic

Deena J. Schmitz, MA, RN, CD, CS
Instructor, Clinical Nurse Specialist
Terrence Cardinal Cooke Health Care Center
New York, NY
Potential for violence/harm to self or others

Craig R. Sellers, MS, RN, CS-ANP
Adult Nurse Practitioner and Director of
   Clinical Operations, Community Health
   Network, Inc.
Adjunct Clinical Instructor
School of Nursing, University of Rochester
Rochester, NY
*Hepatitis viruses A–E, human herpesvirus 6,
progressive multifocal leukoencephalopathy*

Mark Senak, JD
Director of Policy and Planning
AIDS Project Los Angeles,
Los Angeles, CA

Kathy Shook, MS, RN
Clinical Nurse Specialist
San Francisco General Hospital
San Francisco, CA
Anxiety, depression, mania & psychosis

Annette Smerko-Henry, RD, CNSD
HIV Clinical Program Manager
Coram Healthcare
Mt. Prospect, IL
AIDS wasting syndrome

Jill Solomon, MPH
Research Specialist
National Hemophilia Foundation
New York, NY
People with hemophilia

Chuck Spragg, BSN, RN
Branch Manager
Coram Healthcare
Indianapolis, IN
Blastomycosis

JoAnne Staats, MSN, RN, ANP
Director of Early Identification & Intervention
   Services
Primary Care Education & Research
Ambulatory OB-GYN
Bronx-Lebanon Medical Center
New York, NY
*Aphthous ulcers, appendicitis, cholecystitis, ente-
rocolitis & malabsorption: anorectal disease (non-
malignant), generalized peritonitis, hepatic disease, intestinal pathogens, gastrointestinal reflux
& esophagitis, Kaposi's sarcoma, microbial-relat-
ed esophagitis, non-Hodgkin's lymphoma, pancreatic disease, pill-induced esophagitis, sclerosing
cholangitis*

Hopkins D. Stanley, MS, RN
Outpatient Infusion Coordinator
AIDS Activity Division
University of California, San Francisco
San Francisco General Hospital
San Francisco, CA
*Bartonella, Campylobacter, Haemophilus influenzae,
Listeria monocytogenes, Mycobacterium avium
complex, Nocardia asteroides, Pseudomonas
aeruginosa, Rhodococcus equi, Salmonella,
Shigella, Staphylococcus aureus, Streptococcus
pneumoniae*

Joan R. Turner, MS, RN
Coordinator, Pulmonary Research, UCSF
San Francisco General Hospital
San Francisco, CA
*Inflammatory airway disorders, interstitial
pneumonitis, pulmonary neoplastic complications*

Peter J. Ungvarski, MS, RN, FAAN
Clinical Nurse Specialist, HIV Infection
Visiting Nurse Service of New York
New York, NY
*All musculoskeletal complications; aspergillosis,
candidiasis, coccidioidomycosis, cryptococcosis,
general information on fungal diseases, histoplas-
mosis; introduction to opportunistic infections*

Sharon Valente, PhD, RNC, ANP
Assistant Professor
University of Southern California
Los Angeles, CA
*Guilt, hopelessness, powerlessness, social
isolation*

Mary Ann Vitiello-Taylor, MSN, RN, CNS
Project Supervisor, AIDS Resource Center
Visiting Nurse Association of Central Jersey
Asbury Park, NJ
  All cardiac complications

Vida Maria Vizgirda, MS, RN
Doctoral Student, College of Nursing,
Dept. of Medical/Surgical Nursing,
University of Illinois
Chicago, IL
  Disease origin, etiology,
  virology

David Vlahov, PhD, RN
Professor of Epidemiology
School of Hygiene and Public Health
Johns Hopkins University
Baltimore, MD
  Parenteral transmission

Kristin Weaver, MSN, RN, CNSN
HIV Research Nurse
Saint Francis Memorial Hospital
San Francisco, CA
  Dehydration, diarrhea, dysphagia/odynophagia,
  nutritional deficit

Laurie Wojtusik, MSN, RN
Case Manager
VNA of Western Massachusetts
Holyoke, MA
  Homeless people

Vivian L. West, MBA, RN, CRNI
National Director of Nursing
NMC Homecare
Waltham, MA
  Appendix: CVADs

Janice M. Zeller, PhD, RN
Professor, Dept. of Medical Nursing
Associate Professor, Dept. of
  Immunology/Microbiology
Rush-Presbyterian-St. Luke's Medical Center
Chicago, IL
  Normal & abnormal immunology

Section 1

Emergence and Recognition of the Epidemic

The 1980s witnessed the discovery of a new disease, acquired immunodeficiency syndrome (AIDS). AIDS developed into a pandemic, whose impact on the world is unparalleled in modern times. The pandemic started in the 1970s with a period of unrecognized spread of the causative viral infection, human immunodeficiency virus type I (HIV-1). By the mid-1980s at least 100,000 people across five continents had been infected.

AIDS was not recognized as a distinct clinical entity until mid-1981 after clusters of deaths from *Pneumocystis carinii* pneumonia (PCP) and Kaposi's sarcoma (KS) had been reported in young, previously healthy homosexual men in New York City, Los Angeles, and San Francisco. The pandemic's early natural history reflected local and global social transformations that started in the 1960s. Its subsequent evolution resulted from public policies that framed public health responses, including prevention efforts, healthcare delivery, and biomedical research.

Section 1 addresses the first recognition of AIDS, theories of disease etiology, the emergence and transcontinental spread of the causative virus, and the sociocultural context of responses to the disease and those affected.

I. ORIGINS OF THE AIDS EPIDEMIC

A. Recognition of the Disease

1. In the United States
   a. Young homosexual men in New York City, Los Angeles, and San Francisco were diagnosed with PCP and KS from November 1979 to 1981 (CDC, 1981); these were unusual diagnoses
      (1) PCP was usually diagnosed in the immunocompromised (e.g., those taking immunosuppressive drugs)
      (2) KS was usually diagnosed in older men of eastern European or Mediterranean descent, and in people living in equatorial Africa
   b. Associated morbidity and mortality were also unusual
      (1) KS was typically not very aggressive, except in Africa
      (2) PCP was treatable, with good results if there was no continuing cause for immunosuppression
   c. Those affected had no apparent reason for immunodeficiency
   d. The clusters of cases sparked attention because
      (1) Cancer registries routinely tracked KS incidence and mortality, which revealed the unusual demographics, clinical presentations, and fatalities
      (2) PCP incidence had previously been so low that the drug used to treat it (pentamidine) was obtained through the Centers for Disease Control and Prevention (CDC). The sudden rise in orders for pentamidine alerted public health officials.
   e. The summary report published in *Morbidity and Mortality Weekly Report* (*MMWR*) (CDC, 1982) elicited subsequent reports of additional cases
   f. Concomitant with the reported acquired immunodeficiency in previously healthy adult men, pediatric immunologists in separate areas (New York, San Francisco, Los Angeles, Miami) noted increased numbers of infants with unexplained immunodeficiencies
   g. In New York, injecting drug users (IDUs) were seen with a similar constellation
   h. Epidemiologists anticipated the disease syndrome in hemophiliacs and blood-transfusion recipients
   i. Epidemiologists were surprised when disease was reported in Haitian immigrants who were not gay, or IDUs and heterosexual partners of IDUs
2. Around the world (immediately following publication of the CDC report)
   a. Europe: First case reported in France, July 1981
   b. Soon afterwards other cases were identified in other European countries, the Caribbean, and Central Africa (Zaire, Rwanda)
   c. Few cases reported in Asia until the late 1980s
3. Case reports indicated an underlying profound deficiency in cell-mediated immunity, accompanied by a profile of life-threatening opportunistic infections (OIs)

B. Naming the Disease

1. In the United States
   a. Initially called gay cancer, then labelled gay-related immune deficiency (GRID)
   b. CDC adopted the label AIDS in July 1981
2. In Africa it was called *slim disease* because of
   a. The profound wasting manifested
   b. Association of death with progressive weight loss and diarrhea related to gastrointestinal pathogens
3. The etiologic virus
   a. Viruses recovered from people with symptoms were each labelled differently by the scientists involved, until it was verified that all were in fact isolates of the same virus
      (1) Lymphadenopathy-associated virus (LAV): Recovered from the lymph nodes of men with lymphadenopathy; isolated by French scientists led by Luc Montagnier at the Pasteur Institute

(2) Human T-lymphotropic virus type 3 (HTLV III): It infected T lymphocytes and its molecular genetics were similar to two other viruses — studied by American scientists led by Robert Gallo at the National Cancer Institute (NCI), part of the U.S. National Institutes of Health (NIH) — that also infected T lymphocytes

(3) AIDS-related retrovirus (ARV): Isolated by scientists at the University of California in Los Angeles led by Jay Levy

(4) Immunodeficiency-associated virus (IDAV): Isolated from a series of people from identified risk groups whose lab tests demonstrated cell-mediated immunodeficiency

b. The CDC used the dual nomenclature of HTLV III/LAV until the virus was officially named human immunodeficiency virus type 1 (HIV-1) by the international subcommittee for nomenclature in 1986

C. Epidemiologic Investigations to Identify Scope of Epidemic and Uncover Its Etiology

1. CDC established the Kaposi's Sarcoma and Opportunistic Infections (KSOI) Task Force, subsequently renamed KS/AIDS Task Force

2. June 1981: CDC began systematic U.S. surveillance for PCP and KS, publishing weekly surveillance reports for distribution to health departments and concerned agencies

3. September 1982: CDC published first surveillance case definition of AIDS
   a. Definition: Occurrence of disease indicative of at least moderate deficiency in cell-mediated immunity occurring in a person with no known cause for that immunodeficiency
   b. Purpose
      (1) Designed to calculate incidence and prevalence of AIDS in United States

(2) Intended to provide a uniform definition for cases reported through the surveillance system
      (3) Not intended to restrict clinical focus on the condition
   c. World Health Organization (WHO) initially recommended use of the CDC definition for international surveillance despite recognized limited comparability of data from different nations

4. October 1983: AIDS was officially designated reportable (i.e., mandatory to report diagnosis to state/territorial health departments, who then report to CDC) under U.S. public health law

5. Identification of risk groups and epicenters

6. CDC tracked U.S. incidence by gender, race, and mode of exposure, using a hierarchically constructed schema that reflected the respective proportion of cumulative cases in each category at the time it was developed
   a. The system has been criticized as unsatisfactory and even inappropriate. Cases are hierarchically classified in a single category according to the person's whole risk history rather than according to either a specific exposure (possible transmission) incident or the most frequent exposures.
   b. Initially, people from Haiti were included as a separate category
   c. The category of travel to or from an area of high prevalence (Haiti, Africa) was included for a short time

7. Surveillance of seroprevalence of antibodies to HIV began in 1985
   a. Until licensure of test to detect antibodies to virus (March 1985), surveillance depended on clinical reports based on the case definitions and case control and cohort studies that used surrogate immunologic markers; retrospective review of cancer registries, abstracts, and death-certificate data showed KS incidence occurring among never-married men aged between 20 and 50 years, beginning in 1977
   b. Systematic seroprevalence studies
      (1) Retrospective studies (examination of stored sera to identify infection

extant in population before disease manifestations were apparent and subsequent rate of spread within and across risk groups)

    (a) First documented infection occurred in Africa in 1959 (Nahmias et al., 1986)

    (b) Infection rare until mid-1960s in what became the AIDS belt of Africa

    (c) Probably <100,000 infections worldwide before 1982, then >1 million people were infected during the subsequent decade

    (d) Infection believed present in U.S. before 1976, but about 10,000 infections estimated to have occurred by end of 1976

    (e) European epidemic about 3 years behind the U.S. epidemic in terms of magnitude; first cases were people who had lived in Zaire before 1976

  (2) Follow-up ("look-back" studies) in U.S. included pre-1985 blood recipients from donors subsequently diagnosed with AIDS or HIV infection and people who had invasive medical procedures performed by healthcare providers (physicians, surgeons, dentists) who were subsequently diagnosed with AIDS or HIV infection

  (3) Prospective studies in United States

    (a) Cohort studies of noninfected members of risk groups to identify spread of infection

    (b) Following documented exposure (e.g., transfusion) to quantify transmission risks and identify natural history

    (c) Healthcare workers (HCWs): Cross-sectional, retrospective, and prospective studies

    (d) Sentinel surveillance system (also known as family of HIV seroprevalence surveys) begun in 1987–1989 in 41 states, 39 metropolitan areas, and Puerto Rico

      i) To provide standardized, consistent national prevalence data

      ii) To monitor patterns and trends of infection by direct prevention programs to appropriate groups and evaluate effectiveness

      iii) To evaluate reasons for hospitalization by people with unrecognized HIV infection

  c. Confirmed modes of spread

    (1) Sexual (via semen, seminal fluid, vaginal secretions), including artificial insemination

    (2) Blood borne

      (a) Transfusions (blood and blood products, including clotting factors)

      (b) Other organ transplants

      (c) Percutaneous contact with used needles or other sharps that could be contaminated by blood

    (3) From mother to infant before, during, or shortly after birth

8. The pandemic comprised multiple subepidemics in different population groups and in different geographic areas

  a. In 1988, WHO suggested that the uneven worldwide distribution reflected three successive pandemics, which exhibited multiple waves over time (see *Epidemiology of HIV Infection and AIDS*, p. 8)

  b. With successive waves, the pattern descriptions became blurred and then obsolete by the early 1990s

D. Search for Disease Etiology and Origins of Pandemic

1. Theories about the epidemic's emergence and transcontinental spread

  a. Sociocultural context: The natural history of the worldwide pandemic reflected local and global social transformations of the 1960s and 1970s

    (1) Intense urbanization in Africa

    (2) Economic changes that deepened

tears in the basic fabric of social life in developed and developing parts of the world

(3) Unprecedented intercontinental mobility by people from diverse social strata for both business and pleasure

(4) Local and global revolutions in sexual behavior related to various sociodemographic changes

  (a) Changing marriage and fertility patterns

  (b) Changing gender roles in home and labor force

  (c) Gay liberation (more open and visible gay communities, accompanied by political and social activism and assertion of civil rights to express personal sexuality)

(5) Epidemic of drug use in U.S. and Europe

(6) A conservative political climate in 1980s

  (a) Political backlash, partially in reaction to the civil rights movements and atmosphere of sexual freedom of the 1970s

  (b) Reduced funding for numerous government programs, including public health programs

  (c) Implications when AIDS appeared

    i) AIDS was associated in the public's mind with homosexuality and injecting drug use, and dismissed

    ii) The federal government was slow to respond

    iii) Cities were forced to cope on their own

2. 1985: Isolation and identification of a virus (HIV-2) with similar molecular structure and life cycle

E. Responses to the Epidemic and People Affected

1. October 1981: CDC declared the new disease to be an epidemic

a. November 1982: CDC issued prevention recommendations for clinical and laboratory workers

b. 1983: The National AIDS hotline was established

c. Efforts to protect blood supply

  (1) March 1983: U.S. health officials asked people from groups identified as at risk for AIDS (gay and bisexual men, IDUs, Haitian immigrants) not to donate blood

  (2) March 1985: Food and Drug Administration (FDA) required HIV-antibody testing of all donated blood

  (3) The blood-bank industry has been criticized for its failure to warn and lack of an aggressive response

d. 1985: National Institute of Allergy and Infectious Diseases (NIAID) establishes network of AIDS Clinical Trial Units (ACTUs)

e. 1987: CDC recommends universal blood and body fluid precautions (UP) for preventing HIV, hepatitis B virus, and other blood-borne pathogen transmission in healthcare settings

f. October 1987: National information campaign, America Responds to AIDS, begins under direction of C. Everett Koop

g. 1988: CDC requires partnership notification programs as part of its funding for state HIV-prevention programs

h. 1994: CDC proposes named reporting of HIV infection

i. 1993: HIV education in the workplace begins for all federal employees

2. Government attention, funded efforts, and policies varied among countries; many responded with a period of denial, followed by a period of inaction, with the rationale that the magnitude of the problem was exaggerated

a. U.S. Surgeons General reports

  (1) October 1986 : Report on AIDS (requested by President Reagan in February 1986)

  (2) April 1987: Workshop on Children with HIV Infection and Their Families

(3) 1993: Report to the American Public on HIV Infection and AIDS

b. Presidential Commission on the Human Immunodeficiency Virus Epidemic: June 1988—Issued report after holding nationwide hearings

c. December 1, 1988: WHO initiated World AIDS Day

3. In 1981, gay men in New York and San Francisco initiated dissemination of information and informal networks of support services for friends, neighbors, and eventually others affected by what was being referred to as gay cancer

a. There was not always consensus within gay communities or the community-based organizations they founded about either goals and priorities or the most appropriate means to achieve them

b. The gay community's unprecedented response to the urgent needs brought by the epidemic shaped an entirely new social service network, invigorated healthcare consumer activism, and challenged the biomedical control of health

c. The focus on gay men with AIDS directed attention away from nongay people affected by the disease, including those in other marginal or under-served groups

d. Homophobia and other political/public responses

(1) Engendered a view that it was a concern of "others," and not a broad societal threat

(2) Delayed initiating precautions necessary to protect the blood supply (e.g., implementing donor restrictions)

(3) Deterred prevention efforts targeting young adults and adolescents

(4) Contributed to inattention by the media to the growing epidemic

4. Anti-HIV antibody testing

a. March 1985: First tests licensed by the FDA for marketing in the United States

b. Enabled identification of persons who had been infected and thus nonsymptomatic carriers who could transmit the infection to others

5. AIDS-specific services were the norm for program planning and development during the 1980s, but in the 1990s calls for mainstreaming began

6. By early 1987, AIDS public education campaigns had been launched on every continent; denial of the danger of the epidemic continued in relatively unaffected countries

7. Disease trends of the 20th century

a. The postantibiotic era led to a perception by HCWs as well as the general public that infectious disease had been conquered

b. Chronic diseases began to receive priority attention in public health

8. When AIDS appeared

a. Many people believed that a cure for AIDS would soon be discovered

b. The system was unprepared to serve single adults who lived alone and did not have other household members available to assist them with illness or care needs at home

c. Many practitioners, largely inexperienced with large-scale epidemics associated with high mortality, were overwhelmed and fearful of contagion, distrusting the efficacy of infection control practices

d. HCWs were not accustomed to high morbidity and mortality in young adult patients and were unprepared to meet their emotional needs and the emotional impact on the providers themselves

9. Responses of healthcare workers

a. Initially, and for several years, HCWs depended, to a large and unprecedented extent, on community groups for up-to-date information about the epidemic, clinical manifestations, useful treatments, and available resources

b. Professional groups

(1) Infection control practitioners (ICPs) and nurse epidemiologists were quick to respond within their facilities; they played a major role at the beginning of the epidemic as staff educators, policy makers, and spokespeople to avert unwarranted panic among staff and public

(2) Nurses' roles in the early years of the epidemic
  (a) Developing policies within their work settings
  (b) Providing direct patient care and support to people with AIDS (PWAs) and their families, sometimes when others refused to provide care
  (c) Helping develop community-based support services for people affected by AIDS and their families
  (d) Providing education for HCWs and community education for the general public, including those at risk, about infection control and basic care needs
(3) Many gay and lesbian nurses and physicians came out to their co-workers to express solidarity with and support for gay PWAs, and to work toward improving care
(4) Reports of nurses refusing to care for PWAs were rare
(5) Professional organizations
  (a) Position statements by the American Nurses Association (ANA), some state nurses associations, and specialty nursing organizations reflected concerns for patients' rights, nurses' rights and safety, and nurses' ethical responsibilities
  (b) 1986: California Nurses Association developed "Train the Trainer" program, which became a national model for other professional organizations
  (c) 1988: Association of Nurses in AIDS Care (ANAC) founded
  (d) 1988 and 1994: National League for Nursing published guidelines for schools of nursing
  (e) International Council of Nurses (ICN) issued joint statement with WHO on rights and responsibilities of nurses worldwide in caring for HIV-infected people
c. In the mid-1980s, most PWAs were cared for in hospitals
  (1) Many hospitals provided care but were slow to develop appropriate policies for AIDS care
    (a) Inappropriate and unnecessary isolation precautions
    (b) Inadequate education for staff
    (c) Inappropriate HIV-testing without informed consent associated with discriminatory decisions about treatments
  (2) Some hospitals established AIDS-dedicated units
  (3) The long-term care industry was slow to accept a role; many facilities refused admission to PWAs
  (4) By the end of the decade, an increasing proportion of AIDS care was being provided on an outpatient or home care basis
  (5) There remains considerable variation in patterns of use
  (6) A common theme in descriptions of the impact of AIDS is inequality that demonstrates the already sharp differences in health system infrastructures and underlying social, economic, and political supports.

II. EPIDEMIOLOGY OF HIV INFECTION AND AIDS

This section presents a brief discussion of principles followed by definitions of epidemiologic terms. The discussion helps the reader understand and interpret epidemiologic data from the CDC, WHO, and other sources.

Epidemiology specifically related to AIDS covers exposure categories for adults and children. While most of the information is specific to the United States, this section also addresses global concerns and gives information on epidemiology in healthcare workers.

A. Principles and Terms of Epidemiology

1. Evolving definition of *epidemiology*
   a. Classic definition: The study of the distribution of disease (e.g., HIV infection) or physiologic conditions in human populations, and factors (e.g., risk behaviors) that influence that distribution (Lilienfeld & Stolley, 1994). Epidemiology is an applied discipline, involving both content and methods to find systematic answers to health problems.
   b. Clinical epidemiology has expanded the definition to include the study of other aspects of diseases, health conditions, and injuries that occur in health care. It includes clinical issues such as normality/abnormality, diagnosis, frequency, risk, prognosis, and treatment, prevention, and cause (Fletcher, Fletcher, & Wagner, 1988).
2. *Rate:* The measure of the frequency of a phenomenon (e.g., disease, injury) expressed per unit of size of population in which it is observed (MacMahon & Pugh, 1970) at, or over, a certain time. Rate reflects the frequency at which the illness or death occurs in a defined population.
   a. "Use of rates rather than raw numbers is essential for comparison of experience between populations at different times, different places, or among different people" (Last, 1988, p. 11)
   b. To be epidemiologically useful, rates require a numerator (the number of people actually newly affected), a de-

nominator (an estimate of the average number of people in the population able to be affected), and a specified time interval

3. *Morbidity:* "Any departure, subjective or objective, from the state of physiologic or psychologic well-being" (Last, 1988, p. 83). Morbidity is usually expressed as a ratio, proportion, or rate.
4. *Morbidity rates:* Rates that measure the frequency of illness or conditions within specific populations. To be a rate, time and place must always be specified. Common morbidity rates are expressed as
   a. *Prevalence:* The frequency or number of all current cases of a disease, both old and new. Think all when you think of prevalence, and compare with incidence (see below); gives a snapshot of the overall picture.
   b. *Point prevalence:* The frequency of all current cases of disease (e.g., HIV infection or AIDS, old and new) at a given instant
   c. *Period prevalence:* The frequency of all current cases of disease (e.g., HIV infection or AIDS, old and new) for a prescribed time interval. It combines the point prevalence at the beginning of that interval and the new cases that occur during the remainder of the period.
   d. *Incidence:* The rapidity with which diseases or health conditions (e.g., HIV infection) occur or develop over a stated period. Think new when you think of incidence. Incidence and prevalence are frequently confused.

(1) New cases occur either through onset of new disease in the current population, or by immigration of people who are already ill
(2) Incidence provides a direct estimate of the risk of developing a disease or health condition during a given interval
(3) Incidence compares development of disease in different populations or looks at the relationship between etiologic factors and the disease
e. *Relationship between incidence and prevalence*: Incidence rate (risk of getting) × duration = prevalence
f. *Attack rate*: A special incidence rate (usually expressed as a percentage) when the risk for development of a given attribute or event is limited, especially in epidemics. It is usually observed for a specified period.
g. *Secondary attack rate*: Reflects the number of exposed people developing a disease (i.e., incidence) within a given range of time, consistent with the incubation period for that condition divided by (among) the number of people exposed to the primary case and susceptible to the disease; in the case of HIV infection, presumably everyone is susceptible; secondary attack rates are used to
(1) Reflect the infectivity of an agent
(2) Indicate the etiologic role of an infectious agent when etiology of a communicable disease is unknown
(3) Evaluate efficacy of a prophylactic agent (e.g., a vaccine)
h. Common problems in morbidity reporting that lead to inaccuracies
(1) Underreporting
(2) Combining categories or changes in definition (e.g., changes in CDC AIDS-defining criteria)
(3) Who is at risk is not always known, thus the denominator can be difficult to determine
(4) Progression of illness: When do you consider someone morbid?
(5) Misuse of incidence vs. prevalence
i. Changes in prevalence
(1) Why prevalence appears to increase

(a) Improved care prevents death
(b) Improved diagnostic methods allow earlier detection
(c) Changes in population
(d) Improved availability of health care
(2) Why prevalence appears to decrease
(a) Immunization
(b) Decreased incidence
(c) Not susceptible to the disease or condition
(d) Death from competing cause
(e) Faster recovery due to improved treatment
(f) More rapid death
j. *Spectrum of disease*: The sequence of events that occurs from the time of exposure to the etiologic agent until death from the disease
(1) May involve both a subclinical phase and a component in which the person is clinically ill
(2) Progression through the entire spectrum is influenced by prevention and treatment measures
5. *Mortality:* The number of deaths; simpler to define than morbidity—it is usually easier to tell if people are alive or dead than to determine if they are sick; sources of mortality data are
a. Death certificates
b. Medical records, insurance and coroner's reports
c. Census data
d. Military data
6. Mortality rates are reported as
a. *Crude mortality rate*: The number of deaths in that group per stated period (usually annual)/number in population (midinterval) exposed to the risk of dying
b. *Specific mortality rates*: Death can be examined by age groups (e.g., pediatric vs. adult AIDS cases), disease-specific groups (e.g., AIDS or non-AIDS HIV), or sex-specific groups
c. Differences in mortality may be compared by time, place, or person
7. *Risk*: Generally refers to the probability of some untoward event (e.g., developing HIV infection after exposure)

a. *Risk factors*: Associated with increased risk of becoming diseased (in the case or morbidity) or dying (in the case of mortality). Risk factors may be in
  (1) Physical (in the environment, e.g., infectious agents such as *Salmonella*)
  (2) Social (e.g., culture, ethnicity)
  (3) Behavioral (e.g., unprotected sex with an HIV-infected or needle-sharing partner)
  (4) Inherited (e.g., primary immunodeficiencies, hemophilia)
b. *Measures of risk*
  (1) Incidence (absolute risk)
  (2) Relative Risk (RR), also called the Risk Ratio
    (a) Formula: Incidence in the exposed/incidence in nonexposed
    (b) RR asks, "How many times more likely to get the disease are exposed vs. nonexposed persons?"
    (c) Tells the degree of risk in those with a characteristic relative to those without it. RR measures strength of association.
    (d) Useful for studies of disease etiology

B. U.S. General HIV Epidemiology (AIDS case definition)

1. AIDS cases are reported to the CDC using a uniform surveillance case definition and case report form for all 50 states, the District of Columbia, U.S. dependencies and possessions
2. Requires both the determination of the case and its reporting by the healthcare provider
3. CDC has modified its AIDS case definition a number of times because of new knowledge about the disease, including a broader range of AIDS-indicator lesions and improved diagnostic tests
  a. After its initial development in 1981, the definition was modified in 1985, 1987, 1993, and 1994

  b. The 1993 revision had the greatest impact on case reporting (CDC, 1994c). It added the conditions of pulmonary tuberculosis (TB), recurrent pneumonia, invasive cervical cancer, and severe HIV-related immunosuppression (defined as CD4+ lymphocyte count of <200/μl or a CD4+ percentage <14 in people with laboratory confirmation of HIV infection).
4. AIDS case surveillance has enabled description of the characteristics of the people at risk for HIV infection and the modes of transmission, which can be used to develop prevention strategies and target healthcare resources (Jones & Curran, 1994). This surveillance is limited by the extent to which cases are completely and accurately reported.
5. The current definition, including conditions, may be found in Appendix A, p. 398

C. Exposure Categories

1. Adult
  a. Hierarchical system: AIDS cases are counted only once. People with more than one reported exposure are counted only in the exposure category that is listed first in the hierarchy. Exceptions are men with a history of both sexual contact with other men and IDUs who make up a separate category (CDC, 1994c).
  b. Major modes of transmission have not expanded beyond those described early in the epidemic. Most cases have occurred through sexual contact, parenteral transmission (drug injection; percutaneous occupational exposure; receipt of infected blood, blood products, organs, or tissues), or perinatal transmission from infected mother (Jones & Curran, 1994).
2. Adult/adolescent
  a. Approximate percentage of cases in each category through December, 1995 (CDC, 1995d)
    (1) Men who have sex with men: 51%
    (2) IDUs: 25%

(3) Men who have sex with men and inject drugs: 7%

(4) Hemophilia/coagulation disorder: 1%

(5) Heterosexual contact: 8%; includes subcategories of sex with IDUs, bisexual males, persons with hemophilia, transfusion recipients with HIV infection, HIV-infected persons (risk not specified)

(6) Receipt of blood transfusion, blood components, or tissue: 1%

(7) Other/risk not reported or identified: 7%

  (a) Other: Healthcare workers and those who acquired HIV in the healthcare setting

  (b) Risk not reported or identified: Persons under investigation, lost to follow-up, declined interview, or not reporting one of the exposures listed after interview

3. Children (under 13 years old)

a. Approximate percentages of cumulative cases in the U.S. through 1995 (CDC, 1995d)

(1) Hemophilia/coagulation disorder: 3% of cumulative cases through 1995 (1% of pediatric cases reported in 1994)

(2) Mother with/at risk for HIV infection: 90% (92% of new pediatric cases reported in 1994); breastfeeding increases the risk of perinatal transmission by 14%

(3) Receipt of blood transfusion, blood components, or tissue: 5% (3% of pediatric cases reported in 1994)

(4) Sexual abuse: Not reported within CDC categories

D. Trends in AIDS Occurrence

1. AIDS information from 1981–1995 reveals important changes in the nature of the HIV epidemic, but note that for all men, male-to-male sexual contact remains the most frequently reported mode of HIV exposure and accounts for the greatest proportion of cases

2. Although many previously infected gay men will progress to AIDS and new infections are occurring in this population, het-erosexual transmission is becoming more important with certain populations at much increased risk

a. Young, disadvantaged, African-American and Hispanic women living in northeastern inner cities and the rural south

b. The major source of transmission for women has been male IDUs, especially for women with multiple partners (Buehler, Petersen, & Jaffe, 1995)

3. Increases in recent years have leveled off, largely because there are fewer new cases among men who have sex with men, although there have been some recent increases noted among young homosexual men

4. A second major change has occurred in the lower proportionate increase in cases among groups or areas that have accounted for the majority of AIDs cases in the past

a. Even though men comprise the largest proportion of AIDS cases, there has been a rapid increase in the number of cases in women

b. Case reports among men who have sex with men and among IDUs have leveled off. In contrast, heterosexual transmission is the most rapidly increasing exposure group with a 17% increase during 1991 and 1992 (Buehler et al., 1995).

5. Minority communities have experienced the greatest impact of the AIDS epidemic

a. For African Americans and Hispanics, AIDS rates are approximately 4 times and 3 times greater than among whites

b. Nearly 80% of AIDS cases attributed to drug injection are among African Americans or Hispanics (Buehler et al., 1995)

c. The number of cases in the exposure category of injecting drug use is higher for black and Hispanic males than for other racial/ethnic groups, and is close to the number of cases in the category of men who have sex with men

6. Geographic comparisons (CDC, 1995d)

a. The 10 states reporting the highest AIDS case rates per 100,000 population for

1995: District of Columbia, New York, Florida, New Jersey, Maryland, Connecticut, Delaware, California, Nevada, Georgia
   b. The 10 metropolitan areas with the highest AIDS case rates per 100,000 population for 1995: Jersey City, San Francisco, New York, Miami, Fort Lauderdale, Newark, West Palm Beach, San Juan (Puerto Rico), Baltimore, New Haven
   c. The epidemic has spread from its beginnings in major metropolitan areas to affect smaller cities and rural areas
7. HIV transmission related to transfusion of blood and blood products has been virtually eliminated is the United States

E. HIV-Related Mortality
(for those deaths in which it is recognized and acknowledged that HIV infection was responsible)

1. For all age groups in combination in 1992, HIV infection was the 8th leading cause of death
2. Among all U.S. 25- to 44-year-olds, the age group most heavily affected, HIV infection became the leading cause of death (CDC, 1995d). For this age group, HIV infection accounted for 23% of all deaths in men, 11% of all deaths in women.
3. In a short time, what was originally a small outbreak among gay men in a few discontiguous locations has become a major killer of relatively young Americans
4. In terms of mortality, the impact of HIV infection has been greatest in large metropolitan areas

F. HIV Seroprevalence, Earlier Disease

1. AIDS case reporting information is less helpful in following current trends because of the 7- to 10-year period between infection and AIDS diagnosis in any one person
2. Surveillance of early HIV infection (before AIDS) is more useful for determining community patterns of prevalent HIV infection

G. Infection in Women

1. Women represent the fastest growing group of people with HIV
   a. In 1995, of the new cases reported, >23% were women (CDC, 1995d)
   b. Estimates suggest that women represent almost half of all new infections worldwide with the majority of transmission occurring before age 25; worldwide, 3,000,000 women will die from AIDS in the 1990s
   c. The medical community is still learning about the course of infection, care, and consequences of transmission among women
   d. The possibility of having both HIV-infected children and healthy orphans relates to infection in women of childbearing age
   e. At least 50% of cases of HIV infection in women have been reported since 1989, an indication that infection among women is increasing (Stine, 1993)
   f. By December 1995, women comprised >16% of the cumulative adult cases of AIDS in the United States (CDC, 1995d)
2. Epidemiologic information specific to women
   a. Primary prevention of infection in women assures a healthy infant and mother—infants are born without the disease and mothers live to care for them
   b. Transmission patterns
      (1) The rate of heterosexual transmission is increasing
         (a) The number of women infected through this route surpasses the number of men
         (b) Accounts for about 8% of total AIDS cases and 37% of all female cases
         (c) The number and proportion of women acquiring HIV from heterosexual contact with male IDUs, male bisexuals, and men infected through blood products comprise the largest number of HIV-infected women of childbearing age

(d) Numbers of women with AIDS acquired through heterosexual transmission continue to increase (37%, compared with 3% for men)

(2) Injecting drug use

(a) The major route of HIV transmission for women since the beginning of the epidemic

(b) About 65% of women have been infected through needle sharing or the use of sex for drugs (CDC, 1995d)

3. Biologic vulnerability places women at risk

a. Sperm releases a higher dose of HIV than does vaginal fluids (dose-response relationship)

b. Epithelium of vagina and cervix are directly infected

c. Menstrual cycle causes pH of the vagina to be less acidic, more hospitable to HIV

4. Ethnic and racial composition: Twice as many African-American women as white or Hispanic women are infected (CDC, 1991a)

5. Testing of women: Median time range between last testing among those who have been previously tested and the first positive test is 0.5 months to 24 months (Stine, 1993)

H. Pediatric AIDS

1. Pediatric cases make up about 1.5% of the total number of reported AIDS cases in the United States, a number that approximates the incidence of childhood cancer

2. Significance of the problem

a. 6,948 pediatric AIDS cases in the U.S. reported through 1995 (CDC, 1995d); one sixth of total pediatric AIDS cases were reported in 1994

b. For infants and young children, AIDS is among the 10 leading causes of death (U.S. estimates of 10,000–20,000 cases of HIV in children)

c. It is likely to be among the leading 5 causes of death within the next 3–4 years

3. Transmission categories specific to children

a. Blood and blood products

(1) Almost all transmission of HIV to the hemophiliac population occurred before mid-1985 (Stine, 1993)

(2) Through 1995, 3% of cases were hemophiliac children who had received contaminated blood or blood products; another 5% were nonhemophiliac children transfused with contaminated blood

b. Vertical transmission

(1) At least 90% of infected children received the virus from HIV-infected mothers (CDC, 1995d)

(2) Rate of transmission from mother to child believed to range from 14.4% to about 40%, with the average being 20%–30% without intervention (European Collaborative Study, 1992)

(3) Through 1995, 90% of 6,948 pediatric AIDS cases resulted from the vertical transfer of HIV from an infected mother to her fetus or to her newborn as it passed through the birth canal (CDC, 1995d)

(4) Little information documented which factors influence vertical transmission from mother to fetus; mother's clinical and immunologic status may be important

c. Breast milk

(1) Newborns can become infected through breast milk—3 cases reported among infants of women who became infected by blood transfusions immediately following birth (Curran et al., 1988)

(2) Number infected by breast milk has not been determined

d. Other/risk not reported or identified: About 1% of pediatric cases determined (CDC, 1995d)

4. Prognosis

a. About 58% of children reported to the CDC through 1987 have died, half within 9 months of diagnosis (Rogers, 1988)

b. Improved medical care means children are now living longer

c. Many HIV-infected children are orphans because family members are infected with HIV

I. Exposure Among Health Professionals

1. In 1994 the CDC listed 42 documented cases of U.S. healthcare workers who acquired HIV infection via occupational exposure; another 91 were listed as possible cases of occupational transmission. A few of those infected have progressed to AIDS, and some have died
   a. About 100,000 needle-stick injuries are reported in the United States each year
   b. Transmission rate of HIV appears to be about 0.3% to HCWs exposed to patients with HIV; most of these are from needle-stick injuries.
2. Persons at risk: Nurses (largest group of exposed HCWs), surgeons and OR personnel, lab technicians, dentists

J. Global Patterns

1. The HIV/AIDS epidemic affects all countries of the world
   a. International travel and cultural variations have had a dynamic effect
   b. HIV is unstable and continues to intensify in both areas already affected and in communities previously spared
   c. The disease is becoming more complicated as time passes because of overlapping transmission modes and numbers of persons infected and affected
2. Significance of the problem
   a. Greatest number of HIV-infected people are in the developing world. Sub-Saharan Africa has 68% (about 8.8% of the adult population) of the world's cases vs. 9% in North America, and 8% in Latin America (Mann, Tarantola, & Better, 1992).
   b. Estimates in January 1992 put the numbers infected with HIV as 11.8 million adults and 1.1 million children (8.77 million in sub-Saharan Africa) (Mann et al., 1992)
3. International patterns of spread: Three broad and distinct patterns of HIV transmission were initially identified world

wide; a combination pattern was added later
   a. Pattern I (predominant in North America, western Europe, Australia, New Zealand, and the urban areas of South America during the 1970s)
      (1) HIV began to spread extensively during the mid- to late-1970s, primarily among homosexual and bisexual men
      (2) Perinatal transmission low because relatively few women had been infected
   b. Pattern II (also emerged in the late 1970s, evolved in sub-Saharan Africa and some areas of Latin America and the Caribbean)
      (1) Transmission primarily heterosexual with 25% of the persons in the 20–40 age group; estimated that 90% of female sex workers became infected
      (2) Perinatal transmission apparent: 5%–15% of pregnant women were infected by the late 1980s
   c. Pattern III: Even though HIV infection had not penetrated populations in Eastern Europe, the Middle East, North Africa, and countries in Asia and the Pacific Islands, indigenous spread occurred among sex workers and persons with HIV drug habits in these regions (Mann et al., 1992)
   d. Pattern I/II (Latin America and parts of the Caribbean)
      (1) Emerged in the late 1980s
      (2) In areas where original transmission was among men having sex with men, heterosexual transmission began to increase
   e. Present patterns: By the early 1990s, the global epidemic trends had changed significantly, and the paradigm of geographic patterns was no longer so clear (Mann et al., 1992)
      (1) Heterosexual transmission is continuing in both developing countries and the developed world
      (2) In Latin America, more heterosexual and perinatal transmissions are being reported

(3) In Asia, there is an explosion of cases resulting from heterosexual and IDU transmissions
(4) Limited resources cause life span of HIV-infected persons to be much shorter in developing countries
(5) Many countries have no systematic screening and the numbers of HIV-infected people remain unknown

K. The Future

1. All the world's nations feel the impact both economically and morally as cost of care becomes a burden.
2. Agencies charged with caring for infected persons and international agencies working to stop the epidemic have seen challenges to precious resources and to human capabilities.

Section 2

Pathophysiology of HIV/AIDS

The information that follows provides a basic understanding of the clinical and therapeutic approaches to HIV infection and AIDS. The section begins with a review of general virology and specific aspects of virology in relation to HIV, followed by an overview of the normal immune system and immune alterations found after infection with HIV. Transmission of HIV is considered next along with the natural history of the disorder and HIV testing.

I. VIROLOGY: A GENERAL REVIEW

A. Retroviridae
(Retroviruses, RNA viruses)

1. Taxonomy (Cullen, 1993)
   a. Retroviruses can be classified into sub-groups based on their pathogenic potential
      (1) Oncovirus (transforming) subgroup: Induces neoplastic disease in vivo
         (a) Human T-lymphotrophic virus-I (HTLV-I)
         (b) Human T-lymphotrophic virus-II (HTLV-II)
         (c) Feline leukemia virus (FeLV)
         (d) Simian T-lymphotrophic virus (STLV)
      (2) Lentivirus (Lentiviridae) subgroup or slow virus: Characteristic lengthy incubation period; lacks neoplastic potential
         (a) HIV Type 1 (HIV-1)
         (b) HIV Type 2 (HIV-2)
         (c) Simian immunodeficiency virus (SIV)
         (d) Feline immunodeficiency virus (FIV)
   b. Classification also based on the pattern of viral gene regulation in the infected cell
      (1) Simple retroviruses (encode ≤4 gene products with no regulatory proteins)
         (a) FeLV
         (b) Simian sarcoma virus (SSV)
      (2) Complex retroviruses (encode at least 5 gene products, of which at least 1 is a regulatory protein)
         (a) HIV-1
         (b) HIV-2
         (c) HTLV-I/II
         (d) SIV
         (e) STLV
2. Unique properties (Kaplan, 1989)
   a. Genes encoded in 2 single-stranded RNA (RNA viruses)
   b. Transcription of genetic message is reversed: RNA to DNA, vs. DNA to RNA
   c. Reverse transcriptase enzyme responsible for transcribing RNA into DNA
   d. Three common genes: env, pol, gag
   e. Able to incorporate viral DNA into host cell nuclear genome
   f. Incorporated retroviral DNA can be activated to produce exogenous budding viruses
   g. Conserved structure (Essex & Kanki, 1988)
      (1) Internal core proteins most conserved or common among viruses within the group
      (2) Envelope glycoproteins least conserved or more distinct for each virus within the group
3. Species-specific retroviruses
   a. Human retroviruses (Kaplan, 1989)
      (1) HTLV-I
         (a) Etiologic agent of acute T-cell leukemia (ATL) and T-cutaneous lymphoma
         (b) Endemic to southern islands of Japan, parts of United States, most of Caribbean, northern South America, Africa
      (2) HTLV-II
         (a) Two isolates associated with hairy-cell leukemia
         (b) One isolate from hemophiliac with a peculiar immune deficiency state
      (3) Human T-lymphotrophic virus-V (HTLV-V)
         (a) Associated with mycosis fungoides
         (b) Less aggressive form of T-cell infection
      (4) HIV-1: Most prevalent in the world
      (5) HIV-2: Primarily localized to Africa
   b. Animal retroviruses
      (1) STLV
         (a) Identified in Japanese macaque (monkey)
         (b) Identified in Asian and African Old World monkeys and apes
      (2) SIV (Essex & Kanki, 1988)
         (a) SIVmac identified in captive Asian macaques and linked to inducing AIDS-like disease (Simian AIDS [SAIDS])

(b) SIVagm identified in 30%–70% of wild African green monkeys with no evidence of SAIDS

(3) FIV
(a) Isolated in 1987
(b) Found in domestic cats with chronic AIDS-like pathology: Immunosuppression, opportunistic infections (OIs)
(c) Similar to HIV in morphology and biochemistry, but distinct antigenically

c. Similarities between human and animal retroviruses
(1) HTLV-I/II and STLV
(a) Both viruses transform T cells into a cancerous state
(b) High level of cross-reactivity (recognition of viral proteins on one virus by antibodies [Abs] elicited to the proteins of the other virus)
(c) 90%–95% homology in genome nucleotide sequence of both viruses (Essex & Kanki, 1988)
(2) HIV and SIV
(a) Both viruses infect CD4+ subset of lymphocytes
(b) Both are cytopathic to CD4+ cells
(c) Cross-reactivity of human antibodies from AIDS patients with SIV protein epitopes
(d) Almost identical organization of structural and regulatory genes, with exception being vpx gene of SIV missing in HIV; HIV vpu gene missing in SIV (Essex & Kanki, 1988)

B. Human Immunodeficiency Virus

1. Viral classification
a. HIV belongs to the family of retroviruses because
(1) Has reverse transcriptase activity
(2) Its genome is found on RNA
(3) Has gag, pol, and env genes common to all retroviruses
b. HIV belongs to lentiviridae subfamily
(1) Does not have oncogenic potential
(2) Has a period of latency or nonproductive expression of integrated HIV proviral DNA
c. HIV also a complex retrovirus
(1) Has 6 additional genes identified in its genome
(2) At least 2 of the 6 encode for regulatory proteins
d. Other characteristics
(1) Can infect CD4+ receptors, particularly T4 lymphocytes
(2) Inserts its genetic material into host DNA, creating permanent infection

2. Structure
a. Size/shape
(1) Slightly >100 nm in diameter
(2) General appearance of a dense cylindrical core surrounded by a lipid envelope
b. "Envelope" or outer membrane
(1) Lipid membrane acquired during budding from plasma membrane of the infected host cell
(2) Embedded within the lipid membrane are discrete glycoproteins referred to as "knobs" or "spikes"
(a) Spike/knob is an outer glycoprotein, gp120, anchored to a transmembrane scanning glycoprotein, gp41
(b) Entire gp120 structure and amino terminus of gp41 are exposed on the virion's cell surface
(c) Amino acid sequences in gp120 divided into regions of conserved (C) and variable (V) domains (Planelles, Li, & Chen, 1993)
(d) V3 loop of gp120 is the Ab binding site
c. Viral core
(1) Core protein, p17, embedded on inner leaflet of the lipid envelope adjacent to a protein core
(2) Core is a protein coat composed of 2 major proteins, p24 and p15
(3) p17, p24, and p15 are cleaved from a polyprotein precursor p55
d. Viral core components
(1) Enzymes necessary for viral life cycle

(a) Reverse transcriptase transcribes viral RNA template into a viral DNA

(b) Integrase or endonuclease integrates proviral DNA into host cell's DNA

(c) Protease cleaves large precursor viral polyproteins into smaller active proteins or glycoproteins

(2) Genome or genetic material: Approximately 10 kilo-base pairs in length (Fauci, 1988)

(3) Three structural genes

(a) Gag: Encodes core proteins and partial information for protease enzyme

(b) Env: Encodes surface gp120 and transmembrane gp41

(c) Pol: Encodes reverse transcriptase (p66), integrase, and partial information for protease

(4) Six additional viral regulatory genes (AIDS 89 Summary, 1990; Pavlakis, 1992)

(a) Nef: Encodes for Nef protein believed to be involved in regulation of viral replication

(b) Vpr: Encodes for Vpr protein

(c) Vpu: Encodes for Vpu protein, which may be involved in enhancing viral release from the host cell

(d) Vif: Encodes for Vif protein

(e) Tat: Encodes for Tat protein

 i) Positive regulatory gene: Increases rate of its own synthesis and that of env, pol, and gag genes

 ii) Essential for viral replication and expression

(f) Rev: Encodes for Rev protein

 i) Positive regulatory gene

 ii) Believed to control amount of messenger RNA available for protein translation

(g) Long terminal repeat (LTR) regions

 i) Located at the 5′ and 3′ ends of genome and flank

genes encoding for structural proteins

 ii) Critical component for viral integration into host cell's genome

 iii) Contains promoter and enhancer elements recognized by cellular and possibly viral transcription factors

3. HIV life cycle: Divided into 2 phases (Haseltine, 1992)

a. Establishing infection in a host cell

(1) HIV and host cell attach

(a) Attachment is via high-affinity binding of viral gp120 to CD4 surface molecule of T4 helper/inducer lymphocytes, monocytes, macrophages

(b) Region located between amino acids 40 and 82 on CD4 recognized by gp120 as the binding site

(2) HIV penetrates host cell

(a) Process of internalization not completely clear; appears to be membrane-to-membrane fusion of HIV and host cell

(b) Fusion appears to be mediated by V3 region of gp120 and hydrophobic spike at gp41 amino terminus (Weiner, 1992)

(c) Following fusion, the viral protein core uncoats itself and releases HIV genome and enzymes into host cell's cytoplasm

(3) Viral gene transcription

(a) Reverse transcriptase transcribes viral RNA to viral DNA in host cell's cytoplasm

(b) Two linear strands of DNA synthesized into double-helix configuration

(c) Single-stranded RNA template degraded by viral ribonuclease H

(d) Some of double-stranded DNA joined together to form a closed circle while other strands remain in linear form

(e) Circular viral DNA inserted into host cell's genome by integrase while proportion of linear viral DNA may remain in the host cell's cytoplasm

(4) Latency

  (a) Host cell is in a quiescent state

  (b) Period of nonproductive expression of the integrated proviral DNA

b. Active productive infection or active budding of new virion

(1) Active viral assembly

  (a) Infected host cell is activated by antigens, mitogens, or cytokines

    i) Activation of the host cell induces a protein, NF-kβ, which binds to specific segments on genes to initiate transcription of the host cell's DNA (Nabel, 1993)

    ii) NF-kβ will also interact with binding sites in the LTR regions of the HIV DNA and initiate transcription of the viral DNA (Rosenberg & Fauci, 1991)

  (b) Proviral DNA is transcribed into mRNA which is then transported out of the nucleus into the cytoplasm

  (c) mRNA codons are then translated into amino acid sequences for the polyprotein precursors located in the viral protein core and the virion envelope

  (d) Protease modifies (cleaves) the larger polyproteins initially produced into the active protein subunits, p24, p15, p17, gp120, gp41 needed for assembly of new virion

(2) Viral budding

  (a) Virion core with HIV RNA, modified proteins, and enzymes is assembled at plasma membrane of the host cell

  (b) Final mature virion formed via budding through plasma membrane

  (c) gp120 and gp41 incorporated into the outer lipid membrane

4. HIV subtypes

a. HIV-1

b. HIV-2

(1) Endemic to West Africa

  (a) Serologic detection in AIDS cases in Portugal with previous history of living in Africa

  (b) Serologic detection in asymptomatic Senegalese prostitutes (Essex & Kanki, 1988)

(2) Associated with inducing AIDS

c. Similarities between subtypes

(1) Both are retroviruses belonging to the lentivirus subfamily

(2) Humans are hosts for both viruses

(3) Both infect host cells bearing CD4 surface molecule

(4) Both exhibit variations or mutations in strains within each subtype

d. Differences between subtypes

(1) Genetic difference localized to

  (a) Absence of vpu gene in HIV-2 genome

  (b) Presence of the regulatory gene vpx in HIV-2 genome whose function is unknown (Essex & Kanki, 1988)

(2) Structural difference

  (a) Located in env genes

  (b) Amino acid sequence differs in structure of the envelope glycoproteins for HIV-1 and HIV-2

  (c) Requires differential serum detection of both virion

(3) HIV-2 appears to be less virulent, possibly has a longer period of clinical latency; serologically and genetically more closely related to SIV

5. Mutation of HIV

a. Mutations during HIV replication result in strains with genetic and biologic variability (diversity) (Connor & Ho, 1992)

b. Genetic diversity

(1) Mutations introduced into HIV genome during reverse transcription

(2) Gag and pol gene nucleotide sequences are relatively conserved during transcription

(3) Env gene nucletide sequence is the site of the greatest variability during transcription

(4) Changes in env gene nucleotide sequence result in
  (a) gp120 variable domain, V3, site of the highest frequency for mutation
  (b) Variation of amino acid sequences within the V3 region has been associated with viral mutants produced both in vitro and in vivo
    i) Associated with changes in viral tropism for certain cell types
    ii) Changes in susceptibility of virus to neutralization by Abs
    iii) Changes in virus's ability to induce syncytium formation

c. Biologic diversity
  (1) Changes in the viral genome during transcription may influence biologic function of the virus
    (a) Different kinetics of replication
    (b) Preferential infectivity of certain cell types (tropism)
    (c) Induction of cytopathic effects
    (d) Susceptibility to virus neutralization by antibodies
  (2) Biologic functional changes seen in variants can be divided into early and late stages of disease (Planelles et al., 1993)
  (3) Typical attributes of early isolates obtained from asymptomatic individuals
    (a) Slow replication kinetics
    (b) Non-syncytium inducing
    (c) Tropic for primary cells but not for transformed T-cell lines in vitro
  (4) Isolates from later stages of disease
    (a) Include characteristics seen in early isolates
    (b) Able to infect immortalized T-cell lines in vitro
    (c) Show high rates of replication
    (d) Syncytium inducing

d. Extent of diversity across infected individuals (Planelles et al., 1993): Viral nucleotide sequences will vary among isolates from different AIDS patients, from an individual at different stages of disease, from different tissues within one person

C. Etiology of AIDS

1. Nonviral agents
  a. Identified nonviral substances as possible etiologic agents of AIDS from behaviors associated with early AIDS cases (Essex, 1992)
    (1) Frequent exposure to sperm
    (2) Rectal exposure to sperm
    (3) Use of amyl or butyl nitrates ("poppers")
    (4) Exposure to foreign proteins and tissue antigens in blood
  b. Proposed profound immunosuppression results from
    (1) Frequent exposure to immunostimulatory doses of the nonviral substances
    (2) Chronic immune stimulation leading to exhaustion of the immune system
2. Transmissible agent
  a. Support for an infectious or transmissible agent in the etiology of AIDS was gathered from early epidemiologic surveillance of AIDS cases
    (1) AIDS appeared to be a new disease
    (2) AIDS cases identified early on were reported in a limited geographic area, Africa, which then spread
    (3) Affected homosexual men, intravenous drug users (IDUs), and blood/blood-product recipients were also susceptible to communicable diseases
    (4) Pattern of distribution of AIDS cases closely resembled the presentation and distribution of hepatitis B virus (HBV)
      (a) Transmission of hepatitis could serve as a representative model for transmission of an infectious agent in AIDS (De Cock, 1984)

(b) Hepatitis B also transmitted by homosexual contact, blood exchange, contaminated needles (Weber, 1984)

(5) AIDS in IDUs with no previous history of homosexuality indicated that the etiologic agent could not be something intrinsically linked to homosexuality (Fauci, 1984)

b. Proposed that the infectious agent could be a virus because (Essex, 1992)

(1) Cytomegalovirus (CMV) was already associated with a less severe immunosuppression in kidney

(2) Epstein-Barr virus (EBV) is a lymphotrophic virus

(3) HBV is known to occur in elevated rates in both homosexuals and blood-product recipients

3. Retrovirus

a. Support for a retroviral agent as the etiology of AIDS was based on information regarding HTLV

(1) HTLV only human retrovirus known to have T-cell tropism

(2) HTLV altered T-cell function

(3) HTLV and AIDS agent had the same transmission routes

(a) Sexual contact

(b) By blood

(c) From mother to baby

(4) HTLV caused a nonlethal immunosuppression

(5) HTLV induced disease after a long latency period

(6) HTLV-I is endemic to Haiti and Africa, areas with a high incidence of AIDS (Norman, 1985)

(7) FeLV, animal T-cell retrovirus, also causes an immunosuppression (Norman, 1985)

(8) Infection with HTLV-1 also associated with relatively high rates of OIs (Norman, 1985)

b. Evidence to support a variant of HTLV as the etiology of AIDS

(1) Infection of T cells in culture with HTLV was associated with T-cell proliferation and transformation; lymphocytes from AIDS cases were dying in culture

(2) Serologic detection of Abs to HTLV envelope proteins in AIDS cases with no detection of Abs to HTLV-I structural core proteins

(3) Serologic detection of Abs to HTLV-I envelope antigens in AIDS cases; however, few cases where able to isolate the virus itself

4. HIV

a. HIV isolated and characterized as etiologic agent of AIDS by three independent groups

(1) Montagnier's group at the Pasteur Institute, Paris, called it lymphadenopathy-associated virus (LAV)

(2) Gallo's group at National Cancer Institute of Health, National Institutes of Health, called it HTLV-III

(3) Levy's group in San Francisco, CA, called it AIDS-associated retrovirus (ARV)

b. All three viruses were isolate variants

c. Support for HIV as etiologic agent in AIDS

(1) HIV does infect and is cytotoxic to CD4 cells in vitro

(2) Cells other than lymphocytes/peripheral blood monocytes, such as brain tissue macrophages, which are susceptible to and infected by HIV in AIDS patients are also infected by HIV in vitro (AIDS 89 Summary, 1990)

D. Origin of AIDS

1. Possible origins of the etiologic agent of AIDS

a. Mutation of an existing agent produced a variant that became a more virulent strain

b. The infectious organism may be a recombinant of an organism that previously was infecting people without causing disease, or the disease had a different clinical presentation

c. The new infectious agent was introduced from an isolated group with host resistance to the agent's lethal effects

d. The new infectious agent crossed over from another species into man (Essex, 1992)
   (1) Original host for the infectious agent was probably a primate
   (2) Simian retrovirus, STLV, isolated from African chimpanzees and green monkeys has genetic similarity with human retrovirus HTLV (Essex & Kanki, 1988)
   (3) Blood-borne animal viruses crossed over to man and caused Lassa fever, Marburg disease, Ebola hemorrhagic fever
   (4) In 1984, reports of captive macaque monkeys with AIDS-like syndrome, simian AIDS (Essex & Kanki, 1988)
   (5) SIV isolated in captive macaques and in wild African green monkeys
   (6) SIV and HIV are approximately 50% related at the nucleotide sequence level
   (7) People infected with HIV-2 have Abs that are crossreactive with SIV (Essex & Kanki, 1988)

2. The site of origin for AIDS was probably Africa
   a. High incidence of Kaposi's sarcoma (KS) in U.S. AIDS patients; KS is endemic in parts of Africa—aggressive types seen (Weber, 1984)
   b. Reported cases of AIDS in Europe with previous history of residence in sub-Saharan Africa
   c. STLV with the greatest genetic similarity to HTLV isolated from African chimpanzees and green monkeys (Essex & Kanki, 1988)
   d. SIV with the greatest similarity to HIV isolated from African green monkeys (Essex & Kanki, 1988)
   e. Ebola and Lassa fever viral illnesses were first recognized in Africa (De Cock, 1984)

E. Other Theories

1. Role of arthropods as a vector for HIV transmission has not been proven
   a. Reports that HIV survives in bedbugs (Lyons, Jupp, & Schoub, 1986)
   b. Mosquitoes
2. Opposition to HIV as the etiology of AIDS
   a. Massive immune suppression and dysfunction seen in AIDS patients cannot be directly related to HIV infection of CD4 cells because the quantity of infected CD4 cells is too small to produce the profound immunosuppression
   b. Support to discount this reasoning comes from polymerase chain reaction (PCR) analysis (a method that detects small amounts of viral DNA in host cells), which has found that far larger numbers of CD4 cells are infected than in earlier estimates—1 in 100 cells infected vs. 1 in 10,000 (AIDS 89 Summary, 1990)
   c. HIV is not the causative agent of AIDS because it does not follow typical patterns for infectious disease
      (1) Equally distributed among the sexes, whereas AIDS is predominantly male
      (2) Etiologic agent is both abundant and active in a specified tissue during active disease; low titers make it difficult to isolate the virus in AIDS
      (3) Typically see disease within days or weeks after infection is established and prior to having mounted an immunity, whereas in AIDS see antiviral immunity develops prior to active disease (Duesberg, 1991; Lindenmann, 1994).

II. THE IMMUNE SYSTEM

A. Normal Immunology

1. Cells of the immune system
   a. Granulocytes
      (1) Cells of the myeloid lineage that can be characterized by dense cytoplasmic granules
      (2) Neutrophils
         (a) Major phagocytic cells in the blood
         (b) Represent approximately 60% of circulating leukocytes (white blood cells)
      (3) Basophils
         (a) Participate in allergic reactions
         (b) Represent approximately 1% of circulating leukocytes
         (c) Involved in early inflammatory reactions
      (4) Eosinophils
         (a) Participate in modulation of inflammatory responses
         (b) Represent approximately 5% of circulating leukocytes
   b. Mononuclear phagocytes
      (1) Agranular cells of the myeloid lineage that populate the blood and tissue compartments
      (2) Exhibit multiple functions including phagocytosis, antigen presentation, secretion, and target cell killing
      (3) Monocytes
         (a) Found within the blood; represent 5%–10% of blood leukocytes
         (b) Undergo differentiation into macrophages upon leaving the circulatory compartment
      (4) Macrophages
         (a) Large phagocytic cells found in the brain (microglial), skin (Langerhans), spleen, liver, lungs (alveolar), and lymphoid tissues that participate in local immune responses
         (b) May be free (in blood) or fixed (permanently located in specific organs such as Kupffer cells in liver)
   c. Lymphocytes
      (1) Major participants in specific immune reactions
      (2) Represent 5%–10% of circulating leukocytes
      (3) B cells
         (a) Antibody-producing cells
         (b) Represent approximately 10% of lymphocytes in peripheral blood
         (c) Major lymphoid cell in lymphoid organs outside of the blood
      (4) T cells
         (a) Can serve as either effector cells or regulatory elements of the immune system
         (b) Represent 70%–90% of all circulating lymphocytes
         (c) Found in lesser amounts in lymphoid tissues
      (5) Natural killer cells
         (a) Non-B, non-T lymphocytes
         (b) Represent 5%–15% of circulating lymphocytes
         (c) Kill virus and tumor targets
2. Organs of the immune system
   a. Primary lymphoid organs (sites of immune cell development and maturation): Bone marrow, thymus
   b. Secondary lymphoid organs (dense localizations of immune cells; sites of immune activation): Lymph nodes, spleen, mucosal lymphoid system, bone marrow, gut-associated lymphoma tissue
3. Nonspecific immunity
   a. Physical, mechanical, chemical, and microbial barriers: Skin, mucous membranes, soluble factors, natural flora
   b. Phagocytosis
      (1) Particle uptake by cells of the granulocytic and mononuclear phagocytic lineages
      (2) Protective mechanisms against invading bacteria
   c. Inflammatory response
      (1) Increased blood flow to site of injury
      (2) Increased capillary permeability
      (3) Accumulation of phagocytic cells

4. Specific immunity
   a. Antigens
      (1) Agents capable of eliciting immune responses
      (2) Can be comprised of multiple antigenic determinants
      (3) Elicit activation of specific immune cells (e.g., B and T lymphocytes)
   b. Antibodies (immunoglobulins)
      (1) Basic structure
         (a) Fab region (recognizes antigenic specificity)
         (b) Fc region (activates complement and binds to phagocytic cells)
      (2) Isotypes
         (a) Determined by heavy chain of antibody molecule
         (b) Blood levels
            i)   IgG (600–1600 mg/dl)
            ii) IgM (50–250 mg/dl)
            iii) IgA (80–350 mg/dl)
            iv) IgD (<125 units/ml)
            v)   IgE (0–30 mg/dl)
      (3) Function
         (a) Opsonize and agglutinate bacteria
         (b) Neutralize viruses and bacteria
         (c) Limit colonization of mucosal surfaces by bacteria
         (d) Facilitate antibody-dependent cellular cytotoxicity
   c. Primary vs. secondary immune response
      (1) Latency
         (a) Primary response demonstrates a long lag time
         (b) Secondary response occurs rapidly after exposure to antigen
      (2) Strength
         (a) Primary response is weak
         (b) Secondary response produces high titers of antibody
      (3) Duration
         (a) Primary response is transient
         (b) Secondary response is long lasting
      (4) Antibody isotype
         (a) Primary response is characterized by IgM
         (b) Secondary response: IgG predominates

5. Regulation of immune response
   a. Antigen-presenting cells (may include mononuclear phagocytes and B cells)
   b. T helper/inducer cells (initiate development of specific immune response)
   c. T suppressor/cytotoxic cells (terminate an immune response; participate in killing of virally-infected and tumor cells)
6. Humoral immunity
   a. B-cell involvement
      (1) Proliferation to antigen
      (2) Differentiation into plasma cells
      (3) Generation of memory cells
   b. Response to bacterial antigens
   c. Antibody effector mechanism
      (1) Opsonization of bacteria
      (2) Activation of complement
7. Cell-mediated immunity
   a. T-cell and macrophage involvement
   b. T-cell proliferation to antigen
   c. T-cell differentiation
      (1) Inducer of delayed type hypersensitivity (DTH) response
      (2) Cytotoxic effector
   d. Response to virally infected target cells, tumor cells, intracellular pathogens
   e. DTH response
      (1) T helper/inducer cells generate cytokines to activate macrophages
      (2) Macrophages destroy intracellular pathogens
   f. Antitumor and antiviral responses
      (1) T helper/inducer cells generate cytokines to activate T cytotoxic cells
      (2) T cytotoxic cells destroy tumor or virally-infected cells
8. Natural killer cells
   a. May become activated by T helper/inducer-derived cytokines to generate lymphokine activated killer cells
   b. Antitumor and antiviral response
      (1) Lyse target cells following direct binding to altered cell membrane
      (2) Lyse antibody-coated targets through antibody-dependent cellular cytotoxic mechanism
9. Complement system
   a. Complement components
   b. Classical vs. alternative pathway

c. Biologic consequences of complement activation
   (1) Generation of opsonins
   (2) Enhancement of inflammation: Chemotaxis, anaphylatoxins, viral neutralization, cell lysis
10. Measurement of immunologic status
   a. Quantification of cell populations
      (1) Complete white blood cell count (WBC) with differential
         (a) Total WBC in adults: $5-10 \times 10^3$ cells/mm^3 blood
         (b) Differential cell counts determined by percentages of types of WBCs
      (2) Lymphocyte subset analysis using specific monoclonal antibodies to cell surface markers (CD markers reflect cell clusters of differentiation)
         (a) B cells (CD19, CD20, CD22): Identify approximately 10% of all blood lymphocytes
         (b) T cells (CD3, CD5): Identify approximately 70%–75% of all blood lymphocytes
            i) T helper/inducer cells (CD4): Identify approximately 45% of blood lymphocytes
               a) CD4+ TH1 cells facilitate cell-mediated immune reactions
               b) CD4+ TH2 cells facilitate humoral immune reactions
            ii) T cytotoxic/suppressor cells (CD8): Identify approximately 25% of blood lymphocytes
         (c) Natural killer cells (CD16, CD57): Identify approximately 15% of all blood lymphocytes
   b. Granulocytes/mononuclear phagocytes
      (1) Particle phagocytosis
      (2) Bacterial killing
      (3) Migration to inflammatory stimulus
   c. Humoral immune response
      (1) Serum antibody levels
      (2) Lymphocyte proliferation to specific antigens or mitogens: Evaluated in

culture by measuring incorporation of ^{3}H-thymidine into cellular DNA
      (3) Production of specific antibody to antigenic challenge: Measured followed in vivo or in vitro challenge with antigen
   d. Cell-mediated immunity
      (1) DTH skin testing: Involves innoculation of antigens into the skin to detect previous exposure of the immune system; if immune recognition occurs, inflammation becomes apparent at 48–72 hours
      (2) Lymphocyte proliferation to specific antigens or mitogens: Measured in culture as above
      (3) Antitumor cytotoxicity: Evaluation of target cell lysis in culture
   e. Natural killer cell activity: Antitumor cytotoxicity (see above)

B. Altered Immunologic Status Following HIV Infection

1. CD4 T helper/inducer cells
   a. Target for infection by HIV
   b. Progressive decline in cell numbers over course of disease
   c. Progressive loss in proliferation and cytokine secretion by TH1 cells that promote cell-mediated immune responses
   d. Excessive activation of TH2 cells that promote generation of humoral immune responses
   e. Reduced reactivity to DTH skin test antigens
2. CD8 T cytotoxic/suppressor cells
   a. Increase in cell numbers during acute infection
   b. Decline in numbers at time of AIDS diagnosis
   c. Increased expression of activation markers on cell surface that correlates with stage of illness
   d. Diminished HIV-specific cytotoxic lymphocyte activity
3. Natural killer cells
   a. Conflicting reports of changes in cell numbers
      (1) CD57-positive cells elevated in early illness but reduced in AIDS

        (2) CD16-positive cells reduced at all stages of disease

    b. Reduced cytotoxicity that correlates with disease progression (may reflect reduced levels of cytokines)

4. B lymphocytes
   a. Expression of activation markers on cell surfaces
   b. Elevated levels of immunoglobulins
   c. Reduced specific humoral immune response to immunization associated with late stages of illness

5. Mononuclear phagocytes
   a. Targets for infection by HIV
   b. Decreased migration to inflammatory stimuli
   c. Diminished phagocytosis and bacterial killing

6. Granulocytes: No consistent alterations reported.

III. TRANSMISSION OF HIV INFECTION

A. Routes of Transmission

1. Sexual contact
   a. Male-to-male: Anal-receptive sexual intercourse places the person at greatest risk for exposure to the virus
   b. Male-to-female: High risk of transmission
   c. Female-to-male: Risk of transmission not as high as male-to-female contact
   d. Female-to-female: Low risk of transmission much lower than either male homosexual or heterosexual
2. Blood borne
   a. Parenteral exposure
      (1) Sharing unsterile needles or other drug paraphanelia
      (2) Unsterile invasive instruments
      (3) Occupational exposure to needle sticks/sharps by healthcare workers
   b. Transfusion with contaminated blood and blood products: Transmission rates in developed countries have declined since blood banks initiated stringent policies and procedures on screening blood for HIV
   c. Mucocutaneous exposure to blood or other infected body fluids
3. Vertical transmission: Perinatal transmission from mother to infant prenatally, intrapartum, postpartum (several documented cases of vertical transmission of HIV from mother to infant via breast-feeding)
4. Unproven routes
   a. Casual contact with an HIV-infected person (e.g., via hugging, bathing, feeding)
   b. Casual, horizontal household contact between uninfected and infected household members; a few cases are believed to have resulted from household contact, but in general this is not considered another type of transmission
   c. Insect vectors

B. Disruptions of Physiologic Barriers (Trauma impairing natural mucosal barrier of the genitalia may enhance transmission of HIV)

1. Trauma related to sexual practices (e.g., open lesions) may present a portal of entry for HIV in the uninfected partner
   a. Anal intercourse
   b. "Dry" sex: A lack of natural lubrication (or if partners do not use an artifical lubricant) may cause tears in the mucosal barrier
   c. Partners using sexual toys
   d. "Fisting" (one sexual partner inserts a fist into the rectal canal or vaginal vault of the other partner)
   e. Douching (vaginal or rectal)
   f. Atrophic vaginitis: A decrease in the natural lubrication of the vagina as women age
2. Trauma to the mucosal membranes of the female genitalia related to the use of contraceptive methods
   a. Vaginal barrier mechanical methods may traumatize the vaginal epithelium
   b. Oral contraceptives may cause changes to the vaginal and cervical epithelium; cervical erosion is common
   c. Intrauterine devices (IUDs) may cause endometrial trauma
3. Other trauma
   a. Tampons are under investigation as a cause of trauma to the mucosal membranes
   b. Sexually transmitted diseases (STDs) (e.g., syphilis, herpes simplex type II, STDs causing chancroid, *Chlamydia trachomatis*, gonorrhea) result in genital ulcerations that interrupt the natural mucosal barriers
   c. Menstrual-cycle shedding of the uterus lining may make the woman more susceptible to HIV infection; conversely, the infected woman who is menstruating may place her partner at greater risk of infection during unprotected sex

C. Biologic Disturbances

1. Level of infectivity: As a person's level of infectivity increases, the potential risk of transmitting HIV to another person also increases
   a. Antigenemia is associated with increased infectivity
   b. Infectivity increases as the person progresses through the disease
   c. A decline in the CD4 count resulting in altered immune function (due to increased viral replication and increased levels of infectious virus in the body fluids)
   d. Detection of the p24 antigen indicates increased infectivity
2. Alterations of lymphocytes
   a. Concomitant STDs cause the immune system to circulate more lymphocytes to the area of infection in the genital tract; it is postulated that the increased lymphocytes to the area are prime targets for infection, leading to harboring and transportation of the virus to other lymphocytes
   b. Oral contraceptives affect a person's hormonal environment
      (1) Synthetic sex steroids may modify the immune response
      (2) Oral contraceptives may suppress some aspects of the immune response
   c. Circulating IgG antibodies to sperm (antisperm antibodies)
      (1) Sperm and seminal plasma are immunosuppressive; under normal circumstances they inhibit lymphocyte activation
      (2) The antisperm antibodies bound to sperm are potent gamma-interferon inducers and are less effective in inhibiting lymphocyte proliferative responses, a change that could lead to the activation instead of the inhibition of lymphocytes
      (3) The female genital tract has an increased number of lymphocytes being directly exposed to HIV-infected semen (Witkin, 1990)

d. The use of alcohol, illicit (recreational) drugs, or tobacco has been associated with suppression of lymphocyte function/number
3. Other biologic factors: One study (Fischl, Fayne, & Flanagan, 1988) found a greater incidence of transmission among men who were uncircumcised

D. Behaviorial Factors

1. Risk group: Rates of transmission from IDUs are higher than from bisexual men or men infected from contaminated blood products
2. Number of sexual partners: The greater the number of sexual partners, the greater the potential exposure to HIV
3. Types of sexual activities (Schram, 1990)
   a. High-risk sexual practices
      (1) Receptive anal/vaginal intercourse with ejaculation and without a condom
      (2) Insertive anal/vaginal intercourse without a condom
      (3) Receptive/insertive anal intercourse with withdrawal prior to ejaculation
      (4) Receptive/insertive vaginal intercourse with spermicidal foam but without a condom
      (5) Receptive/insertive anal/vaginal intercourse with a condom
   b. Sexual practices with some risk of HIV transmission
      (1) Oral sex with men with or without ejaculation
      (2) Oral sex with women
      (3) Oral sex with men with pre-ejaculation; with no ejaculation or pre-ejaculation fluid
   c. Sexual practice with some risk depending on intactness of mucous membranes and other factors
      (1) Mutual masturbation with external or internal touching
      (2) Sharing sex toys
      (3) Anal or vaginal fisting
4. Drug use can lead to engaging in high-risk behaviors
   a. Alcohol (diminishes a person's inhibitions)

b. Use of mood-altering drugs (either illicit or prescription)
5. Bisexuality can be a hidden behavior

E. Perinatal Disturbances

1. Intrauterine transmission from the mother to the developing fetus (can occur during each trimester)
   a. Circulatory interface: Structures within the fetus—syncytiotrophoblast, a fused basal lamina, and an endothelial cell monolayer—interface with maternal blood; as all nutrients pass through this interface between the mother and fetus it is presumed that infectious agents pass through also
   b. Cellular interface: The amnion is permeable to molecules, which may include HIV
   c. Cytokines (e.g., tumor necrosis factor [TNF]) released locally in sites of placental inflammation may serve to increase HIV replication and promote transmission across the placenta)
2. Intrapartum exposure of the infant
   a. Theorized to occur though direct muco-cutaneous exposure to the virus during delivery or ascending infection during labor
   b. Swallowing of infected amniotic fluid could provide a significant dose of virus to the newborn
3. Postpartum exposure of the infant through breast milk
4. Maternal factors influencing the rate of HIV transmission from mother to infant
   a. p24 antigenemia of the mother
   b. Low CD4 number
   c. Advanced disease stage either during pregnancy or within months of giving birth
   d. Absence of maternal antibody to specific HIV epitopes, certain maternal antibodies may have a neutralizing effect in preventing transmission
   e. Episiotomy may expose the newborn to infected blood as the infant passes through the birth canal

5. Placental factors
   a. Placental morphology changes during gestation; different placental cells may have disparate susceptibilities to HIV infection, implying that the risk of infection changes with placental changes
   b. Virus transmission might occur by passage of cell-free virus through the placental barrier by active Fc receptor-mediated transport of HIV immune complexes (Mofenson & Wolinsky, 1992)
   c. Maternal co-infections associated with chorioamnionitis could impair the integrity of the placenta
6. Virologic factors
   a. Viral phenotype and genotype may differ in degrees of virulence
   b. Site of viral expression may be more or less active within certain blood or mucous membrane tissue
7. Obstetric factors
   a. Increased length of ruptured membranes correlates with increased risk of transmission
   b. Mode of delivery
      (1) Cesarian section may decrease risk of transmission (not statistically significant)
      (2) C-section may have increased risks to mother associated with trauma, wound healing
   c. Invasive fetal monitoring
      (1) May increase risk by violating integrity of baby's skin/scalp and provide opportunity for infection
      (2) Consider in context of HIV risk vs. benefit of monitoring to infant
8. Neonatal factors
   a. Individual genetic and immune responses may differ
   b. Birth order in multiple births—increased risk for first born in vaginal delivery
   c. Immaturity of infant's GI tract may allow transmission from swallowed amniotic fluid/breast milk
   d. Prematurity associated with increased risk of transmission

F. Cofactors

1. Vertical transmission
   a. Co-infections of the mother during pregnancy
   b. Smoking tobacco or taking illicit drugs may alter the placental barrier, enhancing the transport of the virus across the placental membrane
2. Parenteral transmission
   a. Risk of seropositivity increases as the number of persons with whom needles are regularly shared increases
   b. Number of injections by the IDUs increases risk of exposure
   c. Intrinsic immunosuppressive properties of the drugs used
   d. IDUs themselves may have many immunologic abnormalities
   e. IDUs may have antigenic overload
   f. Consequent immunosuppression due to multiple infections from the use of non-sterile water, contaminated diluents, impure narcotics, and blood- and dirt-contaminated needles (Ginzberg et al., 1985); also includes coincident viral infections such as HBV
   g. IDUs may have chemical immunosuppression due to physician- and self-prescribed use of antibiotics for their numerous infections (Ginzberg et al., 1985).
   h. Malnutrition: Drug and alcohol use have a direct appetite-suppressing effect; alcohol can also lead to impaired absorption of food
3. Sexual transmission
   a. Malnutrition (most common cause of T-cell immunodeficiency worldwide is protein-calorie malnutrition)
   b. Use of IV or recreational drugs (e.g., volatile nitrites)
   c. Exposure to prescription drugs
   d. Allergic disorders
   e. Stress (may have an immunologic component)
   f. Age: Older adults have natural loss of resistance
   g. Frequent use of antibiotics may lead to chemical immunosuppression
   h. Exposure to allogeneic semen and sperm
   i. Multiple infections (e.g., syphilis, parasitic diseases) may cause antigenic overload and stimulation, causing a chronic stress to the immune system
   j. Douching or enemas before sexual intercourse
4. Possible role of cofactors in disease susceptibility and progression
   a. Increase the likelihood of being infected after exposure
   b. Additive effect
   c. Deterministic effect
   d. Synergistic role
   e. Facilitative role
   f. Enhance antigenic overload and stimulation
   g. Affect lymphocytes
   h. Depress lymphocyte function/number.
   i. Potentiate circulation of lymphocytes to a site that is a portal of entry for the virus (e.g., STDs in the genital tract).

IV. NATURAL HISTORY OF HIV INFECTION AND AIDS

A. Primary Infection (0–12 weeks)
Virus infects cells, thereby activating immune system. Immune system clears the virus to the lymphatic organs where rapid growth occurs, leading to a viral burst back into circulation. Physical manifestations of the viral burst are similar in character and duration to mononucleosis. As more immune mechanisms are initiated the amount of circulating virus declines until most of the virus is sequestered in lymphatic tissue, where it continues to replicate at a relatively constant rate.

1. Viral activity
   a. Immune activation results in rapid clearing of circulating virus by dendritic cells to lymphatic organs, where rapid growth leads to burst of virus back into circulation
   b. The virus infects CD4+ lymphocyte cells of the central nervous system (CNS), bone marrow, and lymphoid tissue (nodes, lamina propria, thymus), including CD4 progenitor cells
   c. Circulating virus levels rise rapidly during first 6 weeks as reflected in p24 antigen, plasma HIV reverse transcriptase polymerase chain reaction (RT-PCR), and branched DNA (bDNA) testing, then decline
   d. The sharp decrease in circulating virus quantities results from
      (1) Proliferation of activated T lymphocytes, especially CD8 cytotoxic T lymphocytes (CTL)
      (2) Filtering and mechanical trapping of virions, infected CD4+ lymphocytes, and HIV antibody conjugates in lymphoid tissue
      (3) Activation of classical and alternate pathways of the complement cascade
      (4) Increased interferon-alpha (IFN-α) levels acting directly against HIV or causing retrafficking of lymphocytes
2. Immune activity

   a. Phagocytic effect
      (1) CD4 expressing monocyte lineage cells (monocytes, macrophages, microglia) are seeded
      (2) Antibody production begins as macrophages present HIV antigens to CD4+ lymphocytes
      (3) Macrophage activation results in increased levels of neopterin (a breakdown product of macrophage activation) and increased secretion of IFN-α, TNF-α, IL-6
      (4) Natural-killer (NK) cell activity diminishes while numbers and phenotype remain relatively normal (possibly related to alterations in normal CD4+ lymphocyte inductive signals)
   b. Humoral effect
      (1) Proliferation of large numbers of B cells and clones (polyclonal)
      (2) B cells manufacture anti-HIV antibodies (detectable at 2–5 weeks) following presentation of HIV antigens to CD4+ lymphocytes and other immune cells
         (a) Antibodies are produced to envelope, core, and regulatory gene proteins
         (b) Antibodies may be specific to a single HIV strain or multiple strains
         (c) Antibodies are produced associated with antibody-dependent cellular cytotoxicity (ADCC) (NK cells bearing anti-HIV antibodies)
      (3) B cells become hyporesponsive to common antigens and mitogens
      (4) B cells secrete inflammatory cytokines TNF-α, IL-1, IL-6, IL-10, and elevated amounts of immunoglobulin (Ig)
   c. Cell-mediated effect
      (1) CD4 expressing T lymphocytes are seeded and express activation markers on their surface
      (2) Activated CD4+ lymphocytes secrete IL-2, IFN, TNF, IL-4, activat-

ing both B lymphocyte production of antibody and CD8+ cytolytic cells
- (3) Sharp decline in CD4+ lymphocyte counts from 1,000–500/μl
- (4) CD8+ lymphocyte proliferation
- (5) Initiation of CD4+ lymphocyte depletion by accelerated apoptosis (early cell death) induced by cross-linking of CD4 receptors resulting in CD4+ cell death on subsequent activation and other mechanisms
- d. Lymphoid organ effect
  - (1) Lymph node germinal cell formation and hyperplasia
  - (2) Seeding of thymic epithelial cells, thymocytes and beginning of thymic degeneration
3. Miscellaneous immune response
  - a. Initial increase (first 6 weeks) then decrease in levels of β-2 microglobulin expressed in association with major histocompatibility complex Class I (MHC-I), indicating an increase in cell turnover
  - b. Degree of immunodeficiency: Mild to moderate (CD4+ lymphocyte counts 500–1,000/μl)
4. Clinical manifestations
  - a. Acute retroviral syndrome (presentation similar to mononucleosis)
    - (1) Common symptoms: Fever, arthralgias, myalgias, lymphadenopathy, pharyngitis, anorexia, weight loss, and rash lasting 1–4 weeks
    - (2) Rare and more severe manifestations: Meningitis, encephalitis, peripheral neuropathy, and myelopathy

B. Clinical Latency (12 weeks–8 years) Virus is present primarily in lymphatic tissue where it continues to replicate and stimulate the immune system. Stimulation results in a chronic immune activation, which further undermines the immune system. Virus continues a slow spread to vulnerable cells throughout the body. Responses to diagnostic skin tests (DTH) may diminish. Clinical symptoms of disease are usually absent or mild.

1. Viral activity
  - a. A self-perpetuating viral cycle consists of persistent viral replication, persistent immune activation, immunoregulatory cytokine level elevations or dysfunctions, and viral spread to uninfected tissue and cells
  - b. Viral replication continues at a relatively constant rate primarily in lymphoid organs (e.g., thymus, lymph nodes, lamina propria)
2. Immune activity
  - a. Phagocytic effect
    - (1) Monocyte lineage cells act as reservoirs of HIV and replicate virus in intracytoplasmic vacuoles, as well as outward at the plasma membrane; vacuolar caching may conceal the virus from the immune system
    - (2) Infected macrophages, while secreting decreased amounts of IFN-α, may also infect naive CD4+ lymphocytes in the course of normal antigen presentation
    - (3) Neutrophils exhibit defects in chemotaxis, bacteriocidal effects, phagocytosis
    - (4) NK cells exhibit an increasing defect in release of cytotoxic factors
  - b. Humoral effect
    - (1) Decrease in the number of B cell clones (oligoclonal)
    - (2) HIV buds off cells, taking with it portions of cell walls including membrane-bound restriction factors that protect human cells from attack by complement and cytotoxic cells (another mechanism by which virus may be concealed from the immune system)
    - (3) Autoantibodies to neutrophils and platelets are produced
  - c. Cell-mediated effect
    - (1) HIV-specific CD8+ CTLs are manufactured but become less effective against HIV possibly due to escape mutations by the virus, which are no longer recognized, or to the ability of HIV-tat to decrease Class I MHC expression

(2) Gradual attrition of CD4+ lymphocytes occurs through multiple mechanisms
   (a) Viral infection and cell death (single cell killing)
   (b) Immune-mediated mechanisms of cell death (theoretical—e.g., syncytia formation)
   (c) HIV-specific immune responses including HIV-specific CTLs, antibody-dependent cellular cytotoxicity (ADCC), NK cell killing
   (d) Autoimmune mechanisms involving class reactivity between antigens of HIV and self
   (e) Anergy related to inappropriate cell signaling via CD4 – gp120 interaction
   (f) Superantigen-mediated deletion or anergy (theoretical and controversial)
   (g) Apoptosis
  d. Lymphoid organ and cytokine effect: Continuation of effects initiated during primary infection process
3. Degree of immunodeficiency: Mild (CD4+ lymphocyte counts 500 – 750/μl)
4. Possible clinical manifestations
  a. Psychosocial: Depression and anxiety related to HIV-positive status
  b. Persistent generalized lymphadenopathy (PGL)

C. Early Symptomatic HIV Disease (8–10 years)

The rate of viral replication on a cellular level remains relatively constant, but the immune system's waning ability to control virus results in greater amounts in circulation. Signs and symptoms of disease progress from mild to moderate, begin to interfere with activities of daily living and quality of life; responses to diagnostic skin tests may disappear.

1. Viral activity: Viral replication rate relatively constant but increasingly detectable in circulation as lymphoid microenvironment deteriorates
2. Immune activity
  a. Phagocytic effect: Phagocytic integrity erodes, but without clinical manifestations
  b. Humoral effect
    (1) HIV-specific antibody declines
    (2) B-cell elevations continue, but number of clones continues to decline
    (3) Continued increase in autoantibody levels to neutrophils and platelets
  c. Cell-mediated effect: Decline in anti-HIV CTL activity
  d. Lymphoid organ and cytokine effect
    (1) Decreased trapping of virus
    (2) Increased secretion of proinflammatory cytokines continues
  e. Degree of immunodeficiency: Moderate (CD4+ lymphocyte counts 200 – 500/μl)
3. Clinical manifestations
  a. Increase in occurrence or onset of diseases such as PGL, oral candidiasis, persistent vaginal candidiasis, TB, oral hairy leukoplakia, shingles (varicella zoster [VSV]), thrombocytopenia, *Molluscum contagiosum*, cervical and rectal dysplasia, KS
  b. Development of anergy to skin tests

D. Advanced HIV Disease (AIDS) (10–11 years)

Immune system mechanisms for virus control fail, resulting in large amounts of virus in circulation. Immune system activation continues. Clinical manifestations include lean body mass loss and wasting syndrome. OIs occur as cellular immunity fails. Death usually results from infection, neoplasm, or wasting.

1. Viral activity: Continues as in early symptomatic disease
2. Immune activity
  a. Phagocytic effect: Continues as in early symptomatic disease
  b. Humoral effect
    (1) Levels of antibody to HIV core proteins decrease as antigen levels increase

(2) Levels of antibody to HIV envelope core protein remain relatively stable

(3) Anergy to de novo antigens is relatively complete

c. Cell-mediated effect

(1) Decrease in anti-HIV CTL activity

(2) Decrease and elimination of components of the CD4+ lymphocyte repertoire that mediate immune response to specific OI-associated organisms (theoretical)

d. Lymphoid organ and cytokine effect

(1) Lymphoid involvement continues as in early symptomatic disease

(2) Increasing proinflammatory cytokine levels

(3) Decreasing antiviral cytokine levels

e. Degree of immunodeficiency: Profound (CD4+ lymphocyte counts 0–200/µl)

3. Clinical manifestations

a. OIs due to depleted CD4+ lymphocytes (site specific or disseminated)

(1) Viral infections: CMV, HSV, VSV, progressive multifocal leukoencephalopathy (PML)

(2) Bacterial infections: *Mycobacterium avium* complex (MAC), *M. tuberculosis* (MTB), other atypical *Mycobacterium* infections

(3) Protozoal infections: *P. carinii* (although some believe it is a fungus), toxoplasmosis, *Cryptosporidium*, isosporiasis

(4) Fungal infections: Candidiasis (including oral thrush), cryptococcosis, histoplasmosis, coccidioidomycosis

b. Other bacterial infections due to leukopenia and monocyte macrophage dysfunction

(1) Pneumonias from streptococci, *Hemophilus influenzae, Pseudomonas aeruginosa, Klebsiella pneumoniae*, staphylococci, *Rhodococcus equii*

(2) Gastroenteritis from *Shigella flexneri, Salmonella, Campylobacter, Clostridium difficile* toxin

(3) Skin infections due to *Rochalimaea quintana, Bartonella bacilliformis* (bacillary angiomatosis), staphylococci, streptococci

(4) Meningitis due to *Listeria monocytogenes*

(5) Sinusitis due to streptococci, *P. aeruginosa*, staphylococci, *H. influenzae*, other anaerobes

(6) Disseminated infections due to salmonella, streptococci, bacillary angiomatosis, *P. aeruginosa, Escherichia coli*, other enterobacteria

c. Neuropsychiatric pathology

(1) Adjustment disorders (with anxious or depressed mood)

(2) Affective disorders (major depression, bipolar disorder)

(3) Cognitive disorders (impaired memory, concentration, confusion, mental "slowing," hallucinations)

(4) Behavioral disorders (apathy, withdrawal, agitation)

(5) Anxiety disorders

(6) Organic disorders (e.g., AIDS-related dementia, infections of the CNS)

d. Neoplastic processes (lymphoma, KS, cervical dysplasia, high-grade cervical tumors)

e. Wasting syndrome possibly mediated by increased levels of TNF-α

f. Other manifestations

(1) Anergy to antigenic stimulation

(2) Hematologic abnormalities due to multiple factors (bone marrow suppression, autoantibody levels, disease, pharmacokinetic activity or interactions)

(3) Other organ system disorders

E. HIV and AIDS Disease Staging

1. Public Health Service CD4+ Lymphocyte Categories

a. Early-stage disease: CD4+ lymphocyte count ≥500/µl

b. Middle-stage disease: CD4+ lymphocyte count 200–499/µl

c. Late-stage disease: <200/µl

2. Public Health Service Revised Classification System for HIV Infection (Adolescents and Adults) (see Appendix A, p. 398)

a. Category A: One or more of the following conditions in the presence of

documented HIV infection; conditions listed in B and C must not have occurred
(1) Asymptomatic HIV infection with CD4+ lymphocyte count ≥500/μl
(2) Persistent generalized lympha-denopathy with CD4+ lymphocyte count 200–499
(3) Acute (primary) HIV infection with accompanying illness or history of acute HIV infection and with CD4+ lymphocyte count <200/μl

b. Category B: Symptomatic conditions that are not included among conditions listed in Category C and that meet at least one of the following criteria
(1) Conditions are attributed to HIV infection or are indicative of a defect in cell mediated immunity
(2) Conditions are considered by physicians to have a clinical course or require management that is complicated by HIV infection, e.g.
(a) Bacillary angiomatosis
(b) Oropharyngeal candidiasis (thrush)
(c) Vulvovaginal candidiasis (persistent, frequent, or poorly responsive to therapy)
(d) Cervical dysplasia (moderate or severe) or cervical carcinoma in situ
(e) Constitutional symptoms such as fever (>38.5°C) or diarrhea lasting >1 month
(f) Oral hairy leukoplakia
(g) HSV involving at least 2 distinct episodes or >1 dermatome

(h) Idiopathic thrombocytopenia purpura (ITP)
(i) Listeriosis
(j) Pelvic inflammatory disease (PID), particularly with tubo-ovarian abscess
(k) Peripheral neuropathy

c. Category C
(1) Clinical conditions listed in the AIDS surveillance case definition for classification purposes
(2) Once a Category C condition has occurred the person will remain in Category C

3. Walter Reed Staging Classification is used at some facilities
4. Staging systems
a. To be clinically useful a staging system must describe the progression of disease and correspond to available management and treatment strategies
b. At present, only the staging of patients by CD4 count offers an appropriate correspondence to disease progression and permits recommendations for the initiation of antiretroviral treatment and primary prophylaxis for some OIs
c. One key deficit in AIDS care is the current lack of widely available direct markers of viral activity and the consequent heavy dependence on surrogate markers for staging; recent work published on the development of direct markers suggests that patient staging based on individual assessment of viral activity, as well as immune status, will be available in the near future
d. Pediatric staging: See p. 375.

Section 3

HIV Counseling and Testing

The detection of HIV antibodies in the blood was the first step in the establishment of HIV counseling and testing programs. Such counseling and testing programs eventually included pretest counseling, which offered the opportunity to explore with individuals what the results of HIV testing (whether positive or negative) might mean to them. It also included posttest counseling for those who tested positive or negative, which included content on prevention in ways that would be meaningful for individual patients. Various issues surrounding anonymous and confidential testing have been important in such programs. The types of HIV tests available and the associated counseling are discussed in this section.

A. Issues Concerning Counseling and Testing

1. HIV can affect anyone, therefore healthcare providers need to address risk factors and perceptions about personal risk with *every* patient

2. People being tested for HIV antibodies face many complex issues. HIV counseling needs to offer up-to-date information and an opportunity to explore concerns sensitively. These two essential elements *must be* done in person as they form an important first step in assisting those who have HIV deal with their disease.

3. Receiving the results of a positive HIV antibody test is the beginning of a process of learning to live with HIV that may be filled with the potential of discrimination in employment, housing, insurance coverage, medical care, and loss or estrangement from family, friends, co-workers. In addition, people with HIV deal with taboos concerning sexual identity, drug use, sexual behavior, and death. All contribute to the stigma that confronts people with HIV.

4. Understanding these issues and being sensitive to cultural and linguistic differences are key in developing trusting and successful partnerships with patients

5. If a patient's primary language is not English, and even if the patient understands a little English, the provider should offer information and allow for questions in the patient's primary language, using a translator when appropriate. Avoid using family members as translators.

6. The provider also must consider cultural, ethnic, religious, class, sexual orientation, and sex differences and avoid passing judgment on the patient's reaction to the illness, lifestyle, or behavior. HIV, like other diseases, highlights variables that exist among different cultures — for example, reactions to pain, views of male/female roles, the importance and inclusion of family, or reluctance to access available support.

7. Differences are also manifested when discussing or describing sexual behaviors. It is helpful to ask people how they describe sexual behaviors and use common non-medical terms. Cultural, ethnic, religious, and gender factors can have an impact on men's reluctance to use condoms, or a couple's reluctance about contraception in general. Some women may have difficulty discussing sexual matters with any man, including the healthcare provider (and vice versa).

8. Women, often the primary caregivers in families, may experience heightened anxiety around being ill and may not come to terms with the severity of their illness. Concerns about bearing children, as well as caring for children and spouse, may interfere with their own care.

9. Knowing how a patient became infected may be helpful in understanding issues facing the patient. However, it may take time and the development of a trusting relationship for the patient to share this information. Finally, it is important for providers to identify their own biases so they can approach the patient with a nonjudgmental attitude. Only then will the door open to working with the patient on his or her health and well-being.

B. Risk Assessment Tool: Making the Decision to Test

1. Consider all adult and adolescent patients potentially at risk
   a. Assumptions cannot be made that patients are not engaging in behaviors that put them at risk regardless of their marital status, class, race, residence, age, gender, or assumed sexual orientation
   b. Interview the patient alone and give assurance that everything discussed will be held in strict confidence. Be aware that confidentiality and reporting laws vary from state to state.
   c. Your comfort in discussing issues nonjudgmentally will facilitate the patient's

ability to respond honestly and completely

2. Ask the patient the following questions to help determine whether HIV antibody testing is indicated

   a. Have you been sexually active within the last 10 years? with men, women, or both?

   b. How many sexual partners have you had in the past 12 months? If multiple, were any of these partners well known to you?

   c. Have you talked with your partner(s) about their risk for HIV?

   d. Have you had intercourse (anal/vaginal) without a condom during this time?

   e. Do you understand what safer sexual practices are? (Ask for description; correct any misinformation.)

   f. Do you use safer sex practices now? If so, how long have you been doing this? Do you use condoms **every** time you have intercourse? oral sex?

   g. Do you use drugs or drink alcohol? Are you able to practice safer sex consistently even when using these substances?

   h. Do you believe your partner(s) may be (at risk of being) HIV infected? Have they had other sexual partners, used needles, tested positive, had a previous sexual partner who was infected, received blood transfusions or blood products?

   i. Have you used needles within the last 10 years? Did you ever share needles, cookers, or other drug paraphernalia?

   j. Are you using needles now? If yes, are you cleaning your works? How? Have you had clean/sober time? Are you interested in a treatment program?

   k. Have you or any of your partners received a transfusion of blood or blood products before 1985? If so, when and where?

3. The more risk behaviors people engage in, the greater the risk they are infected. However, any risk behavior is cause for concern.

C. HIV Testing

Two methods currently in use— antibody and antigen testing

1. Antibody testing

   a. HIV antibody test

      (1) A blood test that can show if a person is infected with HIV; the test should be preceded by pretest counseling

      (2) It takes from 1–3 weeks to get the test results; results should be given in person at a posttest counseling session

   b. Enzyme-linked immunoabsorbent assay (ELISA): Initial test for HIV infection

      (1) HIV antigens are coated onto wells of a culture plate

      (2) Patient's serum is added to wells; any HIV antibody contained in serum binds to antigens

      (3) Anti-human HIV antibody (which is bound to a protein) is added

         (a) Binds only if HIV antibody is present

         (b) This protein brings about a reaction (color change) when a final substance is added

         (c) If color change is strong enough (measured by spectrophotometer) the test is considered positive; this is routinely repeated to confirm positive result

      (4) ELISA is very sensitive (picks up almost all positive) but not completely specific (a few of the positives are false positives); therefore, patients are not given results solely based on ELISA results

   c. Western blot: Confirmatory test for HIV infection

      (1) Very specific, but labor intensive; performed only on those tested positive by ELISA

      (2) A mixture of HIV antigens are put on a gel, separated by molecular weight, and transferred ("blotted") to nitrocellulose paper incubated with serum samples; any HIV

antibodies present bind to the antigens
(3) An anti-HIV antibody protein is added
(4) A colorless substance is added that, if it reacts with the attached anti-HIV antibody, will produce a colored band on the strip; characteristic patterns of colored bands are seen with HIV infection
d. Patients with positive ELISA and positive Western blots are said to be HIV seropositive
e. HIV window period
(1) The 1- to 3-month period after HIV exposure but before formation of antibodies in amounts detectable by ELISA; those who test negative have either not been exposed to the virus or have not yet seroconverted
(2) ELISA test 3–6 months after exposure: If the patient tests negative and is in a monogamous relationship with an HIV-negative or low-risk partner, the negative test result is likely accurate
(3) However, if the person has a negative result but has reported significant risk, consider that the person may not yet have formed antibodies but may be within the window period
(a) For low risk, retesting is recommended at 6 months
(b) For higher risk, repeat testing at 6 months and 1 year
2. Antigen testing
a. Polymerase chain reaction (PCR)
(1) Can detect HIV-1 nucleic acid sequences in a DNA form, as proviruses integrated into the chromosomes of infected cells, or as RNA synthesized in infected cells that are actively expressing viruses, or within virus particles present in the cell free plasma
(2) Labor intensive and extremely costly
b. Branched DNA (bDNA) assay
(1) Designed to measure the amount of

HIV RNA in plasma of infected patients
(2) Recently developed technology that uses highly sensitive probes to detect and quantify RNA sequences
(3) Test is reproducible and relatively simple to perform
c. The cost of both PCR and bDNA assay is a major factor determining use or nonuse of these tests; only available in selected sites that are often part of medical and research settings
d. p24 antigen
(1) Measure of HIV-produced proteins
(2) Identifies the presence of the HIV protein but may not accurately gauge the amount of HIV in a person's blood (viral burden)
e. HIV blood culture
(1) Culturing is labor intensive; results vary from laboratory to laboratory
(2) Cost is lower than previously mentioned tests; reliability also low
3. See *Clinical Management of Pediatric HIV Patients*, p. 375, for testing parameters and interpretation of results in children

D. HIV Counseling and Testing Options

1. It is essential that the patient who is pregnant, symptomatic, or has just had a baby has a medical evaluation as soon as possible. People tested anonymously who have a positive result usually have to be retested in a confidential setting in order to document the test result, which can delay medical evaluation and treatment.
2. Confidential testing
a. The advantage of confidential counseling and testing done in the medical setting is that necessary medical care and services can be provided or arranged
b. HIV counseling and testing information, including the test result, is recorded in the patients's medical record; in most states the result is protected by law from unauthorized disclosure. Laws around HIV test results

change frequently and vary from state to state; it is essential you know the law in your state.

3. Anonymous testing
   a. Anonymous counseling and testing is usually available through state departments of health HIV counseling and testing programs and some public STD clinics
   b. No personally identifying information is asked at any time
   c. Records and blood specimens are identified by code numbers only and are reported using the same code numbers
4. If the patient requests counseling from another provider, give specific assistance and directions for locating counseling and testing programs

E. Informed Consent

1. The patient's written informed consent is a prerequisite should a patient choose to have HIV testing
   a. The patient must give voluntary consent to testing
   b. The patient must read (or have been read in their first language) and sign an informed consent before performing an HIV-related test, which indicates circumstances under which and classes of persons to whom disclosure of HIV-related information may be required, authorized, or permitted
   c. Give the patient sufficient opportunity to ask any questions
2. Capacity to consent means that a person, regardless of age, has the ability to understand and appreciate the nature and consequences of a proposed healthcare service (e.g., HIV antibody testing), and to make an informed decision concerning the HIV antibody test
   a. If there is any doubt whether the patient has the capacity to consent (due to mental incompetence, lack of understanding, altered mental status due to medication, effects of anesthesia, intoxication) or is consenting due to external pressures (involuntary), do not perform the test

   b. If you believe the patient temporarily lacks capacity to consent, defer the discussion
      (1) Document in the medical record that a test was not done at this time and the rationale
      (2) If the patient legally lacks the capacity to consent, contact the person lawfully authorized to consent to health care for the patient; provide counseling to both persons

F. Disclosure

1. Remind patient of the state law that applies
   a. Either it is mandated that HIV-positive tests be reported or it is not
   b. In a state that prohibits disclosure without consent, inform patients of appropriate fines and legal recourse
2. The patient who has signed a disclosure form under law has the right to withdraw consent at any time

G. Pretest Counseling

1. HIV counseling and testing are becoming a routine part of care in more and more healthcare settings
   a. Healthcare providers need to discuss risk behaviors as an important part of overall health assessment
   b. Healthcare providers need to advise patients that interventions early in the spectrum of HIV disease can have significant impact on the quality and length of life
2. Tell the patient that your discussion about HIV will remain confidential in the same way that all other discussions do (laws permitting)
3. Ask the patient if s/he has a previous history of HIV counseling and testing
4. Assess patient's knowledge of HIV/AIDS and provide information as needed; define HIV/AIDS as needed
   a. HIV is the virus that causes a disease called AIDS
      (1) HIV infection occurs after a person is exposed to the virus and it begins

to weaken the immune system
  (2) The body initially tries to fight the virus by creating antibodies that are found in the blood
  (3) An HIV test of blood can identify that HIV antibodies are present in the bloodstream
  b. The immune system is the part of the body that protects a person from infection; when the immune system is weakened, a body cannot fight off infections
  (1) The immune system is made up of white blood cells and antibodies whose job it is to fight infection
  (2) HIV attacks one kind of white blood cell called the CD4+ lymphocyte cell, a very important cell in the immune system
5. Explain that the most serious consequence of HIV infection is the progression to AIDS
  a. It can take ≥10 years for a person with HIV infection to develop AIDS
  b. Most people who are infected with HIV do not appear ill and may not know they have been exposed
  c. Symptoms do not generally appear until a person's immune system is already weakened
6. Provide information on HIV transmission and prevention
  a. HIV is transmitted when an uninfected person engages in risk behaviors with an infected person; the HIV virus can be transmitted as a result of
  (1) Sexual intercourse (vaginal or anal) without a condom, or incorrectly using a condom
  (2) Sharing needles, works (cotton-coke caps), cookers, spoons, and other drug-injecting paraphernalia
  (3) Oral sex (vaginal, penile) with a partner that has genital or oral lesions/sores, bleeding gums, or menstrual blood
  (4) During pregnancy, birth, or breast-feeding if the women is HIV infected
  b. The risk of HIV transmission increases when a person is exposed to multiple partners, particularly multiple HIV-infected partners
  (1) A previous history of STDs or cur-

rent diseases can increase the risk of transmission
  (2) Exposure to only one HIV-infected partner can result in HIV infection
7. Safer sex
  a. Safer sexual practices involve sexual partners keeping their blood, semen, pre-ejaculate, and vaginal secretions from entering each other's bodies
  b. Differing sexual behaviors carry different levels of risk depending on how likely they are to allow blood, semen, pre-ejaculate, and vaginal secretions to enter a partner's body
  c. Understanding levels of risk is important for making informed choices about how much risk is acceptable
  d. The most important means of reducing risk of transmission is wearing latex condoms for anal or vaginal sex
  (1) Use a water-based (e.g., K-Y jelly), not an oil-based lubricant
  (2) Never store condoms in a glove compartment or back pocket because they can dry out
  (3) When putting a condom on, leave space at the tip for semen
  (4) Remove the condom immediately after ejaculation
  (5) Using condoms with spermicide such as nonoxynol-9 may offer additional protection; nonoxynol-9 can cause irritation, so it is helpful first to try it on the wrist
  (6) Be consistent in use, proper application, and the need for the condom to remain intact (helped by using a water-based lubricant)
  e. No barrier method, including condoms, can guarantee 100% protection as product failure or incorrect use may occur
  f. Most sexual practices are considered less risky than unprotected anal or vaginal sex
  (1) All forms of oral sex, and sexual activity where there is a possibility of blood or semen entering the body through broken skin, pose some risk
  (2) Latex barriers (condoms, male and female; gloves, finger cots) further reduce this risk

g. Even if both partners are infected, they should practice safer sex to prevent reinfection

h. A mutually monogamous relationship between uninfected partners carries no risk of infection; however, monogamy is not always assured and one partner may already be infected

8. Levels of safer sex

a. Absolutely safe: Abstinence, dry kissing, masturbation, oral sex on a man with a condom, oral sex on a woman with a dental dam, rimming (oral-anal) with a dental dam, finger sex wearing latex gloves or finger cots, external water sports (urinating on someone), touching, massage, fantasy

b. Reasonably safe: Wet kissing, vaginal or anal intercourse with a condom

c. Risky: Oral sex on a man without a condom, masturbation on open/broken skin, oral sex on a woman without a barrier, rimming without a barrier

d. High risk: Vaginal or anal intercourse without a condom, oral sex with a woman while she has her period, internal water sports, fisting without gloves and lubricant

e. Harmful to your judgment: Recreational drugs, alcohol

9. Sharing needles and paraphernalia

a. Seek needle-exchange program

b. Cleaning injection equipment with disinfectants (e.g., bleach) does not guarantee inactivation of HIV

c. Disinfectants do not sterilize injection equipment, but consistent and thorough cleaning of shared injection equipment with undiluted bleach should reduce transmission of HIV; the following steps are believed to be the best procedures for disinfection with bleach

   (1) Always clean injection equipment (needles, syringes, works) immediately after use and just before reuse, even if equipment package is new

   (2) Before using bleach, wash out the needle and syringe by filling them several times with clean water (reduces the amount of blood and other debris in the syringe); take

works apart and rinse with water after bleach

   (3) Use full-strength liquid household bleach (not diluted bleach); keep it in a container that does not allow light to pass through (sunlight reduces the strength of bleach)

   (4) Completely fill the needle and syringe with bleach at least 3 times; leave the bleach in the syringe for at least 30 seconds (the longer HIV is exposed to the bleach, the more likely it will be inactivated)

d. Needles purchased on the street should never be considered clean, even if packaged

10. Other risk-reduction practices

a. Do not share razors, toothbrushes, tattoo needles, body-piercing needles, and similar implements

b. If you are HIV infected do not donate blood, organs, sperm, or other body tissues

c. Use a bleach solution to clean blood and other body fluid spills

d. Review risk of transmitting HIV in pregnancy or by breastfeeding

11. Casual contact

a. HIV cannot be spread by casual contact (e.g., shaking hands, using public rest rooms, hugging, eating or drinking from common utensils or dishes, sneezing or coughing, being in the company of an HIV-infected person)

b. HIV has been isolated from saliva, tears, and urine; however, there is no documented case of HIV transmission from any of these body fluids

c. Dry kissing (closed lips), except in the presence of open sores or lesions on the mouth, is considered safe; deep kissing (open mouth, wet) poses a risk if lesions or blood are present in the mouth

H. Posttest Counseling

1. Test result: Ensure the patient receives the test result in person

2. Review risk-reduction issues discussed during pretest counseling session; be

Table 3.1   HIV-Positive Posttest Counseling

Review the following information with HIV-positive patients in the posttest counseling session.

- Your immune system protects you from infection through white blood cells and antibodies. Keeping your immune system healthy is crucial.

- Being HIV positive is not synonymous with having AIDS.

- HIV is a virus that causes AIDS and damages the immune system and other cells in your body.

- Your test is positive for HIV antibodies. That means the virus is living in your body and you can give it to other people through blood, semen, and vaginal secretions.

- One of the cells most damaged by the AIDS virus is called the CD4+ cell. CD4+ cells play an important role in maintaining your immune system.

- HIV is a chronic, manageable disease, and there are different stages of the disease. Generally, the more damaged your immune system, the more likely you are to develop symptoms and infections. It is possible to have a very damaged immune system and yet have few or no symptoms. However, at that point you are very susceptible to infections. You need to have a medical evaluation to determine the condition of your immune system.

- When you are first infected, you may have few or no symptoms because you have little or no damage to your immune system.

- As the virus stays in the body longer, it tends to damage the immune system. This damage can lead to development of symptoms.

- Whether or not you have symptoms, you are considered infected and infectious (able to give the virus to others) for life.

- Normally, your CD4+ cells are between 600 and 1,000. As the virus damages your immune system, your CD4+ cells begin to drop. Usually people don't develop symptoms until their CD4+ cells fall below 400.

- Taking care of yourself can affect the course of your disease:
  - Good nutrition (cook meat and eggs well)
  - Stay away from people with colds and flu
  - Sleep
  - Exercise
  - Wear gloves when changing cat litter
  - Decrease stress
  - Drugs and alcohol can damage your immune system.

- Infection control
  - Don't share your toothbrush or razor—they may have blood on them.
  - It is okay to wash laundry and dishes with other people's. Use 1 part bleach to 10 parts water to clean blood spills on surfaces.
  - Inform sexual and needle-sharing partners (you can get assistance in doing this).
  - Do not donate blood, sperm, organs, or other body tissues. HIV may be transmitted in pregnancy, at birth, or through breast milk.

- Diagnostic testing: It is important to know the level of damage the virus may have done to your immune system. Until further diagnostic tests are performed, it is not possible to know how much damage, if any, the virus has done. You also should be screened for infections for which you are at risk. Your blood will be screened to assess immune system damage and the presence of other infections such as sexually transmitted diseases and TB.

- Treatment options: Based on your level of disease and your underlying health, you may be offered a variety of antiviral and prophylactic medications to prevent infections. You should also have a yearly flu vaccine and a one-time pneumococcal vaccine.

- Identifying support: Make a plan for those in your life with whom you will share this information and how you will share it. Services such a support groups, buddies, benefit application assistance, etc., are available through community based AIDS service organizations. Provide list if available.

aware that the patient's ability to absorb this information will be reduced at this time because of anxiety

3. Begin posttest counseling by providing the test result

  a. Show the patient the lab slip with the recorded test result

  b. Give the patient time to react to the test result and encourage the patient to express feelings and concerns

  c. Address the patient's immediate concerns

4. Meaning of negative test result

  a. A negative HIV test result almost always means that the patient in not infected; provide full explanation

    (1) The patient who has not engaged in risk behavior in the past 6 months is most likely not infected with HIV

      (a) S/he was not exposed to HIV

      (b) The patient was exposed to HIV but did not become infected

    (2) If the patient is a new mother and is not infected, the baby is not infected

  b. If the patient has engaged in risk behavior in the past 6 months, the patient may be infected with HIV but may not yet have produced antibodies

    (1) People usually produce antibodies within 6–12 weeks after infection

      (a) Some people take longer (≥6 months); a very small number of infected people may never produce antibodies to HIV

      (b) Discuss retesting for HIV antibody, when appropriate, based on the patient's risk history

    (2) Explain to the new mother that if she is infected but her result is negative, her baby may also be infected but not yet have HIV antibodies; if the mother is retested and the result is positive, the baby should also be tested

  c. Explain that a negative test result does not mean the person is immune to infection; exposure to HIV always presents a risk for infection

  d. Again review transmission and risk-reduction practices, including safer needle and sexual practices

5. Meaning of postive test result

  a. All people who are antibody positive (whether symptom free or ill) are considered infectious to others by various routes; antibody positivity is not synonymous with having AIDS

  b. Review the HIV-Positive Posttest Counseling information outlined in Table 3.1, on the facing page

  c. Refer to *Wellness Strategies*, p. 327.

Section 4

Clinical Manifestations and Treatment of HIV Disease in Adults

This section provides a comprehensive overview of clinical manifestations and treatments in the care of adult patients with HIV disease. It outlines the medical treatments for HIV, features immune-based therapies, and reviews opportunistic diseases, as well as organ system complications. Appendix B, *Common Medications Used in Treating the Patient With HIV/AIDS*, and Appendix C, *The FDA Drug-Approval Process*, contain additional relevant information.

Figure 4.1 Targets for Interruption

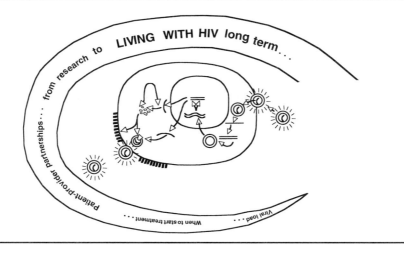

I. MANAGEMENT OF HIV INFECTION

A. Suppression of HIV Disease with Antiretrovirals

1. Targets of drug intervention that coincide with the life cycle of HIV
   a. Agents that impede binding and entry of HIV into the host CD4 cell
      (1) Low-molecular-weight sulfated polysaccharides
      (2) Antibodies to HIV or host-cell receptors: Immunoadhesions
         (a) rCD4 molecules connected to the Fc portion of an antibody (rCD4-IgG or rCD4-IgM)
         (b) Proposed mechanism of action is antibody-mediated phagocytic engulfment
         (c) Kills HIV-1 virus
         (d) Crosses placental barrier—may play a role in preventing transmission of HIV disease to the fetus
      (3) Recombinant soluble CD4 (rCD4)
         (a) Does not kill HIV virus
         (b) Inhibits binding and replication of HIV-1 in vitro by attaching to gp120 on the viral capsid
         (c) Clinical effectiveness is doubtful
      (4) CD4-conjugated exotoxins
      (5) Hypericin
         (a) Natural pigment found in the plants of genus *Hypericum*
         (b) Mechanism of action is not completely understood
         (c) Anti-HIV activity may result from the compound's ability to increase the rigidity of the retroviral capsid; this prevents the release of the reverse transcriptase, thus inhibiting infectivity
   b. Agents that inhibit reverse transcriptase
      (1) Nucleoside analogs
         (a) Result in DNA chain termination
         (b) See Table 4.1 for specific agents
      (2) Nonnucleoside reverse-transcriptase inhibitors
         (a) Majority of drugs still in clinical trials
         (b) Rapid emergence of HIV resistance precludes a role for these compounds as single agents
      (3) See Table 4.2 for specific agents
   c. Agents that inhibit transcription and translation
      (1) Ro 24-7429
         (a) Structurally related to the benzodiazepines
         (b) Evaluations conducted in asymptomatic and mildly symptomatic patients
         (c) No demonstrated antiretroviral activity
         (d) Tat protein remains a plausible target for the inhibition of HIV
      (2) GLQ223
         (a) Ribosome-inactivating protein
         (b) Derived from the root of the Chinese cucumber
         (c) Found to have activity against HIV in both T lymphocytes and macrophages in vitro
         (d) Drug remains investigational
   d. Agents that inhibit viral maturation and budding
      (1) Secondary processing of viral polyproteins after translation require modification (e.g., glycoprotein of HIV, gp120, must be trimmed of excess glucose residues for HIV to bind to the host cell)
      (2) Specific agents: Castanospermine and N-butyldeoxynojirimycin
         (a) Inhibitors of glycosylation
         (b) Block HIV infection in vitro
         (c) Clinical studies underway
   e. Protease inhibitors (e.g., saguinavir, indinavir, ritonavir)
      (1) Virus-encoded protease is responsible for cleaving precursor polypeptides
      (2) Active during late stages of HIV replication
      (3) Protease is required for the production of mature budding infectious virions; therefore protease inhibitors render the virions noninfective

Table 4.1   Nucleoside Analogs

Drug	Actions
Zidovudine (AZT) (Retrovir [Burroughs-Welcome])	• Has demonstrated survival/natural history benefit (clinical efficacy) • Initial drug of choice • Useful as monotherapy when CD4+ lymphocyte counts are ≤500/μl • Raises CD4+ lymphocyte counts and suppresses viral load • Demonstrated effect is approximately 20 months after initiation of therapy • Can also be used in combination therapy with other antiretroviral agents
Didanosine (ddl) (Videx [Bristol-Myers Squibb])	• Indicated for patients with advanced HIV infection who are intolerant of AZT therapy or who have demonstrated significant clinical or immunologic deterioration during AZT therapy • Demonstrated clinical activity rather than clinical efficacy (survival, natural history) • Transient rise in CD4+ lymphocyte counts • Suppresses HIV viral replication • Can be used as monotherapy or in combination therapy
Zalcitabine (ddC) (Jovod [Roche])	• Indicated for patients with advanced HIV infection (CD4+ lymphocyte counts ≤300/μl) who have demonstrated significant clinical or immunologic deterioration • Demonstrated clinical activity rather than clinical efficacy (survival, natural history) • Transient rise in CD4+ lymphocyte counts • Suppresses HIV viral replication • Used in combination therapy with AZT
Stavudine (d4T) (Zerix [Bristol-Myers Squibb])	• Indicated for use in adults with advanced HIV infection who are intolerant of approved therapies or who have significant clinical or immunologic deterioration • Demonstrated clinical activity rather than clinical efficacy (survival, natural history) • Transient rise in CD4+ lymphocyte counts • Suppresses HIV viral replication • Stavudine's lower affinity for thymidine kinase (an enzyme) may represent a therapeutic advantage over AZT
Azidouridine	• Less potent than AZT • No demonstrated clinical efficacy • May be ineffective in patients with AZT-resistant strains of HIV secondary to cross-resistance • May not be of any value in combination regimens secondary to its inability to prevent emergence of resistant isolates
Lamivudine (3TC)	• Clinical trials currently in process • Preclinical studies have demonstrated lamivudine to be well tolerated

Table 4.2 Nonnucleoside Reverse-Transcriptase Inhibitors

Drug	Actions
Foscarnet	• Currently indicated for use in the treatment of CMV retinitis and not approved for the treatment of HIV • Pyrophosphate analogue • Inhibits the DNA polymerase of human herpes viruses and the reverse transcriptase of HIV • Has been found to have additive effect with AZT against HIV in vivo
TIBO Compounds and Nevirapine	• Structurally related to the benzodiazepines • Potent inhibitors of HIV in vitro • No convincing evidence of clinical antiretroviral effect • Nevirapine has potent activity against HIV • Clinical trials done with Nevirapine as a single agent and in combination with AZT • Reductions in HIV antigen levels demonstrated • Nevirapine-resistant isolates of HIV develop rapidly, therefore role of this drug as a single agent is questionable.
Atevirdine and Delavirdine	• Block HIV-1 replication in vitro • Clinical trials in progress

(4) Poor oral absorption, which renders these compounds unstable
(5) Several compounds have been approved by the FDA
(6) Given in combination with other antiretroviral agents

f. Other agents: Interferon-alpha
(1) Protein produced by peripheral blood mononuclear cells with at least 15 different subtypes
(2) Each subtype protein interacts with specific cell-surface receptors
(3) Modulation of many other cellular proteins is produced; these proteins are responsible for inducing molecular changes in immune effector cells
(4) Initially used to treat KS; antiretroviral effect was recognized
(5) Is not used as single agent antiretroviral therapy because of its limited efficacy

g. Combination therapy
(1) Goals: Exploit several targets in the HIV replicative cycle, minimize toxicities, and decrease the emergence of resistance

(2) A variety of agents is used in combination
2. Future directions of antiretroviral therapy
a. This is an ever-changing, dynamic area of clinical practice; practice patterns vary widely and new agents are expected to be introduced
b. The initiation of antiretroviral therapy may occur early in the course of HIV disease because of the new understanding of viral kinetics

B. Immune System Enhancement/Restoration

1. Increased understanding of the immunopathologic aspects of HIV disease and the modest benefit currently available from antiretroviral therapies has increased the interest in immune-based therapies
2. Goals for immune-based therapies
a. Enhance immune competence
(1) Improve CD4 function and increase CD4+ lymphocyte count
(a) Inhibit apoptosis
(b) Restore glutathione levels

(2) Cellular therapies
    (a) Transplantation of stem cells
    (b) Transfusion of peripheral blood lymphocytes
    (c) Ex vivo expansion of lymphocyte subsets
(3) Replace deficient cytokines (e.g., IL-2)
(4) Enhance anti-HIV immune response (passive or active immunization)
  b. Inhibit host-derived cofactors of viral replication
  c. Inhibit host mechanism that causes complications of HIV disease
  d. Improve immunity for treatment/prevention of opportunistic complications as treatment is lifelong, cure is not achieved, and recurrences are common
    (1) Passive immunization (specific neutralizing antibodies)
    (2) Active immunization (better adjuvants to therapy)
    (3) Cytokines
    (4) Cytokine antagonists
    (5) Strategies under investigation include use of specific neutralizing monoclonal antibodies in cytomegalovirus treatment
3. Rationale for targeting host factors in pathogenesis
  a. It may be possible to interrupt the cycle in which HIV infection causes the expression of factors that stimulate viral replication
    (1) Example: Proinflammatory cytokines — possible agents under study include pentoxifylline and thalidomide, which inhibit tumor necrosis factor (TNF-2)
    (2) Factors that stimulate viral replication can result from opportunistic infections (OIs)
  b. There is a possible role for immunosuppression in some clinical situations — for example, corticosteroids are currently in use as treatment or treatment adjuvants in the following conditions
    (1) Moderate to severe *Pneumocystis carinii pneumonia* (PCP)
    (2) Immune thrombocytopenia (ITP)
    (3) Severe aphthous ulcers

    (4) Rheumatoid complications
4. Status of general approaches under development
  a. Limited success of methods aimed at exerting a primary effect on the HIV-infected individual's immune system
  b. Strategies still under study
    (1) Postinfection therapy in HIV-seropositive patients to control HIV infection
    (2) Postexposure prophylaxis to prevent HIV infection or disease
5. Ideal qualities of an immune-based therapy
  a. Stimulate long-lived HIV-neutralizing antibody
  b. Stimulate durable HIV-specific T-helper responses
6. Vaccine development
  a. Requirements of an HIV vaccine
    (1) Induce neutralizing antibody to prevent infection
    (2) Induce lymphokines (i.e., interferon) to limit the spread of infection
    (3) Induce cell-mediated immunity, especially cytotoxic T cells, to ensure recovery from infection
    (4) Induce long-term memory T and B cells, to ensure sustained protection
  b. Approaches
    (1) Attenuated live virus
    (2) Inactivated whole virus
    (3) Recombinant live virus
    (4) Native virus subunits
    (5) Recombinant virus subunits
    (6) Synthetic peptides
    (7) Anti-idiotypes
    (8) Passive immunization
  c. Obstacles to the development of an HIV vaccine
    (1) The properties of HIV as a lentivirus, which allow it to escape immune surveillance, present a major challenge in developing effective HIV vaccines
      (a) Antigenic variation: Extreme genetic variations occur in lentivirus gene sequences and thus in viral antigens, both over time in an infected person and among isolates obtained from

different people (HIV mutates at a rate ±1,000 times greater than influenza A virus)

(b) Integration of viral DNA: The immune system may not detect cells infected with a retrovirus if the infecting virus is present as viral DNA integrated into the host cell DNA but not expressed

(c) Cell-associated transmission of HIV: HIV is transmitted in HIV-infected lymphocytes and macrophages via sexual contact and exposure to infected blood; HIV vaccines must therefore protect against intracellular as well as cell-free HIV and must confer protection at genital mucosal surfaces

(d) Infection and destruction of crucial CD4 cells: A vaccine must prevent the persistent infection or depletion of CD4+ lymphocytes that perform essential roles in the host immune system; high-affinity CD4+ receptors for HIV cell binding include the CD4+ or T4 lymphocytes, monocytes, and macrophages

(e) Neurotropism of HIV: A successful vaccine must protect against HIV infection of the CNS, an immunoprivileged site relatively insulated from systemic immune defense mechanisms

(f) Antibody enhancement of infection: HIV vaccines should not induce antibodies that might exacerbate rather than limit disease following infection

(g) Failures of antibodies or cell-mediated immunity to eliminate HIV: There is no evidence that any infected person ever recovers, eliminates all latent virus, and remains immune to reinfection. Therefore, a vaccine will need to prevent infection from being established.

(2) Uncertainties about requirements necessary to establish protective immunity

(a) The nature of protective immunity in the animal lentivirus models or in HIV-infected humans is unclear

(b) Perhaps a vaccine-induced immunity extant prior to infection to induce complete protection from infection or to suppress viral replication and delay onset should infection occur

(3) Shortcomings of experimental vaccines in animal models

(a) Low efficacy and late breakthroughs

(b) Lack of reproducibility

(c) Limited strength of protection

(d) Duration of protection <1 year

(e) No proven protection against widely divergent isolates

(f) No protection shown against genital mucosal infection

(g) Lack of practicality

(h) Safety not proven

(4) Social, economic, political, moral, and legal issues

(a) Protection against multiple strains, not simply strains common in Western Europe or North America where pharmaceutical companies clearly perceive most commercial benefit

(b) Discrimination against those testing HIV positive when antibody presence may result from vaccination

(c) Altruism vs. the potential for harm to vaccine research subjects

(d) How to test for efficacy of the protective mechanism without exposure to the virus and risk of infection

(e) Access to clinical vaccine trials

(f) Maintaining public confidence

7. Gene therapy: The introduction of new genetic material into the cells of a patient, with resulting therapeutic benefit

a. Intracellular protection ("intracellular immunization") as a strategy

(1) Protein-based strategies: The gene

product is a protein
(a) Transdominant proteins
   i) Altered (mutant) viral proteins that compete with natural viral regulatory proteins
   ii) When incorporated instead are non- or dysfunctional
(b) "Suicide" genes (e.g., thymidine kinase gene with ganciclovir): Insertion of genes that under the specific influence of HIV, or when triggered by corresponding drugs, become expressed in high levels and cause toxic chemical processes within the cell, killing the cell and decreasing viral load
(c) Intracellular toxins
   i) Delivery of a toxin that is activated by the incoming virus
   ii) The toxin inhibits protein synthesis acting to destroy the infected cells and decreasing viral spread
   iii) Example: Diphtheria toxin
(d) Intracellular immunogen (single-chain antibodies): Antibodies placed directly into the cell, which bind to and inhibit processing of viral structural proteins, reducing the number of viral particles formed
(2) RNA-based strategies: The gene product is a RNA molecule
(a) Ribozymes—catalytic RNAs that cut or cleave RNA molecules through enzyme-like activity
   i) Prevent formation of genetic sequences crucial to the viral replication cycle
   ii) May work at multiple points in the HIV life cycle, theoretically wherever there is a RNA intermediate
(b) Antisense oligonucleotides—RNA sequences that bind to important RNA sites in a comple-

mentary (mirror-image) manner
   i) Prevent translation of the RNA chain by ribosomes
   ii) Elicit a response by enzymes (RNAases) that degrade the RNA.RNA duplex
(c) RNA decoys—short pieces of RNA that mimic the natural binding regions to which HIV-stimulating proteins bind
   i) Flooding the cell with decoys (fakes) causes the stimulating proteins to be misdirected away from their normal (i.e., stimulatory) targets
   ii) Examples: TAR decoys, RRE decoys (TAR is the binding site for tat; RRE is the binding site for rev; tat and rev are stimulating proteins)
(3) Immune enhancement
(a) Generation/adoptive transfer of HIV-specific cytotoxic T cells: Genetic modification of CD8+ lymphocytes with a universal receptor to target more specifically and kill HIV-infected cells, thus lowering viral burden
(b) Cytokine genes—intracellular cytokines
   i) When activated by viral antigens, could mediate direct immune responses
   ii) Potentially have fewer side effects than parenterally administered cytokines
   iii) Example: IL-2
(c) Direct DNA injection into tissue ("naked" DNA)
   i) Purified DNA constructs that can evoke cellular and humoral immune responses when injected into tissue
   ii) Preferable to live virus vaccines for HIV
   iii) Example: HIV gp120 envelope lycoprotein

b. Issues in gene therapy
  (1) Vectors
    (a) A carrier; the means by which the new genetic material, toxin, or therapeutic chemical is transported to the cell of interest
    (b) Types of vectors
      i) Viruses
        a) Target and attach naturally to certain types of cells by splicing the new genetic material to the targeting portions of these viruses
        b) The natural attachment and cell penetration abilities of the virus are used to inject the gene through the cell membrane
        c) Examples: Murine retroviruses, HSV, adenovirus, parvovirus, adeno-associated virus
      ii) Liposomes
        a) Encapsulate therapeutic genetic material, toxins, and therapeutic chemicals by a lipid membrane that can be targeted to certain cells by coupling them with specific antibodies
        b) Enter the cell and deliver the product via endocytosis (phagocytosis)
    (c) Safety
      i) Replication-competent retrovirus (RCR)
        a) Genetically altered viral vectors have the potential to eliminate reproductive capability
        b) Potential ability to recombine with other available viral genes to reestablish reproductive capabilities
        c) Potential to cause leukemias and lymphomas
      ii) Cellular mutation
        a) Incorporation of foreign genetic material into the genome of the host cell
        b) Potential to activate an oncogene or inactivate a tumor-suppressive gene, thus initiating cancerous changes
  (2) Target cells
    (a) Peripheral blood cells
      i) Genetic alterations effective only as long as the mature cell lives
      ii) Examples: CD4+ lymphocytes, CD8+ lymphocytes
    (b) Stem cells
      i) Bone marrow vs. peripheral blood
      ii) Cells replicate, making genetic alterations longer lasting
    (c) Ex vivo vs. in vivo alteration of cells
  (3) No appropriate animal models for preclinical experimentation
  (4) FDA has established guidelines regarding patient participation in more than one gene therapy trial and life-long monitoring to protect the patient and to study the long-term effect of genetic manipulation

C. The Use of Surrogate Markers to Evaluate HIV Treatment and Efficacy

1. CD4 counts are not accepted because they are not predictive of clinical response
2. Viral load measures (see Appendix D, *Selected Adult Laboratory Values*, p. 421) are becoming the preferred surrogate marker in certain areas of the country, but are not widely available
3. Clinical endpoints in HIV disease (e.g., survival, time to progression of disease)— OIs, etc.
4. Surrogate markers are also used to stage HIV infection

D. General Management of HIV Opportunistic Infections

1. General information
   a. OIs are caused by a diverse spectrum of pathogens, many ubiquitous in nature
   b. Rarely cause disease in immunocompetent individuals
   c. In many instances, the OI is the secondary reappearance or reactivation of a previously acquired pathogen
   d. Rarely curable; at best, brought under control during the initial acute episode, which may be more severe and the course of treatment more prolonged in a person with AIDS
   e. May have atypical presentation
   f. Atypical sites of infection are common
   g. Relapse after treatment and the development of resistant disease are common
2. Epidemiologic studies and clinical research
   a. Development of antibiotic therapy to prevent the two most serious OIs—PCP and infection from *Mycobacterium avium* and *M. intracellulare*
   b. Primary prophylaxis: Preventing initial illness episode
   c. Secondary prophylaxis: Long-term suppressive (maintenance) therapy after an illness episode
      (1) Often required in order to prevent an acute recurrence episode
      (2) With the continued use of antibiotics, can result in drug-resistant strains of the infecting organism; in some instances, a different antibiotic will be needed for treatment
   d. Single infections are rare
   e. Concurrent or consecutive infections with different organisms are common
   f. Most infections related to severe immunodeficiency occur with CD4+ lymphocyte counts of <200/µl
   g. In the presence of a limited immune response infecting organisms flourish, resulting in a high density of organisms in the infected tissue(s)
      (1) The initial treatment period (±14–21 days) is longer than that for an infection in an immunocompetent person
      (2) Clinicians should be aware that in any underlying immunodeficiency an impaired inflammatory response develops; an infection may be developing while the patient is afebrile (give careful attention to self-reported signs and symptoms)
3. A description of and treatment for the manifestations of the most common bacterial, fungal, viral, and parasitic infections that affect HIV/AIDS patients follow; refer to Tables 4.4 and 4.5 for prophylaxis regimens.

II. BACTERIAL INFECTIONS

A. Mycobacterium Tuberculosis

1. Specific etiologic agent and disease process
   a. Bacterial *Mycobacterium tuberculosis* (MTB) infection (asymptomatic)
      (1) A person with TB coughs a droplet nucleus carrying MTB into the air
         (a) Droplets can also be aerosolized by singing or talking
         (b) Droplets can remain airborne for up to 48 hours
      (2) The contact inhales the droplet into the respiratory system where it reaches the alveoli and infection is established
      (3) The droplet is then picked up and distributed throughout the body by macrophages and encapsulated in tubercules
      (4) During initial 2–8 weeks, cell-mediated hypersensitivity is established, resulting in a positive TB skin test (PPD, Mantoux)
   b. When immune system can no longer contain the infection the bacteria proliferate, most often in the lungs
      (1) This is the disease state of TB, in contrast to the initial infection
      (2) Can also activate in extrapulmonary sites (e.g., miliary TB, involvement of the lymphatic system, CNS, soft tissue, bone marrow, liver, other viscera)
   c. Most cases of TB in HIV-infected patients are due to the reactivation of dormant infection as a result of diminished cell-mediated immunity.
   d. TB that is resistant to at least two of the first-line pharmaceutical agents is called *multidrug-resistant TB* (MDR-TB); it has a much higher fatality rate and a shorter interval between diagnosis and death than the nonresistant form of the disease
2. Risk, transmissibility, and source of infection
   a. Characteristics of source patient
      (1) Concentration of acid-fast bacilli in sputum
      (2) Frequency and force of patient's cough
      (3) Presence of cavitation in chest x-ray
      (4) Compliance of patient with therapy
      (5) Adequacy of anti-TB therapy
   b. Environmental characteristics
      (1) Volume of air in common between source and contact
      (2) Concentration of infected droplet nuclei in that air
      (3) Duration of exposure between source and contact
      (4) Degree of air ventilation or recirculation
      (5) Presence of ultraviolet lights or air filters
   c. Characteristics of contact
      (1) Host factors (e.g., age, health status in general, immunologic status)
      (2) Physical closeness and duration of time spent with source
      (3) Prior infection with MTB
   d. Nosocomial outbreaks of TB have occurred in healthcare settings (e.g., clinics, inpatient units, substance-use treatment facilities, AIDS residential facilities) and prisons
      (1) Patients with diminished cell-mediated immunity (e.g., HIV-infected patients, diabetics) are at increased risk of manifesting TB (the disease) once they become infected
      (2) Undetected TB in patients increases the risk of TB exposure to the other patients, staff, and visitors
      (3) Nosocomial outbreaks that have involved MDR-TB have high fatality rates, with death ensuing within several months; most of the MDR-TB outbreaks have involved HIV-positive patients and staff
3. Frequency and distribution
   a. An estimated 10 million people in the U.S. are infected with MTB; 1 million U.S. people are infected with HIV; the magnitude of future problems depends on the overlap
   b. Blinded HIV seroprevalence in TB clinics
      (1) A median HIV seroprevalence of 3% (range 0%–46%)

(2) Highest incidence is in cities with a high number of AIDS cases

  c. Demographics: Greatest increases in the incidence of TB in groups with highest prevalence of AIDS
    (1) African Americans
    (2) Hispanics 25–44 years old

4. Relationship to natural history of HIV disease
  a. Incidence of TB in patients with AIDS is almost 500 times that of the general population
  b. TB can occur much earlier in the course of HIV infection
  c. May be the initial manifestation of HIV infection
  d. Risk of activation in HIV-positive person infected with TB is 8%–10% per year vs. 7%–10% per lifetime for HIV-negative person infected with TB
  e. Prevalence: Because of laws protecting the confidentiality of HIV status, information on the HIV status of people with TB in the U.S. is incomplete (missing/unknown for 67% of TB patients aged 25–44 years in 1993)
  f. The clinical presentation of TB in HIV-infected patients varies somewhat, depending on the severity of immunosuppression (Schecter, 1994)
    (1) In earlier stages of HIV (CD4+ lymphocytes >300/µl), presentation tends to resemble that in people without immunodeficiency; pulmonary disease is most common
    (2) When the patient's CD4+ lymphocyte count is <200/µl, the features of TB are often atypical, with a much greater frequency of extrapulmonary involvement and diffuse pulmonary disease without cavitation
    (3) Patients with advanced HIV disease more often have miliary TB and involvement of the lymphatic system, CNS (parenchymal, meningeal), soft tissue, bone marrow, liver, and other viscera

5. Morbidity and mortality
  a. No mortality data available specifically for TB/HIV

  b. Chemotherapy has reduced the mortality rate by 94% since 1953
  c. Fatality rates increase with age, malnutrition, underlying medical conditions like cancer or HIV, presence of MDR-TB
  d. Mortality rates are higher in African Americans than in whites

6. Early detection, prevention, prophylaxis
  a. Anyone with HIV should receive skin testing with PPD and two antigens (e.g., *Candida*, mumps, tetanus toxoid) to determine PPD status and anergy
  b. HIV patients (regardless of age) with a positive PPD or a history of positive PPD and who have not been previously treated should receive prophylactic isoniazid (INH) after chest x-ray and clinical evaluation to rule out active disease; HIV-infected patients with a PPD reaction ≥5 mm who do not have TB should receive prophylaxis with INH for 12 months
  c. HIV patients who are anergic should be considered for prophylaxis after obtaining a careful history to assess their risk for possible past exposure to TB; most patients with symptomatic HIV disease do not react to the PPD (i.e., are anergic), making diagnosis of TB difficult
  d. Early detection of disease depends on having a high degree of suspicion when a person with HIV, no matter what the demographic group, presents with symptoms of TB
  e. Healthcare facility infection control standards
    (1) Active case finding and disease surveillance
      (a) Patients scheduled to receive aerosolized pentamidine should first have a chest x-ray to rule out TB
      (b) TB control programs administered by infectious disease expert
      (c) Most healthcare workers who work with AIDS patients receive a PPD test every 6 months (per agency policy)
    (2) Use of fitted respiratory masks with small micron filtration (also called particulate respirators)

(3) Use of hepafilters, room air exchanges of 6/hour, and possibly recessed ultraviolet light sterilization

(4) Use of isolated rooms with doors closed and precaution signs posted

f. Patients with HIV disease and TB who have positive findings in sputum or bronchoscopy specimens are infectious and their contacts should be screened for TB and given prophylaxis when indicated (Schecter, 1994)

(1) HIV-positive contacts should be evaluated for anergy using at least two control antigens such as mumps and *Candida* or tetanus toxoid

(2) Clinicians should give INH to anergic contacts despite negative PPD skin responses

(3) Clinicians must rule out active TB before initiating prophylaxis

(4) HIV-positive contacts to patients with MDR-TB should receive prophylaxis with 2 drugs (e.g., pyrazinamide and ethambutol or ofloxacin, among others) to which the organism from the index patient is susceptible

g. HIV-infected people should be advised that certain activities and occupations (e.g., volunteer work; employment in healthcare facility, correctional institution, shelter) may increase the likelihood of exposure to TB

h. Because HIV-infected people are at risk for peripheral neuropathy, those receiving INH should also receive pyridoxine

7. Signs and symptoms: Vary with severity of immunosuppression

a. Pulmonary TB

(1) Productive cough or hemoptysis

(2) Fever and night sweats

(3) Weight loss

b. Extrapulmonary TB (clinical presentation depends on the site); usually includes the constitutional symptoms mentioned above

8. Diagnosis

a. Tests/procedures

(1) PPD

(2) Chest x-ray

(3) Smear and culture of sputum or any other body fluids or tissue (may be obtained by bronchoscopy or biopsy)

b. Differential diagnoses: Any other infectious pulmonary process caused by MAC, CMV, or other bacteria or viruses

9. Treatment

a. Prophylaxis: INH, for 1 year (unless known exposure to or infection with a drug-resistant strain)

b. Treatment (pulmonary and extrapulmonary)

(1) First-line drugs are INH plus pyridoxine, rifampin, pyrazinamide, ethambutol, and streptomycin

(2) After initial 2 months on 4 drugs, the regimen is adjusted according to drug sensitivities

(3) If the organism is pansensitive, the patient will continue on a combination of INH and rifampin (available in combination as Rifamate)

(4) Duration of treatment varies, depending on several factors

(5) Given the importance of adherence to a lengthy multidrug treatment period for cure (and to prevent the creation of drug-resistant strains), added treatment-related support; examples are directly observed therapy (DOT), outreach workers visiting patients, combining services (e.g., methadone treatment with TB therapy), and possibly even confining the patient to a TB-treatment facility (state laws permitting)

c. MDR-TB: Choice of drugs requires consultation with public health authorities

10. Laboratory results and other indices to monitor for side effects, adverse effects, and response to therapy

a. Pulmonary TB

(1) Monitor patients monthly for symptoms of liver problems

(2) Have liver function tests (LFTs) drawn at initiation of therapy and monthly thereafter, due to hepatotoxicity of some anti-TB drugs (e.g., INH)

(3) Rifampin can cause anemia, thrombocytopenia, or leukopenia, so CBC

should be drawn monthly
  (4) Pyrazinamide can cause hyperurice-
      mia; monitor for symptoms of gout,
      have uric acid drawn if indicated
  (5) Ethambutol can cause optic neuri-
      tis; perform a baseline eye examina-
      tion and monitor the patient closely
      for symptoms
  (6) Obtain sputum smear and culture
      monthly to monitor effectiveness of
      treatment for pulmonary TB
  b. Extrapulmonary TB: The site dictates
     the feasibility and usefulness of follow-
     up specimens
11. Importance of patient adherence to effect
    a cure and prevent the spread of TB
  a. TB is the only infection associated with
     HIV with such important implications
     for public health
  b. The responsibility of monitoring com-
     pliance rests with the local or state
     health department, which will have
     information about TB trends in a spe-
     cific area and resources for compliance
     (1) Culturally and linguistically appro-
         priate outreach workers and public
         health nurses
     (2) Availability of educational materi-
         als, incentives, and a program for
         directly observed therapy
  c. Most states have a process for dealing
     with patients who are unable or
     unwilling to take their medication
  d. In most states, the healthcare provider
     (HCP) is responsible for reporting a
     suspected case of active TB
  e. Under no circumstances should a HCP
     be managing a case of active TB unless
     s/he is working closely with the appro-
     priate health department

B. Mycobacterium Avium Complex

1. Specific etiologic agent and disease process
  a. *M. avium* complex (MAC, a term coined
     as a result of the AIDS epidemic) con-
     sists of *M. avium* and *M. intracellulare*
     and other strains that await definitive
     classification
  b. Historically these organisms have been

difficult to isolate
  c. Probably a primary acquisition rather
     than reactivation of previous infection,
     resulting most likely from underlying
     immune dysfunction/compromise
     (Havlir & Ellner, 1995)
     (1) Asymptomatic colonization of the
         respiratory or GI tract is probably an
         essential step in the disease process;
         respiratory colonization is unusual
         in patients with CD4+ lymphocyte
         count >100/µl
     (2) *M. avium*-infected macrophages can
         evade host defense by inactivation
         of normal intracellular killing mech-
         anisms; cytokines from infected
         monocytes may contribute to
         mycobacterial evasion of host
         immune system
     (3) Monocytes infected with HIV may
         enhance intracellular replication of
         M. avium
     (4) Widespread replication results first
         in intermittent bacteremia and
         metastatic seeding
2. Risk, transmissibility, and source of infection
  a. *M. avium* and *M. intracellulare* are ubiq-
     uitous saprophytes in the environment
     (1) Have been isolated from soil, nat-
         ural water, municipal water sys-
         tems, food, house dust, domestic
         and wild animals
     (2) Animals are probably not an impor-
         tant reservoir for human infection
     (3) Environmental isolates are probably
         source of most human infections;
         colonization probably results from
         inhalation or ingestion of organism
     (4) *M. avium* is probably more virulent
         than *M. intracellulare*
  b. Historically, MAC has been known as
     an uncommon cause of pneumonia,
     especially in men with chronic lung dis-
     ease; it has shown little virulence in the
     normal host
3. Frequency and distribution
  a. Distribution of MAC isolate serologic
     types differs in the environment, AIDS
     patients, and non-AIDS patients
     (1) 90% of MAC isolates from AIDS

patients are serogroups 1, 4 or 8, which indicate *M. avium*

(2) *M. avium* isolates from AIDS patients have been shown to be more virulent compared to in vitro and animal model isolates

(3) Current studies are underway to establish the relationship between environmental and clinical isolates; serogroups 4 and 7 frequently recovered from fresh and heated water supplies

b. MAC organisms are the most common cause of nontuberculous mycobacterial disease

c. Incidence in AIDS patients is underreported and probably occurs in 15%–24% of this population

4. Relationship to natural history of HIV disease

a. MAC prevalence has increased dramatically as a direct result of the AIDS epidemic; before AIDS epidemic, *M. avium* and *M. intracellulare* infection was uncommon

b. Disseminated MAC (DMAC) infection is a common bacterial complication of AIDS

c. DMAC disease tends to occur in late-stage HIV infection and is not a common AIDS-defining diagnosis; median CD4+ lymphocyte count at time of diagnosis is <60/μl

d. Reported MAC infection in AIDS patients is increasing — probably reflects better and more widespread availability of diagnostic procedures, along with better characterization of natural history and increasing long-term survival of AIDS patients

5. Morbidity and mortality

a. Several large retrospective studies strongly suggest that DMAC negatively impacts morbidity and mortality in AIDS patients

b. Because DMAC infection is generally concomitant with other infections or neoplasms, it is difficult to ascribe constitutional symptoms and organ dysfunction to any single entity in HIV-infected patients; *M. avium* infection is

rarely considered a direct cause of death

c. Profound anemia may be a negative prognosticator

d. Untreated disease is progressive; median survival ranges from 2–7 months from diagnosis

6. Early detection, prevention, prophylaxis

a. Lifelong prophylaxis with rifabutin is recommended for consideration for AIDS patients with a CD4+ lymphocyte count <75/μl (Kaplan et al., 1995)

(1) Clarithromycin or azithromycin is recommended for patients intolerant of rifabutin

(2) There is substantial clinical uncertainty regarding the ultimate role of MAC prophylaxis for patients with advanced HIV infection

(3) DMAC and active TB should be ruled out before prophylaxis is initiated

b. AIDS patients with CD4+ lymphocyte counts <50/μl should have routine screening blood cultures drawn; current data do not support routine screening of respiratory secretions or stool

7. Signs and symptoms

a. DMAC infection is association with both GI and systemic symptoms

(1) Highly unusual in non-HIV-infected patients or HIV-infected patients with CD4+ lymphocytes >100/μl

(2) GI manifestations

(a) Chronic diarrhea and abdominal pain

(b) Chronic malabsorption

(c) Extrabiliary obstructive disease that can result in jaundice secondary to periportal lymphadenopathy

(3) Systemic manifestations

(a) Fever (with or without night sweats), malaise, and weight loss often associated with anemia and neutropenia

(b) Unexplained skin lesions may reflect systemic infection in immunosuppressed host

(4) Splenohepatomegaly and lymphadenopathy are common

(5) Alkaline phosphatase level may be

elevated and transfusion-dependent anemia may be present

b. Pulmonary manifestation as pneumonia is rare for diagnosis of pneumonia; see *Pulmonary Complications*, p. 151

8. Diagnosis
   a. DMAC disease
      (1) Most commonly affected organs are blood, bone marrow, liver, spleen, lymph nodes, but MAC has been recovered from a wide variety of other organs; reflects disseminated hematogenous spread
      (2) Isolation from blood is the most reliable and common method for diagnosis
          (a) Nearly all AIDS patients with invasive MAC infection have positive mycobacterial blood cultures
          (b) Blood cultures may be intermittently positive in early infection, and several sets may be necessary to establish diagnosis
      (3) Bone marrow/tissue biopsies offer advantage over blood cultures for showing acid-fast bacillus (AFB) presence or granuloma weeks before blood cultures turn positive; histopathologic studies of involved organs generally show absent or poorly formed granulomas and chronic inflammation with AFB within macrophages
      (4) Radiographic imaging studies or endoscopic procedures may assist in diagnosis; GI tract appears to be more common entry portal compared to pulmonary tract
          (a) Lesions most commonly found in duodenum
          (b) Biliary obstruction, abdominal lymphadenophy commonly found
   b. For pulmonary disease, recovery of MAC from an isolated sputum or bronchial washing alone is not sufficient for diagnosis; MAC can colonize healthy individuals and is common in patients with underlying chronic pulmonary disease
          (1) Two or more positive sputum or bronchial cultures and the presence of pulmonary cavitation not attributable to any other disease process is considered sufficient for diagnosis if the patient has pulmonary symptoms
          (2) In HIV-infected patients producing sputum, AFB-positive smears may represent infection or coinfection with *M. tuberculosis*; therapy should be directed at *M. tuberculosis* until definitive diagnosis is made
   c. Differential diagnosis: Evaluate patients in whom *M. avium* and *M. intracellulare* cannot be isolated for other causes such as nonbacilliformic *Bartonella*, lymphoma, TB, fungal disease, CMV, enteric bacteremias, and AIDS-wasting syndrome

9. Treatment: Standard TB drugs are unable to inhibit MAC activity completely at achievable plasma concentrations
   a. Optimal therapy is probably a combination of a macrolide (e.g., clarithromycin) and other antimycobacterial agents; current recommended combination therapy is either clarithromycin or azithromycin with one or more of the following agents
      (1) Ethambutol
      (2) Rifabutin
      (3) Ciprofloxacin
      (4) Clofazimine
   b. Therapy is bacteriostatic and therefore lifelong; combination therapy is important to prevent/delay emergence of resistance associated with clinical deterioration

10. Laboratory results and other indices to monitor for side effects, adverse effects, and response to therapy
    a. Symptoms of fever, night sweats, malaise frequently respond to therapy within 2–8 weeks of initiating therapy
       (1) Weight loss, diarrhea, and elevated alkaline phosphatase levels respond less frequently to therapy
       (2) Anemia seldom responds to therapy and patients may be given erythropoietin, if indicated

(3) Patients may not tolerate therapy because of rash, GI symptoms, neutropenia, and other side effects

(4) Repeat blood culture after 4–8 weeks of therapy may be useful for ascertaining microbiologic response

b. Multiple complex drug interactions may occur

(1) Rifabutin and rifampin use can result in altered metabolism of oral contraceptives, warfarin, phenytoin, methadone, AZT; patients receiving methadone therapy should be closely observed for symptoms of withdrawal and will need a methadone dosage increase

(2) Blood counts of patients with DMAC infection on potential myelosuppressive agents (e.g., ganciclovir, trimethoprim + sulfamethoxazole [TMP-SMX]) should be closely monitored

(3) Give careful consideration to potential toxicity, drug interactions, and the effect of adding another drug to patients with advanced HIV infection

11. Patient education: Discuss risks and benefits of prophylactic therapy

C. Salmonella

1. Specific etiologic agent and disease process
   a. Non-spore-forming and motile gram-negative rods that grow under aerobic or anaerobic conditions; divided into 7 serotypic subgroups; subgroup 1 contains most of the serotypes pathogenic for humans
   b. Infection is associated with enterocolitis, enteric fever, or bacteremia
   (1) Ingested organisms must pass from the mouth to stomach and small intestine to cause infection
      (a) Acid barrier is first line of defense against enteric infection; a lack of or decrease in stomach acidity may lower the inoculum necessary for infection
      (b) Secretory products of the intestines, pancreas, and gall

bladder are probably an important second line of defense against infection
      (c) Microfold or M cells overlying the Peyer's patches are the probable initial target
      (d) Can also induce normally non-phagocytic cells to internalize organism
   (2) Mucosal invasion of small bowel and enterotoxin elaboration probably result in diarrhea
   (3) Survival within macrophages allows for disseminated spread via the blood stream
   (4) Enteric fever probably results from endotoxin enhancement of local inflammatory responses at tissue infection sites
   c. Although rare, can occur as meningitis
   d. A small percentage of infected patients may develop a chronic carrier state (persistence of *Salmonella* in stool or urine)
2. Risk, transmissibility, and source of infection
   a. *S. typhi* and *S. paratyphi* colonize only humans; transmitted through proximity with infected individuals
   (1) Children <1 year lack acquired immunity and are at highest risk of infection
   (2) Immunocompromised hosts are at increased risk for infection and for invasive disease
   b. Nontyphoidal *Salmonella* is widely disseminated in the environment and is intimately associated with animals
   (1) Poultry and poultry products, primarily eggs, constitute principle reservoir; approximately half of U.S. chickens are culture positive
   (2) Neonates and infants are at high risk for infection from recently or chronically infected mothers, family members, or other infants
   c. In most cases, humans acquire *Salmonella* by ingesting contaminated food or water; direct fecal-oral route is rare, but possible
   d. Patients with certain types of GI alterations are at increased risk for salmonellosis

(1) Achlorhydria or antacid abuse
(2) Alterations in endogenous intestinal flora for unknown reasons, antibiotic use, or recent intestinal surgery
(3) Chronic GI disease (e.g., inflammatory bowel disease, malignancies)
3. Frequency and distribution
   a. Typhoidal *Salmonella* infection remains a global health problem
      (1) Higher incidences reported in countries with rapid population growth, increased urbanization, inadequate water supplies/sanitation/healthcare systems, overcrowding
      (2) Not endemic in the U.S.
         (a) Most reported cases related to foreign travel
         (b) Most domestically acquired cases traceable to a chronic carrier
   b. Incidence of reported nontyphoidal *Salmonella* cases on the rise in the U.S.
      (1) Most reported outbreaks occur in the home
      (2) Second most common location of reported outbreaks is in institutions (cross-infection especially common in medical institutions)
   c. Seasonal variation reported worldwide; peak incidences correspond to warm weather
4. Relationship to natural history of HIV disease
   a. Salmonellosis in HIV-infected patients is generally nontyphoidal; recurrent bacteremia, with or without clinical enteritis, has a higher incidence in AIDS patients
   b. *Salmonella* bacteremia was a commonly reported AIDS-defining OI in the 1980s
      (1) Often associated with clinical signs and symptoms of gastroenteritis
      (2) Relapses were common, sometimes even with appropriate antibiotic suppressive therapy
   c. *Salmonella* is now less common and relapses are unusual; decreased incidence has been attributed to the antibacterial activity of AZT and TMP-SMX
   d. Typhoid fever mortality rate may

increase from the AIDS epidemic
5. Morbidity and mortality
   a. Outbreaks of typhoid fever in developing countries associated with high morbidity and mortality, especially infection from antibiotic-resistant organisms
   b. Although *Salmonella* gastroenteritis is associated with substantial morbidity in AIDS patients, directly associated fatality is uncommon
6. Early detection, prevention, prophylaxis
   a. Most caregivers recommend that HIV-infected patients avoid obvious sources of salmonellosis (see *Infection Control*, p. 363)
      (1) Avoid undercooked or raw poultry products, unpasteurized dairy products
      (2) Wear gloves while cleaning animal cages and disposing of feces
      (3) Discourage reptiles as pets
      (4) Travelers to endemic countries should consider typhoid vaccination, although it is generally not recommended
   b. Caregivers should employ good hand-washing technique
   c. Household contacts of HIV-infected people with salmonellosis should be evaluated for asymptomatic carriage of *Salmonella*
7. Signs and symptoms
   a. Classically, salmonellosis is divided into discrete syndromes of enterocolitis, enteric fever, and bacteremia; however, clinically these syndromes often overlap
   b. Enterocolitis is indistinguishable from manifestations of other GI pathogens (see *GI System Complications*, p. 169)
      (1) HIV-infected patients generally present with fever, chills, and non-bloody/nonmucoid diarrhea
      (2) Onset is usually within 48 hours after ingesting contaminant
      (3) Diarrhea may vary from mild to fulminant
      (4) Abdominal cramping, nausea, headache, myalgias may or may not be present
   c. Enteric fever is a severe systemic illness characterized by abdominal symptoms

followed by fever

   (1) Diarrhea with vague constitutional symptoms without fever may be initial present complaint

   (2) Abdominal symptoms usually resolve before onset of fever

   (3) Symptoms are generally insidious; may be present for weeks

   (4) Neuropsychiatric manifestations (typhoid state) may be present (delirium and muscle twitching; coma and lethargy)

  d. Salmonellosis may present as a debilitating, febrile illness without GI referable symptoms

   (1) Diarrhea has been absent in about half the reported cases (Miller, Hohmann, & Pegues, 1995); stool cultures may be negative

   (2) *Salmonella* appears to have a propensity for infecting endothelial sites (e.g., aorta, myocardial tissue)

8. Diagnosis

  a. Send stool specimens for C&S, examination for ova and parasites (primarily *Cryptosporidium, Isospora belli*, amoebas)

   (1) If stool cultures are negative or patient has bloody diarrhea, anoscopic or sigmoid exam for direct lesion culture may be indicated; biopsy may or may not be performed

   (2) Stained fecal smear may be indicated (PMN leukocytes usually present)

   (3) <5% of immunocompetent patients with GI symptoms have positive blood cultures, although blood cultures may be indicated in at-risk populations; neonates can develop bacteremia and AIDS patients develop recurrent bacteremia

  b. Enteric fever generally results from *S. typhi* (typhoid fever); a milder form may result from *S. paratyphi* A, B, or C (paratyphoid fever)

   (1) Differential diagnosis: Malaria, amoebic liver abscess, visceral leishmaniasis, viral syndromes

     (a) Recent history of travel to tropical areas

     (b) Incubation period 5–21 days after ingestion of organism

   (2) Fever pattern is nondiagnostic

   (3) Patients may present with faint, salmon-colored maculopapular rash on trunk (organisms may be cultured from punch biopsy of lesions)

   (4) Abdominal pain with deep palpation and hepatosplenomegaly

   (5) Definitive diagnosis requires isolation of *S. typhi, S. paratyphi* from patient

     (a) Blood cultures about 50%–70% sensitive

     (b) Bone marrow cultures about 90% sensitive

     (c) Stool string cultures have much lower sensitivity

  c. Perform tests/procedures for patients with suspected recurrent bacteremia

   (1) CBC with differential and platelets, PT-PTT, blood chemistry

   (2) Draw blood cultures from two separate sites, including a central line if present, before starting antibiotics

   (3) Culture suspected infection sites (if any) before starting antibiotics

   (4) Start IV fluid using large-bore catheter

9. Treatment

  a. Ciprofloxacin is considered the optimal therapy for HIV-related *Salmonella* infections; patients with GI symptoms may require IV fluid and electrolyte repletion

  b. Chloramphenicol or quinolone antibiotics are treatment of choice for enteric fever

   (1) TMP-SMX and ampicillin can be used as alternative therapy

   (2) Neuropsychiatric manifestations of typhoid fever may be treated with high-dose glucocorticoids

  c. Treat patients with suspected bacteremia with an IV antipseudomonal beta-lactam (e.g., imipenem) combined with an aminoglycoside (e.g., tobramycin) until sensitivities are known

10. Laboratory results and other indices to monitor for side effects, adverse effects, and response to therapy

  a. Monitor patients with *Salmonella*

infection closely for dehydration and electrolyte imbalance from diarrhea and vomiting
  (1) Fluid balance
  (2) May require IV repletion
  b. Monitor HIV-infected patients for recurrent or persistent disease
11. Patient education: See *Infection Control*, p. 363

D. Staphylococcus Aureus

1. Specific etiologic agent and disease process
  a. Gram-positive bacterium characterized by individual cocci occurring singly, in pairs, or in short chains
  b. Basic anatomic lesion induced is a pyogenic exudate or abscess that occasionally becomes the seeding point of bacteremia and sepsis
2. Risk, transmissibility, and source of infection
  a. Nasal carriage is the most common reservoir, occurring in 20%–40% of adults
    (1) Healthcare providers (HCPs), insulin-dependent diabetics, patients on chronic hemodialysis, and IDUs may have higher carriage rates than the general population
    (2) Transmission to compromised patients probably via HCPs
  b. Carriers transfer organism from nasal passages to skin
  c. Trauma provides portal of entry for subsequent local and possible systemic infection
3. Frequency and distribution: Clustering of cases of methicillin-resistant *S. aureus* have been described with increasing frequency in the U.S. (most incidence reported in large tertiary care hospitals)
4. Relationship to natural history of HIV disease
  a. In HIV-infected patients, *S. aureus* results more frequently in soft-tissue infection, bacteremia, and sepsis than in the general population
  b. Secondary site infections occur more frequently than in non-HIV-infected historical controls

  c. Possible increased carriage rates in HIV-infected patients may play an important factor in the pathogenesis of serious bacterial infection
  d. Increased incidence of bacteremia/sepsis is associated with the use of central venous access devices (CVADs)
5. Morbidity and mortality
  a. Untreated bacteremia in neutropenic patients is fatal
  b. Septic shock is associated with a 50%–70% mortality rate
6. Early detection, prevention, prophylaxis
  a. Patients at high risk for infection should observe good skin care
  b. Inspect CVAD sites frequently for signs and symptoms of infection (see Appendix E, *CVADs*, p. 424)
7. Signs and symptoms
  a. Skin/soft-tissue infections
    (1) Can present as exfoliative disorder (Ritter's disease/staphylococcal scalded skin syndrome)
      (a) Fever, irritability, skin tenderness, and eruptions in skin folds, perianal, and oral areas seen initially
      (b) Development of flaccid blisters/skin erosion within 24–48 hours of onset
    (2) Can present as toxic shock syndrome (TSS)
      (a) High fever and profound/refractory hypotension
      (b) Erythroderma followed by desquamation, especially on palms and feet
      (c) Profuse diarrhea, mental confusion, renal failure
  b. Complaints of fever with chills/rigors
    (1) Obtunded, may complain of joint pain
    (2) Presence of obvious source of localized infection (e.g., wound infection, cellulitis, CVAD/peripheral IV site)
    (3) Fever/chills and signs of localized infection may be diminished or absent in profoundly neutropenic patients
    (4) Presence of petechiae on digits and extremities, subconjunctival hemorrhages

c. Patient may present with endocarditis (see *Cardiac Complications*, p. 49)
   (1) Tachycardia with or without gallop/murmurs
   (2) Pericardial friction rub occasionally heard
d. Patient may present with osteomyelitis (intense pain in a metaphyseal area with normal overlying skin)

8. Diagnosis
   a. *S. aureus* is a common cause of skin and soft-tissue infection; TSS occurs primarily in young women, but can present in men and children
      (1) Abrupt onset of symptoms during menses with vaginal hyperemia/discharge
      (2) Abrupt onset of symptoms following an invasive procedure without signs of infection at wound site
   b. Bacteremia/sepsis most often associated with IV catheter/drug use
      (1) HIV-infected patients with bacteremia or sepsis may present with or without fever or neutropenia
      (2) All acutely ill patients should receive fever workup
   c. Perform tests/procedures for patients with suspected bacteremia and invasive disease
      (1) CBC with differential and platelets, PT-PTT, blood chemistry
      (2) Draw blood cultures from two separate sites, including a central line if present, before starting antibiotics
      (3) Culture suspected infection sites (if any) before starting antibiotics
      (4) Start IV fluid using large-bore catheter
   d. *S. aureus* is most common cause of bacterial endocarditis
      (1) Diagnosis made by positive blood cultures in absence of primary extracardiac sites of infection
      (2) ECG and other cardiac studies for presence of valvular vegetation are indicated
   e. Differential diagnosis: If *S. aureus* is not recovered from appropriate cultures, disease may be from *Haemophilus influenzae, Streptococcus pneumoniae, K.*

pneumonia, P. aeruginosa, or a noninfectious etiology

9. Treatment: Treat patients with suspected bacteremia with an IV antipseudomonal beta-lactam (e.g., imipenem) combined with an aminoglycoside (e.g., tobramycin) until sensitivities are known; monitor closely febrile, neutropenic, or seriously ill patients for signs of sepsis and shock

10. Patient education
    a. Teach at-risk patients signs and symptoms of infection
    b. Ensure proper care of CVADs
    c. Emphasize hand washing
    d. Maintain skin integrity

E. Streptococcus Pneumoniae

1. Specific etiologic agent and disease process
   a. *S. pneumoniae* (previously designated *Diplococcus pneumoniae*)
   b. Bacterial adherence to pharyngeal cells and subsequent colonization is essential step of disease production
      (1) Can invade eustachian tubes, sinuses, bronchi if normal mechanisms of rapid clearance are impaired
      (2) Invasion can result in pneumonia, sinusitis, meningitis, otitis media (primarily in children) of abrupt onset, profound toxicity, fulminant course
   c. Results in disease from capacity to replicate in host tissues and generate intense inflammatory response
      (1) Resistant to phagocytosis in immunologically naive or impaired hosts
      (2) Can destroy or inhibit function of phagocytic cells
      (3) Activates complement, resulting in intense inflammatory response
      (4) Produces few toxins; does not commonly result in bacteremia/sepsis

2. Risk, transmissibility, and source of infection: Pneumococci are common inhabitants of the human upper respiratory tract and can be isolated in 5%–70% of the normal adult population
   a. Rate of asymptomatic carriage varies with age, environment, and presence of

upper respiratory infection (URI)
b. Vector is extensive, close person-to-person contact via droplets; higher incidence associated with crowded living conditions (e.g., homeless shelters, daycare centers)
3. Frequency and distribution
   a. Pneumococcal pneumonia is the most common community-acquired pneumonia in the general population (Musher, 1995)
      (1) More common in men then woman
      (2) Incidence 3–4 times higher in people >40 years old
      (3) Commonly associated with influenza virus
      (4) IDU associated with a higher incidence
   b. Incidence of infection is seasonal, probably reflects periods of increased time spent indoors
      (1) Increased infection associated with months children are in school
      (2) Decreased infection during months when average temperature remains above 80°F
4. Relationship to natural history of HIV disease: Population-based studies suggest pneumococcal pneumonia and bacteremia respectively occur 10–100 times more frequently in patients with HIV disease than in age-matched populations (Musher, 1995)
   a. *S. pneumoniae* common early in the course of HIV; probably related to humoral immune deficiency
      (1) Antibody function may be deficient early on in HIV disease
      (2) Complement function appears altered early on in HIV disease, resulting in decreased clearance of opsonized *S. pneumoniae*
   b. AIDS patients with significant CD4+ lymphocyte depletion appear to have higher incidences of complications (e.g., bacteremia, empyema) and mortality rates than non-HIV-infected populations
   c. Smoking/IDU patients, especially with low CD4+ lymphocyte counts, are at increased risk for infection

   d. Recurrent disease occurs more commonly among HIV-infected patients than in controls with invasive pneumococcal disease
5. Morbidity and mortality
   a. 5% fatality rate from pneumococcal pneumonia in general population: bacteremia develops in about 20%–25% of cases
   b. 20% fatality rate in bacteremic pneumococcal pneumonia; higher risk associated with additional extrapulmonary site of infection
      (1) Fatality rate approximately 60% with coexistence of CNS infection
      (2) Mortality among the HIV infected is probably similar to non-HIV-infected populations
6. Early detection, prevention, prophylaxis
   a. Immunization generally recommended with 23-valent pneumococcal polysaccharide vaccine
      (1) No data currently available on actual use; several vaccine failures have been reported (Musher, 1995)
      (2) Current studies examining preventive approaches using newer vaccines and prophylactic antibiotics
   b. PCP prophylaxis with TMP-SMX may decrease risk of infection
   c. Patients at risk should avoid crowds or those possibly infected
7. Signs and symptoms
   a. Presentation of pneumonia in HIV-infected populations is similar to general population (see *Pulmonary Complications*, p. 151); complaints of fever, productive cough, chills, dyspnea, pleuritic chest pain
      (1) Acute onset of generally <1 week
      (2) Hypoxia/hypocarbia reflect disease severity and underlying lung disease
   b. Sinus presentation: See *Sinusitis*, p. 156
8. Diagnosis
   a. Most HIV-infected adults with pneumococcal bacteremia present with pneumonia (see *Pulmonary Complications*, p. 151); most common source of bacteremia in HIV-infected adults

b. *S. pneumoniae* may also present as sinusitis and rarely as meningitis, pericarditis, endocarditis, brain abscess, and mediastinitis

c. Perform tests/procedures for patients with suspected bacteremia
   (1) CBC with differential and platelets, PT-PTT, blood chemistry
   (2) Draw blood cultures from two separate sites, including a central line if present, before starting antibiotics
   (3) Culture suspected infection sites (if any) before starting antibiotics
   (4) Start IV fluid using large-bore catheter

d. Differential diagnosis: If *S. pneumoniae* is not recovered from appropriate cultures, disease may be from *H. influenzae*, *Pseudomonas aeruginosa*, *Klebsiella pneumoniae*, *S. aureus*, or a noninfectious etiology

9. Treatment
   a. Penicillin G remains antimicrobial agent of choice
   b. Treat patients with suspected bacteremia with an IV antipseudomonal beta-lactam (e.g., imipenem) combined with an aminoglycoside (e.g., tobramycin) until sensitivities are known; monitor febrile, neutropenic, or seriously ill patients closely for signs of sepsis/shock
   c. Patients with sinusitis may require decongestants and antihistamines with antimicrobial agents; surgical drainage may be required in refractory cases

10. Laboratory results and other indices to monitor for side effects, adverse effects, and response to therapy
    a. Patients with persistent fever and tachycardia failing to respond to therapy or worsening after initially responding may have coexisting OI
    b. Reports of the increase in drug-resistant *S. pneumoniae* raise concerns about excessive and inappropriate antibiotic use and emphasize the importance of antimicrobial-sensitivity testing of all invasive pneumococcal isolates

11. Patient education: Discuss increased probability of pneumococcal pneumonia with newly diagnosed HIV-infected patients
    a. Instruct about signs and symptoms

b. Advise to avoid crowds or close contact with infected individuals during seasonal outbreaks
c. Discuss pros and cons of pneumococcal vaccination

F. Syphilis

1. Specific etiologic agent and disease process
   a. Spirochete, *Treponema pallidum*, causes a chronic systemic infection
   b. Can infect any organ, including the CNS, eyes
   c. Immune response involves humoral and cellular immunity
   d. Extreme variability in clinical presentations
   e. Usually 3-week incubation
   f. Sexually transmitted from infectious lesions
      (1) Chancre: Primary syphilis
         (a) Usually painless
         (b) May be painful in anorectal area
      (2) Mucous patch: Oral, genital
      (3) Condyloma lata: Secondary syphilis groups of flat-topped papules often found in the moist orogenital areas
   g. Other routes
      (1) In blood from infected persons
      (2) Via the placenta from mother to fetus (congenital syphilis)
   h. Dissemination via lymphatic system to regional lymph nodes, then via bloodstream
   i. Abnormalities in CSF in 15%–40% with primary and secondary syphilis

2. Risk, transmissibility, and source of infection: Approximately 30%–50% of early syphilis contacts become infected

3. Frequency and distribution: Highest incidence of syphilis in U.S. in 40 years in 1990 — 18 cases per 100,000; coincides with increasing HIV infection

4. Relationship to natural history of HIV disease
   a. May have false-negative syphilis treponemal serologic test
   b. May have false-negative or delayed positive nontreponemal serologic test
   c. Natural history of syphilis possibly altered in HIV infection

(1) Increased frequency of early neurosyphilis with HIV, especially with conventional doses of penicillin

(2) Slower resolving cutaneous lesions

   d. Assessing effectiveness of treatment may be problematic using serologic testing

   e. Increased time for serologic tests to return to normal after treatment

5. Morbidity and mortality

   a. Fulminant neurosyphilis may cause death

   b. Untreated syphilis

     (1) 25% will experience one or more relapses during the first year

     (2) 50% of patients show CSF abnormalities during the secondary stage

6. Early detection, prevention, prophylaxis

   a. History

     (1) Exposure, high-risk activities

     (2) Previous infection

     (3) Uncertain treatment

   b. Physical examination: Evidence of primary or secondary infection; yearly screening

   c. Prevention

     (1) Identify and treat contacts

     (2) Identify, screen, and counsel those at risk (all pregnant women)

     (3) Promote use of barrier methods for sexual contacts

     (4) Use latex gloves and other precautions when performing clinical exams

     (5) Use appropriate and adequate antimicrobial treatment

   d. Prophylaxis: Not applicable

7. Signs and symptoms

   a. Primary syphilis (early or infectious stage)

     (1) Painless ulcer 2–6 weeks after exposure (on genitalia, perianal area, rectum, pharynx, tongue, lip, or elsewhere)

     (2) Frequently nontender enlargement of regional lymph nodes

     (3) The same as in non-HIV infected

     (4) No constitutional symptoms

     (5) If untreated, lasts 3–6 weeks

   b. Secondary syphilis (early or infectious)

     (1) Occurs 1–5 months after exposure

     (2) Represents disseminated disease

     (3) Generalized maculopapular skin rash, 75%–100%; typically nonpruritic

     (4) Constitutional symptoms, 60%–90%

     (5) Generalized adenopathy, 50%–85%

     (6) Mucous membrane lesions, 5%–30%

     (7) Condylomata lata, 5%–25%

     (8) Alopecia, 5%–20%

     (9) CNS involvement

     (10) Focal complaints associated with hepatitis, osteitis, arthritis, or iritis

     (11) Early latent (infection duration <1 year): 90% of relapses occur within the first year

     (12) Late latent (infection duration ≥1 year): Usually accompanied by a rising titer in quantitative serologic tests

   c. Tertiary syphilis

     (1) Progressive inflammatory disease

     (2) Cutaneous lesions: Multiple nodular, ulcerative, or solitary "gummas"

     (3) Cardiovascular signs and symptoms

     (4) Neurosyphilis

     (5) Develops 5–50 years after onset of infection

8. Diagnosis

   a. Goals

     (1) Identify and treat infected patients

     (2) Establish stage of disease

     (3) Identify and treat contacts

   b. Darkfield microscopic examination of fresh exudate for spirochetes

     (1) Requires special equipment

     (2) Fluid expressed from lesion contains *T. pallidum* by immunofluorescence or darkfield microscopy in >70% of chancres

   c. Nontreponemal serologic tests

     (1) Provide indirect, imprecise, and presumptive method of diagnosis

     (2) Serologic test often positive 1–2 weeks after noting primary lesion

     (3) Measure antibodies; nonspecific

     (4) Easy, rapid, inexpensive

     (5) Used primarily for screening

     (6) Valuable to monitor response to therapy

(7) Rapid plasma reagin (RPR)
(8) Venereal Disease Research Lab (VDRL)
    (a) Positive 4–6 weeks after infection
    (b) May be low or negative in late disease
d. Treponemal antibody tests
  (1) Increased sensitivity; useful to identify false-positive nontreponemal tests
  (2) Fluorescent treponemal antibody absorption (FTA-ABS): Most sensitive
  (3) *T. pallidum* hemagglutination assay (TPHA)
e. Biopsy of skin lesions for primary and secondary cases
f. CSF evaluation: Routinely evaluate in all HIV-infected patients with any form of syphilis
9. Treatment
  a. HIV may alter response to treatment
  b. Requires maximal doses of appropriate antibiotics
  c. Primary and secondary syphilis (without clinical evidence of neurosyphilis)
    (1) Benzathine penicillin G once
    (2) Doxycycline for 14 days for penicillin-allergic patients; confirm allergy and consider desensitization
  d. Latent syphilis (with normal CSF evaluation)
    (1) Benzathine
    (2) Penicillin G weekly for 3 successive weeks
  e. Neurosyphilis
    (1) Aqueous crystalline penicillin G for 14 days, *or*
    (2) Aqueous procaine penicillin G daily for 14 days, *plus* probenecid for 14 days, *plus* benzathine penicillin G after the above regimen
  f. Caution patients regarding Jarisch-Herxheimer reaction prior to treatment (inflammatory reaction sometimes induced by treatment)
  g. Treatment alternatives: The efficacy of regimens with amoxicillin, tetracyclines, and cephalosporins is unknown
10. Laboratory results and other indices to monitor for side effects, adverse effects, and response to therapy
  a. Serologic titers
    (1) Nontreponemal titers should fall fourfold by 4 months in primary and secondary syphilis, by 6 months in early latent syphilis
    (2) Repeat testing at 3- to 6-month intervals after treatment until results are normal
    (3) Persistent elevated nontreponemal titers despite treatment or fourfold increase
      (a) Rule out reinfection
      (b) Repeat treatment
    (4) Immune dysfunction may cause titers to inappropriately fall, especially in late HIV
    (5) In high titer disease, RPR may always remain positive
  b. Cerebrospinal fluid testing
    (1) Usually returns toward or to normal in 1–3 months
    (2) Monitor q3–6mos after treatment until results are normal; low titer may persist
11. Patient education
  a. Stress importance of medication compliance
  b. Counsel regarding safer sexual practices
  c. Encourage patients to report signs and symptoms (e.g., headache, rash, genital lesions) to HCP immediately

G. Campylobacter

1. Specific etiologic agent and disease process
  a. Motile, non-spore-forming, comma-shaped, gram-negative rods: Slower then usual growth of enteric flora under microaerobic conditions
    (1) Stool specimens usually identifiable on plating media within 24–48 hours, but atypical specimen may take up to 96 hours
    (2) Blood cultures may take up to 2 weeks
  b. Small intestine infected initially, spreading to jejunum, ileum, and colon, occasionally resulting in bacteremia and sepsis

(1) Clinical enteric manifestations of all *Campylobacter* are essentially the same; *C. jejuni* is considered prototypical for enteric infection
(2) The most important factors involved in disease development appear to be the amount of organism reaching small intestine and host immunity to specific organism ingested
(3) Acid barrier is first line of defense against enteric infection; a lack of or decrease in stomach acidity is associated with lowering the required infectious dosage
(4) Mucosal invasion of small bowel and enterotoxin elaboration probably results in diarrhea
c. Can occasionally result in bacteremia and sepsis
(1) Contains, produces, and secretes toxins implicated as pathogenic factors resulting in sepsis and shock
(2) *C. fetus* is more common cause of bacteremia; possibly resistant to bactericidal activity in normal human serum
2. Risk, transmissibility, and source of infection
a. Spread worldwide; animal reservoir probably the primary source of infection
(1) Meat from infected animals frequently contaminated with intestinal contents during slaughter; nearly all commercially raised poultry is infected with *C. jejuni*
(2) Infected animal excretion may contaminate soil or water
(3) Most human infections probably result from consumption of contaminated food or water
b. Spread can be fecal-oral from person-to-person or animal-to-person
c. Anal sexual practices associated with increased risk for infection
d. Immunocompromised people are at increased risk for severe and recurrent infection
3. Frequency and distribution
a. In developed countries prevalence is <1% in healthy individuals
(1) Incidence peaks in children <1 year

old and in people 15–29 years old
(2) Infections occur year round, sharply peaking in summer and early fall
(3) *Campylobacter* infections are probably more common than *Salmonella* or *Shigella* infections
b. In developing countries, *C. jejuni* commonly isolated from healthy individuals
(1) Infections especially common in the first 5 years of life
(2) Acute diarrheal illness experienced by travelers frequently associated with *Campylobacter* infections
4. Relationship to natural history of HIV disease
a. In HIV-infected patients, gastroenteritis from *Campylobacter* may be severe enough to result in bacteremia via hematologic spread
b. Chronic *Campylobacter* infection can persist over months despite therapy
(1) Corresponds with failure of humoral response to infection
(2) *C. jejuni* most commonly isolated from HIV-infected patients
5. Morbidity and mortality
a. Rarely a direct cause of mortality in immunocompetent people
b. Fatalities usually result from severe dehydration
6. Early detection, prevention, prophylaxis
a. *C. jejuni* is susceptible to freezing or drying temperatures, pasteurization, standard chlorine-treated water
b. Avoid obvious sources of *Campylobacter*
(1) Unpasteurized milk and cheeses
(2) Undercooked meat, especially poultry
(3) Excretions of infected animals
(4) Untreated water when camping or backpacking
7. Signs and symptoms
a. Acute enteritis is the most common presentation of *C. jejuni* (see *GI System Complications*, p. 169; *Diarrhea*, p. 205)
(1) Diarrhea, malaise, fever, abdominal cramping
(a) Prodromal constitutional symptoms common 12–24 hours before onset of intestinal symptoms

(b) Symptoms may last from 1 day to 1 week, or longer

(2) Frequency of stool can be ≥10/day; initially, stools may be loose or watery; as illness progresses, stools may become frankly bloody with tenesmus

(3) Abdominal cramping improved by defecation

(4) Abdominal cramping or fever may be only symptom of infection

b. Bacteremia is uncommon and usually seen in association with acute enteritis

(1) Can present as prolonged relapsing fevers, chills, and myalgias without an obvious source of infection

(2) Although rare, secondary seeding to an organ can occur, sometimes resulting in a fulminant and fatal course

8. Diagnosis

a. Should be considered in any patient with acute diarrheal illness, especially if duration >1 week (see *GI System Complications*, p. 169)

(1) Send stool specimen for culture and sensitivity and examination for ova and parasites, *Cryptosporidium*, and *I. belli*

(a) Single negative culture does not rule out infection

(b) Direct microscopic exam of fecal material can yield presumptive diagnosis within 2 hours

(2) Anoscopic or sigmoidoscopic exam and direct lesion culture may be indicated if stool cultures are negative or patient has bloody diarrhea

(a) Examination of affected tissues shows a diffuse, bloody, edematous and exudative enteritis

(b) Biopsy may or may not be performed

(3) Stained fecal smear may be indicated

b. Perform tests/procedures for patients with suspected bacteremia

(1) CBC with differential and platelets, PT-PTT, blood chemistry

(2) Draw blood cultures from two separate sites, including a central line if present, before starting antibiotics

(3) Culture suspected infection sites (if any) before starting antibiotics

(4) Start IV fluid using large-bore catheter

9. Treatment

a. Infection is usually self-limited in immunocompetent patients, requiring no therapy; symptoms gradually improve over several days

b. HIV-infected patients should receive antimicrobial therapy based on susceptibility testing

(1) Erythromycin is treatment of choice

(2) Ciprofloxacin can be alternative therapy

c. Patients with suspected bacteremia should receive an IV antipseudomonal beta-lactam (e.g., imipenem, piperacillin) combined with an aminoglycoside (e.g., tobramycin) until sensitivities are known

(1) Oxygen may be needed to maintain adequate tissue saturation

(2) Closely monitor febrile, neutropenic, or seriously ill patients for signs of sepsis, shock

10. Laboratory results and other indices to monitor for side effects, adverse effects, and response to therapy: Monitor patients for dehydration and electrolyte imbalance from diarrhea and vomiting

a. Maintain adequate oral intake

b. May require IV repletion

11. Patient education

a. Discuss risks and preventive measures

b. Avoid obvious sources of *Campylobacter*

c. Use safer sexual practices

d. Refer to *Infection Control*, p. 363

H. Shigella

1. Specific etiologic agent and disease process

a. Small nonmotile and nonencapsulated gram-negative rods of the *Enterobacteriaceae* family

b. Virulent *Shigella* invades intestinal tissue, multiplies, and subsequently destroys the mucosa, resulting in bacillary dysentery

(1) Mucosal destruction and manifestations are usually self-limiting

(a) Toxin elaboration plays a role in local mucosal destruction

(b) Infection is superficial, rarely penetrating beyond the mucosa

(2) Occasionally proceeds to bacteremia and sepsis

(3) Produces a neurotoxin that is suspected to play a role in pathogenesis in clinical disease

c. Infection with strains of enterotoxin-producing *E. coli* can result in clinical illness indistinguishable from shigellosis and is considered an agent of bacillary dysentery; nearly all shigella-like *E. coli* possess somatic antigens related to *Shigella* serotypes

2. Risk, transmissibility, and source of infection

a. Bacillary dysentery is the most communicable of the bacterial diarrheas; source is usually fecal

(1) Person-to-person transmission via oral-fecal route

(2) Can occasionally be spread by contaminated food or water (particularly important vector in developing countries where sanitation principles may not be adhered to)

(3) Flies may be an important vector—dysentery rates in warm countries appear to be directly related to fly populations

(4) Anal sexual practices associated with increased risk of infection

(5) Requires only a relatively small inoculum to produce disease readily in healthy adults

b. Primarily a diarrheal disease in children of school age or younger (often acquired by adults from their children)

c. Malnourishment leads to increased risk for more severe disease and complications

3. Frequency and distribution

a. Infection rate is higher both during warmer season and in warmer climates

b. Outbreaks are cyclic

(1) Suggests that each generation is infected and survivors rendered immune with outbreaks recurring in nonimmune offspring

(2) Infection rates are highest in infants and younger, preschool-age children

4. Relationship to natural history of HIV disease: Bacteremia from shigellosis, usually rare in the non-HIV-infected population, is not uncommon in HIV-infected patients

5. Morbidity and mortality: Mortality is unusual except in the elderly and in malnourished children

6. Early detection, prevention, prophylaxis: Major prerequisite in transmission is degree of contact with infectious material and personal hygiene

a. Good hand-washing techniques and personal hygiene between infected patients and susceptible persons is best prevention

b. High-quality water source sanitation is requisite

c. Household contacts of HIV-infected people with shigellosis should be evaluated for asymptomatic carriage of *Shigella*

7. Signs and symptoms

a. Dysentery clinical course reflects an intestinal tract infection that progresses from small to large bowel (see *GI System Complications*, p. 169)

(1) Initially presents as fever and abdominal cramping followed by voluminous watery stool reflecting infection of the small bowel

(2) Followed by decreasing fever and increasing number of smaller volume stools

(3) Bloody mucoid stools with fecal urgency and tenesmus may develop in a few days, reflecting infection of the colon

(4) Fever may be present or absent and patient may exhibit varying degrees of toxemia

b. Invasive disease and resultant bacteremia occur more frequently in HIV-infected patients

8. Diagnosis

a. Shigellosis should be considered in any patient with acute diarrheal illness associated with toxemia and systemic disease, especially if illness lasts longer than 48 hours

(1) Stool specimen for C&S and examination for ova and parasites (primarily *Cryptosporidium, I. belli,* amoebas)

(2) Anoscopic or sigmoid exam for direct lesion culture may be necessary if stool cultures are negative or patient has bloody diarrhea; biopsy as needed

(3) Stained fecal smear may be performed (prevalence of PMN leukocytes)

(4) Differential diagnosis: *Salmonella, S. aureus,* enterotoxin-producing *E. coli, Campylobacter, Cryptosporidium, E. histolytica, I. belli,* MAC, CMV

b. Perform tests/procedures for patients with bacterial infection

9. Treatment

a. Although shigellosis is usually self-limited, antibiotics are often recommended to shorten its course and decrease the period of fecal excretion of the bacteria

b. HIV-infected patients may require a prolonged course of TMP-SMX, ampicillin, or a quinolone

c. Intestinal motility may be important in recovery from infection and prevention of mucosal invasion (antidiarrheal agents may worsen bacillary dysentery and should be avoided)

d. Treat patients with suspected bacteremia with an IV antipseudomonal beta-lactam (e.g., imipenem) combined with an aminoglycoside (e.g., tobramycin) until sensitivities are known

10. Laboratory results and other indices to monitor for side effects, adverse effects, and response to therapy

a. Fluid and electrolyte balance

b. May require IV repletion

11. Patient education

a. Discuss sources of infection and prevention with HIV-positive patients

(1) Stress importance of personal hygiene and hand washing

(2) Avoid individuals with shigellosis, if possible

(3) Practice safer sex

b. Discuss need for safe water supply with patients traveling to areas with substandard public sanitation

c. Refer to Table 10.3, *Reducing the Risk of/Preventing Exposure to Opportunistic Pathogens,* p. 371

I. Haemophilus Influenzae

1. Specific etiologic agent and disease process

a. *H. influenzae,* a pleomorphic gram-negative bacterium requiring special growth factors supplied by erythrocytes

b. Invasion of respiratory epithelium can manifest as chronic bronchitis, otitis media, sinusitis, and conjunctivitis; may potentially lead to systemic bacteremia resulting in sepsis, meningitis, epiglottitis, pneumonia and empyema, septic arthritis, cellulitis, and osteomyelitis

(1) Respiratory tract infections generally result from unencapsulated of nontypable strains; a common and substantial problem in adults; probably secretes factors that both facilitate attachment to human buccal epithelial cells and slow down ciliary activity of epithelial cells

(2) Encapsulated, type b strain is more virulent and responsible for most invasive disease; probably enters blood stream more readily that other strains for rapid hematogenous spread

2. Risk, transmissibility, and source of infection

a. *H. influenzae* colonizes the human respiratory tract in approximately 80% of the population (but does not cause disease)

b. Transmission is via airborne droplets or direct contagion with secretions

c. Invasive infections rare in healthy adults

(1) Higher incidence of pneumonia in patients >50 or with primary pulmonary disease, malignancy, or alcoholism

(2) Associated with conditions significantly impairing host immune function

(3) Prior nasopharyngeal infection with

influenza and viruses potentiates bacteremia

(4) Occurrence of meningitis correlates with duration and intensity of bacteremia

(5) IDU associated with increased frequency of infection

3. Frequency and distribution
   a. Disease mainly seen in children; associated with seasonal outbreaks
   b. Outbreaks of type b systemic infections have occurred in closed populations
   c. Occurrence in adults often related to coexisting age or other illness parameters such as IDU, alcoholism, malignancy, immune deficiency, age >50, and pulmonary disease

4. Relationship to natural history of HIV disease
   a. HIV-infected patients are at higher risk for infection because of underlying immune dysfunction
   b. *Haemophilus* species are responsible for 18.8%–55.5% of all HIV-associated bacterial pneumonias (Moxon, 1995)
      (1) Can occur in early stages of HIV disease
      (2) Patients with pulmonary KS or concomitant PCP are at higher risk
      (3) Smokers or IDUs, especially with low CD4+ lymphocyte counts, are at increased risk for infection
      (4) 14% of pneumonias in HIV-infected patients have been associated with bacteremia

5. Morbidity and mortality: Annual occurrence rate of invasive *H. influenzae* infection is 2.8 per 100,000 HIV-infected men in San Francisco, compared to 0.5–1.7 per 100,000 adults in the general population (Steinhart, Reingold, Taylor, Anderson, & Wenger, 1992)

6. Early detection, prevention, prophylaxis
   a. HIV-infected patients should avoid crowds or close contact with infected individuals during seasonal outbreaks
   b. Although *H. influenzae* type B vaccine has been recommended for patients with HIV-disease, no clinical data support its efficacy
      (1) Antibody response dependent on

residual cellular immune function

(2) Affords no protection against the more common nontypable strains

(3) PCP prophylaxis with TMP-SMX may decrease risk of infection

7. Signs and symptoms
   a. Presentation of *H. influenzae* in HIV-infected patients is similar to that in general population (see *Pulmonary Complications*, p. 151)
      (1) Fever of 38°–39°C, productive cough, dyspnea, and pleuritic chest pain
      (2) Increased WBC with shift to left
      (3) Lobar, patchy, or diffuse infiltrates on chest x-ray
   b. *H. influenzae* most commonly presents as pneumonia, but can also present as sinusitis
      (1) May involve one or more sinuses
      (2) Symptoms can range from mild coryza with facial discomfort to severe headache, cough, and bacteremia/sepsis

8. Diagnosis
   a. For the usual pulmonary workup, see *Pulmonary Complications*, p. 151
   b. Patients with sinus complaints may require nasal exam (see *Sinusitis*, p. 156)
   c. Perform tests/procedures for patients with suspected bacteremia
      (1) CBC with differential and platelets, PT-PTT, blood chemistry
      (2) Draw blood cultures from two separate sites, including a central line if present, before starting antibiotics
      (3) Culture suspected infection sites (if any) before starting antibiotics
      (4) Start IV fluid using large-bore catheter
      (5) Draw additional special blood cultures
   d. Differential diagnosis: *S. aureus, S. pneumoniae, K. pneumoniae, Pseudomonas aeruginosa*, or a noninfectious etiology

9. Treatment
   a. See *Pulmonary Complications*, p. 151
   b. Treat patients with suspected bacteremia or meningitis with an IV antipseudomonal beta-lactam (e.g., imipenem) combined with an amino-

glycoside (e.g., gentamicin) until sensitivities are known

   c. Patients with sinusitis: See *Sinusitis*, p. 156

10. Patient education: Discuss increased probability of *H. influenzae* pneumonia with newly diagnosed HIV-infected patients

   a. Instruct about signs and symptoms of pneumonia

   b. Advise to avoid crowds or close contact with infected individuals during seasonal outbreaks

   c. Discuss pros and cons of *H. influenzae* type b vaccination

J. Pseudomonas Aeruginosa

1. Specific etiologic agent and disease process

   a. Gram-negative rod occurring singly, in pairs, or in short chains; grows under aerobic conditions on a wide variety of media

   b. Opportunistic pathogen and immune disruption/underlying dysfunction are essential step in disease process

     (1) Produce and secrete factors implicated in both aiding penetration of tissue and impairing host defenses; result in tissue destruction and systemic spread

     (2) Produce and secrete toxins implicated in systemic symptoms and shock

2. Risk, transmissibility, and source of infection

   a. *P. aeruginosa* is isolated from soil, water, plants, and animals; reservoir can be wherever moisture is found

   b. Human colonization is rare, but can occur at moist sites (perineum, axilla, ears, respiratory and GI tracts); much higher incidence in hospitalized patients

   c. Rarely causes disease in healthy people

     (1) Infections tend to be nosocomial and associated with severe neutropenia, disruptions of mucocutaneous barriers, and alterations in normal flora

     (2) Patients receiving antibiotic therapy and patients with repeated/chronic hospitalization are at higher risk

3. Frequency and distribution: Primarily a nosocomial pathogen

   a. Discrete hospital-acquired outbreaks usually traceable to specific reservoirs (e.g., respiratory equipment)

   b. Leading cause of nosocomial pneumonia

   c. Pathogen most often associated with intensive care unit infections

4. Relationship to natural history of HIV disease: Associated with increasing incidences of bacteremia, pneumonia, sinusitis, and soft-tissue and bone infections, primarily in HIV-infected patients

   a. Primarily occurs in patients with CD4+ lymphocyte counts <100/μl

   b. Increased incidence associated with the presence of CVAD, systemic corticosteroids, or myelosuppressive therapy

5. Morbidity and mortality

   a. Bacteremic *Pseudomonas* pneumonia is a fulminant disease with death typically occurring 3–4 days in 33%–66% of reported cases (Lerner, 1995)

   b. Pseudomonal infections associated with high relapse rates in those who survive initial infection

   c. In a study of 32 AIDS patients with *P. aeruginosa* infection (Shepp, Tang, Raumaundo, & Kaplan, 1994), median survival from time of diagnosis was 80 days

     (1) All patients with pneumonia lived <250 days from time of diagnosis

     (2) Only 9% of patients with nonpulmonary infections were alive 250 days after diagnosis

6. Early detection, prevention, prophylaxis

   a. Good hand washing before and after patient contact

   b. Proper observation and care of CVAD and peripheral IV sites (see Appendix E, *CVADs*, p. 424)

   c. Proper disinfection of all hospital equipment

   d. Controversial is whether antiretroviral therapy may delay onset of *P. aeruginosa* infection by favorably altering the immune function in AIDS patients (Lerner, 1995)

7. Signs and symptoms: Primarily manifest in severely debilitated patients as pulmonary infection or bacteremia; can also present as a wide variety of conditions (e.g., endocarditis, sinusitis, skin/soft-tissue and other infections)
   a. Pneumonia, see *Pulmonary Complications*, p. 151
      (1) Fever, chills, severe dyspnea, purulent sputum of fulminant nature
      (2) Severe systemic toxicity
      (3) Chest x-ray reveals bronchopneumonia with distinctive nodular infiltrates that resembles *S. aureus* pneumonia
   b. Bacteremia occurs primarily in immunocompromised patients
      (1) Complaints of fever with chills/rigors
      (2) Confused or obtunded, toxic-appearing patient
      (3) Presence of obvious source of localized infection (e.g., skin lesions, wound infection, cellulitis, CVAD/peripheral IV site)
      (4) Underlying infection of respiratory, GI, or urinary tract
   c. Endocarditis: Febrile patient with cardiac murmur with history of IDU or CVAD (see *Endocarditis*, p. 148)
   d. May present as sinusitis
      (1) Symptoms may range from mild coryza with facial discomfort to severe headache, fever, cough, bacteremia/sepsis
      (2) May involve one or more sinuses
   e. Ear infections that present as complaints of itchy or painful ear with discharge
   f. Rapidly developing corneal ulceration may be bacterial keratitis
   g. Skin/soft-tissue presentation
8. Diagnosis
   a. For the usual pulmonary workup for pneumonia, see *Pulmonary Complications*, p. 151
      (1) Almost always exclusive to patients with compromised local respiratory or systemic host defense
      (2) Pneumonia is commonly associated with bacteremia
   b. Perform tests/procedures for patients with suspected bacteremia
      (1) CBC with differential and platelets, PT-PTT, blood chemistry
      (2) Draw blood cultures from two separate sites, including a central line if present, before starting antibiotics
      (3) Culture suspected infection sites (if any) before starting antibiotics
      (4) Start IV fluid using large-bore catheter
   c. Endocarditis common in IDUs
   d. For patients with sinus complaints, see *Sinusitis*, p. 156
   e. Skin/soft-tissue presentation
   f. Differential diagnosis: If *P. aeruginosa* is not recovered from appropriate cultures, disease may be from *S. aureus, S. pneumoniae, K. pneumoniae, H. influenzae,* or a noninfectious etiology
9. Treatment
   a. For treatment of pulmonary disease, see *Pulmonary Complications*, p. 151
   b. Treat patients with suspected bacteremia with an IV antipseudomonal beta-lactam (e.g., imipenem) combined with an aminoglycoside (e.g., gentamicin) until sensitivities are known
   c. Patients with sinusitis may require decongestants and antihistamines in additional to antimicrobial agents
   d. Uncomplicated nonbacteremic/septic infections may be treated with oral quinolones (e.g., ciprofloxacin)
10. Laboratory results and other indices to monitor for side effects, adverse effects, and response to therapy: Monitor patients treated for *P. aeruginosa* pulmonary infections closely for relapses after completion of therapy
11. Patient education
    a. Teach at-risk patients signs and symptoms of infection (and to report any to nurse or doctor), hand-washing techniques
    b. Instruct on proper care of CVADs (see Appendix E, p. 424)

K. Bartonella

1. Specific etiologic agent and disease process
   a. *Bartonella* (previously designated

Rochalimaea) are slow-growing, small, gram-negative, slightly curved rods

b. Genus-level relation between former *Rochalimaea* and *B. bacilliformis* established after identification of AIDS-associated clinical syndromes and additional related pathogens

c. *B. quintana* and *B. henselae* have been associated with bacillary angiomatosis (BA), bacillary peliosis hepatitis, and bacteremia; basic anatomic lesion induced is vascular in nature and can become the seeding point for disseminated disease, bacteremia, and sepsis

d. Cat scratch disease can result from infection with *A. felis* or, more commonly, from *B. henselae* infection

2. Risk, transmissibility, and source of infection

a. Body louse is only known source of *B. quintana*

(1) Outbreaks of trench fever associated with poor sanitation and personal hygiene

(2) No known nonhuman vertebrate reservoir

b. Ticks and fleas may be vector for *R. henselae* based on epidemiologic associations and identification from cat-associated fleas

(1) BA from *B. henselae* in HIV-infected patients is strongly associated with recent history of cat scratches/bites, especially from kittens

(2) Absence of cat exposure in one third of patients with BA or peliosis hepatitis suggests other sources of infection

(3) Cat fleas or other insects may be a vector

(4) Direct contact with soil may be another source of infection

3. Frequency and distribution

a. *B. quintana* and *B. henselae* believed to be globally epidemic

b. Cat scratch disease more frequent in immunocompetent people

(1) 80% of cases occur in people <21 years old

(2) Most common cause of chronic benign adenopathy in children and young adults

4. Relationship to natural history of HIV disease: BA and hepatitis occur primarily in AIDS patients, although cases have been reported in immunocompetent people

5. Morbidity and mortality

a. Undiagnosed or untreated disease may result in gradually progressive illness and death from local complications or overwhelming disseminated infection

b. Up to 2% of patients with *Bartonella* bacteremia may develop complications involving CNS, liver, spleen, lung, bone, skin

6. Early detection, prevention, prophylaxis

a. Maintenance of good sanitation and personal hygiene

b. Avoidance of tick- and flea-infested environments

c. Cat/kitten scratches and bites have only been associated with BA (see *Infection Control*, p. 363)

7. Signs and symptoms

a. Bacillary angiomatosis

(1) Cutaneous presentation

(a) Multiple or single reddish, vascular, cutaneous, or subcutaneous lesions of varying appearance

(b) Lymph nodes may have firm, nontender nodules

(c) Constitutional symptoms: poor appetite, vomiting, weight loss

(2) Patients present with extracutaneous involvement of a variety of internal organs

(a) Constitutional symptoms: poor appetite, vomiting, weight loss

(b) Multiple cutaneous lesions may develop

(c) Lymph nodes may have firm, nontender nodules

b. Bacillary peliosis: GI symptoms of nausea, vomiting, diarrhea or abdominal distension accompanied by fever, chills, and hepatosplenomegaly are most common presentation

c. Bacteremia

(1) Sudden onset of chills and fevers with nonspecific findings (e.g., headache, eye pain, rash) and no obvious site of focal infection

(2) HIV-infected patients may present with insidious development of recurrent fevers of gradually higher elevations and no obvious site of focal infection

(3) Malaise, fatigue, anorexia, weight loss

d. Cat scratch disease (most common presents as lymphadenopathy)

(1) Usually preceded by erythematous papule or pustule at inoculation site

(2) Lymphadenopathy usually resolves spontaneously within several months

(3) May present with cutaneous lesions

(4) Relatively uncommon in HIV-positive patients

8. Diagnosis

a. Special blood cultures and serologic tests should be drawn for *Bartonella*

b. Cutaneous BA presentation

(1) Lesion can closely resemble KS; should be biopsied

(2) Histopathologic findings of vascular proliferation and a myxoid stroma containing a mixture of inflammatory cells and granular clumps identifiable as bacillary organisms with Warthin-Starry staining or electron microscopy

c. Extracutaneous BA infection (e.g., bone, respiratory, GI): Radiographic imaging studies and biopsy are indicated

d. Bacillary peliosis may develop concomitantly with cutaneous BA or bacteremia; involves the liver, sometimes within spleen and lymph nodes; radiographic imaging studies and biopsy indicated

e. Perform tests/procedures for patients with suspected bacteremia

(1) CBC with differential and platelets, PT-PTT, blood chemistry

(2) Draw blood cultures from two separate sites, including a central line if present, before starting antibiotics

(3) Culture suspected infection sites (if any) before starting antibiotics

(4) Start IV fluid using large-bore catheter

(5) Draw additional special blood cultures and serologic tests for *Bartonella*

f. Cat scratch disease: Lymph node biopsy may be indicated

9. Treatment

a. Erythromycin current treatment of choice for BA, bacillary peliosis hepatitis, and *Rochalimaea* bacteremic syndrome

(1) Excellent responses have also been obtained with doxycycline in patients intolerant of erythromycin

(2) Ciprofloxacin can be effective

b. Treatment of choice for cat scratch disease is not clear

c. HIV-positive patients may require weeks to months of therapy

d. Patients with recurrent disease may require lifelong maintenance therapy

10. Laboratory results and other indices to monitor for side effects, adverse effects, and response to therapy

a. Positive serologic results from indirect fluorescent antibody testing should be carefully interpreted within the clinical context; meaning of results is still vague and requires further clinical investigation

b. If non-bacilliformis *Bartonella* is not recovered from patients with fever of unknown origin, disease may be from fungi such as *Cryptococcus neoformans, H. capsulatum,* or *Coccidioides immitis;* bacteria such as MAC and *Listeria monocytogenes;* or viral infections

c. Patients may initially respond to therapy with fever, myalgia, and constitutional symptoms

(1) Monitor HIV-infected patients closely for response to therapy and recurrent disease

(2) Relapse is common; may involve a different presentation of infection

11. Patient education: See *Infection Control*, p. 363

L. Listeria Monocytogenes

1. Specific etiologic agent and disease process
   a. Gram-positive rod that is motile at room temperature and is hemolytic
   b. Grows under aerobic conditions on enrichment media; often difficult to isolate; specimens should be delivered to lab promptly
   c. Monoclonal antibodies, PCR, and DNA probe techniques currently being developed
   d. Can invade the eye and skin of humans after direct exposure, although portal of entry is usually not evident
      (1) Patients become bacteremic
      (2) T-lymphocytes and monocytes are important host defenses
      (3) Secretes listeriolysin O, which disrupts cell membranes
      (4) Bacteremia may seed CNS tissue, resulting in meningitis; has a predilection for CNS tissue, especially meninges
2. Risk, transmissibility, and source of infection
   a. Has been isolated from soil, dust, animal feed, water, sewage, and almost every type of animal cultured (including asymptomatic humans)
   b. Infection is classically associated with patients with cellular immunity dysfunctions
   c. Risk factors include pregnancy, immunosuppression, malignancy, organ transplantation
   d. Vectors have been traced to unpasteurized milk and contaminated or undercooked meat
3. Frequency and distribution
   a. Annual U.S. incidence of listeriosis estimated at 0.7 per 100,000
   b. Associated with food-related epidemics
   c. Incidence of listeriosis higher in summer months
   d. Most U.S. cases occur in urban areas
4. Relationship to natural history of HIV disease
   a. Prevalence of symptomatic infection in AIDS patients has been estimated at 1,300 per million compared to 3.6–7.1 per million in the general population; mortality rate is extremely low (Armstrong, 1995)
   b. Although listeriosis is associated with cellular immunodeficiency, *L. monocytogenes* is uncommon in HIV-infected patients
5. Morbidity and mortality: Mortality rate is lower in adults than in children
6. Early detection, prevention, prophylaxis: For HIV-infected people, some healthcare professionals recommend that patients avoid foods associated with outbreaks of listeriosis (e.g., raw meats, unpasteurized milk, soft Mexican-style cheeses)
7. Signs and symptoms
   a. Most common presentation of *L. monocytogenes* in HIV-infected patients is bacteremia or meningitis/cerebritis, with or without bacteremia; presentation is generally subacute but may be fulminant
      (1) The only signs of meningitis may be low-grade fever and personality change
      (2) Cerebritis may present with headache, fever, and varying degrees of paralysis resembling a CVA
   b. Focal infections may include ulcerative skin lesions, purulent conjunctivitis, acute anterior uveitis, lymphadenitis
   c. May appear as an infection during pregnancy
      (1) Presents with symptoms of influenza, pyelonephritis, septic abortion
      (2) Neonates may become infected during or after birth
      (3) May result in increased reproductive loss
8. Diagnosis
   a. Perform tests/procedures for patients with suspected bacteremia
      (1) CBC with differential and platelets, PT-PTT, blood chemistry
      (2) Draw blood cultures from two separate sites, including a central line if present, before starting antibiotics
      (3) Culture suspected infection sites (if any) before starting antibiotics
      (4) Start IV fluid using large-bore catheter

b. Differential diagnosis includes other bacterial infections, cryptococcal meningitis, and CNS lymphoma
9. Treatment
   a. Either IV ampicillin or penicillin given alone or in combination with an aminoglycoside (e.g., gentamicin) is considered appropriate therapy
   b. IV TMP-SMX may provide adequate additional therapy
   c. Treat patients with suspected bacteremia with an IV antipseudomonal beta-lactam (e.g., piperacillin) combined with an aminoglycoside (e.g., gentamicin) until sensitivities are known
10. Laboratory results and other indices to monitor for side effects, adverse effects, and response to therapy: Relapses are uncommon
11. Patient education
    a. Discuss possible sources of infection with HIV-infected patients, particularly with HIV-infected women of childbearing age
    b. For kitchen and food safety, see Table 10.3, *Reducing the Risk of/Preventing Exposure to Opportunistic Pathogens*, p. 371

M. Nocardia Asteroides

1. Specific etiologic agent and disease process
   a. Weakly gram-positive soil-borne actinomycete characterized by filamentous growth and true branching; predominant human pathogen of *Nocardia* species
   b. Infection results in suppurative necrosis and abscess formation typical of pyogenic infections
      (1) Most commonly infects the respiratory tract; decreased bronchociliary clearance or bronchial obstruction predisposes patient to colonization
      (2) Neutrophils inhibit spread but do not kill *Nocardia*
      (3) Activated macrophages/CD4+ lymphocytes capable of killing *Nocardia*; may be resistant to oxidative burst
   c. May seed extrapulmonary infections

2. Risk, transmissibility, and source of infection
   a. *N. asteroides* is found in soil, dust, and decaying organic matter; most commonly infects humans through respiratory tract, although GI tract is also susceptible
   b. Not spread via animal or human contact
   c. Primarily an opportunistic infection
      (1) Chronically immunocompromised patients are at great risk (particularly associated with cellular immunity dysfunction)
      (2) Patients with chronic pulmonary infection are at great risk; respiratory colonization occurs in patients with malignancy, TB, cystic fibrosis, asthma, bronchitis, allergic aspergillosis
      (3) Infection rarely occurs unless steroid therapy is present
3. Frequency and distribution: Men affected more commonly then women; infection has occurred in all ages
4. Relationship to natural history of HIV disease
   a. Only 0.19%–0.3% of AIDS patients have been reported as developing nocardiosis (Lerner, 1995)
   b. May be underreported because of misdiagnosis and the difficulty in making a diagnosis
   c. Use of TMP-SMX as PCP prophylaxis/treatment and sulfadiazine as treatment for toxoplasmosis may obscure it as a complication of AIDS
   d. Nocardiosis is not an index diagnosis of AIDS
5. Morbidity and mortality
   a. Reported mortality rate from pulmonary nocardial infection is 15% in healthy people (Lerner, 1995)
   b. Higher mortality rate seen in patients
      (1) Receiving corticosteroid therapy or otherwise immunocompromised
      (2) With acute infection or with disseminated disease involving two or more noncontiguous organs or the CNS
   c. Death is always from sepsis, brain abscess, or overwhelming pneumonia

d. Corticosteroid therapy appears to be a significant factor in mortality

6. Signs and symptoms
   a. Presents as an acute, subacute, or chronic suppurative pulmonary infection
      (1) Nonspecific symptoms (e.g., anorexia, weight loss, productive cough, pleural effusion, dyspnea, hemoptysis)
      (2) Tends to have a pronounced pattern of remission and exacerbations
   b. May present as extrapulmonary infection with a wide variety of manifestations; most commonly presents as soft-tissue or nervous system infection

7. Diagnosis
   a. Pulmonary lesions are often multiple, confluent abscesses, although single coin lesions and miliary patterns have been described (Lerner, 1995)
      (1) Radiographic findings include fluffy infiltrates, irregular densities, subpleural plaques, single or scattered nodules, or reticular infiltrates; lower lobes more commonly involved
      (2) May be found with concurrent infections of PCP, *Aspergillus*, *Cryptococcus*, or *M. tuberculosis*
      (3) Untreated pulmonary infection may clear spontaneously, obscuring source of subsequent metastatic infection
   b. Should be suspected in all high-risk patients with soft-tissue swelling, abscesses, or CNS manifestations in conjunction with current or recent chronic/subacute pulmonary infection
      (1) CNS infections reported in one third of cases
      (2) Needle biopsy of cerebral mass may be indicated in AIDS patients, even those with confirmed pulmonary nocardiosis, because of potential for multiple concomitant disease processes
   c. Perform tests/procedures for patient with suspected bacteremia
      (1) CBC with differential and platelets, PT-PTT, blood chemistry
      (2) Draw blood cultures from two separate sites, including a central line if present, before starting antibiotics
      (3) Culture suspected infection sites (if any) before starting antibiotics
      (4) Start IV fluid using large-bore catheter

8. Treatment
   a. Sulfanomides are mainstay of therapy
   b. Antimicrobial susceptibility studies can select alternative therapies for sulfonamide failure/intolerance (e.g., Minocycline, TMP-SMX)
   c. Variable and chronic nature of infection generally requires maintenance therapy
   d. Surgical intervention may be necessary
   e. Patients with suspected bacteremia should be treated with an IV antipseudomonal beta-lactam (e.g., piperacillin) combined with an aminoglycoside (e.g., tobramycin) until sensitivities are known

9. Laboratory results and other indices to monitor for side effects, adverse effects, and response to therapy
   a. Patients receiving high-dose sulfonamides should maintain high fluid intake to avoid renal/urinary complications (preventable by administration of oral sodium bicarbonate for urine alkalinization)
   b. Monitor patients for relapse and exacerbations
   c. Non-primary-site metastatic infectious lesions can appear despite sulfonamide treatment and maintenance therapy
   d. Monitor febrile, neutropenic, or seriously ill patients closely for signs of sepsis and shock

10. Patient education: Discuss risks of infection with immunocompromised patients receiving steroids

N. Rhodococcus Equi

1. Specific etiologic agent and disease process
   a. *R. equi* (previously designated *Corynebacterium equi*) are gram-positive, nonmotile, non-spore-forming rods

b. Pathology is a slowly progressive lobar infiltrate and consolidation that results in cavitary pneumonia; probably acquired through respiratory tract

c. Occasionally disseminates and can develop into bacteremia/sepsis and metastatic infection

2. Risk, transmissibility, and source of infection
   a. *R. equi* resides in soil and is a well-known pathogen in domestic animals
   b. Rarely pathogenic in humans
   c. Severely immunocompromised patients are at risk for this disease, particularly chronic alcoholics and people with malignancies receiving cytotoxic therapies

3. Relationship to natural history of HIV disease
   a. *R. equi* is an unusual pathogen in HIV-infected patients; may precede the onset of an AIDS-defining diagnosis
   b. Bacteremic pneumonia is more frequently reported in AIDS patients

4. Morbidity and mortality: Prognosis is poor

5. Signs and symptoms
   a. HIV-infected patients most commonly present with pneumonia; insidious onset of fatigue, fever, and nonproductive cough
   b. May present as an extrapulmonary infection

6. Diagnosis
   a. For the usual pulmonary workup, see *Pulmonary Complications*, p. 151; chest x-ray often shows evidence of cavitary lesions

b. Perform tests/procedures for patient with suspected bacteremia
   (1) CBC with differential and platelets, PT-PTT, blood chemistry
   (2) Draw blood cultures from two separate sites, including a central line if present, before starting antibiotics
   (3) Culture suspected infection sites (if any) before starting antibiotics
   (4) Start IV fluid using large-bore catheter

7. Treatment
   a. Pulmonary presentation may not be recognized and specific therapy started early enough to change disease course
   b. Optimal antimicrobial therapy for *R. equi* infections is unknown
      (1) In vitro, erythromycin and rifampin are the most active agents
      (2) Treat patients with suspected bacteremia with an IV antipseudomonal beta-lactam (e.g., imipenem) combined with an aminoglycoside (e.g., tobramycin) until sensitivities are known
   c. Patients may need lung resection as therapeutic adjunct

8. Laboratory results and other indices to monitor for side effects, adverse effects, and response to therapy
   a. Patients may relapse despite therapy
   b. Patients with persistent fever and tachycardia despite antibiotic therapy should have suppurative complications ruled out.

III. FUNGAL DISEASES

A. General Information

1. Systemic fungal infections occur as manifestations in the late stages of HIV disease, generally when CD4+ lymphocyte counts are <200/μl
2. Advances in diagnostic techniques and newer treatments, combined with clinicians' awareness of the threat of fungal infections, have significantly reduced related morbidity and mortality
3. Regional differences are noted: A patient's travel history and places of residence are clinically relevant (histoplasmosis, coccidioidomycosis, and blastomycosis have a higher incidence in regions where these mycoses are endemic)
4. Local fungal infections resulting from *Candida albicans* commonly occur in the oral cavity, skin, and esophagus; oral candidiasis is a proven predictor of AIDS development independent of CD4+ lymphocyte counts
5. The following fungal infections are currently considered AIDS-defining diagnoses
   a. Cryptococcosis (extrapulmonary)
   b. Candidiasis of the bronchi, trachea, lungs, or esophagus
   c. Histoplasmosis (disseminated or extrapulmonary)
   d. Coccidioidomycosis (disseminated or extrapulmonary)
6. Aspergillosis, designated as an AIDS-indicator disease in 1981, was removed in 1987 because of the low incidence of diagnosis

B. Candidiasis

1. Specific etiologic agent and disease process
   a. *Candida*: Yeastlike fungi that exist in unicellular forms
   b. More than 80 species of *Candida*, but only 8 are clinically important
   c. Most common species seen in HIV disease is *C. albicans*
      (1) *C. albicans* is ubiquitous; has been found in soil, food, inanimate objects, and hospital environments
      (2) Albicans is considered a commensal organism that is found on teeth, gingiva, oropharynx, vagina, large intestine, and skin
2. Risk, transmissibility, and source of infection
   a. Most *Candida* infections seen in HIV disease are endogenous and related to the interruption of normal host defense mechanisms (immunodeficiency, damaged or diseased skin or mucous membranes, indwelling IV devices, pressure monitoring devices, urinary catheters, drug therapy)
   b. Human-to-human transmission
      (1) Mother-to-child after vaginal delivery
      (2) Balanitis in uncircumcised men who have sex without a condom
      (3) Nosocomial transmission in congregate healthcare settings
3. Relationship to natural history of HIV disease
   a. Infections caused by *C. albicans* are estimated to occur in 75%–90% of HIV-infected people during the course of HIV disease
      (1) The likelihood of mucosal *Candida* infection increases with a progressive decrease in CD4+ lymphocyte counts, although oral candiasis has been reported in primary HIV infection
      (2) Studies have demonstrated that
         (a) Oral candidiasis is an accurate predictor of HIV disease progression and the development of other AIDS-related infections
         (b) Vaginal candidiasis in HIV-infected women has been found even with high CD4+ lymphocyte counts
   b. Candidiasis of the bronchi, trachea, or lungs as an initial AIDS-defining diagnosis occurs in 1%–2% of HIV-infected patients
   c. Esophageal candidiasis, as an initial AIDS-defining diagnosis, occurs in 8%–15% of HIV-infected patients
   d. Candida vaginitis is often the first

condition seen in HIV-infected women; data on the incidence of vaginal candidiasis is probably falsely low as many women may self-treat with over-the-counter (OTC) medications; clinicians treating women should explore the possibility of HIV disease following diagnosis of vaginal candidiasis with no explanation (e.g., the woman is not taking broad-spectrum antibiotics)

   e. Candidiasis should be considered a sentinel disease; its presence without an identifiable explanation should alert the clinician to explore the possibility of HIV disease

4. Early detection, prevention, prophylaxis
   a. *Candida* organisms are common on mucosal surfaces and skin
   b. No measures available to reduce exposure to these fungi
   c. Routine primary prophylaxis is not recommended

5. Signs and symptoms
   a. Oral
      (1) Erythematous, smooth red patches on the hard or soft palate, buccal mucosa, or dorsal surface of the tongue (often seen in asymptomatic patients)
      (2) Angular cheilitis produces erythema, cracks, and fissures at the corners of the mouth (considered by some to be a prognostic indicator for the development of AIDS)
      (3) Pseudomembranous patches appear as removable white plaques on any oral mucosal surface (often seen in patients with AIDS); complaints of dysphagia or odynophagia in the presence of oral candidiasis should alert the clinician that esophageal candidiasis may also be present
   b. Esophageal
      (1) Most frequently associated with dysphagia (see *Dysphagia/Odynophagia*, p. 207)
      (2) Other complaints include odynophagia (painful swallowing and retrosternal pain)
      (3) Absence of oral candidiasis does not

preclude the possibility that candida esophagitis may be present
   c. Vulvovaginal
      (1) Characterized by complaints of intense pruritus of the vulva with a curdlike vaginal discharge
      (2) Typically, the labia, vulva, and perineum are erythematous
   d. Intertrigo
      (1) Can occur at any site where the proximity of skin surfaces provides a warm, moist environment (e.g., groin, axillae, under/around the breasts)
      (2) Complaints are of burning and pruritus
      (3) Bright red appearance; slightly eroded eruption with wrinkled surfaces
   e. Paronychia (inflammation of the tissues surrounding the nails or the nail itself); primary complaint is tenderness
   f. Other: Related to site of infection (trachea, bronchi, lungs, heart, CNS, eyes, joints, testes); although rare, disseminated candidiasis may occur late in the course of AIDS

6. Diagnosis
   a. Definitive diagnosis of candidiasis
      (1) Made by gross inspection, by endoscopy, or by microscopy on a specimen of affected tissue
      (2) Although diagnosis by culture will tell the species, the distinction between infection and colonization in body sites where *Candida* is normally present is not always clear
   b. Differential diagnosis
      (1) With oral candidiasis, rule out oral hairy leukoplakia
      (2) With esophageal candidiasis accompanied by odynophagia, rule out esophageal viral lesions

7. Treatment
   a. Site-specific treatment strategies
      (1) Oral
         (a) Nystatin vaginal tablets dissolved slowly in the mouth
         (b) Nystatin oral pastilles
         (c) Clotrimazole
         (d) Ketoconazole

(e) Fluconazole until the lesion disappears
  i) Increasing reports of fluconazole-resistant *Candida* in patients exposed to this drug
  ii) Use of fluconazole for minor fungal infections, accompanied by the development of drug resistance, will preclude its use for more severe fungal infections (e.g., for maintenance therapy should cryptococcosis develop)
  iii) Nystatin-triamcinolone topical cream, clotrimazole topical cream, or ketoconazole topical cream can be used for angular cheilitis
(2) Esophageal
  (a) Ketoconazole
  (b) Fluconazole
(3) Vulvovaginal
  (a) Clotrimazole topical cream
  (b) Ketoconazole, followed by 5-day courses each month for 6 months for refractory cases
  (c) Fluconazole can be used for the most refractory cases, but increasing reports of drug resistance means its use should be limited
(4) Intertrigo: Clotrimazole topical cream, although other topical antifungal may be used
(5) Paronychia: Imidazole topical cream
(6) Other
  (a) Initial treatment of disseminated or internal-organ infection will usually require amphotericin B, with or without 5-flucytosine
  (b) For long-term suppressive therapy, ketoconazole or fluconazole may be prescribed
8. Laboratory results and other indices to monitor for side effects, adverse effects, and response to therapy
  a. Nystatin (local, oral, topical): No special laboratory tests required
  b. Clotrimazole
    (1) Local, oral, AST [SGOT] (as indicated)
    (2) Topical: No special laboratory tests required
  c. Ketoconazole
    (1) Oral: Liver function tests (as indicated)
    (2) Topical: No special laboratory tests required
  d. Fluconazole
    (1) Serum creatinine and BUN (as indicated)
    (2) Liver function tests (as indicated)
  e. Amphotericin B
    (1) Serum magnesium and potassium levels (twice weekly)
    (2) CBC and platelet count (weekly)
    (3) Serum creatinine and BUN (q2d while dosage is increased and then at least twice weekly)
  f. Flucytosine
    (1) ALT [SGPT], alkaline phosphatase, AST [SGOT], bilirubin, creatinine, BUN (before and frequently during therapy)
    (2) Serum flucytosine concentration
  g. Recurrent mucocutaneous candidiasis will be problematic throughout the course of HIV disease, especially when antibiotic therapy is prescribed to treat the numerous infections that will occur; clinicians should therefore assess HIV-infected patients routinely for mucocutaneous candidiasis by oral and skin exam, paying particular attention to the genital area, upper thighs, and under the breasts
9. Patient education
  a. Establish a daily oral hygiene routine that is atraumatic to mucosal surfaces
  b. Establish a daily skin care regimen to maintain the integrity and cleanliness of skin surfaces
  c. Add yogurt (at least 8 oz/day) that contains *Lactobacillus acidophilus*, especially when any antibiotic therapy is ordered
  d. Teach correct use of medications to minimize drug-resistant strains and to enhance bioavailability

C. Cryptococcosis

1. Specific etiologic agent and disease process
   a. *Cryptococcus neoformans:* A yeastlike fungus, ubiquitous in nature and with a worldwide distribution
   b. Found in pigeon droppings; can be retrieved in nesting places, soil, fruit, and fruit juices
   c. The organism can remain viable for up to 2 years in desiccated pigeon feces
   d. Infection is easily acquired from the environment
      (1) The organism is aerosolized and inhaled
      (2) After being inhaled, the organism settles in the lungs where it can remain dormant or spread to other parts of the body, particularly the CNS
      (3) In immunocompetent hosts the infection is usually contained; in immunodeficient patients extrapulmonary disease may result
2. Risk, transmissibility, and source of infection
   a. In people with HIV disease infection most probably occurs from reactivation of latent infection; it is associated with progressive immunodeficiency
   b. No documentation exists for either person-to-person or animal-to-person transmission
   c. In people with HIV disease, infection from *C. neoformans* is more commonly seen among IV drug users, ethnic minorities, and in the south-central United States; there is no explanation for this distribution
   d. A higher incidence of this disease appears in HIV-infected individuals who smoke due to impaired pulmonary defenses (Forthal et al., 1992)
3. Frequency and distribution: Cryptococcosis is the most prevalent life-threatening fungal infection seen in persons with HIV disease
4. Relationship to natural history of HIV disease
   a. Cryptococcosis usually occurs in advanced HIV disease

   b. Current estimates are that 5%–13% of patients with AIDS develop cryptococcosis (Coker et al., 1993)
5. Morbidity and mortality
   a. Left untreated, cryptococcosis is fatal in those infected with HIV
   b. Even when treated, the estimated mortality for people with AIDS is substantial
6. Early detection, prevention, prophylaxis
   a. Routine screening of HIV-infected people with the cryptococcal antigen test (CRAG) is controversial and not currently recommended, given false-positive and false-negative results
   b. Prevention
      (1) Although HIV-infected people cannot avoid exposure to *C. neoformans* completely, avoiding sites that are likely to be heavily contaminated (e.g., with pigeon droppings) may reduce risk of infection
      (2) Cessation of tobacco smoking may also reduce the risk of disease
   c. No recommened prophylaxis
7. Signs and symptoms
   a. Onset of cryptococcal disease
      (1) Usually insidious
      (2) Waxing and waning presentation often results in a delay in medical diagnosis
   b. Pulmonary cryptococcosis: Usually manifested by fever, cough, dyspnea, and pleuritic chest pain
   c. CNS cryptococcal infection: Most common site
      (1) Causes disease in both brain and meninges so the term "cryptococcal meningitis" is a misnomer; the correct term is "cryptococcal meningoencephalitis"
      (2) Signs and symptoms
         (a) Fever, malaise, headaches, stiff neck, focal deficits, seizures
         (b) Diarrhea may also be present
         (c) Underlying immunodeficiency may cause fever to be greatly muted (either absent initially or low grade)
   d. Other manifestations: Related to the site of infection (bone marrow, kidneys,

liver, spleen, lymph nodes, heart, oral cavity, prostate, skin, bones, adrenals, thyroid)
8. Diagnosis
   a. Cryptococcal antigen titers and fungus cultures of the blood and CSF (obtained via lumbar puncture); sputum culture
   b. Most clinicians will perform an imaging study (computed tomography [CT] scan or magnetic resonance imaging [MRI]) before performing a lumbar puncture to rule out toxoplasmosis or lymphoma of the CNS, which can produce similar symptoms
   c. Differential diagnosis: Rule out other CNS space-occupying lesions or infections (e.g., syphilis, toxoplasmosis, primary lymphoma of the brain)
9. Treatment
   a. Primary prophylaxis not recommended for cryptococcal infection
   b. Acute therapy for the initial infection
      (1) Amphotericin B over 6–12 weeks, with or without 5-flucytosine (adjusted for renal insufficiency that may develop), *followed by*
      (2) Fluconazole for 8–10 weeks or itraconazole
   c. Maintenance suppressive therapy (secondary prophylaxis)
      (1) Fluconazole, *or*
      (2) Itraconazole, *or*
      (3) Amphotericin B
   d. Management
      (1) Relieve the symptoms of increased ICP (in the absence of obstructive hydrocephalus); serial lumbar punctures
      (2) When this strategy proves insufficient, a lumbar drain, ventriculostomy, or placement of a ventricular-peritoneal shunt
      (3) Administration of acetazolamide and corticosteroids remains controversial
10. Laboratory results and other indices to monitor for side effects, adverse effects, and response to therapy
   a. Amphotericin B
      (1) Serum magnesium and potassium levels (twice weekly)
      (2) CBC and platelet count (weekly)
      (3) Serum creatinine and blood urea nitrogen (BUN) (every other day while dosage is increased, then at least twice weekly)
      (4) Shivering or rigors: See *Fever and Night Sweats*, p. 211
   b. 5-flucytosine
      (1) Serum alanine aminotransferase (ALT [formerly SGPT]), alkaline phosphatase, aspartate aminotransferase (AST [formerly SGOT]), bilirubin, creatinine, and BUN (before and frequently during therapy)
      (2) Serum flucytosine concentration
   c. Fluconazole
      (1) Serum creatinine and BUN (as indicated)
      (2) Liver function tests (as indicated)
   d. Itraconazole
      (1) Serum potassium (as indicated)
      (2) Liver function tests (as indicated)
      (3) Interacts with rifampin and rifabutin, resulting in impaired absorption—thus the concomitant use of these agents as prophylaxis or treatment for mycobacterial infections should be avoided
   e. Repeated lumbar punctures
      (1) Will be performed for CSF cultures
      (2) To evaluate efficacy of treatment
   f. Relapse
      (1) Despite continued maintenance suppressive therapy, relapse will occur in some patients as evidenced by the reappearance of symptoms
      (2) Usually requires retreatment, often with other agents

D. Histoplasmosis

1. Specific etiologic agent and disease process
   a. *Histoplasma capsulatum*: A fungus that is part of the intestinal flora of birds and bats and exists in the soil
   b. *H. capsulatum* spores are aerosolized and inhaled
      (1) In the lung the organisms multiply and disseminate to the reticuloendothelial system, involving the liver, spleen, and lymph nodes

(2) In immunocompetent people who have the ability to mount an appropriate immune response, the infection is usually controlled by CD4+ lymphocyte mediated immunity

(3) In a immunodeficient person the pathologic process continues and the person develops progressive disseminated histoplasmosis

2. Risk, transmissibility, and source of infection
   a. In the U.S., the major endemic areas are the middle, central, and south central states
   b. Histoplasmosis that occurs in HIV-infected patients who live outside endemic areas is considered to be reactivation of previously acquired infection
   c. Histoplasmosis that occurs in HIV-infected patients in endemic areas is due either to reactivation of previously acquired infection or to reinfection from constant exposure

3. Frequency and distribution
   a. In the south, endemic areas extend to Alabama in the east and to southwest Texas in the west, continuing into Mexico, the Caribbean, and Central and South America
   b. In the north, endemic areas extend into Ontario and Quebec
   c. Indianapolis, IN, and Kansas City, MO, are referred to as hyperendemic (high incidence) areas

4. Relationship to natural history of HIV disease
   a. Usually occurs in the more advanced stages of HIV disease
   b. In nonendemic areas it represents reactivation of previously acquired infection (e.g., cases seen in New York City have been reported in people who previously lived in Puerto Rico)
   c. In endemic areas the incidence as an AIDS-defining illness is about 5% of total cases of histoplasmosis; in hyperendemic areas the incidence increases to 25%

5. Morbidity and mortality: Untreated progressive disseminated histoplasmosis in HIV patients is fatal; treatment has reduced the mortality to <10% but relapse is common (Lee & Täuber, 1994)

6. Early detection, prevention, prophylaxis
   a. Routine screening for histoplasma antigens is of little value in endemic areas—most people will test positive with no predictive value for future development of disease
   b. Primary prophylaxis for histoplasmosis is not recommended

7. Signs and symptoms
   a. Cough accompanied by fever is the most common initial presentation, along with hepatosplenomegaly
   b. Lymphadenopathy
   c. Skin lesions and oral ulcers in some patients
   d. Fatigue, weight loss, abdominal pain, and diarrhea may also be reported
   e. Common laboratory abnormalities are anemia, leukopenia, thrombocytopenia
   f. Other: Related to site of infection (eyes, CNS, heart, pancreas, prostate)

8. Diagnosis
   a. Because symptom presentation is nonspecific, diagnosis may be difficult, especially in nonendemic areas where this diagnosis may not be suspected; ask where the patient has lived/visited in the past in order to prevent delay in diagnosing patients who do not live in endemic areas
   b. The most reliable method of diagnosis is by culture of the organism from blood or tissue specimens
   c. Bone marrow or tissue biopsy for histopathologic evaluation also possible
   d. Differential diagnoses: Rule out other pulmonary opportunistic infections, beginning with tuberculosis

9. Treatment
   a. Acute therapy for the initial infection
      (1) Itraconazole; for meningeal or septic histoplasmosis this is not a recommended initial therapy (amphotericin B should be used)
      (2) Amphotericin B
   b. Maintenance suppressive therapy (secondary prophylaxis)
      (1) Amphotericin B
      (2) Itraconazole

10. Laboratory results and other indices to monitor for side effects, adverse effects, and response to therapy
    a. Itraconazole
       (1) Serum potassium (as indicated)
       (2) Liver function tests (as indicated)
       (3) Itraconazole interacts with rifampin and rifabutin, resulting in impaired absorption
    b. Amphotericin B
       (1) Serum magnesium and potassium levels (twice weekly)
       (2) CBC and platelet count (weekly)
       (3) Serum creatinine and BUN (every other day while dosage is increased and then at least weekly)
       (4) Shivering or rigors: Prevention and control during amphotericin infusion (see *Fever and Night Sweats*, p. 211)
11. Other important issues
    a. Instruct patients relocating from endemic to nonendemic areas to tell their primary care providers where they have lived in the past
    b. HIV-infected patients who have not traveled to endemic areas may be advised against such travel

E. Coccidioidomycosis

1. Specific etiologic agent and disease process: *Coccidioides immitis* fungus was originally identified in the United States as the etiologic agent of a self-limiting disease seen frequently in California, known as *San Joaquin Valley fever* ("valley fever")
2. Risk, transmissibility, and source of infection
    a. *C. immitis* mycelia grow in the soil during rainy seasons; during the dry season they develop into resistant spores and become airborne
    b. Wind and mechanical disruption of the soil (e.g., earthquakes) increase airborne distribution
    c. In patients who reside outside endemic areas infection can result from travel to these areas, laboratory exposure, or inhaling spore-contaminated fomites (e.g., soil, cotton, packing material,

museum artifacts) transported from endemic areas
    d. After inhalation of the spores, primary pulmonary infection is contained in the lungs in immunocompetent people; in immunodeficient patients, fulminant, disseminated infection can involve the skin, meninges, lymph nodes, and liver
3. Frequency and distribution
    a. *C. immitis* is endemic to some areas of Arizona, California, Nevada, New Mexico, Texas, and Utah
    b. Skin testing in endemic regions reveals that up to one third of residents have had a primary infection due to *C. immitis*
4. Relationship to natural history of HIV disease
    a. In HIV-infected patients living in nonendemic areas, coccidioidomycosis is due to reactivation of previously acquired infection; in infected patients living in endemic areas, reactivation of previously acquired infection is believed to be the cause of disease although constant exposure and reinfection may play a role
    b. HIV-infected patients going from nonendemic to endemic areas have been reported to acquire disease shortly after arriving in endemic regions
    c. Coccidioidal infection usually develops in HIV-infected patients with a CD4+ lymphocyte count <250/μl
    d. In endemic areas, coccidioidomycosis can be a frequent complication of advanced disease (e.g., in Arizona coccidioidal disease occurs in 25% of patients with HIV disease)
5. Morbidity and mortality: Mortality is related to the type of infection (Fish et al., 1990)
    a. Better prognosis for localized lung infection
    b. Guarded for meningitis
    c. Poor for disseminated infection (with a median survival of 1 month)
6. Early detection, prevention, prophylaxis
    a. Routine screening with skin testing is not recommended; studies have shown that a positive skin test has no predictive value in the development of coccidioidal infection
    b. No recommended prophylaxis

7. Signs and symptoms
   a. Usually nonspecific; include malaise, fever, cough, fatigue
   b. Other: Related to site of infection (skin, CNS, lymph nodes, liver, spleen, kidneys, adrenal glands, peritoneum)
8. Diagnosis
   a. The major problem in patients with HIV disease is the lack of suspicion of coccidioidomycosis in nonendemic areas; ask where the patient has lived/visited in the past in order to prevent delay in diagnosing patients who do not live in endemic areas
   b. Diagnosis is made by microscopy, culture, or direct examination of affected tissues or fluid from those tissues (bronchoscopic, blood, bone marrow, lymph node, urine, and liver specimens)
   c. *C. immitis* is extremely infectious and may be easily spread in laboratory settings; warn lab staff that coccidioidomycosis is suspected so they can take appropriate precautions
   d. Differential diagnoses: Rule out other pulmonary opportunistic infections, beginning with TB
9. Treatment
   a. Acute therapy for the initial infection: Amphotericin B
   b. Maintenance suppressive therapy (secondary prophylaxis)
      (1) Amphotericin B
      (2) Fluconazole
      (3) Itraconazole
10. Laboratory results and other indices to monitor for side effects, adverse effects, and response to therapy
    a. Amphotericin B
       (1) Serum magnesium and potassium levels (twice weekly)
       (2) CBC and platelet count (weekly)
       (3) Serum creatinine and BUN (weekly)
    b. Fluconazole
       (1) Serum creatinine and BUN (as indicated)
       (2) Liver function tests (as indicated)
    c. Itraconazole
       (1) Serum potassium (as indicated)
       (2) Liver function tests (as indicated)
11. Patient education

   a. Instruct regarding correct use of medications to minimize risk of drug interactions
   b. See Table 10.3, *Reducing the Risk of/Preventing Exposure to Opportunistic Pathogens*, p. 371, for travel instructions

F. Aspergillosis

1. Specific etiologic agent and disease process
   a. *Aspergillus*: A fungus found in soil and water, in various foods, and in decaying vegetation
   b. During the reproductive stages, spores are formed and aerosolized
   c. Although more than 300 species of *Aspergillus* have been identified, only a few have been implicated in disease in humans, most notably *A. fumigatus, A. niger*, and *A. flavus*
2. Risk, transmissibility, and source of infection
   a. Principal mode of transmission: Airborne, often entering the respiratory tract or, sometimes, the operative site
   b. Secondary mode of transmission: Through contact with the skin or a wound
      (1) Additionally, reports are increasing of nosocomial transmission related to inadequate ventilation systems in healthcare facilities
      (2) Other routes of transmission: Contaminated IV solutions, contaminated marijuana
   c. After spores are inhaled, colonization in the alveoli can lead to invasive disease
3. Frequency and distribution: The incidence of aspergillosis in people infected with HIV is increasing. Identified risk factors include recurrent bouts of pneumonia and marijuana smoking.
4. Relationship to natural history of HIV disease
   a. *Aspergillus* is truly ubiquitous and has a worldwide distribution
   b. Disease due to *Aspergillus* tends to occur in advanced stages of HIV infection
      (1) Also associated with severe immunodeficiency, neutropenia, and concomitant pulmonary disease

(2) Most cases of HIV-associated aspergillosis occur in patients with coexisting OIs rather than as an isolated fungal infection

(3) Treatment of these OIs with broad-spectrum antibiotics, corticosteroids, and antineoplastic agents, increases the risk of aspergillosis

5. Morbidity and mortality
   a. Estimated incidence is approximately 0.7% (Pursell, Telzak, & Armstrong, 1992)
   b. Mortality due to invasive disease, even with treatment, is considered to be high

6. Early detection, prevention, prophylaxis
   a. No recommended prophylaxis for aspergillosis
   b. Despite its rarity, invasive aspergillosis should be included in the differential diagnosis of patients with advanced HIV disease and pulmonary or systemic signs of illness

7. Signs and symptoms
   a. Invasive pulmonary disease: Fever, dyspnea, nonproductive cough, pleuritic chest pain, hemoptysis (rare)
   b. Broncho-obstructive disease: Breathlessness, cough, fever, chest pain
   c. Extrapulmonary: Relate to site of infection (CNS, maxillary sinuses, heart, esophagus, kidneys, pancreas)

8. Diagnosis of aspergillosis should be made by microscopy and culture for fungi
   a. Although clinicians are encouraged to collect appropriate specimens from sputum, blood, bone marrow, and organ tissues (based on the patient's symptoms), this fungus is often difficult to detect; in some instances a definitive diagnosis is only arrived at postmortem
   b. Only an estimated 10%–30% of patients with invasive pulmonary aspergillosis have positive findings on sputum culture, whereas bronchoalveolar lavage will yield a positive result in most infected patients
   c. Differential diagnoses: Rule out other pulmonary OIs, beginning with TB

9. Treatment
   a. Experience in the treatment of invasive aspergillosis is limited and the appro-

priate length of therapy has not been determined
   b. Current recommendations
      (1) Amphotericin B
      (2) Some clinicians recommend the addition of rifampin for additive or synergistic effects with amphotericin
      (3) Recommendations for maintenance suppressive therapy are not available

10. Laboratory results and other indices to monitor for side effects, adverse effects, and response to therapy
    a. Amphotericin B
       (1) Serum magnesium and potassium levels (twice weekly)
       (2) CBC and platelet count (weekly)
       (3) Serum creatinine and BUN (every other day while dosage is increased and then at least weekly)
    b. Rifampin: Liver function tests as indicated

11. Patient education
    a. Teach measures to prevent or control shivering or rigors during amphotericin B infusions (see *Fever and Night Sweats*, p. 211)
    b. Educate about risks of acquiring aspergillus from smoking marijuana (baking may kill spores)

G. Blastomycosis

1. Specific etiologic agent and disease process
   a. *Blastomycosis:* A systemic endemic fungal disease caused by the dimorphous *B. dermatitides*, a fungus found in soil
      (1) Primary acute pulmonary blastomycosis occurs when the fungus is inhaled
         (a) Acute phase may be nonapparent, mild, or mimic influenza
         (b) Progression may result in a localized chronic pulmonary infection or extrapulmonary disease arising from lymphatic or hematologic dissemination
      (2) Extrapulmonary disease occurs in most patients
         (a) Most often involves skin, bones, joints, genitourinary tract, CNS

(b) May appear as deep cutaneous ulcers

b. *B. dermatitides* described as a spherical or elliptical, thick-walled multinucleated yeast

2. Risk, transmissibility, and source of infection
   a. Infection acquired by inhalation; incubation period ±45 days
   b. History of living, past or present, in an endemic area
   c. May have contracted fungus years before it became clinically manifested; reactivation occurs up to 3 years after primary blastomycosis

3. Frequency and distribution
   a. Natural habitat of *B. dermatitides* has been isolated in humid areas from soil with a high organic content, an animal waste-product component, and an acid pH
      (1) In North America, found in areas surrounding the Mississippi, Missouri, and Ohio rivers and extending to Canada (Quebec, Ontario, Manitoba)
      (2) Also found in India, Africa, Europe, and the Middle East
   b. Has been reported infrequently in patients with HIV, but rising number of reports of coinfection with HIV indicate *B. dermatitides* may be an increasing problem
   c. Relevant points of interest in reported cases of blastomycosis
      (1) Patients lived or have lived in endemic regions
      (2) Reactivation may be possible explanation for increase in number of cases

4. Relationship to natural history of HIV disease
   a. Blastomycosis possible in early stage of HIV disease
   b. Usually found in coinfected patients with CD4+ lymphocyte counts <200/μl
   c. Not an AIDS-defining infection, according to CDC guidelines
   d. CNS involvement occurs 5%–10% more frequently than in non-HIV-infected patients

5. Morbidity and mortality
   a. The patient coinfected with HIV disease and blastomycosis can have an aggressive disease process
   b. Mortality rate high even with proper diagnosis and treatment
      (1) Mortality rate for coinfected person: 40%–54% (5 times the mortality rate in non-AIDS population)
      (2) Many patients who have died from other causes had evidence of persistent blastomycosis
   c. Multiple organ and CNS involvement common

6. Early detection, prevention, prophylaxis
   a. Patients who should be evaluated for blastomycosis
      (1) History of residence in endemic region
      (2) Patients with pneumonia or pleural effusions of undetermined origin
      (3) Include blastomycosis in the differential diagnosis when evaluating patients with HIV
   b. Laboratory should be aware of possible atypical presentation of *B. dermatitides* in tissues
      (1) Morphology possibly altered in vivo as a result of treatment
      (2) Immune status of patients with HIV/AIDS may provide an environment in which the fungus has grown in an unusual conformation
   c. No prophylaxis

7. Signs and symptoms
   a. Primary lesions are in lung(s) following respiratory infection
      (1) Acute form may be nonapparent or mild, or may mimic influenza, bronchitis, pneumonia
      (2) Lesions may be unilateral or bilateral, appearing as nodular infiltrates or pneumonic consolidation, with or without cavitation
      (3) Clinical manifestations: Chills, fever, cough, SOB, pleuritic chest pain
   b. Progression of primary lung infection may lead to chronic disease state
      (1) May result in localized chronic pulmonary infection or extrapulmonary disease

(2) Extrapulmonary disease occurs in most patients
  (a) Usually involves skin, bone, joints, genitourinary tract, CNS
  (b) Skin lesions appear raised but enlarged and potentially ulcerating
  (c) CNS involvement may exhibit as changes in neurologic status
8. Diagnosis
  a. Pulmonary
    (1) Chest x-ray abnormalities: Lobar infiltrates, lesions, nodules, interstitial changes, patchy alveolar patterns
    (2) Pleural effusions, cavitary lung lesions
    (3) Culture of sputum
    (4) Bronchoalveolar lavage (BAL)
  b. Skin: Culture, skin biopsy
  c. Prostate: Urine culture
  d. CNS: Brain biopsy
  e. Serum: Check for *B. dermatitides* antibody with IgG
9. Treatment
  a. Amphotericin B is drug of choice for initial therapy
    (1) Multiple organ involvement, including CNS, warrants aggressive early intervention
    (2) CD4+ lymphocyte-depleted patients with HIV and CNS blastomycosis may respond better to amphotericin B than to ketoconazole and itraconazole
    (3) Controversy surrounds changing therapy from amphotericin B to azole therapy after patient has responded to initial therapy of amphotericin B
  b. Ketoconazole and itraconazole are efficacious for treating blastomycosis in immunocompromised patients without CNS involvement
    (1) Primary therapy with azole not usually recommended
    (2) Carefully monitor patient for signs of disease progression from treatment failure with attention to signs and symptoms of CNS involvement
    (3) Neither drug has significant CNS penetration
    (4) Initiate amphotericin B if disease progression is noted
    (5) Azole drugs poorly absorbed in decreased gastric acidity
    (6) If azole therapy chosen to follow amphotericin B therapy, treat at least 6 months with no clinical evidence of disease progression
  c. Maintenance therapy
    (1) Lifetime maintenance therapy recommended for patients successfully treated
    (2) Use oral ketoconazole or itraconazole
    (3) Fluconazole is not a potent antifungal agent against *B. dermatitides*
10. Laboratory results and other indices to monitor for side effects, adverse effects, and response to therapy
  a. Amphotericin B: Potassium level
  b. Azole therapy: Gastric absorption
  c. Monitor for progression of disease, including CNS involvement
11. Patient education
  a. Reactivation is possible; stress importance of compliance with drug therapy
  b. Tell patients to inform nurse or physician of changes in mental status and new skin lesions or other physiologic changes.

IV. VIRAL INFECTIONS

A. Cytomegalovirus

1. Specific etiologic agent and disease process
   a. Cytomegalovirus (CMV), is a DNA, member of the herpesvirus group, latent in monocytes
   b. Clinical presentation varies depending on the organ system involved
2. Risk, transmissibility, and source of infection
   a. 40%–60% of the U.S. population have antibodies to CMV
   b. Generally a subclinical infection or may produce a flulike illness
   c. Primary transmission mode from pediatric populations or via sexual activity
3. Frequency and distribution: >90% of gay men have antibody and >50% shed virus in semen or urine
4. Relationship to natural history of HIV disease
   a. Disseminated disease generally not seen until CD4+ lymphocyte counts <50/µl
   b. Many AIDS patients have persistent CMV viremia
      (1) Frequent complication is retinochoroiditis, a progressive disease that can lead to blindness
      (2) CMV enteritis, esophagitis, hepatitis, pancreatitis, peritonitis
      (3) Hepatobiliary sclerosis may be due to CMV
      (4) Pneumonitis may be caused by CMV though in most cases other disease-causing organisms are isolated; its role in primary pulmonary disease is controversial
      (5) CMV can cause encephalitis, ventriculitis, or a rapidly progressive polyradiculopathy
5. Morbidity and mortality: Common cause of morbidity and mortality in end-stage patients
6. Early detection, prevention, prophylaxis
   a. Possible prophylaxis with oral ganciclovir when CD4+ lymphocytes fall below 50/µl; remains controversial as only preliminary data are available
   b. Patients use visual grid to detect vision changes; routine ophthalmology exams for any visual changes
   c. Avoid giving CMV+ blood products to a patient with no history of CMV infection
   d. Inform HIV patients of increased risk of acquiring CMV via sexual contact and when caring for young children in child care centers
7. Signs and symptoms
   a. Retinitis: "Floaters," scotoma, visual complaints
   b. Enteritis: Diarrhea, dyspepsia
   c. Esophagitis: Odynophagia
8. Diagnosis
   a. Retinal exam detects cotton-wool patches, hemorrhages; following vascular pattern is pathognomonic for CMV retinitis
   b. In GI disease, endoscopy with biopsy reveals ulcerations, biopsy reveals typical intranuclear inclusions
   c. Histologic diagnosis is the gold standard: tissue cultures may be positive but are not specific for active disease
   d. CMV buffey-coat
      (1) Indicates active viremia, not active disease
      (2) Urine cultures sensitive for CMV shedding, not for active disease
   e. CMV serologies are not helpful in determining the presence of active disease
9. Treatment: All therapies require induction and continued maintenance except for GI disease
   a. Ganciclovir effective with retinitis; outcome is more variable with other body systems
      (1) Induction: 14–21 days, depending on clinical response and patient tolerance; parenteral administration only
         (a) Relapse rates with GI disease may not be as frequent; further study is needed to determine best regimen
         (b) Intraocular implants for "local" treatment of retinitis have been effective; however, morbidity

associated with extraocular disease is still a concern, therefore oral ganciclovir is recommended

(2) Maintenance

(a) Retinitis: Recommended lifelong therapy

(b) "Stable" retinitis: Oral ganciclovir; absorption is poor

(3) Toxicity

(a) Bone marrow suppression most common, resulting in severe neutropenia; avoid concomitant AZT administration

(b) Hepatotoxic

(c) Seizures; psychiatric manifestations

(d) Nephrotoxic

b. Foscarnet

(1) Induction: Parenteral administration only; central line recommended due to risk of severe phlebitis (if given via peripheral line drug must be a greater diluent)

(2) Maintenance

(a) Nephrotoxicity may be cumulative

(b) Monitor renal function closely

(3) Toxicity

(a) Nephrotoxic: additional hydration (1–2 L/day) necessary to minimize nephrotoxicity

(b) Hypo/hypercalcemia

(c) Hepatotoxic

(d) Seizure

(e) Bone marrow suppression (uncommon)

(f) Penile ulcers

(4) Confers greater longevity (4 months on average) in comparative trials with ganciclovir in patients with retinitis but has greater toxicity

10. Laboratory results and other indices to monitor for side effects, adverse effects, and response to therapy

a. Monitor renal function, electrolytes, calcium, magnesium, CBC with differential

b. Serial ophthalmic exams

11. Patient education

a. Self-administration of medications; arrange for ganciclovir infusion therapy

b. Teach use of visual grid for high-risk patients

c. Arrange for home care, visual-aid devices if patient sustains visual loss

B. Varicella Zoster Virus

1. Specific etiologic agent and disease process

a. Varicella zoster virus (VZV) is a member of the herpesvirus group

(1) Primary VZV infection is called chicken pox

(2) Latent in dorsal root ganglia

(3) Herpes zoster represents reactivation of a previously acquired infection; a common condition in older adults

2. Risk, transmissibility, and source of infection

a. Risk of transmission via cutaneous exposure to serum inside vesicle to a varicella-naive person (never had the primary infection)

b. Can be transmitted via aerosolized infected droplets

c. The acute primary infection (varicella) commonly occurs during childhood and is usually self-limiting; in adults it can be more severe; in HIV patients it can be life-threatening

3. Frequency and distribution

a. Recurrent episodes of zoster can occur in HIV-positive people

b. Risk of developing zoster increases with age

4. Relationship to natural history of HIV disease

a. Frequently occurs in HIV-infected patients with symptomatic disease; however, it is not currently believed to correlate with progression of asymptomatic infection to AIDS

b. Unusual presentation is common in severe immunodeficiency

5. Morbidity and mortality

a. Zoster eruptions in HIV-infected patients can be extensive and locally destructive and become secondarily infected

b. Zoster can be disseminated with life-threatening complications; pneumonia, hepatitis, or encephalitis may be fatal

c. Acute pain (burning, stabbing) frequently occurs; a chronic pain syndrome (postherpetic neuralgia) can be a severe and disabling complication
6. Early detection, prevention, prophylaxis: People who are varicella naive (especially those of advanced age, who are debilitated, pregnant women) should avoid patients with chicken pox or herpes zoster. If they are exposed to chicken pox or zoster, they should be given zoster-immune globulin (VZIG) within 96 hours.
7. Signs and symptoms: Clinical presentation vesicular, sometimes bullous lesions associated with serpiginous ulcers
   a. May be one unilateral dermatome, or polydermatomal; multidermatomal involvement is diagnostic for Class C disease
   b. Lesions may be very painful; in the asymptomatic patient clinical presentation and natural history are fairly typical when compared to the immunocompetent host
   c. Rarely will cause disseminated disease in immunocompromised patients; anorexia, fever, cough may indicate dissemination, a potentially fatal complication
8. Diagnosis: Immunofluorescent assay (IFA) (detection of virus antigens), culture
   a. Less sensitive than HSV cultures
   b. Tzanck prep helpful, sensitivity is better
   c. Check for acyclovir resistance if indicated clinically
   d. Characteristic clinical presentation
9. Treatment
   a. High-dose acyclovir
      (1) Best response if initiated within 72 hours of outbreak
      (2) Parenteral therapy in disseminated or severe infection; maintenance dose may be required in AIDS patients with recurrent VZV
   b. Famciclovir: Shown to decrease the incidence of post-herpetic neuralgia in the elderly; clinical implications in patients with AIDS is unknown
   c. Foscarnet
   d. Ganciclovir
   e. Vauciclovir now available

10. Laboratory results and other indices to monitor for side effects, adverse effects, and response to therapy
    a. Maintain strict isolation until all lesions are crusted; hospitalization may be necessary
    b. Local lesion care is required as open lesions can develop superimposed bacterial infections
    c. Pain management for both acute illness and postherpetic neuralgia
11. Patient education
    a. Teach local wound care
    b. Emphasize need for strict isolation
    c. Counsel varicella-naive visitors or staff not to enter the patient's isolation room
    d. Refer to *Pain*, p. 229, and *Impaired/Risk for Impaired Skin Integrity*, p. 222

C. Herpes Simplex Virus

1. Specific etiologic agent and disease process
   a. Herpes simplex virus (HSV) is a member of the herpesvirus group; during acute primary infection, it becomes permanently latent in the dorsal route ganglia
      (1) Following orolabial infection, HSV becomes latent in the trigeminal ganglia; after genital or anorectal infection, HSV becomes latent in the sacral ganglia (Erlich, Safrin, & Mills, 1994)
      (2) Stimuli (e.g., trauma, ultraviolet light) to the sensory nerve may reactivate latent HSV; during reactivation, virus replication occurs within the ganglia and progeny virions travel peripherally along sensory nerves to the mucosal or epithelial surface, innervated by the reactivated ganglion; active virus replication at the cutaneous surface then produces clinical signs and symptoms (Erlich et al., 1994)
   b. Mucocutaneous very common, particularly perianal infection in gay men; 90% of gay men have antibody to HSV-2
   c. Cutaneous also common; often have atypical appearance in immunocompromised individuals

d. Despite the close relationship of the two viruses, HSV-1 and HSV-2 have different epidemiology patterns and usual routes of transmission (Erlich et al., 1994)
   (1) Initial HSV-1 often occurs in childhood with infection developing as a result of direct inoculation of infected droplets from orolabial or nasal secretions on to susceptible mucosal surfaces; many initial infections are subclinical
   (2) Initial HSV-2 is acquired from sexual activity; can be asymptomatic
2. Risk, transmissibility, and source of infection
   a. Transmission occurs via person-to-person contact with lesions that are shedding virus; can also result from contact with symptom-free excreters
   b. The risk for HSV-1 increases with crowded living conditions and low socioeconomic status
   c. The risk for HSV-2 usually begins at puberty with the onset of sexual activity and increases with the number of different sexual partners
3. Frequency and distribution
   a. High rates of HSV-2 prevalence have been found in prostitutes, sexually active homosexual men (who have higher rates than sexually active heterosexual men), adults of lower socioeconomic status, and people attending STD clinics
   b. Both HSV-1 and HSV-2 are common in HIV-infected people due to high rate of HSV infection worldwide
4. Relationship to natural history of HIV disease
   a. Usually represents reactivation in AIDS patients
   b. Lesions, which are frequently ulcerative, may be atypical in appearance; sites will vary
   c. May also present as esophagitis, proctitis, perianal or anorectal disease; passive rectal intercourse is associated with an increased risk of HSV-2 anorectal infection
   d. Rarely the cause of encephalitis in patients with AIDS

5. Morbidity and mortality
   a. Acyclovir-resistant HSV infections may become life-threatening (see *Impaired/ Risk for Impaired Skin Integrity*, p. 222)
   b. HSV recurrences can become more frequent or severe in patients as the immune system deteriorates
6. Early detection, prevention, prophylaxis
   a. Avoid contact with any open lesions
   b. Practice safer sex to avoid contact with open lesions and to prevent exposure to symptom-free excreters
   c. In light of the high incidence of recurrent HSV outbreaks following resolution of acyclovir-resistant HSV infection, consider chronic prophylaxis if complete healing is achieved
7. Signs and symptoms
   a. Recurrent orolabial herpes: May have 1- to 2-day prodromal sensations (of paresthesias, itching, tingling) at site of impending eruption, followed by painful vesicular lesion that becomes an ulcer; fever, phalangitis, and cervical lymphadenopathy may be present
   b. Recurrent genital herpes: May have 1- to 2-day prodromal sensations at site of pending eruptions; begin as papules that advance to vesicles, rapidly unroof and form shallow ulcerations; local itching and tenderness often present
   c. Esophagitis: Dysphagia, odynophagia
   d. Proctitis: Anorectal pain, perianal ulcerations, rectal discharge, fever
8. Diagnosis
   a. Culture
   b. Endoscopy when indicated
   c. Differential diagnoses for genital ulcerations: Syphilis, chancroid, scabies, mucocutaneous candidiasis, venereal warts, amongst others
9. Treatment
   a. Acyclovir
      (1) Oral: Increase dose per clinical response (AIDS patients often require higher doses than immunocompetent patients)
         (a) Bioavailability of drug is low
         (b) Maintenance therapy may be needed if breakthrough is frequent or if bouts are severe

(2) Parenteral: Use for severe outbreaks or if disseminated disease is suspected

b. Foscarnet
   (1) Available by compassionate release for acyclovir-resistant infections (see *CMV*, p. 94)
   (2) Dosage usually lower than for CMV
   (3) Will probably required lifelong therapy, though may relapse with acyclovir-sensitive phenotype

c. Ganciclovir
   (1) Active against herpes simplex
   (2) Not usually treatment of choice due to its higher potential for toxicity

d. Famciclovir: Licensed for treatment of varicella zoster virus but has activity against HSV; studies underway

e. Vidarabine
   (1) Licensed prior to acyclovir
   (2) Toxicity is usually unacceptable in adults having questionable efficacy
   (3) Must be given parenterally

10. Laboratory results and other indices to monitor for side effects, adverse effects, and response to therapy
    a. Toxicity related to acyclovir
       (1) Usually well-tolerated when given orally
       (2) Bone marrow suppression
       (3) Renal insufficiency
       (4) Hepatotoxic
       (5) Seizure
    b. Monitor for superimposed bacterial or fungal infection on ulcerated HSV disease
    c. There is risk for nosocomial transmission of HSV-1 and HSV-2 from infected patients to healthcare staff
       (1) Use barrier precautions when examining oral, genital, or anal lesions and for activities that involve exposure to excretions such as mouth care, suctioning, vaginal care
       (2) Herpetic whitlow can occur if barrier precautions and meticulous hand washing are not implemented

11. Patient education
    a. Care of mucocutaneous lesions for comfort: See *Impaired/Risk for Impaired Skin Integrity,* p. 222
    b. Safer sex practices, avoidance of skin-to-lesion contact
    c. See *Anorectal Signs and Symptoms,* p. 201, *Dysphagia/Odynophagia,* p. 207

D. Hepatitis Viruses A–E

The hepatitis viruses are a diverse group of hepatotropic viruses — that is, they all infect liver cells preferentially; for their similarities and differences, see Table 4.3.

E. Progressive Multifocal Leukoencephalopathy

1. Specific etiologic agent and disease process
   a. Progressive multifocal leukoencephalopathy (PML) is caused by a human papovavirus, JC virus (JCV), a slow-growing, neurotropic DNA virus, first isolated in 1971, which causes selective demyelination in the CNS (family Papovaviridae, genus *Polyomavirus*)
   b. Small foci develop in subcortical white matter in the brain; coalescence of small lesions leads to formation of larger lesions; affected areas may be in both hemispheres, the cerebellum and brain stem, and, rarely, in the spinal cord
   c. PML is a subacute or chronic progressive illness most often characterized by focal neurologic findings and mental status/personality changes
   d. No clear data to show that HIV and JCV infect the same cells in AIDS patients with PML; JCV and HIV may be directly mutually interactive
   e. At present, no illness has been associated with acute or primary JCV infection

2. Risk, transmissibility, and source of infection
   a. Primary JCV transmission with infection is thought to be by the respiratory route during childhood
   b. JCV may reside in the kidneys and or in B lymphocytes during the latency period
   c. No known animal reservoirs

Text continues on p. 107

Table 4.3 The Hepatitis Viruses A to E

Hepatitis A	Hepatitis B	Hepatitis C	Hepatitis D	Hepatitis E
Specific etiologic agent and disease process				
• Hepatitis A virus (HAV) • Frequently referred to as *infectious* hepatitis • HAV, a picornavirus, is a single-stranded RNA virus, which causes an acute or sub-acute, self-limiting infection of the liver • Incubation period: 2–7 weeks (mean 28 days) • Humans are the primary reservoir	• Hepatitis B virus (HBV): a member of the hepadnavirus family • A small, double-stranded DNA virus; the Dane particle • Previously known as *viral* or *serum* hepatitis; hepatitis-associated antigen (HAA), and Australia antigen; discovered in 1965 • Incubation period: 2–3 months (range 45–180 days) • Also a cause of immune complex disease (e.g., polyarteritis, glomerulonephritis)	• Hepatitis C virus (HCV): an RNA virus • A member of the flavivirus family, discovered in the mid-1970s • Previously called non-A, non-B hepatitis (NANB), or post-transfusion hepatitis • Strong tendency for progression to chronic hepatitis with a waxing and waning course • Incubation period: 20–90 days (average 50 days)	• Hepatitis D virus (HDV): a small, single-stranded RNA virus • Also known as delta (δ) hepatitis, in the hepadnavirus family • Discovered in 1977 • HBV is required to initiate infection and package HDV RNA into infectious particles • HDV may shorten the incubation period of HBV and increases the severity of HBV disease • HDV infection may persist after the acute phase	• Hepatitis E virus (HEV): a single-stranded RNA virus, otherwise untyped; discovered in the early 1980s • Also known as epidemic-, waterborne-, or enterically transmitted-non-A, non-B hepatitis (ET-NANBH) • Incubation period: 30–40 days • Resolution of acute illness occurs within a few weeks
Risk, transmissibility, and source of infection				
• Transmitted via the fecal-oral route and through close personal contact • Found in the feces of infected individuals • Spread of HAV infection readily accomplished by contamination of food and water with feces • Recurrent epidemics common • Crowding and poor sanitation contribute to the risk of HAV epidemics • Not transmissible to a fetus	• Enters the body through a break in the skin or mucous membranes • Transmission is via contaminated needles, transfusion of blood or blood products, sexual contact, or transplacentally • Communicable weeks before development of symptoms through acute clinical phase • Chronic carriers (HBsAg positive) are infectious for life	• Percutaneous exposure to contaminated blood, blood products • Frequently transmitted by IDUs who share their works • Role of sexual transmission not well understood, although multiple sexual partners is a risk factor for HCV infection; sexual contact is probably not an efficient means of infection	• In areas of high HBV endemicity (Africa, southern Italy, South America), HDV transmission is via sexual and parenteral contact • In areas of low HBV endemicity (U.S.), transmission is limited to groups with frequent percutaneous blood exposure (IDUs, hemophiliacs) • HDV seroprevalence is variable in Southeast Asia	• Infection is through ingestion of fecally contaminated water • Fecal-oral transmission • Person-to-person communicability unclear • Period of communicability unknown • Soldiers stationed in endemic areas may be at particular risk

continued

Table 4.3 *Continued*

Hepatitis A	Hepatitis B	Hepatitis C	Hepatitis D	Hepatitis E
• Contaminated shellfish represent an additional source of infection		• Communicable from about 1 week after exposure into chronic stage	• No evidence to support fecal-oral or waterborne transmission	

Frequency and distribution

Hepatitis A	Hepatitis B	Hepatitis C	Hepatitis D	Hepatitis E
• Worldwide • Cases in women and men are equivalent • Case frequency is reported as 9 per 100,000 population • Actual incidence is probably higher due to the large number of subclinical, and therefore, nonserologically diagnosed cases	• Worldwide • 200,000 primary HBV infections per year • 300 million HBsAg carriers • Prevalence varies among risk groups - Gay men: 60%–70% - IDUs: 5%–15% - Hemophiliacs: 3%–53% • More cases in women than in men	• Worldwide, but overall incidence low (U.S. 0.6%, Japan and southern Europe1.5%) • Most common among IDUs, hemodialysis patients, hemophiliacs (as high as 60%–70% infection rate) • Host range is limited to humans and chimpanzees • 150,00 new HCV infections per year	• Worldwide, most readily spread in households that include a HBV carrier; distribution closely parallels that of HBV infection • Approximately 5%–84% of HBsAg positive patients are infected with HDV, depending on sample studied - Gay men: 15% - IDUs: 25%–91% - Hemophiliacs: 34%–53%	• May be widespread; however no documented indigenous cases in U.S. • Majority of outbreaks in Asia, Africa, Mexico, and other developing countries due to crowding and poor sanitation; Americans traveling in these areas have brought the infection home with them • Outbreaks are both sporadic and epidemic • Occurs equally in men, women, and children

Relationship to natural history of HIV disease

Hepatitis A	Hepatitis B	Hepatitis C	Hepatitis D	Hepatitis E
• Many gay men and people from developing countries have a history of past exposure to HAV, so the prevalence of anti-HAV IgG seropositivity is correspondingly high in HIV-positive people from these populations	• HIV and HBV both transmitted sexually and by sharing contaminated needles • Reports of failure to develop protective antibody after vaccination in HIV infected people are high (perhaps as high as 40%–80%)	• Recently, new cases of HCV infection have been reported after treatment with IVIG used to treat thrombocytopenia • Not generally transmitted from mother to fetus; however, coinfection with HIV may increase transmission risk	• As sexual transmission and contact with infected body secretions is primary mode of transmission of both HIV and HBV, infection with HDV is also a risk • Coinfection with HDV and HIV leads to a worsening of liver disease	• Since HEV infection may cause severe disease in pregnant women, it is possible that the immune suppression associated with HIV might lead to more serious disease than would otherwise be expected

Table 4.3 Continued

Hepatitis A	Hepatitis B	Hepatitis C	Hepatitis D	Hepatitis E
• HIV is not known to adversely affect the course of acute HAV infection, nor does HAV have any known impact on the progression of HIV disease	• In some high risk groups, 50%–75% of HBsAg-positive are also HIV positive • Patients with advanced HIV/AIDS are at higher risk of becoming chronic carriers than HIV negative people (Broder, Merigan, & Bolognesi, 1994) • HIV and HBV may infect the same liver cells, thus adding to viral reproduction and failure of the immune response to clear acute HBV infection • HIV may also cause reactivation of HBV replication (Broder et al., 1994)	• Hemophiliacs with HCV and HIV coinfection may prematurely progress to fulminant hepatitis and liver failure, some as quickly as within 3 years of onset	• HIV has also been shown to decrease the antibody response to HDV and episodes of reactivation with elevated transaminases has been reported	• This relationship is currently speculative; no actual cases reported to date

Morbidity and mortality

Hepatitis A	Hepatitis B	Hepatitis C	Hepatitis D	Hepatitis E

• Usually subclinical in children, may be acute in adults, but rarely causes a fulminant hepatitis
• HAV does not cause a persistent infection or a chronic carrier state
• Both icteric and non-icteric HAV infections possible
• HAV infection results in a solid immune response and confers lifetime immunity from further infection
	• Most HBV infections are self-limiting, and resolve within 6 months; 25% are acute icteric illnesses
	• Chronic active hepatitis (CAH): 10% of acute infections persist as chronic infection (carrier state)
	  - LFT elevations and HBsAg persist >6 months
	  - HBeAg persisting >10 weeks also predicts persistent infection
		• Chronic HCV hepatitis develops within 9–48 months in >60% of the HCV infected (may be 70%–90%)
		• Chronic HCV infection may progress to cirrhosis and hepatocellular carcinoma, usually up to 20 years after initial infection
		• Chronic HCV and alcohol abuse may act synergistically in the development of chronic liver disease
			• Superinfection of chronic HBV carrier results in a severe acute hepatitis, with frequent and rapid progression to cirrhosis
			• Risk of hepatocellular carcinoma is not strongly associated with HDV infection
				• No known chronic carrier state
				• No associated chronic illness
				• Carries a high mortality rate in pregnant women due to fulminant hepatitis and disseminated intravascular coagulation (10%–20% fatality rate); mechanism unknown
				• It is not known whether HEV infection confers lifelong immunity

continued

Table 4.3 *Continued*

Hepatitis A	Hepatitis B	Hepatitis C	Hepatitis D	Hepatitis E
• Mortality from fulminant HAV infection remains high (probably >50%) • Case fatality rate reported as 0.015%	- 10% of persons with CAH progress to liver cirrhosis or hepatocellular carcinoma • Chronic persistent hepatitis (CPH) is not considered progressive • HBV causes more than 10,000 hospitalizations and 250 deaths per year (due to fulminant hepatitis and hepatic failure)	• Chronic HDV infection occurs in about 90% of patients • Little evidence to suggest that HCV is capable of causing a fulminant hepatitis • May be the cause of about 13,000 deaths per year from chronic liver disease		

Early detection, prevention, prophylaxis

Hepatitis A	Hepatitis B	Hepatitis C	Hepatitis D	Hepatitis E
• Serologic evidence of acute infection (anti-HAV IgM); routine screening of asymptomatic individuals is not recommended • Individuals (see *Other important information*, below) may be passively immunized with Ig • Ig is effective for both pre- and postexposure prophylaxis • Prevention is best accomplished by personal hygiene, sanitation measures avoiding fecal contamination of water and food; safer sex practices (avoiding oral-anal sexual contact—"insertive rimming")	• Screening of people at risk for anti-HBs and HBsAg as part of baseline and annual evaluation • Screening of donor blood • HBV vaccination is highly recommended and effective (90%–95% of people successfully develop protective antibody—anti-HBs) • Vaccination of all infants and 10-year-olds is hoped to significantly reduce the incidence of HBV infections over the next 20 years • Prior infection with HBV with development of anti-HBs confers life-long immunity to reinfection • Vaccine nonresponders	• Screening people at risk, for serologic evidence of HCV infection • Screening of donor blood • No vaccination available at present • Unfortunately, about 0.3%–0.7% of blood transfusions continue to be HCV infected as current antibody screening tests do not detect all infectious donors • The use of predonation, auto transfusion with salvaged blood decreases or eliminates transfusion-associated risk	• HDVAg cannot be detected until HBsAg begins to circulate as an early marker of HBV infection • Prevention of HDV infection closely follows prevention of HBV infection by the currently available HBV vaccines	• No recommendations for routine screening • Prevention of HEV infection is incumbent on strict sanitation practices in endemic areas and where overcrowding occurs (military camps, refugee camps) • No vaccine currently available

Table 4.3 *Continued*

	Hepatitis A	Hepatitis B	Hepatitis C	Hepatitis D	Hepatitis E
	• Food handlers must be excluded from work until the illness has resolved • HAV vaccine (FDA approved 2/95) is recommended for those traveling to HAV-endemic areas. Vaccine may be administered concurrently.	may receive a second 3-dose series; 50% may develop antibody • Anti-HBc may be the only marker between disappearance of HBsAg and appearance of anti-HBs (window period)			

Signs and symptoms

	Hepatitis A	Hepatitis B	Hepatitis C	Hepatitis D	Hepatitis E
	• Acute onset of malaise (80%) or fatigue, anorexia, weight loss (82%), abdominal pain, transient fever, headache, N&V • Occasional myalgias and arthralgias, rash • Jaundice (84%) and hepatomegaly (87%) • Dark-colored urine, clay-colored stools common • Epigastric or RUQ pain may occur • Cholestasis (fever, marked pruritus due to elevated bilirubin, prolonged jaundice) is more common than in HBV infection	• Insidious onset of anorexia, abdominal pain, nausea and vomiting, mild fever, headache and malaise • Occasional arthralgias, rash • Jaundice • Severity varies widely, from subclinical to fulminant • Right upper quadrant tenderness is not unusual, and may be associated with hepatomegaly	• Insidious onset of anorexia, nausea and vomiting, and jaundice • Course similar to HBV, and may be milder than acute HBV infection, but may also be more prolonged • 75% of cases are anicteric	• Insidious onset of anorexia, abdominal pain, nausea and vomiting, mild fever, headache and malaise • Occasional arthralgias, rash • Jaundice • A more severe or fulminant course of hepatitis is seen in HBV-HDV coinfection • 14% of cases of fulminant hepatitis due to HBV infection are also positive for HDVAg • 20%–60% of people with chronic HDV infection progress to cirrhosis within 2–6 years	• Sudden onset of fever, malaise, nausea and vomiting, headache, abdominal pain, and anorexia • Variable severity; ranges from a mild illness of 7–10 days duration to a rare, severely disabling condition lasting several months • Jaundice, hepatomegaly may occur • Clinical course is similar to HAV infection

Diagnosis

	Hepatitis A	Hepatitis B	Hepatitis C	Hepatitis D	Hepatitis E
	• Histology: Focal necrosis of hepatocytes, Kupffer cell proliferation, acidophilic bodies, ballooning degeneration	• Histology: Similar, but more pronounced, as in HAV • Tests/procedures; elevated LFTs and bilirubin; positive	• Histology: Abnormal hepatocytes (vacuoles, tubules, and proliferated endoplasmic reticulum) and inflammatory	• Histology: See HCV • Tests/procedures: Serologic test for anti-HDV IgG is readily available	• Histology: Hepatitis necrosis • Tests/procedures: Elevated LFTs (particularly ALT), positive serologic markers for

continued ➧

Table 4.3 *Continued*

Hepatitis A	Hepatitis B	Hepatitis C	Hepatitis D	Hepatitis E

• Tests/procedures
  - Elevated LFTs particularly aminotransferases (ALT, AST), at >2.5 times the upper limits of normal
  - Serologic marker for acute HAV infection is anti-HAV IgM (RIA)
• Staging: Not applicable
• Differential diagnosis
  - Acute viral hepatitis infections
  - Chronic active or persistent hepatitis
  - Chemical-, drug-, or alcohol-induced hepatitis
  - Leptospirosis
  - Obstruction
• liver biopsy may be warranted in severely ill patients
	serologic markers (see standard infectious disease texts for descriptions and time course of serologic markers)
	  - HBsAg: HBV surface antigen
	  - Anti-HBs: HBV surface antibody
	  - Anti-HBc IgM: HBV core antibody IgM
	  - HBeAg: HBV e antigen
	  - Anti-HBe; HBV e antibody
	  - Liver biopsy
	• Staging
	  - Acute HBV infection
	  - Persistent HBsAg 10% (chronic active hepatitis 30%, chronic persistent hepatitis 70%)
	• Differential diagnosis: See HAV
		infiltrates on liver biopsy
		• Tests/procedures
		  - Elevated LFTs (ALT), positive serologic markers
		  - First generation: ELISA
		  - Second generation: Recombinant immunoblot assay (RIBA), more sensitive and specific, detects core protein antibody and nonstructural protein antigens of HCV
		  - An experimental HCV RNA PCR is in development
		  - Liver biopsy
		• Staging
		  - Acute HCV infection
		  - Chronic active HCV liver disease
		• Differential diagnosis: See HAV
			• Staging
			  - Concurrent acute HBV-HDV infection
			  - Chronic δ hepatitis diagnosed by presence of HBsAg, anti-HDV
			• Differential diagnosis:
			  Other than in research, HDV testing is warranted only in cases of known acute or chronic fulminant HBV hepatitis
				HEV (anti-HEV IgM, IgG), although commercial tests are not readily available
				• Staging: None known
				• Differential diagnosis: See HAV

Treatment

Hepatitis A	Hepatitis B	Hepatitis C	Hepatitis D	Hepatitis E

• Primary prophylaxis: Passive immunization with injection of immune globulin (see *Other important information*, below)
• Secondary prophylaxis: Ig injection is frequently offered by local health departments to patrons exposed to HAV-infected food handlers or food sources
	• Primary prophylaxis: HBV vaccination has been available since 1981; monitor donor blood supply for HBsAg
	• Secondary prophylaxis:
	Postexposure treatment with hepatitis B immune globulin (HBIG) for single, percutaneous exposures and infants born to HBsAg-positive mothers
		• Primary prophylaxis: No vaccination available at present; monitor donor blood supply for HCV and elevated LFTs; heat treat clotting factor concentrates
		• Secondary prophylaxis: None known
		• Acute treatment
		  - Supportive (see previous descriptions)
			• Primary prophylaxis: No vaccination available at present, although prevention of primary HBV infection by vaccine theoretically prevents HDV infection
			• Secondary prophylaxis: None known
			• Acute treatment
			  - Supportive (see previous descriptions)
				• Primary prophylaxis: Clean water supply, sanitary disposal and handling of feces; no vaccine currently available
				• Secondary prophylaxis: None known
				• Acute treatment: Supportive only (see previous descriptions)
				• No specific antiviral therapy currently recommended

Table 4.3 *Continued*

Hepatitis A	Hepatitis B	Hepatitis C	Hepatitis D	Hepatitis E
• Acute treatment - Supportive care: Maintain adequate caloric intake and balanced diet, rest, fluids, diet based on palatability, avoidance of alcohol; bed rest is not required and has concomitant risks - Hospitalization only for severe illness, as in fulminant hepatitis, encephalopathy, bleeding • Maintenance: Not required	• Acute treatment - Supportive care: See HAV - INF-α - Corticosteroids have been used, but less favorable outcomes may result (e.g., may accelerate HBV replication) - Other antiviral agents (Ara-A) have been studied • Maintenance - INF-α for chronic hepatitis - Equivocal reduction of chronicity	- INF-α 3/week for 6 months results in ALT reductions in 40%–70% of patients, although more than half relapse within the first few months • Maintenance - Benefit of INF-α for chronic hepatitis or prevention of liver cancer are unknown at present - Long-term response rate may be as low as 20%	- INF-α qd or 3/week; discontinue treatment if ALT decreases within 3 months, otherwise continue for up to a year • Maintenance: May continue with INF-α 3/week for 12 months	• Maintenance: Not applicable since chronic state unknown

Laboratory results and other indices to monitor for side effects, adverse effects, and response to therapy

Hepatitis A	Hepatitis B	Hepatitis C	Hepatitis D	Hepatitis E
• Serial LFTs and bilirubin, PT, albumin/globulin • Serum anti-HAV IgM is usually gone by 6 months after infection • Serum anti-HAV IgG usually persists for life	• Serial LFTs and bilirubin, PT, albumin/globulin • Serial serologies to note development of anti-HBs, anti-HBc, or persistence of HBsAg and HBeAg after 6 months • INF-α therapy is associated with low-grade fevers and arthralgias after each injection for the first 2–3 weeks of therapy; other side effects include fatigue, diarrhea, depression • Concomitant use of NSAIDs will often ameliorate the side effects associated with INF-α therapy	• Serial LFTs and bilirubin, PT, albumin/globulin • SGOT elevated for >6 months associated with persistent anti-HCV RIBA may warrant GI referral for liver biopsy and possible treatment with INF-α • See HBV for care of patient on INF-α	• Anti-HDV IgM persists in people with unremitting or progressive liver disease but declines or disappears in patients whose disease improves or resolves • Anti-HDV IgM peaks at about 20 days after infection, and is gone by about 60 days after infection • Anti HDV IgG starts to appear about 20 days after infection; usually peaks by day 40–50	• Serial LFTs and bilirubin, PT, albumin/globulin • See previous discussions of fulminant hepatitis caused by other viruses

continued

Table 4.3 *Continued*

Hepatitis A	Hepatitis B	Hepatitis C	Hepatitis D	Hepatitis E
	• Patients should be followed closely for support in self-injection techniques, as well as proper handling of contaminated sharps			

Other important information and patient education

Hepatitis A	Hepatitis B	Hepatitis C	Hepatitis D	Hepatitis E
• Susceptible individuals who would benefit from passive immunization (see package insert for dosing recommendations) - Travelers to endemic areas - Close personal contacts (household, sexual) of people with HAV infection - Day care center staff where diapered children attend - Patrons when a hepatitis A-infected food handler or food source is identified • Passive immunization confers immunity for 4–6 months, takes 2 weeks to develop protective antibody • Active immunization with HAV vaccine now available (see manufacturer recommendations for vaccine candidates and schedule information)	• Safer sex practices, limiting numbers of sexual partners, use of latex condoms, not sharing tooth brushes, razors • Use of needle-exchange programs is recommended for active IDUs • The high cost of HBV vaccine (around $180 for the series) may be the primary factor limiting widespread use • Anti-HBs is the only marker detectable in people who have been vaccinated against HBV • HCWs not responding to vaccination (i.e., no detectable anti-HBs) must be treated with HBIG for HBV exposures • For care of HBV-positive needle-sticks, the reader is urged to seek out readily available resources elsewhere	• USPHS recommends not sharing toothbrushes, razors • Universal blood and body fluid precautions (UP) are appropriate • No current recommendations address sexual and perinatal transmission • New techniques for solvent-detergent treatment of blood products inactivates contaminating viruses • No reports of HCV infection from IM immune-globulin products	• Perinatal transmission of HDV, although not extensively studied, does not appear to be very efficient • As noted above, preventing HBV infection by vaccination or UP is effective as prevention against HDV infection as well	• Health education must include emphasis on avoiding fecal contamination of water sources • Travelers to endemic areas should take special precautions to avoid contaminated water supplies

d. JCV also found in uroepithelial cells, B lymphocytes in bone marrow and spleen, and in peripheral blood lymphocytes

e. Only patients with a high degree of immunosuppression (e.g., late-stage HIV disease, lymphoproliferative diseases, patients treated with immunosuppressive therapies) are likely to develop PML

3. Frequency and distribution
   a. JCV infection is widespread in the general population
   b. 4%–5% of patients with advanced HIV disease will develop PML
   c. PML has been seen primarily in AIDS patients ages 20–50
   d. PML may be more prevalent in gay and bisexual men than in IDUs

4. Relationship to national history of HIV disease
   a. PML was described in AIDS patients as early as 1982
   b. PML is presumed to be a consequence of reactivation of latent JCV infection when the patient becomes profoundly immunosuppressed
   c. It is speculated that infected B-lymphocytes carry JCV across the blood-brain barrier into the brain

5. Morbidity and mortality
   a. In most cases there is a progressive decline over a period of months (rarely more than 4–6) until death
   b. There are reports of improvement and stabilization of disease in biopsy-proven PML patients following intrathecal cytosine arabinosine

6. Early detection, prevention, prophylaxis
   a. Primary prophylaxis
      (1) No current recommended regimen; seroprevalence of JCV is very high in urban populations
      (2) Low-dose heparin sulfate may be of some use in reducing transport of JCV-infected B lymphocytes across the blood-brain barrier; may theoretically be of value as a preventive strategy
   b. Routine screening for presence of JCV in AIDS patients is not done, given the

slow growth of the virus in tissue culture
   c. No special precautions required

7. Signs and symptoms
   a. PML presents typically with a focal neurologic deficit, evidenced as a visual disturbance, cognitive abnormality, or weakness
      (1) Weakness is found in most patients, hemiparesis in many; ataxia, hemisensory deficit, bradykinesia, and rigidity also occur
      (2) Neuro-ophthalmic lesions may occur, with cortical blindness manifesting in late-stage disease
      (3) Severe dysarthria, dysphasia, and dystonia are a consequence of basal ganglia lesions
   b. Other manifestations of PML
      (1) Decreased attention and memory
      (2) Confusion
      (3) Personality change
      (4) Dementia
      (5) Diplopia
      (6) Mono-, hemi-, or quadriplegia
      (7) Sensory deficits (face, arm numbness)
      (8) Headache, vertigo, seizures, coma
      (9) Alien hand syndrome
   c. A protracted clinical course is typical (acutely altered consciousness or other signs of acute encephalitis are unusual)

8. Diagnosis
   a. Histology
      (1) Triad of multifocal demyelination; inclusion-bearing, swollen, oligodendrocyte nuclei; and bizarre pleomorphic, lobulated hyperchromatic astrocytes
      (2) Oligodendrocyte inclusions are JCV nucleocapsids
      (3) Inflammation not usually significant
   b. Tests/procedures
      (1) Clinical presentation of focal neurologic findings
      (2) Neuroimaging (brain MRI with and without gadolinium enhancement) is highly suggestive of the diagnosis
         (a) Lesions tend to be nonenhancing; range in size from 1 mm to several centimeters; predominate

in parieto-occipital lobes, but may be anywhere
  (b) Mass effect not usually present
  (c) MRI is superior to CT, as white-matter lesions are often adjacent to the cortex and most evident on T2-weighted images
  (d) Neurologic deficits should correlate with the neuroimaging findings, although the patient may appear worse than evidenced by the scan
  (3) Brain biopsy necessary for definitive diagnosis; stereotactic brain biopsy may be useful for easily accessed lesions
  (4) Diagnosis often confirmed at autopsy
  (5) EEG usually shows diffuse and nonspecific slowing
  (6) Because of the high prevalence of JCV in the population, serology (serum or CSF) is not useful as a diagnostic test
  c. Differential diagnosis: Cerebral toxoplasmosis, primary CNS lymphoma, AIDS dementia complex, CMV encephalitis, HSV encephalitis, VZV encephalitis, neurosyphilis, MTB
9. Treatment
  a. No currently accepted treatment for PML
  b. Some studies have investigated treatments in patients with nucleoside analog antiretrovirals (AZT), gamma-interferon, cytosine arabinoside, and IUDR (NSC-39661)
  c. Other drugs have undergone laboratory testing (cytosine b-D arabinofuranoside, camptothecin)
  d. Further experimental investigations are underway; refer patients to experimental protocols whenever available
10. Laboratory results and other indices to monitor for side effects, adverse effects, and response to therapy
  a. Rapid progression of dementia, weakness, and other physical symptoms
  b. Loss of function, mobility, self-care capacity; decreased ability to effectively communicate with others

  c. The impairments progress rapidly and patients may ultimately develop seizures and lapse into coma shortly prior to death
11. Patient education
  a. Critical to support and counsel patient and significant others with regard to expected course
    (1) Urgent arrangements for home care, hospice, or nursing home placement are necessary due to the rapidly progressive nature of PML
    (2) Planning with advance directives is of paramount importance
    (3) Anticipatory grief counseling and arranging for a peaceful death with dignity in the presence of loved ones
  b. See *Grief and Loss*, p. 253, *Powerlessness*, p. 267

F. Epstein-Barr Virus

1. Specific etiologic agent and disease process
  a. Epstein-Barr virus (EBV) thought to cause infectious mononucleosis (IM), EBV infection, Burkitt's lymphoma, nasopharyngeal carcinoma, chronic fatigue syndrome (CFS), oral hairy leukoplakia; latent EBV infection reappears in the immunosuppressed or with advancing age
  b. Belongs to the herpes group of viruses: Classified as human herpesvirus 4 from the subfamily of gammaherpesvirinae (variable growth cycle, lymphoproliferative, establish latent infections in the lymphoid tissue)
  c. Gains access to body through oropharynx
  d. Infects B lymphocytes (have specific receptors for EBV)
    (1) Causes rapid replication and multiplication, which results in corresponding increase in the number of T-suppressor lymphocytes, which try to inhibit B cell growth
    (2) T cells may identify and attack EBV-infected latent cells, releasing EB nuclear antigen (EBNA), leading to development of antibodies

(3) Other B lymphocytes develop spontaneous lysis, release EBNA, and perpetuate infection

(4) Primary sites of replication are epithelial cells of the oropharynx, parotid gland, uterine cervix

e. Following infection, the virus disseminates by viremia or by circulating B cells

2. Risk, transmissibility, and source of infection: Transmission is by intimate (oral, sexual) contact

a. EBV occasionally transmitted through blood transfusions

b. EBV is shed continuously in the saliva of IM-infected people during the first 3–6 months

c. Years later 5%–20% of healthy people still shed the virus in their saliva (increases to 25%–50% in the immunosuppressed) (Fleisher, 1991)

d. Primary EBV infection is expressed clinically as IM infection, usually in later childhood or adolescence

e. It is desirable that EBV be contracted in early childhood to prevent clinical infection and the complication of IM as an adult

3. Frequency and distribution

a. EBV distributed globally, infecting populations in every climate

(1) Seropositivity dependent on socioeconomic factors; densely populated areas at greater risk and have greater seroconversion

(2) Less densely populated areas show less seropositivity until the age of puberty and intimacy

b. Estimates of rate of infection with EBV producing IM vary

(1) Socioeconomic factors of age, population density, and economic affluence determine incidence rate of IM

(2) IM develops sporadically over various age groups according to ages of highest risk for oral contact

(a) Incidence higher in adolescents of high school age and in college age youths

(b) Epidemics are common where eating utensils are shared

(3) Seropositivity with EBV does not necessarily lead to IM; EBV infection is often silent, leaving only seropositivity and risk of latent clinical expression

4. Relationship to natural history of HIV disease

a. EBV expressed in oral hairy leukoplakia as the EBV replicates itself on the tongues of HIV-positive patients

b. EBV is suspect as cause of CFS that is prevalent and debilitating in HIV infection and AIDS; research (Miller, 1991) shows that some people with acute CFS do not develop antibodies to the EBV antigen EBNA-1 (could be the pathology present in the HIV-infected)

c. EBV infection can be fatal in patient with HIV/AIDS and in the severely immunosuppression by causing complication illnesses (e.g., lymphoma)

d. Increased risk of EBV-induced lymphoproliferative disease resulting in multiclonal lymphomas, diffuse polyclonal lymphomas, lymphocytic interstitial pneumonitis, and oral hairy leukoplakia

e. Lymphomas often do not resemble Burkitt's in HIV infection

5. Morbidity and mortality

a. Secondary infections with *Streptococcus* are common in the nose and throat

b. Mortality uncommon in the healthy and infrequent in the immunosuppressed client

c. Death can occur in the immunosuppressed

6. Signs and symptoms

a. Early symptoms: Fever, malaise, pharyngeal pain, headaches, sore throat, nausea, vomiting, abdominal pain, and myalgia

b. Major signs of IM are fever (most common), pharyngitis, adenopathy, and splenomegaly

c. Possible complications

(1) Neurologic: Rare cases of Guillain-Barré syndrome, encephalitis, neuritis, optic neuritis, depression (common), and psychosis (rare)

(2) GI: Hepatitis (frequent) due to infiltration of the liver by lymphocytes, mesenteric lymphadenopathy, abdominal pain

(3) Hematologic: Aplastic anemia, pancytopenia, thrombocytopenia, abnormal platelet function

(4) Cardiac: Disturbances in conduction, dysrhythmias, cardiomyopathy

7. Diagnosis
   a. EBV serology provides a definitive diagnosis of primary EBV infection; diagnosis and serologic status are determined by the presence or disappearance by time line of antibodies against parts of the EBV antigen
      (1) Viral recovery does not distinguish between new and prior infections
      (2) EBV can be recovered in the saliva of seropositive, healthy people as well as people with IM
   b. Specific for diagnosing IM are the heterophil antibody (HA) test and WBC 10,000–20,000 U/L, lymphocytosis absolute count and a percentage above 50%, atypical lymphocytes on smear (10% and 20% of WBCs), and absolute and relative neutropenia
   c. Differential diagnosis of IM made by the combination of clinical presentation and a positive HA test
      (1) HA negative: Other conditions cannot be ruled out until the EBV-specific serology defines EBV infection
      (2) Rule out: CMV, toxoplasmosis, viral hepatitis, rubella, and streptococcal pharyngitis (Fleisher, 1991)

8. Treatment (general)
   a. Bed rest during the acute phase (1–4 weeks); alternate rest periods with mild activity in recuperating phases
   b. Acetaminophen for antipyretic
   c. Avoidance of physically strenuous activity until spleen returns to normal
   d. Brief corticosteroid therapy for inflammation, fever, tonsilar hypertrophy, and lymphadenopathy in the more severely ill
   e. Acyclovir is administered with some benefit

9. Laboratory results and other indices to monitor for side effects, adverse effects, and response to therapy
   a. WBC, differential
   b. LFTs

c. Renal, cardiovascular and respiratory systems status

10. Patient education
    a. Disease process
    b. Virus transmission
    c. Health maintenance: Medications, diet, avoid extremely heavy physical activity. avoid stress, avoid oral contact with others

G. Human Herpesvirus 6

1. Specific etiologic agent and disease process
   a. Human herpesvirus 6 (HHV-6) is a gamma herpesvirus (same subfamily as Epstein-Barr virus, HHV-4), a large, slow-growing DNA virus
   b. Initially named human B-lymphotropic virus (HBLV); discovered in 1986 from blood of patients with lymphoproliferative disorders
   c. HHV-6 is the etiologic agent for exanthem subitum (roseola infantum), which is also called rose rash of infancy, or sixth disease
   d. Closely related to CMV, but cross-reactivity between HHV-6 and CMV antibodies has not been observed
   e. There are two subtypes, HHV-6a and HHV-6b

2. Risk, transmissibility, and source of infection
   a. HHV-6 is probably a common agent, transmitted by blood and saliva
   b. Shares epidemiologic features with other herpes group viruses
   c. Incubation period after acute infection is about 10 days (range 5–15 days)

3. Frequency and distribution
   a. Most people acquire antibodies to HHV-6 in the first year of life
   b. The virus appears to be ubiquitous, as evidenced by the high prevalence of antibody in the general worldwide population
   c. Incidence may be highest in the spring

4. Relationship to natural history of HIV disease
   a. HHV-6 may be a cofactor for progression of HIV disease by up-regulating the HIV long terminal repeat segment

and enhancing HIV expression in at least one tissue culture system (Stoeckle, 1995)

b. Epidemiologic studies do not yet support a significant role for HHV-6 and acceleration of HIV infection in vivo (Stoeckle, 1995)

c. May be the cause of some B cell lymphomas

d. HHV-6a is thought to be associated with chronic fatigue syndrome and HIV

5. Morbidity and mortality: No data available

6. Early detection, prevention, prophylaxis
   a. No known prophylaxis or prevention
   b. Detection by demonstration of anti-HHV-6 IgM and IgG

7. Signs and symptoms
   a. Primary infection: Exanthema subitum is a benign disease in infants (6–24 months) characterized by a high fever and a faint, nonpruritic maculopapular rash that begins on the trunk and spreads to rest of body; acute illness usually lasts 3–5 days
   b. Acute HHV-6 infection has been reported in adults
      (1) Presentation included cervical lymphadenopathy, dull headache, slight fatigue, mild sore throat
      (2) Modest elevations of LFTs (SGOT), moderate leukopenia with increased monocytes and atypical lymphocytes were noted

      (3) Lymphadenopathy lasted 1–3 months

8. Diagnosis
   a. Tests/procedures
      (1) Serology: Detection of anti-HHV-6 IgM and IgG
      (2) Enzyme-linked immunosorbent assay (ELISA)
      (3) Indirect immunofluorescence
      (4) DNA hybridization
      (5) Polymerase chain reaction (PCR)
   b. Differential diagnosis: Other febrile, viral exanthems of childhood, allergic drug reactions; in adults, need to rule out other viral diseases and causes of lymphadenopathy

9. Treatment
   a. Supportive care to include antipyretics for fever, fluids, rest; isolation not required
   b. Adults with acute HHV-6 infection and severe illness may respond to antiviral treatment with both ganciclovir and foscarnet; acyclovir was less effective against HHV-6

10. Patient education
    a. Information and research development about primary and latent HHV-6 infection remains in early stages
    b. A recently isolated new virus, HHV-7, may cause a disease similar to exanthem subitum.

V. PARASITIC INFECTIONS

A. Pneumocystis

1. Specific etiologic agent and disease process
   a. *Pneumocystis carinii,* a unicellular protozoan with DNA structure similar to a fungus
   b. Parasite attaches to pneumocyte, replicates, and invades the epithelium of the lung
   c. Immunosuppressed hosts are unable to mount an alveolar macrophage defense
   d. Pneumonia develops, followed by decrease in lung surfactant
   e. In PWAs, PCP generally represents a reactivation of latent disease or recrudescence of inadequately treated disease
2. Risk, transmissibility, and source of infection
   a. Risk associated with immune function: Higher in those with compromised immune function (HIV, chemotherapy, malnutrition)
   b. Most people have had subclinical infections by age 4
   c. Some evidence that *P. carinii* can be transmitted between rats, but few data to show transmission between humans
3. Frequency and distribution
   a. Worldwide distribution
   b. Endemic in Iran, Korea, and Vietnam; malnourished children most often affected
   c. Among PWAs, PCP is less common in Africa and Haiti
   d. PCP is most common manifestation of AIDS in developed countries; overall, prophylactic regimens have led to a decline in incidence
4. Relationship to natural history of HIV disease
   a. Most common in patients with CD4+ lymphocyte counts <200/μl or with CD4+ lymphocyte percentage <14
   b. Presence of oral thrush or persistent fevers associated with higher incidence of PCP, even with higher CD4+ lymphocyte counts
   c. Asplenic patients may develop PCP earlier in the course of HIV disease
   d. May be seen in third trimester of pregnancy due to physiologic drop in CD4+ lymphocyte count
   e. Patients who are immunosuppressed for other reasons (steroids, chemotherapy) may develop PCP earlier in their HIV course
5. Morbidity and mortality
   a. Early in epidemic, majority of patients developed and succumbed to PCP
   b. In the U.S., still most common AIDS-defining illness among the medically underserved (secondary to lack of prophylaxis)
   c. Up to 60% of HIV-infected people will develop PCP at some point in their illness
   d. Survival
      (1) Mild to moderate PCP, 86%–94%
      (2) Severe infection, 40%–50%
6. Early detection, prevention, prophylaxis
   a. No effective way of eliminating or limiting exposure
   b. Identify those at risk, institute chemoprophylaxis as appropriate
   c. Monitor for signs and symptoms of early disease
   d. Baseline chest x-ray not a standard of practice
   e. Primary prophylaxis: TMP-SMX (preferred therapy)—see Tables 4.4 and 4.5
      (1) Dapsone
      (2) Aerosolized pentamidine inhaled via nebulizer q4–6wks
      (3) Anecdotal/investigational protocols include dapsone/pyrimethamine, meter-dose pentamidine, atovaquone, trimethoprim, parenteral pentamidine
7. Signs and symptoms
   a. Pulmonary disease
      (1) Most common symptoms are low-grade fever, nonproductive cough and dyspnea (initially with exertion, later in illness, at rest)
      (2) Dry rales may be present on auscultation
      (3) Symptoms are insidious and slowly progress over the course of a few weeks

Text continues on page 118

Table 4.4   Prophylaxis for First Episode of Opportunistic Disease in HIV-Infected Adults and Adolescents

Pathogen	Indication	Preventive Regimens First Choice	Alternatives

I. Strongly recommended as standard of care

Pathogen	Indication	First Choice	Alternatives
P. carinii[1]	CD4+ count <200/μl *or* unexplained fever for >2 wks *or* oropharyngeal candidiasis	TMP-SMX, 1 DS po qd (AI)*	TMP-SMX, 1 SS po qd (AI) *or* 1 DS po tiw (AII); dapsone, 50 mg po bid or 100 mg po qd (AI); dapsone, 50 mg po qd, *plus* pyrimethamine, 50 mg po qw, *plus* leucovorin, 25 mg po qw (AI); dapsone, 200 mg po qw, *plus* pyrimethamine, 75 mg po qw, *plus* leucovorin, 25 mg po qw (AI); aerosolized pentamidine, 300 mg qm via Respirgard II nebulizer (AI)
M. tuberculosis[2] Isoniazid (INH)-sensitive	TST reaction of ≥5 mm *or* prior positive TST result without treatment *or* contact with case of active TB	INH, 300 mg po, *plus* pyridoxine, 50 mg po qd x 12 mo (AI); *or* INH, 900 mg po, *plus* pyridoxine, 50 mg po biw x 12 mo (BIII)	Rifampin, 600 mg po qd x 12 mo (BII)
INH-resistant	Same as above; high probability of exposure to INH-resistant TB	Rifampin, 600 mg po qd x 12 mo (BII)	Rifabutin, 300 mg po qd x 12 mo (CIII)
Multidrug-resistant (INH and rifampin)	Same as above; high probability of exposure to MDR-TB	Choice of drugs requires consultation with public health authorities	None
Toxoplasma gondii[3]	IgG antibody to *Toxoplasma* and CD4+ count of <100/μl	TMP-SMX, 1 DS po qd (AII)	TMP-SMX, 1 SS po qd *or* 1 DS po tiw (AII); dapsone, 50 mg po qd, *plus* pyrimethamine, 50 mg po qw, *plus* leucovorin, 25 mg po qw (AI)

continued ▶

Table 4.4   *Continued*

Pathogen	Indication	Preventive Regimens	
		First Choice	Alternatives
II. Recommended for consideration in all patients			
Streptococcus pneumoniae[4]	All patients	Pneumococcal vaccine, 0.5 ml IM x 1(BII)	None
M. avium complex[5]	CD4+ count <75/μl	Rifabutin, 300 mg po qd (BII)	Clarithromycin, 500 mg po bid (CIII); azithromycin, 500 mg po tiw (CIII)
III. Not recommended for most patients; indicated for consideration only in selected populations or patients			
Bacteria	Neutropenia	Granulocyte colony-stimulating factor (CSF), 5–10 μg/Kg SC qd x 2–4w; *or* granulocyte-macrophage CSF, 250 μg/m², IV over 2h qd x 2–4w (CIII)	None
Candida species	CD4+ count <50/μl	Fluconazole, 100–200 mg po qd (C1)	Ketoconazole, 200 mg po qd (CIII)
Cryptococcus neoformans[6]	CD4+ count <50/μl	Fluconazole, 200 mg po qd (B1)	Itraconazole, 200 mg po qd (CIII)
Histoplasma capsulatum[6]	CD4+ count <50/μl, endemic geographic area	Itraconazole, 200 mg po qd (CIII)	Fluconazole, 200 mg po qd (CIII)
Coccidioides immitis[6]	CD4+ count <50/μl, endemic geographic area	Fluconazole, 200 mg po qd (CIII)	Itraconazole, 200 mg po qd (CIII)
CMV[7]	CD4+ count <50/μl and CMV antibody positive	Oral ganciclovir, 1 g po tid (CIII; only preliminary data available)	None
Unknown (herpesviruses?)[8]	CD4+ count <200/μl	Acyclovir, 800 mg po qid (CIII)	Acyclovir, 200 mg po tid/qid (CIII)
IV. Recommended for consideration[9]			
Hepatitis B virus[4]	All susceptible (anti-HBc-negative) patients	Energix-B, 20 μg IM x 3 (BII); *or* Recombivax HB, 10 μg IM x 3 (BII)	None
Influenza virus[4]	All patients (annually, before influenza season)	Whole or split virus, 0.5 ml IM/y (BIII)	Rimantadine, 100 mg po bid (CIII); *or* amantadine, 100 mg po bid (CIII)

continued ▶

Table 4.4 *Continued*

*Letters and Roman numerals in parentheses after regimens indicate the strength of the recommendation and the quality of the evidence supporting it (adapted from Gross, P., Barrett, T., Dellinger, P., et al., 1994, "Purpose of quality standards for infectious diseases," *Clinical Infectious Diseases, 18,* 421):

A Both strong evidence and substantial clinical benefit support a recommendation for use

B Moderate evidence—or strong evidence for only limited benefit—supports a recommendation for use

C Poor evidence supports a recommendation for or against use

D Moderate evidence supports a recommendation against use

E Good evidence supports a recommendation against use

I Evidence from at least one properly randomized, controlled trial

II Evidence from at least one well-designed clinical trial without randomization, from cohort or case-controlled analytic studies (preferably from more than one center), or from multiple time-series studies or dramatic results from uncontrolled experiments

III Evidence from opinions of respected authorities based on clinical experience, descriptive studies, or reports of expert committees

Note: Not all the recommended regimens reflect current FDA-approved labeling. Anti-HBC = antibody to hepatitis B core antigen; biw = twice weekly; CMV = cytomegalovirus; DS = double-strength tablet; qm = monthly; qw = weekly; ss = single-strength tablet; tiw = three times weekly; TMP-SMX = trimethoprim-sulfamethoxazole; and TST = tuberculin skin test. The Respirgard II nebulizer is manufactured by Marquest, Englewood, CO; Energix-B by SmithKline Beecham, Rixensart, Belgium; and Recombivax HB by Merck, West Point, PA.

[1] Patients receiving dapsone should be tested for G6PD deficiency. A dosage of 50 mg qd is probably less effective than a dosage of 100 mg gd. The efficacy of parenteral pentamidine (e.g., 4 mg/Kg/qm) is uncertain. Inadequate data are available on the efficacy and safety of atovaquone or clindamycin/primaquine. Sulfadoxine/pyrimethamine is rarely used because it can elicit severe hypersensitivity reactions. TMP-SMX and dapsone/pyrimethamine (and possibly dapsone alone) appear to be protective against toxoplasmosis. TMP-SMX may reduce the frequency of some bacterial infections. Patients receiving therapy for toxoplasmosis with sulfadoxine/pyrimethamine are protected against PCP and do not need TMP-SMX.

[2] Directly observed therapy is required for 900 mg of INH biw; INH regimens should include pyridoxine to prevent peripheral neuropathy. Exposure to MDR-TB may require prophylaxis with 2 drugs; consult public health authorities. Possible regimens include pyrazinamide plus either ethambutol or a fluoroquinolone.

[3] Protection against *T. gondii* is provided by the preferred antipneumocystis regimens. Pyrimethamine alone probably provides little, if any, protection. Dapsone alone cannot be recommended on the basis of currently available data.

[4] Data are inadequate concerning the clinical benefit of vaccines against *S. pneumoniae,* influenza virus, and hepatitis B virus in HIV-infected persons, although it is logical to assume that those patients who develop antibody responses will derive some protection. Some authorities are concerned that immunizations may stimulate the replication of HIV. Prophylaxis with TMP-SMX may provide some clinical benefit by reducing the frequency of bacterial infections, but the prevalence of *S. pneumoniae* resistant to TMP-SMX is increasing. Hepatitis B vaccine has been recommended for all children and adolescents and for all adults with risk factors for hepatitis B infection.

[5] Data on 500 mg of clarithromycin po bid have been presented but have not yet been thoroughly analyzed. Data on the efficacy and safety of azithromycin prophylaxis are not yet available.

[6] There may be a few unusual occupational or other circumstances under which prophylaxis should be considered; consult a specialist.

[7] Data on oral ganciclovir are still being evaluated; the durability of its effect is unclear. Acyclovir is not protective against CMV.

[8] Data regarding the efficacy of acyclovir for prolonging survival are controversial; if acyclovir is beneficial, the biologic basis for the effect and the optimal dose and timing of therapy are uncertain.

[9] These immunizations or chemoprophylactic regimens are not targeted against pathogens traditionally classified as opportunistic but should be considered for use in HIV-infected patients. While the use of those products is logical, their clinical efficacy has not been validated in this population.

[10] During outbreaks of influenza A.

Source: From "USPHS/IDSA guidelines for the prevention of opportunistic infections in persons infected with human immunodeficiency virus: A summary," by J. Kaplan et al., 1995, *MMWR, 44*(RR-8), 1–33.

Table 4.5   Prophylaxis for Recurrence of Opportunistic Disease (After Chemotherapy for Acute Disease) in HIV-Infected Adults and Adolescents

Pathogen	Indication	Preventive Regimens	
		First Choice	Alternatives
I. Recommended for life as standard of care			
P. carinii	Prior PCP	TMP-SMX, 1 DS po qd (AI)*	TMP-SMX, 1 SS po qd (AI) or 1 DS po tiw (AII); dapsone, 50 mg po bid or 100 mg po qd (AI); dapsone, 50 mg po qd, plus pyrimethamine, 50 mg qw, plus leucovorin, 25 mg po qw (AI); dapsone, 200 mg po qw, plus pyrimethamine, 75 mg po qw, plus leucovorin, 25 mg po qw (AI); aerosolized pentamidine, 300 mg qm via Respirgard II nebulizer (AI)
T. gondii[1]	Prior toxoplasmic encephalitis	Sulfadiazine, 1.0–1.5 g po q6h, plus pyrimethamine, 25–75 mg po qd, plus leucovorin, 10–25 mg po qd–qid (AII)	Clindamycin, 300–450 mg po q6–8h, plus pyrimethamine, 25–75 mg po qw, plus leucovorin, 10–25 mg po qd–qid (AII)
M. avium complex[2]	Documented disseminated disease	Clarithromycin, 500 mg po bid, plus one or more of the following: ethambutol, 15 mg/Kg po qd; clofazimine, 100 mg po qd; rifabutin, 300 mg po qd; ciprofloxacin, 500–750 mg po bid (BIII)	Azithromycin, 500 mg po qd, plus one or more of the following: ethambutol, 15 mg/Kg po qd; clofazimine, 100 mg po qd; rifabutin, 300 mg po qd; ciprofloxacin, 500–750 mg po bid (BIII)
CMV[3]	Prior end-organ disease	Ganciclovir, 5–6 mg/Kg IV 5–7 d/w or 1,000 mg po tid (AI); or foscarnet, 90–120 mg/Kg IV qd (AI)	Sustained-release implants used investigationally
C. neoformans	Documented disease	Fluconazole, 200 mg po (AI)	Itraconazole, 200 mg po qd (BIII); amphotericin B, 0.6–1.0 mg/Kg IV qw–tiw (AI)
H. capsulatum	Documented disease	Itraconazole, 200 mg po qd (AII)	Amphotericin B, 1.0 mg/Kg IV qw (AI); fluconazole, 200–400 mg po qd (BIII)

continued ▶

Table 4.5 *continued*

Pathogen	Indication	Preventive Regimens	
		First Choice	Alternatives
C. immitis	Documented disease	Fluconazole, 200 mg po qd (AII)	Amphotericin B, 1.0 mg/Kg IV qw (AI); itraconazole, 200 mg po bid (AI); ketoconazole, 400–800 mg po qd (BII)
Salmonella species (non-*typhi*)[4]	Bacteremia	Ciprofloxacin, 500 mg po bid for several months (BII)	

II. Recommended only if subsequent episodes are frequent or severe

Pathogen	Indication	First Choice	Alternatives
Herpes simplex virus	Frequent/severe recurrences	Acyclovir, 200 mg po tid *or* 40 mg po bid (AI)	
Candida species (oral, vaginal, or esophageal)	Frequent/severe recurrences	Fluconazole, 100–200 mg po qd (A1)	Ketoconazole, 200 mg po qd (BII); itraconazole, 100 mg po qd (BII); clotrimazole troche, 10 mg po 5x/d (BII); nystatin, 5 x 10^5 U po 5x/d (CIII)

*Letters and Roman numerals in parentheses after regimens indicate the strength of the recommendation and the quality of the evidence supporting it (adapted from Gross, P., Barrett, T., Dellinger, P., et al., 1994, "Purpose of quality standards for infectious diseases," *Clinical Infectious Diseases, 18,* 421):

A   Both strong evidence and substantial clinical benefit support a recommendation for use
B   Moderate evidence—or strong evidence for only limited benefit—supports a recommendation for use
C   Poor evidence supports a recommendation for or against use
D   Moderate evidence supports a recommendation against use
E   Good evidence supports a recommendation against use

I   Evidence from at least one properly randomized, controlled trial
II Evidence from at least one well-designed clinical trial without randomization, from cohort or case-controlled analytic studies (preferably from more than one center), or from multiple time-series studies or dramatic results from uncontrolled experiments
III Evidence from opinions of respected authorities based on clinical experience, descriptive studies, or reports of expert committees from uncontrolled experiments
III Evidence from opinions of respected authorities based on clinical experience, descriptive studies, or reports of expert committees

Note: Not all the recommended regimens reflect current FDA-approved labeling. Anti-HBC = antibody to hepatitis B core antigen; biw = twice weekly; CMV = cytomegalovirus; DS = double-strength tablet; qm = monthly; qw = weekly; ss = single-strength tablet; tiw = three times weekly; TMP-SMX = trimethoprim-sulfamethoxazole. The Respirgard II nebulizer is manufactured by Marquest, Englewood, CO;

[1] Only pyrimethamine/sulfadiazine confers protection against PCP.
[2] The long-term efficacy of any regimen is not well established. Many multiple-drug regimens are poorly tolerated. Drug interactions (e.g., those seen with clarithromycin/rifabutin) can be problematic. Rifabutin has been associated with uveitis, especially when given at daily doses of >300 mg or along with fluconazole or clarithromycin.
[3] Ganciclovir and foscarnet delay relapses by only modest intervals (often only 4–8 weeks). Ocular implants with sustained-release ganciclovir appear promising.
[4] Efficacious eradication of *Salmonella* has been demonstrated only for ciprofloxacin.

Source: From "USPHS/IDSA guidelines for the prevention of opportunitistic infections in persons infected with human immunodeficiency virus: A summary," by J. Kaplan et al., 1995, *MMWR, 44*(RR-8), 1–33.

(4) In smokers, cough may be productive
(5) Pneumothorax may occur (more often in those on inhaled pentamidine or with bullous lung disease)
  b. Extrapulmonary disease
    (1) Uncommon, represents <1% of *P. carinii* infections
    (2) Fevers, night sweats, fatigue, weight loss
    (3) Sites are ocular, GI tract, bone marrow, lymph nodes, liver, spleen
  c. Disseminated disease is rare
8. Diagnosis
  a. Tests/procedures
    (1) Pulmonary: See *Pulmonary Complications*, p. 151
      (a) Sputum for recovery of *P. carinii* organisms
      (b) Bronchoscopy with bronchoalveolar lavage or transbronchial biopsy; specimens examined for organisms as above
      (c) Chest x-ray
        i) Most often shows diffuse, bilateral infiltrates
        ii) Patients who have received aerosolized pentamidine may have greater incidence of apical infiltrates and intraparenchymal cysts
        iii) Normal chest x-ray is seen in ≤10% of patients with PCP
      (d) Lactate dehydrogenase (LDH) often elevated (nonspecific finding)
      (e) Arterial blood gases (ABGs) (looking for hypoxia and alveolar-arterial (A-a) gradient <35 mm Hg)
      (f) Pulmonary function tests measuring diffusing capacity of CO_2
      (g) Gallium scan shows increased uptake in lungs with PCP
    (2) Extrapulmonary disease: Examine tissue suspected to be infected
  b. Staging: Not standard
    (1) Mild to moderate: PaO_2 on RA >70 mm Hg
    (2) Severe: PaO_2 on RA <70 mm Hg

  c. Differential diagnosis
    (1) Bacterial pneumonia (community acquired, mycobacterial)
    (2) Viral pneumonia (CMV, VZV pneumonitis)
    (3) Fungal pneumonia
    (4) Kaposi's sarcoma, lymphoma
9. Treatment
  a. Acute: Duration of treatment is 21 days (may be extended with severe disease); routes of drug administration may change from parenteral to oral, depending on clinical progress
    (1) TMP-SMX
    (2) Pentamidine
    (3) Trimetrexate with leucovorin rescue during length of infusion and 3 days beyond last dose
    (4) Trimethoprim with dapsone
    (5) Clindamycin with primaquine
    (6) Atovaquone
    (7) Steroids are added when infection is severe (usually prednisone in tapering doses)
  b. Maintenance: Reinstitute primary prophylaxis
10. Laboratory results and other indices to monitor for side effects, adverse effects, and response to therapy
  a. Respiratory status
  b. ABGs, chest x-ray
  c. Ambulatory oximetry monitoring: Expect some desaturation with activity during first week of therapy
    (1) Remove nail polish when performing oximetry
    (2) Dapsone may cause methemoglobinemia, which makes oximetry unreliable
  d. Laboratory monitoring of medications: Frequency depends on severity of infection, concomitant medications, and doses of medications
    (1) CBC (for neutropenia, thrombocytopenia associated with sulfas, trimetrexate)
    (2) Glucose-6-phosphate-dehydrogenase (G6PD) screen prior to starting dapsone or primaquine
      (a) Rule out G6PD deficiency, which can lead to hemolytic

anemia after ingesting certain medications

(b) G6PD deficiency is especially common in African Americans and Caucasians of Mediterranean descent

(3) Depending on agent used, monitoring for LFTs, renal panel, pancreatic enzymes, and blood chemistries may be indicated

e. Adverse effects of medications

(1) Sulfa medications most commonly associated with rash, followed by GI symptoms, elevated liver function tests; photosensitivity

(a) HIV-positive patients have a higher incidence of rash than general population with TMP-SMX

(b) Rash does not always indicate allergic reaction in PWAs, so it is sometimes decided to "treat through" the rash with supportive measures (antihistamines, steroids)

(c) Protocols for desensitization to TMP-SMX vary

(2) Parenteral pentamidine: Hypotension, hypoglycemia, pancreatitis

(a) Monitor blood glucose during therapy

(b) Check vital signs during infusion

(3) Primaquine: GI distress, bone marrow suppression

(4) Clindamycin: Diarrhea (often from *C. difficile*) and other GI side effects

(5) Atovaquone: Rash and GI symptoms

(6) Trimethoprim: Rash, fever, GI symptoms, bone marrow suppression increase in BUN/creatinine, bilirubin, and LFTs

f. Interactions

(1) Dapsone best absorbed in the presence of an acid environment; ddI, antacids, or medications that decrease gastric acid secretion (H_2 blockers); must be taken 2 hours apart from dapsone

(2) Decrease in phenytoin levels seen with trimethoprim

(3) Concomitant medications may intensify bone marrow suppression

(4) Atovaquone is optimally absorbed with high-fat meal

(5) Existing peripheral neuropathy due to concomitant medications may worsen with sulfa-based medications, pentamidine

(6) Alcohol ingestion increases risk of pancreatitis with pentamidine

(7) Do not give primaquine if patient is taking (or recently has been on) quinacrine

g. Trimetrexate is structurally similar to methotrexate; precautions used for administering chemotherapy are often observed

h. Precautions for HCWs in contact with aerosolized pentamidine

11. Patient education

a. Correct technique to collect sputum sample

(1) Induction of sputum with nebulized hypertonic saline is often necessary

(2) First morning specimen has highest yield

(3) Prompt fixation is essential

(4) Sputum yield for PCP lower in patients who have received chemoprophylaxis

b. Aerosolized pentamidine

(1) Notify nurse of respiratory symptoms before, during, or after treatment

(2) Metallic taste in mouth can be controlled by sucking on hard candy after treatment

(3) Proper use of nebulizer, per manufacturers' instruction

(4) Premedicate with bronchodilator if ordered; may be needed in patients with asthma, relatively small rib cages, smokers

(5) Major risk involves possible exposure to airborne infections

(a) Active case surveillance for TB for all patients on aerosolized pentamidine

(b) Administer pentamidine in areas

with adequate ventilation (optimally to outside air source) or air filtration systems

(6) Although pentamidine has been described as a respiratory irritant, this has not been frequently reported in HCWs administering pentamidine

    (a) Monitor patients for correct use of nebulizer

    (b) Lack of conclusive data on the effect of pentamidine on HCWs warrants further research

    (c) See *Pentamidine-Induced Hypoglycemia and Diabetes,* p. 187

c. Some researchers have suggested respiratory isolation of those with active PCP (based on an outbreak in a renal transplant unit); however, this is not standard practice

d. Avoid placing a coughing patient with PCP in a hospital room with a patient who is severely immunocompromised due to cancer chemotherapy or renal transplant until active TB is ruled out

e. Most patients with PCP can be successfully treated as outpatients or at home; hospitalization is generally indicated if significant hypoxia, extensive disease, or another intercurrent illness is present

B. Toxoplasmosis

1. Specific etiologic agent and disease process

a. *Toxoplasma gondii,* an obligate intracellular coccidian protozoan

(1) *Oocysts* are formed in cats; may be infectious for a year

(2) *Tachyzoites* infect mammal GI cells, disseminate, and replicate until an immune response is mounted

(3) After immune response, tissue cysts form

    (a) May be found in all cells

    (b) Most common in brain, heart, and striated muscle

    (c) There is evidence that cysts rupture and may cause recurrent asymptomatic infections

(4) In primary infection, oocysts are ingested in contaminated food

(5) In HIV/AIDS, most disease is due to reactivation of dormant tissue cysts

2. Risk, transmissibility, and source of infection

a. Primary infection may occur in anyone coming in contact with organism

b. Reactivation most commonly seen in PWAs with CD4+ lymphocyte count <100/µl

c. Organism most often ingested in undercooked contaminated meats, objects contaminated with organism (e.g., garden produce contaminated with cat feces)

d. Cat feces can sporulate when dry; inhaled spores can cause infection

e. No person-to-person transmission, but can be transmitted via placenta if mother has primary infection

3. Frequency and distribution

a. Worldwide distribution, with higher incidence of latent infection in Africa, Haiti, Europe, Latin America

b. Highest incidence in U.S. seen in Florida (possibly result of Haitian and Latin-American populations)

4. Relationship to natural history of HIV disease

a. Most frequently seen in PWAs with CD4+ lymphocyte count <100/µl, although it has been described in patients with higher CD4+ lymphocyte counts

b. Virtually all will have evidence of previous infection (positive *T. gondii* IgG antibody); infection rare in seronegative patients

5. Morbidity and mortality

a. In PWAs with positive IgG antibody for *Toxoplasma,* estimates of up to 30%–50% will reactivate

b. In PWAs treated for *Toxoplasma* encephalitis, up to 80% will relapse when acute treatment is stopped

6. Early detection, prevention, prophylaxis

a. Screening *Toxoplasma* antibody (IgG); no standard for routine rescreening of seronegative patients

b. Educate to prevent patients acquiring primary infection

c. Primary prophylaxis

(1) No universally accepted primary prophylaxis
(2) Evidence that some regimens used for PCP prophylaxis, particularly TMP-SMX, are effective in preventing reactivation of latent disease

7. Signs and symptoms
a. Cerebral infection
(1) *Toxoplasma* encephalitis most common presentation
(2) Symptoms: Headache, fever, altered level of consciousness or mood, seizures, strokelike symptoms
(3) Symptoms depend on location and size of lesion(s)
b. Pulmonary
(1) Fever, nonproductive cough, shortness of breath
(2) Progresses more rapidly than PCP
c. Ocular: Decrease in vision, eye pain

8. Diagnosis
a. Tests/procedures
(1) Cerebral toxoplasmosis
(a) MRI most sensitive for detecting cerebral lesions
(b) CT less sensitive but can show characteristic round lesions with ring enhancement
(c) Brain biopsy provides definitive diagnosis; empiric therapy generally initiated without biopsy given high morbidity and mortality of this procedure
(2) Pulmonary
(a) X-ray may show diffuse bilateral interstitial infiltrates similar to PCP, along with hilar adenopathy, pleural effusion, or nodular infiltrates
(b) Bronchoscopy or biopsy
(3) Chorioretinitis
(a) Funduscopic exam has characteristic appearance
(b) Fluorescein angiography
(c) Retinal biopsy or vitreal fluid analysis
b. Differential diagnosis
(1) Cerebral: Cerebral lymphoma, extrapulmonary *M. tuberculosis*, cryptococcoma
(2) Pulmonary

(a) Bacterial pneumonia, including community acquired and mycobacterial
(b) Viral pneumonia, including CMV and VZV pneumonitis
(c) Fungal pneumonia
(d) KS, lymphoma
(e) PCP
(3) Ocular: CMV retinitis, ocular PCP

9. Treatment
a. Acute: Pyrimethamine, clindamycin, dapsone, azithromycin, atovaquone, clarithromycin (see Table 4.4, *Prophylaxis for First Episode of Opportunistic Disease in HIV-Infected Adults and Adolescents*, p. 113)
b. Maintenance
(1) Up to 80% of those with cerebral toxoplasmosis will relapse if not on maintenance therapy
(2) No standard maintenance therapy, commonly lower doses of treatment drugs used

10. Laboratory results and other indices to monitor for side effects, adverse effects, and response to therapy
a. Neurologic status, respiratory status
b. Laboratory monitoring of medications
(1) CBC (for neutropenia, thrombocytopenia associated with dapsone, pyrimethamine)
(2) G6PD screen prior to starting dapsone or pyrimethamine to rule out G6PD deficiency, which can lead to hemolytic anemia after ingesting certain medications; G6PD deficiency is especially common in African Americans and people of Mediterranean descent
(3) If patient develops diarrhea while on treatment, collect stool for *C. difficile* toxin
c. Monitor for adverse effects related to medications
(1) Pyrimethamine: GI side effects (administer with food), bone marrow suppression
(2) Sulfadiazine: Rash, drug fever, itching, photosensitivity, hepatic toxicity, bone marrow suppression

(3) Clindamycin, dapsone, ato-
    vaquone: See Appendix B, *Common
    Medications Used in Treating the
    Patient with HIV/AIDS*, p. 401
d. Interactions
    (1) Pyrimethamine: Antifolic acid med-
        ications increase bone marrow
        toxicity
    (2) Azithromycin: Must be taken on
        empty stomach, no concurrent
        antacids
    (3) Clarithromycin: Monitor theo-
        phylline and carbamazepine levels
11. Patient education: Dietary precautions;
    environment/pet exposures (see Table
    10.3, *Reducing the Risk of/Preventing
    Exposure to Opportunistic Pathogens*, p.
    •••)

C. Cryptosporidiosis

1. Specific etiologic agent and disease process
    a. *Cryptosporidium parvum*, a coccidian pro-
       tozoan
    b. Infects epithelial cells of the GI and bil-
       iary tracts and, less commonly, the res-
       piratory tract
    c. When the GI tract is infected, villa atro-
       phy and become inflamed, leading to
       malabsorption and diarrhea
2. Risk, transmissibility, and source of infection
    a. Most commonly transmitted through
       fecally contaminated water or food;
       chlorination has no impact on this
       organism
    b. Oocysts can remain infective out of the
       body for 2–6 months
    c. Has autoinfective capacity; can undergo
       complete life cycle in one host
3. Frequency and distribution
    a. Worldwide distribution; actual preva-
       lence in the general population believed
       to be underreported
    b. Prevalence higher in developing coun-
       tries
4. Relationship to natural history of HIV disease
    a. Incidence increases with degree of
       immunosuppression
    b. Severity of disease increases as CD4+

lymphocyte count decreases
5. Morbidity and mortality
    a. Cryptosporidiosis is an AIDS-defining
       illness in approximately 4% of AIDS
       cases reported to CDC
    b. 10%–20% of people with AIDS (PWAs)
       will develop cryptosporidiosis at some
       point in their illness
6. Early detection, prevention, prophylaxis
    a. High index of suspicion with GI com-
       plaints
    b. Primary prophylaxis
        (1) Good hand washing
        (2) Avoiding or treating contaminated
            water sources
        (3) No chemoprophylaxis available
    c. Minimize chance of exposure
7. Signs and symptoms
    a. Diarrhea, ranging from mild intermit-
       tent to severe, with up to 10 L/day fluid
       loss
    b. Crampy epigastric pain after meals,
       nausea, flatulence, weight loss
8. Diagnosis
    a. Tests/procedures
        (1) Stool for ova and parasites: 3 sam-
            ples advised due to variable shed-
            ding rates
        (2) Stool studies with special stains,
            monoclonal antibodies
        (3) Intestinal biopsy
    b. Differential diagnosis: Diarrhea from
       other parasites; viral etiology: HIV,
       CMV; bacterial etiology: Enteric
       pathogens; diarrhea from *C. difficile*
       toxin
9. Treatment
    a. Acute
        (1) No curative treatment
        (2) Anecdotal reports of response to
            paromomycin
        (3) Reports of isolated partial responses
            to many other drugs such as litraz-
            eral, octreotide acetate
    b. Maintenance
        (1) Diet manipulation: Lactose free, low
            fat, high protein
        (2) Medications to slow GI motility:
            Opiates, Lomotil
        (3) Parenteral fluids, correcting elec-
            trolyte imbalance

(4) Azithromycin, paromomycin, atovaquone: Efficacy not established
10. Laboratory results and other indices to monitor for side effects, adverse effects, and response to therapy
   a. Response to therapy as indicated by decreased/elimination of diarrhea
   b. Laboratory monitoring of medications
   c. Adverse effects related to medications
      (1) Paromomycin: Nausea, vomiting, diarrhea; poor oral absorption
      (2) Azithromycin: See *Toxoplasmosis*, p. 120
   d. Drug interactions
11. Patient education
   a. Avoid infection; see Table 10.3, *Reducing the Risk of/Preventing Exposure to Opportunistic Pathogens*, p. 371
      (1) Boil or filter suspect water (chemical disinfection insufficient)
      (2) Avoid raw milk
      (3) Protect against exposure to animals with diarrhea
      (4) Avoid swimming in pools or bodies of water that may be contaminated
      (5) Use ammonia for household/laundry cleaning (chlorine is ineffective)
   b. Enteric precautions for incontinent patients (vomitus is infectious)
   c. Proper collection of stool specimens
      (1) Parasites are destroyed by refrigeration and contamination with urine, barium, antibiotics (particularly tetracycline and erythromycin), bismuth (present in toilet paper, paper towels, and OTC diarrhea medications), soap, and laxatives
      (2) Stool-containing mucus or blood has a higher parasite yield
      (3) Patients collecting stool samples at home will need gloves, specimen-collecting containers, tongue depressors, and instruction in sanitary disposal of feces

D. Microsporidiosis

1. Specific etiologic agent and disease process
   a. *Enterocytozoan bieneusi,* an obligate intracellular spore-forming protozoan first described in 1985; most of the microsporidiosis seen in AIDS patients is due to *E. bieneusi; Septata intestinalis* can also cause disease in AIDS patients but is less common than *E. bieneusi*
   b. Process is poorly understood; besides the GI tract, these agents can infect the sinuses, kidneys, muscles, biliary tree, bronchi, and conjunctiva
2. Risk, transmissibility, and source of infection
   a. Most frequently reported in travelers to and residents of tropical areas
   b. Little known about transmission; probably ingestion of material contaminated by spores, which can live in the environment for up to 4 months
   c. Organisms have been identified in stool, urine, and sputum
3. Frequency and distribution
   a. Has been found worldwide except in Antarctica
   b. No epidemic or endemic areas identified
   c. Frequency in AIDS patients estimated at 5%–20%
4. Relationship to natural history of HIV disease: Those with CD4+ lymphocyte count <100/μl seem most at risk
5. Signs and symptoms
   a. GI symptoms and diarrhea similar to those caused by *Cryptosporidium*
   b. Not associated with fever unless cholangitis has developed
6. Diagnosis
   a. Tests/procedures
      (1) Difficult to isolate due to small size; ability to detect organism varies because of laboratory quality and experience
      (2) Intestinal biopsy
   b. Differential diagnosis: Cryptosporidiosis
7. Treatment
   a. Acute (no standard therapy)
      (1) Albendazole (investigational drug available through Smith, Kline Beecham) for 1 month showed some response in small study (Eeftinck-Schattenkerk et al., 1991); response to albendazole better in *Septata* than in *E. bieneusi*
      (2) Thalidomide (no longer FDA

approved, available on compassionate use for aphthous ulcers and through some buyers' clubs)
b. Maintenance: Low-fat, low-fiber diet; nutrition support for malabsorption
8. Laboratory results and other indices to monitor for side effects, adverse effects, and response to therapy
   a. Frequency of stools, weight and nutritional status
   b. Laboratory monitoring of medications
      (1) CBC for bone marrow effects
      (2) Liver function tests
   c. Adverse effects related to medications
      (1) Albendazole: Bone marrow suppression, elevated transaminase; occasional alopecia, stomach upset, headache
      (2) Thalidomide: Sleepiness/drowsiness, skin rash, constipation, headache, neuropathy, mood changes, severe birth defects if taken during pregnancy
9. Patient education
   a. Proper collection of stool specimens: See *Cryptosporidiosis,* p. 122
   b. Nutritional counseling to prevent malnutrition, dehydration
   c. Thalidomide: Contraindicated in pregnancy; stress importance of strict birth control in fertile patients (men and women); stress safety measures to ensure household members or other associates of patients on thalidomide do not "borrow" or self-administer thalidomide doses

E. Isosporiasis

1. Specific etiologic agent and disease process
   a. *Isospora belli,* a coccidian protozoan
   b. Oocytes are ingested and mature to sporozoites and then to oocysts; occurs in proximal small intestine
   c. The oocyst is passed into the environment, where it sporulates and becomes infectious
2. Risk, transmissibility, and source of infection: Method of transmission in HIV not completely understood; infected animals, water, or human-to-human transmission are hypothesized

3. Frequency and distribution
   a. Most common in tropics
   b. Endemic in Africa, South America, Asia
4. Relationship to natural history of HIV disease: Risk increases with increase in degree of immunosuppression
5. Morbidity and mortality
   a. 1%–3% of PWAs in U.S. are infected
   b. Probably higher incidence of PWAs with infection, but treated or suppressed by TMP-SMX
6. Early detection, prevention, prophylaxis
   a. High index of suspicion in diarrhea
   b. No accepted prophylaxis
7. Signs and symptoms
   a. Watery diarrhea, crampy abdominal pain, weight loss, occasional low-grade fever
   b. Steatorrhea and eosinophilia may occur
   c. Can develop into disseminated disease
8. Diagnosis
   a. Tests/procedures
      (1) Stool for ova and parasites
      (2) Oocytes present in small bowel biopsy
   b. Differential diagnosis: *Cryptosporidium*
9. Treatment
   a. Acute
      (1) TMP-SMX for 10 days, then for 3 weeks
      (2) Pyrimethamine for 14 days with folinic acid for 10 days
      (3) Diclazuril for 7 days (investigational)
   b. Maintenance
      (1) TMP/SMX
      (2) Pyrimethamine with folinic acid
10. Laboratory results and other indices to monitor for side effects, adverse effects, and response to therapy
    a. Improvement or resolution of diarrhea
    b. Laboratory monitoring of medications, adverse effects related to medications, and interactions: See *Pneumocystis,* p. 112, *Toxoplasmosis,* p. 120
11. Patient education
    a. Observe water and food safety precautions when traveling in endemic areas
    b. For more information, see Table 10.3, *Reducing the Risk of/Preventing Exposure to Opportunistic Pathogens,* p. 371

F. Amebiasis

1. Specific etiologic agent and disease process
   a. *Endamoeba histolytica,* an amoeba
   b. Ingestion of cyst or trophozoite
   c. Trophozoites infect intestinal wall
   d. May disseminate
2. Risk, transmissibility, and source of infection
   a. All people are at risk, but risk is higher in people in institutions or of lower socioeconomic status (crowded conditions), with poor sanitation or hygiene practices, or with oral-anal sexual contact
   b. Transmitted via oral-fecal route; direct contact with contaminated hands, food, water
   c. Cysts can live for months in moist environment; trophozoites die soon after being passed from the body
3. Frequency and distribution
   a. Worldwide distribution
   b. Higher incidence in Mexico and Africa
4. Relationship to natural history of HIV disease: Can occur at any time in the HIV continuum
5. Morbidity and mortality: Course similar to the non-HIV positive
6. Early detection, prevention, prophylaxis: Avoiding ingestion of contaminated food or water
7. Signs and symptoms: Variable
   a. Many are asymptomatic
   b. Range from intermittent diarrhea alternating with constipation to bloody diarrhea
   c. Fevers and chills
8. Diagnosis
   a. Tests/procedures: Stool for ova and parasites
   b. Differential diagnosis: Other enteric pathogens
9. Treatment
   a. Acute
      (1) Metronidazole for 7 days followed by iodoquinol for 21 days
      (2) Metronidazole for 7 days followed by paromomycin for 7 days
   b. Maintenance: None needed

10. Laboratory results and other indices to monitor for side effects, adverse effects, and response to therapy
    a. Resolution of diarrhea
    b. Repeat stool for ova and parasites after treatment to document resolution of infection
    c. Adverse effects related to medications and interactions
11. Patient education
    a. Avoid potentially contaminated water supplies
    b. Water can be treated chemically (with water purification tablets), boiling, or filtering
    c. Need to treat infected partner(s) and asymptomatic cyst passers

G. Giardiasis

1. Specific etiologic agent and disease process
   a. *Giardia lamblia,* a flagellate protozoan
   b. Ingested cysts infect the small intestine
   c. Infection of bile ducts with trophozoites is possible, but not common
   d. In severe cases, nutrient absorption may be impaired
2. Risk, transmissibility, and source of infection
   a. Anyone coming in contact with cysts is at risk, regardless of HIV status; HIV patients are more symptomatic
   b. Transmitted via oral-fecal route
3. Frequency and distribution
   a. In U.S., more common in areas without water filtration
   b. Streams and other outdoor water sources are becoming increasingly contaminated (hence the name "beaver fever")
4. Relationship to natural history of HIV disease
   a. Can occur at any point in the HIV continuum
   b. Not a major cause of AIDS-related diarrhea
   c. More common in gay men (i.e., oral-anal contact)
5. Early detection, prevention, prophylaxis
   a. Educate patient on avoiding infection
   b. Primary prophylaxis: Avoid contact with cysts

6. Signs and symptoms
   a. Often asymptomatic
   b. Diarrhea (may wax and wane), steatorrhea, abdominal cramps, bloating, weight loss
7. Diagnosis
   a. Tests/procedures
      (1) Stool for ova and parasites: 3 samples recommended for best yield because of intermittent shedding of cysts
      (2) Stool for *Giardia* antigen
   b. Differential diagnosis: Cryptosporidium
8. Treatment
   a. Acute
      (1) Metronidazole for 5 days
      (2) Alternative: Quinacrine for 5 days or tinidazole as single dose
   b. Maintenance: None needed
9. Laboratory results and other indices to monitor for side effects, adverse effects, and response to therapy
   a. Resolution of diarrhea
   b. Laboratory results not routinely monitored, although LFTs need to be monitored if used in patients with preexisting liver disease
   c. Adverse effects related to medications
      (1) Metronidazole: Neurologic, hepatic effects in high doses, nausea, vomiting
      (2) Quinacrine: Mild headache, nausea, diarrhea; may turn urine or skin yellow
   d. Interactions
      (1) Metronidazole and alcohol will produce disulfiram-like reaction up to 48 hours after last metronidazole dose
      (2) Metronidazole must not be given to pregnant women during the first trimester
      (3) Metronidazole may interact with barbiturates, cimetidine, phenytoin, lithium
      (4) Quinacrine and primaquine cannot be given concomitantly
10. Patient education
    a. Personal care
       (1) Good hand washing
          (2) Avoid unprotected oral-anal contact
    b. Proper water treatment if camping or using suspect water supplies
       (1) Boiling is most effective, chemical treatment less so
       (2) If traveling in endemic areas: Use bottled water; do not use ice in beverages; eat fruit that has been peeled, not washed; avoid salads and fresh vegetables washed in local (potentially contaminated) water; for additional information, see Table 10.3, *Reducing the Risk of/Preventing Exposure to Opportunistic Pathogens,* p. 371
    c. Enteric precautions for incontinent patients, children in diapers
    d. Report cases to health department, if mandated in your area
    e. Stress need to abstain from alcohol while on metronidazole: Monitor for concomitant medications with alcohol base
    f. Proper collection of stool specimens: See *Cryptosporidiosis*, p. 122

H. Strongyloidiasis

1. Specific etiologic agent and disease process
   a. *Strongyloides stercoralis* or threadworm
   b. Parasite enters through skin; penetration follows exposure to contaminated material (soil, feces)
   c. Circulatory migration to lungs
   d. Larvae migrate from lungs to pharynx
   e. Eggs are laid in GI tract
2. Risk, transmissibility, and source of infection
   a. Transmitted via contaminated soil; autoinfection common
   b. Can be transmitted via oral-anal sexual contact, poor sanitation
   c. Infection and autoinfection possible as long as larvae remain in GI tract
   d. Parasites can remain infective in soil for years
3. Frequency and distribution
   a. Worldwide distribution
   b. More common in tropical and subtropical areas, Southeast Asia

   c. Prevalence in United States: 0.4%–4% in southern states
4. Relationship to natural history of HIV disease: Can occur at any time in HIV continuum
5. Signs and symptoms
   a. Rash where parasite enters skin
   b. Cough if pulmonary involvement
   c. Burning epigastric and abdominal pain, diarrhea (with mucus), nausea, wasting
   d. Eosinophilia
6. Diagnosis
   a. Tests/procedures: Identify *S. stercoralis* in fresh stool or duodenal fluid
   b. Differential diagnosis
     (1) Nematodes (Ascais lumbricoides, Trichinella spiralis)
     (2) Protozoal infections, including isosporiasis
     (3) Inflammatory bowel disease
7. Treatment
   a. Acute
     (1) Thiabendazole for 2 days
     (2) Imervectin for 2 days, repeat in 2 weeks
     (3) Albendazole for 3 days (investigational from Smith, Kline Beecham)
   b. Maintenance: No standard maintenance therapy, though relapse is not uncommon

8. Laboratory results and other indices to monitor for side effects, adverse effects, and response to therapy
   a. Laboratory monitoring of medications
     (1) Thiabendazole: Monitor LFTs
     (2) Albendazole: Monitor CBC and LFTs
   b. Adverse effects related to medications
     (1) Thiabendazole: Frequent incidence of GI side effects, dizziness; less common are itching, drowsiness, headache
     (2) Imervectin: Infrequent, but headache, itching, fever have been reported
     (3) Albendazole: Bone marrow suppression, elevated serum transaminase, occasional alopecia, stomach upset or headache
   c. Interactions
     (1) Thiabendazole: Contraindicated during pregnancy, will increase theophylline levels
     (2) Albendazole: Contraindicated during pregnancy, best absorbed when taken with high-fat meal
9. Patient education: Wear shoes when traveling in tropical and subtropical endemic areas.

VI. MALIGNANCIES

A. Introduction

1. Factors leading to the development of cancer in HIV-positive patients
   a. Breakdown of the immune system: Cell-mediated immunity
   b. Natural killer cells
   c. Decreased immune surveillance: Hypothesis implies that immune impairment increases the likelihood that aberrant cells, produced in the course of cell replication, will proceed to malignant clones and eventually to clinical cancer instead of being eliminated by a healthy immune system
2. KS, NHL, primary CNS lymphoma, and invasive squamous cell cancer of the cervix account for 95% of cancers diagnosed in AIDS patients
3. Human papillomavirus (HPV)
   a. HPV-6/HPV-11 most commonly found in benign condylomas or low-grade squamous intra epithelial lesions
   b. HPV has also been isolated from rectal smears of gay men, unclear what this means
4. Other virally mediated cancers
   a. EBV and nasopharyngeal cancer
   b. HBV and hepatoma
5. Other cancers found in immunocompromised populations that may eventually be seen in the HIV population: Vulvar, anal

B. Kaposi's Sarcoma

1. Specific etiologic agent and disease process
   a. Pathogenesis
      (1) HIV: Tat gene may initiate the process of cell transformation
      (2) IL-6, Oncostatin M are expressed on the cell surface; act synergistically with Tat
      (3) HIV: Tat increases proliferation of Kaposi's sarcoma (KS)-derived spindle cell
      (4) The cell of origin remains unknown; KS may originate from mesenchymal, smooth muscle cell, or fibroblasts
      (5) May be regulated by tumor necrosis factor (TNF)-α and interleukin (IL)-1b
      (6) Oncogene activation; activation of tumor suppressor gene may play a role
      (7) Uncontrolled growth of these cells with attendant neoangiogenesis and inflammatory cell infiltration results in the characteristic histologic appearance
   b. All types of KS are similar microscopically
      (1) Vascular proliferation
      (2) Spindle cell population
      (3) Extravasated red blood cells
      (4) "Benign" appearance
   c. Etiology
      (1) Possible link between immune suppression and KS
      (2) KS in healthy gay men may support theories of
         (a) Sexually transmitted KS virus
         (b) Undetectable HIV (not likely)
      (3) Role of CMV is unclear
      (4) Gay men who used/use "poppers" have an increased incidence of KS
      (5) Identification of new herpes family virus (HHV-8) within the DNA of KS lesion
   d. Classification system
      (1) Classical KS
         (a) Population at risk: Eastern Europeans, older Greek men
         (b) Male-female ratio: Males predominate
         (c) Indolent, slow growing
         (d) Predictable pattern of spread: Involves feet and legs
      (2) Endemic (African) KS
         (a) Population at risk: Young men
         (b) Male-female ratio: Males predominate
         (c) Aggressive lymphadenopathic to indolent
      (3) KS in transplant patients
         (a) Purposefully immune-suppressed population develops this rare cancer

(b) Visceral involvement
(4) AIDS-related KS: Predominantly affects gay men (acquired HIV through sexual transmission)
  (a) Vast majority of patients are male
  (b) Women 4 times more likely to develop KS if they acquired HIV sexually
  (c) Similar to transplant KS in course, aggressiveness
  (d) Ranges from 1% in hemophiliacs to 21% in gay men
2. Relationship to natural history of HIV disease
  a. AIDS-indicator disease in CDC classification
  b. First emerged in 1981 as AIDS epidemic emerged
  c. KS is 20,000 times more likely to occur in the presence of HIV
3. Morbidity and mortality: Median survival once pulmonary KS develops is 10 months
4. Early detection, prevention, prophylaxis
  a. Skin inspection
  b. Safer sex, no poppers
5. Signs and symptoms
  a. Dermatologic
    (1) Multicentric skin lesions
    (2) Localized/disseminated
    (3) Plaque/nodular
    (4) No characteristic site of involvement; may initiate near ears, eyelids, or anywhere on skin surface
    (5) Colors vary from brown to red to purple
  b. Asymptomatic visceral involvement common, especially the oral cavity and GI tract; all organs can be involved, including the brain
  c. Pulmonary: Nonproductive cough, fever, and dyspnea (see *Pulmonary Complications*, p. 151)
    (1) Isolated involvement rare
    (2) May take 1–36 months to manifest symptoms
    (3) Approximately 18%–32% of patients affected
    (4) In some patients the onset of KS can be marked by significant pulmonary

involvement; usually indicates rapid clinical decline
(5) Difficult to distinguish between pulmonary infections and KS in the lung
(6) Approximately one third of all respiratory symptoms and complications that develop in patients with known KS are due to pulmonary KS
6. Diagnosis
  a. Tests/procedures
    (1) Biopsy of suspicious lesion
    (2) Baseline lab work
    (3) Pulmonary KS
      (a) Chest x-ray: Bilateral interstitial or alveolar infiltrates; less commonly a nodular pattern, unilateral or bilateral
      (b) Gallium/thallium scan
      (c) Pulmonary function tests may be helpful in ruling out infectious etiology
      (d) Bronchoscopy usually reveals violaceous plaques in the tracheobronchial tree
      (e) Lesions are submucosal and difficult to biopsy
  b. Staging
    (1) Original staging system first proposed by Laubenstein/Mitsuyasu (Kaplan & Northfelt, 1995)
    (2) CD4+ lymphocyte counts prognostic indicators
    (3) Helper:suppressor (H/S) ratio
    (4) AIDS Clinical Trial Group proposed staging (Kaplan & Northfelt, 1995)
      (a) Good risk (patient has all the following findings)
        i) Tumor: Confined to skin or lymph nodes, or minimum oral disease
        ii) Immune system: CD4+ lymphocyte count ≥200/μl
        iii) Systemic illness: No history of OIs or thrush, no "B" symptoms (i.e., unexplained fever, night sweats, >10% involuntary weight loss, diarrhea persisting >2 weeks), Karnofsky performance status (KPS) ≥70

(b) Poor risk (any one of the following)
  i) Tumor: Tumor-associated edema or ulceration, extensive oral KS lesions, GI KS lesions, KS lesions in other nonnodal viscera
  ii) Immune system: CD4+ lymphocyte count <200/µl
  iii) Systemic illness: History of OIs or thrush or both, "B" symptoms present, KPS <70, other HIV-related illness (e.g., neurologic disease, lymphoma)

7. Treatment
  a. Radiation therapy
    (1) Cosmetic treatment
    (2) Painful localized lesions (e.g., soles of feet)
    (3) Bulky lymph nodes
    (4) Oral lesions
    (5) Photodynamic therapy (hematoporphyrin derivative photodynamic therapy)
  b. Chemotherapy
    (1) Single agents (e.g., vincristine, vinblastine, doxorubicin, bleomycin, oral etoposide)
    (2) Combination chemotherapy (e.g., doxorubicin, bleomycin, vincristine)
    (3) Low dose; monitor counts
  c. Biologic response modifiers
    (1) Interferon-alpha (INF-α)
    (2) INF-α and AZT
    (3) Experimental
      (a) Tecogalan
      (b) Lipsomal agents
      (c) Antiangiogenesis compounds
      (d) Fumagillin derivatives
      (e) Anti-Tat, anti-Oncostatin-M, IL-6 inhibitors
  d. Algorithm for treating patients
    (1) Limited/indolent disease
      (a) Nondisfiguring: Observation, intralesional therapy, liquid nitrogen, argon laser therapy, biotherapy
      (b) Disfiguring
        i) Localized: Radiation therapy (800 cGy), argon laser

      ii) Diffuse: Chemotherapy (single agent or combination therapy)
    (2) Advanced/aggressive
      (a) Diffuse: Chemotherapy
      (b) Localized: Radiation
      (c) Oral/pharyngeal: Radiation, laser, photodynamic therapy
      (d) Pulmonary: Chemotherapy (single agent or combination therapy)
    (3) Cytopenic patients: Vincristine/bleomycin

8. Patient education
  a. Safer sex
  b. Self-administration of INF injections
  c. Clothing and other means to disguise lesions, if desired
  d. Anticipated body-image changes (see *Body Image Disturbance*, p. 247), social isolation (see p. 269)
  e. For more on symptom management, see *Management of Common Symptons, Signs, and Other Responses to HIV Infection/AIDS*, p. 199

C. Non-Hodgkin's Lymphoma

1. Specific etiologic agent and disease process
  a. General population: Suspected viral etiology
  b. HIV-infected population: No causal relationship
    (1) Epstein-Barr virus (EBV) is passenger virus; coincidentally found
    (2) EBV may determine the type of lymphoma
      (a) 100% HIV-related CNS lymphomas are EBV positive
      (b) 80% immunoblastic/large cell lymphomas are EBV positive
      (c) 40% Burkitt's type are EBV positive
    (3) Across all AIDS lymphomas, approximately 33% are EBV positive
  c. Organ transplant patients with non-Hodgkin's lymphoma (NHL) are 100% EBV positive
  d. Pathogenesis: Lympho-hematopoietic malignancies are characterized by the clonal expansion of cells that have been

arrested at a specific development stage of maturation; essentially what remains is a cell that has retained the property of self-renewal and lost the ability to differentiate terminally
   (1) Immune suppression
   (2) Chronic antigenic stimulation of B cells
 e. Activation of cytokine network, increased IL-6 (may provide chronic proliferation for the arrested cells) and IL-10 (nonspecific B-cell growth factors)
   (1) Chromosome translocation c-mycon-cogene results in unregulated transcription
   (2) Malignant cell is a transformed lymphocyte (most likely B cell)
   (3) Maturation stage of lymphocyte determines the characteristics of the lymphoma
   (4) Cytogenic changes may be present
   (5) Malignant cell invades and compromises function of organs, especially bone marrow
   (6) May be polyclonal (aggressive)
 f. Clinical manifestations in HIV-positive patients
   (1) Extranodal disease
   (2) Very aggressive/high grade; intermediate grade
   (3) CD4+ lymphocyte counts higher in small noncleaved cell lymphoma, lower in large cell/immunoblastic lymphoma
   (4) Most patients will present with B symptoms
2. Frequency and distribution: Sharp increase in the number of patients developing NHL after approximately 2 years on AZT
3. Relationship to natural history of HIV disease (clinical manifestations in HIV-positive patients): Suspected to be diagnosed in 4%–10% of patients with AIDS (average approximately 4,700 cases [range 2,900–9,800])
 a. HIV-related NHL tends to be a late manifestation of AIDS
 b. Incidence 60–100 times greater than in the general population
 c. Women are somewhat less affected than men

 d. Incidence increases with age in gays, bisexuals, hemophiliacs
 e. Increased incidence with prolonged survival
 f. IDUs have about half the probability of presenting with NHL compared with gay and bisexual men
4. Early detection, prevention, prophylaxis: Early detection by clinical assessment of signs, symptoms, and physical exam; higher index of suspicion with lower CD4+ lymphocyte counts
5. Signs and symptoms
 a. Rapidly enlarging mass
 b. B symptoms
6. Diagnosis
 a. Tests/procedures: Bone marrow biopsy and aspirate, lumbar puncture, biopsies
 b. Staging
   (1) Determine extent of disease involvement
     (a) History and physical
     (b) Bilateral bone marrow biopsies
     (c) Lumbar puncture
     (d) CT scans (chest, abdomen, pelvis)
     (e) Chest x-ray
     (f) Routine lab work
   (2) Ann Arbor staging
     (a) Stage I: Single lymph node (LN) region or extralymphatic organ (IE)
     (b) Stage II: 2 or more LN regions; same side of diaphragm; extralymphatic organ and one or more LN region (Ie)
     (c) Stage III: LN regions both sides of diaphragm; extralymphatic organ (IIIe); with or without spleen (IIIs or IIIse)
     (d) Stage IV: Diffuse or disseminated involvement
   (3) Grading (determines aggressiveness of the disease)
     (a) Low grade (slow growing, indolent)
     (b) Intermediate grade (somewhat aggressive)
     (c) High grade (very aggressive)
 c. Prognostic factors
   (1) Poor prognosis
     (a) Prior AIDS diagnosis

(b) KPS <70%

(c) Extranodal disease

(d) CD4+ lymphocyte count <100/μl

(2) Good prognosis

(a) No prior AIDS diagnosis

(b) KPS >70%

(c) No extranodal disease

(d) CD4+ lymphocyte count >100/μl

(3) Cyclophosphamide dose

7. Treatment

a. Chemotherapy: Many active agents (e.g., cyclophosphamide, doxorubicin, vincristine, vinblastine, methotrexate, prednisone, dexamethasone, bleomycin); no superior regimen

b. Radiation therapy: Early stage disease, isolated single lesion, cytopenic patient

c. Biologic response modifiers

(1) Interferon

(2) Colony-stimulating factors: Supportive

8. Laboratory results and other indices to monitor for disease progression and response to therapy

a. Chemotherapy side effects

(1) Tumor lysis syndrome: Patients with large tumor burden

(a) Hyperphosphatemia

(b) Hyperkalemia

(c) Hyperuricemia

(d) Hypocalcemia

(2) Neutropenia: Poor bone marrow reserve due to HIV

(3) Mucositis

(4) Flu-like syndrome

(5) Difficult to determine the etiology of some of the side effects; must rule out HIV-related vs. chemotherapy-related cause

9. Patient education: For management of chemotherapy side effects, aggressive symptom management, see *Pulmonary Complications*, p. 151, *Management of Common Symptoms, Signs, and Other Responses to HIV Infection/AIDS*, p. 199

D. Primary Central Nervous System Lymphoma

1. Specific etiologic agent and disease process

a. Pathogenesis: Confusion over cell of ori-

gin, same cell as NHL

(1) Similar to the pathogenesis of systemic NHL

(2) Transformed lymphocyte replicates in enclosed space

(3) Multicentric

2. Frequency and distribution

a. Rare malignancy: 0.3%–2.0% of all lymphomas

b. Increased risk in immunocompromised host

3. Relationship to natural history of HIV disease

(1) Age: 40- to 50-year-olds

(2) In one study, median interval between HIV seropositivity and diagnosis approximately 4 months (Formenti, Gill, & Rarick, 1989)

(3) CD4+ lymphocyte count <75/μl

4. Morbidity and mortality

a. Epidemiology: Immunocompromised host (primary, acquired, iatrogenic)

b. Prognosis poor; median survival 72 days

c. KPS correlated with survival

d. Majority of patients obtain a short-lived improvement in neurologic symptoms

5. Early detection, prevention, prophylaxis: Detection via clinical surveillance of signs and symptoms

6. Signs and symptoms

a. Mean KPS 36%

b. Confusion, lethargy, memory loss

c. Alteration in personality and behavior

d. Hemiparesis, aphasia

e. Seizures

f. Cranial nerve palsy

g. Headache

h. Symptoms present for <2 months

i. Nonspecific signs of increased ICP

7. Diagnosis

a. Brain biopsy necessary

b. CT/MRI: Single or multiple discrete lesions, midline shift

c. CSF: Nonspecific

8. Treatment

a. Surgical intervention usually not practical

b. Radiation therapy: Somewhat responsive, treatment of choice in non-HIV-related CNS lymphoma

c. Chemotherapy: Poor response

9. Laboratory results and other indices to monitor for disease progression and response to therapy
   a. Monitor mental status for abatement of symptoms
   b. Worsening signs of increased ICP mean lack of response to treatment
10. Patient education
   a. Timely implementation of living will, power of attorney, last will and testament: See *Ethical and Legal Aspects,* p. 358
   b. Supportive care/housing arrangements, safety measures: See *High Risk for Ineffective Management of Therapeutic Regimen*, p. 258
   c. Grief and bereavement counseling: See *Grief and Loss,* p. 253

E. Invasive Squamous Cell Cancer of the Cervix

1. Specific etiologic agent and disease process
   a. Etiology
      (1) HSV type 2
      (2) HPV 16/18
   b. Pathophysiology
      (1) Preceded by dysplasia and carcinoma in situ (CIS)
      (2) Arises from the squamocolumnar junction in the cervix
      (3) Invasive when malignant epithelial cells break through the basement membrane and enter the stroma; spreads by direct extension
      (4) Invasion occurs in 1–20 years
2. Relationship to natural history of HIV disease
   a. Cervical immunity may be altered by HIV
      (1) Both humoral and cellular components
      (2) Specific IgA antibodies against HIV can be isolated from vaginal secretions
      (3) Subepithelial T-cells, Langerhans cells in cervix
      (4) Decreased immune surveillance may allow for more rapid replication of HPV
   b. Pap smears may not accurately reflect cervicovaginal disease in HIV-positive women—colposcopy provides a better exam
   c. High prevalence of cervical invasive neoplasia (CIN) in HIV-positive women
   d. No relationship to the traditional (non-HIV) risk factors (e.g., DES [diethylstilbestrol] daughters, pregnancy at a young age)
   e. Apparent relationship between CD4+ lymphocyte counts and CIN; CD4+ lymphocyte counts and recurrent CIN
   f. Poor outcome after cryotherapy: Unsure of best therapy (5-FU)
3. Early detection, prevention, prophylaxis
   a. Encourage all HIV-positive women to have Pap smears q6mon
   b. Instruct patient to notify primary HCW of any vaginal discharge, drainage, painful intercourse
   c. Instruct patient on safer sex guidelines
4. Signs and symptoms
   a. Asymptomatic in early stages
   b. Postcoital bleeding
   c. Intermenstrual bleeding or heavy flow
   d. Symptoms related to anemia
   e. Foul smelling vaginal discharge
   f. Pelvic pain
   g. Hypogastrium, flank, or leg pain
   h. Urinary or rectal symptoms
5. Diagnosis: Pap smear, colposcopy
6. Treatment: Chemotherapy, radiation therapy, surgery
7. Laboratory results and other indices to monitor for disease progression and response to therapy
   a. Symptom management: Mucositis, nausea and vomiting, neutropenia, pain management, difficulties with elimination
   b. Serial GYN exams
8. Patient education
   a. Basic education regarding disease process
   b. Safer sex guidelines
   c. Side effects of treatment
   d. Importance of GYN exams
   e. Emotional support for patient, family, significant other
   f. See *Vaginal Symptoms*, p. 240.

VII. AIDS WASTING SYNDROME

1. Etiology and disease process
   a. Characteristics of AIDS wasting syndrome (AWS)
      (1) Involuntary weight loss of >10% from usual weight in addition to chronic diarrhea (at least 2 loose stools/day for >30 days)
      (2) Documented fever and weakness (≥30 days, intermittent or constant) in the absence of a concurrent illness other than HIV infection that could explain the weight loss
      (3) Disproportionate loss in lean body tissues compared to adipose tissue
   b. Consequences of malnutrition and wasting
      (1) Malnutrition results in immune disregulation with decreases in number and activity of T lymphocytes, B lymphocytes, and macrophages; decreased secretory IgA and natural killer cells, complement activity, and phagocytic function
      (2) Loss in lean muscle leads to functional impairment, decreased quality of life
      (3) Organ dysfunction (GI tract, pulmonary, cardiac, liver, pancreatic, kidney)
      (4) Malnutrition may also affect drug absorption, pharmacokinetics, and the volume of distribution of drugs (Bidlack & Smith, 1984; Kapembwa et al., 1991)
   c. Malabsorption can contribute to wasting and malnutrition
      (1) Small intestinal diseases associated with malabsorption: *Cryptosporidium, I. belli,* microsporidia, *G. lamblia, M. avium* complex
      (2) Role of HIV in diarrhea and malabsorption is controversial; in most patients with suspected HIV enteropathy, a more thorough diagnostic workup reveals another enteric pathogen
      (3) Bacterial overgrowth due to decreases in IgA production, gastric acid secretion, and GI motility can lead to malabsorption
      (4) Malnutrition may result in malabsorption by causing alterations in small intestinal mucosa
      (5) Lactose malabsorption is common due to deficiency of the brush border enzyme lactase
      (6) Fat malabsorption has been detected during all stages of HIV disease and in the absence of enteric pathogens
      (7) Absorption tests often abnormal in HIV-infected people, including C-glycerol-tripalmitin and D-xylose tests
      (8) Vitamin B12 absorption (measured by Schilling test) also often abnormal
   d. Disorders of metabolism contribute to wasting and malnutrition
      (1) HIV infection results in hypermetabolism even in the absence of a secondary infection
         (a) Weight loss does not always occur during periods without acute secondary infections
         (b) Decrease in energy expenditure may explain stable weight in presence of hypermetabolism without increased caloric intake
      (2) Rapid weight loss and marked hypermetabolism may occur during periods of acute secondary infection
         (a) Fever, anorexia, and other GI manifestations or infections contribute
         (b) Without effective treatment of secondary infection, treatment of malnutrition is difficult
      (3) Inappropriate use of substrates
         (a) Abnormal fat metabolism has been observed; increase in hepatic lipogenesis and decrease in lipoprotein lipase with decreased triglyceride clearance and subsequent hypertriglyceridemia
         (b) Hypothesis of futile cycling with oxidation of carbohydrate and protein for energy and preservation of fat stores

(c) Increase in protein catabolism and decrease in protein anabolism leading to negative nitrogen balance

(4) Endocrine disorders: See *Endocrine Complications*, p. 186

    (a) Gonadal dysfunction: Low serum testosterone could result in decreased body weight, lean body mass, and survival

    (b) Adrenal insufficiency common in association with OIs; elevations in cortisol may be associated with severe weight loss

(5) Role of cytokines disputed

    (a) Elevated TNF levels do not correlate with weight loss, but because TNF is secreted in pulsatile fashion, serum assays of TNF often may not be sensitive or accurate enough to detect elevations

    (b) IL-1, TNF, interferon-alpha may all contribute to anorexia, futile cycling of fatty acids, and protein catabolism

e. Causes of AWS typically multifactorial

(1) Decreased nutrient intake

    (a) Due to course of illness, treatment, weakness

    (b) Food avoidance due to diarrhea

(2) Anorexia

    (a) Related to chronic disease

    (b) Resulting from depression due to living with a chronic, terminal illness; isolation; or physical changes in body appearance

    (c) Due to fever

    (d) Medication side effect

(3) Fatigue and debilitation leading to inability to secure and prepare food

(4) Inadequate financial resources due to inability to work and dependence on income from Social Security, disability, or other entitlement programs

(5) Upper GI tract disease leading to symptoms that may severely limit oral intake

    (a) Dysphagia or odynophagia due to oral herpes simplex, gingivitis, thrush or candida esophagus, CMV esophagitis, esophagitis due to inadequate fluid intake when swallowing pills, or KS or NHL in mouth or esophagus

    (b) Nausea, vomiting obstruction, or pain due to KS or NHL in esophagus or stomach

2. Frequency and distribution

a. Named as AIDS-defining illness by CDC in 1987

b. Weight loss of >10% reported in majority of PWAs; an estimated ≥80% of AIDS patients will experience the adverse effects of weight loss and malnutrition (Chlebowski, Grosvenor, Kruger, Tai, & Beall, 1989; Hellerstein, 1994)

c. Increased incidence reported in women, Hispanics, African Americans (possibly from delayed access to health care or drug use)

3. Morbidity and mortality

a. A high risk of mortality if patient is at 66% of ideal body weight or body cell mass 54% of normal (Kotler, Tierney, Wang, & Pierson, 1989); nutritional status is predictive of survival (Guenter et al., 1993)

b. Morbidity: Malnutrition is associated with longer hospital stays, slower healing, increased complications, and impaired responsiveness to treatment

4. Relationship to natural history of HIV disease: More apt to occur as CD4+ lymphocyte count falls and patients develop symptomatic disease

5. Early detection, prevention, prophylaxis

a. Nutrition screening parameters

(1) Unintentional weight loss of >5% from usual body weight

(2) Serum albumin <3.4 mg/dl

(3) GI symptoms

b. Monitor body-weight changes from usual, pre-illness body weight; >10% weight loss at any time or 5% weight loss in <30 days predictive of AWS

(1) Monitor serum albumin: Hypoalbuminemia and body weight predictive of increased morbidity and mortality

(2) Early intervention through nutrition assessment, counseling, and appropriate intervention during early, asymptomatic HIV infection critical

(3) Prevalence of weight loss and wasting means nutrition assessment by a qualified professional essential to all patients infected with HIV

6. Diagnosis
   a. Rule out presence of a concurrent illness other than HIV (e.g., enteric pathogens, CMV esophagitis); the underlying cause of malnutrition must be identified and, if possible, treated to allow nutritional interventions to be effective
   b. Use of anthropometric measurements
      (1) Changes in weight and body mass index
      (2) Gross estimates of somatic protein and body-fat stores using midarm muscle circumference, triceps skinfold, and measurement of muscle strength with hand-grip dynamometer
         (a) Standard measures (normally used for comparison) are not available for HIV-infected patients
         (b) Serial measurements over time are used instead
   c. Bioelectric impedance analysis is a noninvasive measure of body composition
   d. Monitor serum albumin, prealbumin, transferrin, retinol-binding protein, and nitrogen balance as a measure of visceral and somatic protein stores

7. Treatment
   a. Diagnosis and treatment of underlying OIs is essential
   b. Encourage exercise and aggressive symptom management of nutrition-impact symptoms (e.g., anorexia, dysphagia); see *Nutritional Deficit: Weight Loss, Anorexia*, p. 227
   c. Appetite-enhancing agents
      (1) Megestrol acetate (of all agents, has the largest number of studies showing efficacy)
         (a) An antineoplastic, progestational drug
         (b) Results in increased appetite

         (c) Increase in body weight
         (d) Weight gain may be in fat rather than muscle mass
      (2) Dronabinol
         (a) Synthetic delta-9-tetrahydro-cannabinol (THC), active ingredient of marijuana
         (b) May be useful for appetite enhancement, nausea relief, and weight gain
      (3) Cyproheptadine
         (a) Antihistamine with antiseratonergic properties
         (b) Has been reported to increase appetite and weight in cancer patients; further investigation needed to show effectiveness in AIDS patients
      (4) Anabolic agents
         (a) Testosterone
         (b) Patients with AIDS and wasting commonly have lower serum testosterone than patients with similar CD4+ lymphocyte levels, but without wasting
         (c) Supplemental testosterone may result in muscle anabolism and increased weight
      (5) Growth hormone
         (a) Results of two trials using recombinant growth hormone in people with wasting have resulted in short-term gain of lean body mass
         (b) Recombinant growth hormone not approved by FDA for wasting syndrome, and not widely available
      (6) Pentoxifylline (anticytokine agent)
      (7) Nutritional treatments
         (a) Nutritional supplements
            i) Use of supplements may result in weight gain and improved nutritional status
            ii) Most reports are based on uncontrolled trials
         (b) One controlled trial (Chlebowski et al., 1993) compared use of a peptide-based enteral formula to a whole-protein formula. Consumption of 2–3 8-oz servings/

day of peptide-based formula resulted in fewer hospital readmissions and significantly maintained body weight in asymptomatic HIV patients compared to patients who consumed the whole-protein enteral formula.

(8) Enteral feeding
   (a) Indications for use include conditions associated with impaired intake but normal absorptive function (e.g., dysphagia, anorexia)
   (b) Uncontrolled trials have shown nutritional benefits in this group of patients

(9) Parenteral nutrition
   (a) May be beneficial in patients with impaired absorption
   (b) No randomized, prospective studies have been performed

8. Laboratory results and other indices to monitor for disease progression and response to therapy: Nutritional-screening parameters such as weight changes over time, serum albumin, and presence of GI symptoms

9. Patient education
   a. Provide nutritional counseling in a manner appropriate to socioeconomic and cultural status and lifestyle
   b. Refer to a dietitian/nutritional support team
   c. Teach safe food preparation, sanitary kitchen practices (see Table 10.3, *Reducing the Risk of/Preventing Exposure to Opportunistic Pathogens*, p. 371)
   d. Encourage self-care attributes in diet therapies, management of nutritional supplements, and ongoing nutritional repletion
   e. Teach interventions for symptoms that have an impact on nutrition (e.g., anorexia, pain, dysphagia, nausea, taste changes) in order to prevent nutritional depletion (see *Nutritional Deficit: Weight Loss, Anorexia*, p. 227).

VIII. AIDS DEMENTIA COMPLEX

1. Etiology and disease process
   a. AIDS dementia complex (ADC), a term introduced in 1986, describes a subcortical dementia that has a clinical triad of disabling cognitive, motor, and behavioral changes in people with very advanced immunologic deterioration
   b. This is the most common neurologic illness associated with AIDS and is unique to the syndrome; it has been called subacute encephalitis, HIV encephalopathy, and ADC (see *Nervous System Complications,* p. 143, for other neurologic complications)
   c. The precise mechanism by which HIV infection causes dementia has not been determined; autopsy studies have found HIV in the brains of 80% of HIV-infected patients
   d. At the time of seroconversion to HIV, most patients show evidence of HIV infection in the CSF; a few patients develop symptoms referable to this early infection (e.g., headache, encephalitis, meningitis, myelopathy)
   e. Theories for process
      (1) Most prevalent theory: HIV-infected macrophages in the brain replicate, producing neurotoxins that destroy glial cells
         (a) Toxic gene products of HIV may diffuse into areas distant from immediate source of infection
         (b) Infected cells may elaborate toxic substances that are directed against specific cellular elements (e.g., cytokines), or infected cells may release nonspecific toxic substances such as proteolytic enzymes
         (c) Several studies have demonstrated that an HIV glycoprotein, gp120, has a partial sequence homology with the neurotrophic factor neuroleukin and that gp120 can interfere with the activity of neuroleukin
      (2) Direct neurotoxicity: Most studies have failed to demonstrate the destruction of neurons; too few cells appear to be infected to result in global encephalopathy
      (3) Direct cytotoxic effect of the virus on glial cells, with secondary neuronal death resulting from the loss of glial-derived structural or nutritive elements
      (4) ADC results in motor deficits (in contrast, Alzheimer's disease is a cortical dementia, oriented to intellectual deterioration and the higher cortical functions; late stages may include more subcortical deterioration)
2. Frequency and distribution: The exact incidence of ADC is debated; it may have been altered by the introduction of zidovudine (AZT)
3. Relationship to natural history of HIV disease
   a. With rare exceptions, dementia is a late complication of HIV disease, occurring in the setting of systemic symptoms and severe immunosuppression
   b. Data collected on the CARE Unit, AIDS Dementia Unit at St. Mary's Medical Center, San Francisco, and presented at the International Conferences on AIDS in Amsterdam (1992) and Berlin (1993) for 84 patients (St. Mary's Medical Center, 1993) showed
      (1) Mean CD4+ lymphocyte count 45.9/µl (median 25.0, CD4 range 0–380)
      (2) AIDS-index diagnosis at time of admission to CARE Unit (these data predate the 1993 Revised CDC AIDS case definition)
         (a) 31% of patients were diagnosed with dementia (AIDS-defining illness); all other disease processes were ruled out
         (b) Approximately 69% of patients had other AIDS-defining diagnoses such as PCP (28.3%), KS (13.3%), and toxoplasmosis (7.1% at the time of their ADC diagnosis)

138

4. Morbidity and mortality
   a. CARE Unit experience shows HIV-associated dementia, even in advanced stages, can be managed or partially reversed; demographics related to discharge dispositions reveal that of those patients admitted to the CARE Unit with moderate to severe dementia, >50% are rehabilitated and returned to the community, to a lower level of care and support services
   b. Clinical course of ADC is variable; many patients succumb to OIs before dementia becomes marked
   c. Dementia is associated with drastic changes in self-care ability, employment capabilities
5. Signs and symptoms
   a. CNS infection may remain latent throughout the patient's life or may manifest itself in many ways, ranging from extremely subtle changes to global and devastating dementia
   b. ADC is usually a slowly progressive, diffuse, and nonfocal process that may be accelerated by coexisting systemic infection
      (1) Occasionally, patients with worsening ADC during a bout of systemic illness may have substantial improvement after the illness clears
      (2) Metabolic disturbances and some medications can exacerbate symptoms
   c. The target symptoms of ADC are cognitive, behavioral, motor, and affective
      (1) Early manifestations
         (a) Cognitive functions: Forgetfulness and loss of concentration, slowed information processing, impaired attention, sequencing problems, memory loss
         (b) Behavioral: Withdrawal, irritability, apathy, loss of interest in usual activities
         (c) Motor: May show slowing, ataxia, tremor, incoordination, weakness, hyperreflexia, handwriting change
         (d) Affective: Depression, hypomania

      (2) Late manifestations seen along a continuum of severity from early stages as disease progresses, presenting a very complex clinical picture
         (a) Cognitive: Severe memory loss, word-finding problems or speech arrest, dysarthria, severe attention and concentration problems, very poor judgment with little insight into the problems
         (b) Behavioral: Increasing severity of above, plus disinhibition, impetuous actions
         (c) Motor: Incontinence, paraplegia, marked slowing
         (d) Affective: Severe depression, organic psychosis, mania
   d. Progression of ADC characterized by a cyclical severity not usually seen in other dementias; rapidly developing evidence for a neurotoxin for this disease may explain variability of progression and severity
6. Diagnosis
   a. ADC is a diagnosis of exclusion, ruling out all other possible disease processes
      (1) No diagnostic serum, CSF, neuropsychologic, neuroimaging, or electrophysiologic test identifies or predicts ADC
      (2) Most confounding conditions
         (a) CNS infections (e.g., neurosyphilis, cryptococcal meningitis, fungal meningitis, toxoplasmosis, PML)
         (b) Neuropsychiatric disorders (e.g., depression, drug intoxication, delirium)
         (c) Neoplasms (e.g., lymphoma)
         (d) Drug intoxication
         (e) Malnutrition
      (3) DSM-IV criteria for dementia are used in psychiatry to distinguish dementia from other mental status illness and to establish a diagnosis
   b. Tests/procedures
      (1) Neuroimaging helpful to rule out disease processes
      (2) MRI/CT: May be normal in the presence of symptoms, or may show cortical or ventricular atrophy or

diffuse white matter changes or abnormalities (sulci may be widened)

(3) CSF exam: Often critically important to distinguish suspected ADC from potentially treatable CNS infections that may present with similar symptoms

c. Standard diagnostic workup
  (1) CD4+ lymphocyte count and ratio
  (2) Cranial CT or MRI with contrast
  (3) Lumbar puncture
  (4) RPR/VDRL
  (5) Cryptococcal antigen
  (6) Serum toxoplasmosis IgG titer
  (7) Thyroid function studies
  (8) Serum B12 level
  (9) Serum folate level, serum albumin
  (10) CBC and differential
  (11) Chemistry panel

7. Treatment
  a. Antiretroviral drugs
    (1) Cornerstone of ADC therapy
    (2) Aimed at decreasing viral replication in the brain; AZT is known to cross the blood-brain barrier in doses of >1,000 mg/day
    (3) Other antiretrovirals are currently being evaluated for efficacy in treatment of ADC
  b. Prophylaxis and concurrent treatment are continued for PCP, CMV, and other conditions as indicated
  c. Psychotropic drug therapies are adjunct for behavioral management; start in small doses and titrate for target symptom management
    (1) Agitation, anxiety
      (a) Clonazepam
      (b) Haloperidol: Sparing use at LOW doses; significant potential for extrapyramidal side effects can be profound (typically manifested as motor rigidity, dyskinesias)
      (c) Lorazepam; routine doses and as needed
      (d) Buspirone
    (2) Mania/hypomania
      (a) Valproic acid: Valproic acid and lithium carbonate both require therapeutic monitoring, initially helpful to do as inpatient to monitor effects closely
      (b) Carbamazepine rarely used; requires close monitoring for side effects
    (3) Depression: Fluoxetine, pardetine, sertraline, amitriptyline, norpranin
    (4) Psychosis/agitation and impulsivity (also adjunctive use in mania): Haloperidol, chlorpromazine, molindone (depending on severity of symptoms), perphenazine
    (5) Psychomotor slowing: Methylphenidate, dextroamphetamine (watch for irritability, which can be profound)
    (6) Other agents to be monitored and used sparingly
      (a) Benzodiazepines to treat anxiety or insomnia (known to have sedative properties and impair memory)
      (b) Drugs with strong anticholinergic side effects may precipitate delirium
      (c) Amitriptyline can precipitate mania in predisposed patients
  d. See *Delirium*, p. 145, *Altered Mental Status: Delirium*, p. 200, *Potential for Violence/Harm to Self or Others*, p. 265, *High Risk for Ineffective Management of Therapeutic Regimen*, p. 258

8. Laboratory results and other indices to monitor for disease progression and response to therapy
  a. In the early stages of HIV-associated neuromotor disorder, patients can continue to work and function well in the community will require close monitoring for increase in affective, motor, cognitive, and behavioral signs and symptoms (indicating disease progression)
  b. Monitor patient safety

9. Patient education
  a. Caregivers need support and education related to caring for someone with HIV-associated dementia in providing a safe environment; see *Family Caregiver Burden/Strain*, p. 251, *Alterations in Family Functioning*, p. 243
  b. Assist with advance directives, home care, and assisted living referrals
  c. See *Grief and Loss*, p. 253.

IX. HIV-RELATED IDIOPATHIC THROMBOCYTOPENIC PURPURA

1. Etiology and disease process
   a. Definition: A condition without clear pathogenesis that causes a quantitative decrease in the number of circulating platelets
   b. Clinical features
      (1) Platelet count below 150,000/mm^3
      (2) Elevated levels of platelet-associated immunoglobulin and circulating immune complexes
      (3) Normal or increased megakaryocytes in the bone marrow
   c. Pathogenesis
      (1) The physiology of idiopathic thrombocytopenic purpura (ITP) in HIV infection is not fully known
      (2) Hypotheses to explain the pathogenesis of HIV-ITP include
         (a) Circulating immune complexes nonspecifically deposited on platelet membranes, resulting in clearance by the reticuloendothelial system
         (b) A specific immunoglobulin IgG antiplatelet antibody binds to an antigen on the platelet membrane, resulting in platelet destruction
         (c) Direct infection of megakaryocytes by HIV may impair platelet production and contribute to thrombocytopenia
2. Morbidity and mortality: Increased risk of bleeding with resulting anemia
3. Relationship to natural history of HIV disease
   a. Often an early manifestation of HIV infection, occurs before the development of any AIDS-defining condition
   b. Most studies find no association of ITP and progression of HIV-associated disease
   c. Low platelet count resolves spontaneously in some patients as they evolve to overt AIDS
4. Early detection: Through surveillance of routine CBC, as patient is usually asymptomatic
5. Signs and symptoms: Often asymptomatic despite thrombocytopenia (tolerates the thrombocytopenia)
6. Diagnosis
   a. Review history of HIV infection, previous bleeding episodes, current medications (prescription and nonprescription)
   b. Clinical exam
      (1) Petechiae, bruising, ecchymosis
      (2) Active bleeding from nose, gums, bladder, bowel, or vagina
      (3) Active bleeding from sites of invasive procedures
      (4) Mild splenomegaly may be present
   c. Laboratory findings
      (1) Platelet count <150,000/mm^3
      (2) Peripheral blood smear reveals a dearth of platelets with occasional large forms
      (3) Bone marrow biopsy may reveal an increased number of megakaryocytes, typical of platelet consumption
      (4) Prolonged bleeding times: PT and PTT
   d. Differential diagnoses
      (1) Rule out any other cause of low platelet production or peripheral platelet destruction before applying the diagnosis of ITP to a patient with a low platelet count (see *Potential for Bleeding: Thrombocytopenia*, p. 234)
      (2) Bone marrow biopsy to exclude cytoxic or alcohol-related drug effects or the presence of lymphoma or OIs that would result in reduced megakaryocytes
      (3) The findings of platelet-associated immunoglobulin or immune complexes strengthens the diagnosis of HIV-related ITP; however, it is neither significant nor necessary for the diagnosis
7. Treatment
   a. Reserved for patients with platelet counts <20,000/mm^3 or with clinically significant symptoms (recurrent epistaxis, gingival or subconjunctival bleeding, GI hemorrhage)
   b. Low-dose interferon-alpha (INF-α)

therapy recommended for hemophiliacs with HIV-ITP because of the substantial related morbidity and mortality associated with bleeding

c. Standard therapies
   (1) AZT considered first-line treatment for HIV-related thrombocytopenia; can raise platelet counts while simultaneously providing antiviral activity
   (2) Therapy provides immunodulatory and antiviral action that may be responsible for prolonged platelet survival; long-term maintenance therapy with a lower INF-α dose is often necessary
   (3) ddI has been beneficial for some patients who are either refractory or intolerant to AZT
   (4) Prednisone for patients with severe thrombocytopenia or bleeding; immunosuppressive effects of corticosteroid therapy in HIV-positive patients are of concern
   (5) High-dose IV gamma globulin produces a rapid rise in platelet count, but effect is usually short lived; use is therefore limited to acute episodes of life-threatening bleeding or before surgical procedures or dental extractions in patients with low platelet counts (<30,000/mm³)
   (6) Anti-Rh immunoglobulin (Anti-D Ig, WinRho) has been shown to produce a response, but is not usually sustained and its use may be limited by hemolysis
   (7) Splenectomy for patients who have been refractory to other treatment modalities; concerns surround possible immunosuppressive effects of splenectomy in patients with HIV
   (8) Platelet transfusions generally not indicated in patients with thrombocytopenia of immune origin; however, transfusions may be used in emergencies
   (9) A potential future therapy is a hematopoietic growth factor, megakaryocyte growth and development factor (MGDF) to stimulate platelet production

8. Laboratory results and other indices to monitor for disease progression and response to therapy
   a. Institute measures to decrease risk of complications of thrombocytopenia
   b. Notify physician of platelet count <50,000/mm³ or presence of active bleeding
   c. Monitor for complications related to thrombocytopenia
      (1) Assess lab findings for evidence of ITP progression or bleeding, with resultant decrease in platelets, Hgb and Hct
      (2) Assess skin for evidence of increased petechiae, bruising, or ecchymosis

9. Patient education
   a. Risk factors for thrombocytopenia and bleeding
   b. Signs and symptoms of bleeding to report to a member of the healthcare team
   c. Measures to decrease risk of bleeding
   d. Avoidance of pharmacologic agents that inhibit platelet production or function
   e. Critical changes in patient assessment parameters to report to physician (signs and symptoms of active bleeding from any site)
   f. Review therapy for ITP
      (1) Medications (indication, administration, side effects)
      (2) Lab monitoring (indications, significance of results)
      (3) Splenectomy: Prepare for surgical procedure and provide pre/postop teaching
   g. Effects of ITP on life-style, ADL, self-concept
   h. Effective mechanisms for coping with alterations in ADL such as work and leisure, self-care, sexual practices.

X. NERVOUS SYSTEM COMPLICATIONS

A. Primary HIV Infection of the Brain (HIV encephalitis, AIDS encephalopathy)
See *AIDS Dementia Complex*, p. 138

B. Common Intracranial Opportunistic Infections
See *Toxoplasmosis*, p. 120, *Cryptococcosis*, p. 86

C. Progressive Multifocal Leukoencephalopathy
See p. 98

D. CNS Malignancies
See *Non-Hodgkin's Lymphoma*, p. 130, *Primary Central Nervous System Lymphomas*, p. 132

E. Neurosyphilis
See *Syphilis*, p. 67

F. Peripheral Neuropathies
1. Etiology and disease process
   a. Most commonly detected in HIV disease
      (1) Distal symmetrical polyneuropathy (DSP or DSPN); also known as predominantly sensory neuropathy (PSN)
      (2) Toxic neuropathy related to INH (particularly when used without pyridoxine), ddI, ddC, d4t, vincristine
   b. Other neuropathies in HIV
      (1) Polyradiculitis
      (2) Vacuolar myelopathy
      (3) Inflammatory demyelinating polyneuropathies (acute or chronic)
      (4) Mononeuritis multiplex
   c. Non-HIV-related causes of neuropathy
      (1) Tarsal tunnel syndrome
      (2) Diabetes mellitus
      (3) Alcoholism
      (4) Vitamin B12 deficiency
      (5) Herpes zoster

2. Frequency and distribution: Clinically in more than one third of PWAs
3. Relationship to natural history of HIV disease: May occur at any time during disease process with an increase noted with declining CD4+ lymphocyte count
4. Morbidity and mortality
   a. Peripheral neuropathies are common and disabling
   b. Pathologically present in nearly all AIDS patients
5. Early detection, prevention, prophylaxis
   a. Assess for risk factors, assess for signs and symptoms
   b. Attempt to correct metabolic or nutritional causes
   c. Identify potential neurotoxic agents; discontinue or reduce doses of any such currently used agents
6. Signs and symptoms
   a. Numbness
   b. Paresthesias (spontaneous sensations of tickling or tingling)
   c. Dysesthesias (pain associated with sensations that are not ordinarily painful, which tend to ascend symmetrically from the soles of the feet and gradually affect the legs and hands)
   d. Hyperesthesia (sensory stimuli felt more keenly than normal)
   e. Hyperalgesia (exquisite tenderness to touch)
   f. Burning
   g. Diminished or absent reflexes
   h. Motor weakness less common in DSPN/PSN
7. Diagnosis
   a. Generally made on basis of history and physical exam
      (1) History compatible with predominantly sensory dysfunction
      (2) Physical exam notable for abnormal sensory findings in the feet, reduced or absent knee jerks
   b. Electrodiagnostic studies (electromyography, nerve conduction studies) rarely used to make a clinical diagnosis
   c. Exclude other etiologies

8. Treatment
   a. Pain management (for more detail, see *Pain*, p. 229)
      (1) Tricyclic antidepressants (amitriptyline, nortriptyline)
      (2) Analgesics
          (a) Acetaminophen, NSAIDs
          (b) Mild opioids (codeine, oxycodone)
          (c) Potent opioids (methadone, long-acting morphine)
      (3) Anticonvulsants (carbamazepine, phenytoin)
      (4) Antidysrhythmics (mexilitine, IV lidocaine may be used as a predictor test)
      (5) Topical capsaicin may be tried after a trial of analgesics
   b. Protection from trauma
   c. Heat or ice
   d. Use of prosthetics
   e. Relaxation techniques: See *Therapeutic Touch*, p. 329, *Acupuncture*, p. 333, *Massage*, p. 343
   f. Vitamins, herbal therapy
   g. Counterstimulation provided by routine use of support stockings and TENS
9. Patient education
   a. Notify HCP of apparent or increasing signs/symptoms
   b. Avoid tight footwear
   c. Walk short distances only
   d. Avoid standing for long periods
   e. Soak feet in ice water periodically

G. Cerebrovascular Complications

1. Etiology and disease process
   a. Majority unexplained
   b. Direct effect of virus(es) on vascular endothelium postulated
   c. Hypercoagulable state postulated
   d. Infectious agents: Syphilis, CMV, herpes zoster, TB, toxoplasmosis, subacute bacterial meningitis, marantic meningitis (associated with wasting)
   e. Hypertension
   f. Kaposi's sarcoma
2. Frequency and distribution
   a. Increased 300-fold in comparison with non-HIV-infected age group (Hollander, 1991)
   b. Up to 34% of AIDS patients have evidence of cerebral infarction on autopsy (Engstrom, Lowenstein, & Bredesen, 1989)
   c. Incidence varies with unique risk factors
3. Relationship to natural history of HIV disease
   a. Some patients present initially with stroke syndrome
   b. Cerebral complications are related to development of disease progression, OIs
4. Morbidity and mortality
   a. Increasingly recognized as causing focal deficits in HIV-positive people
   b. Typical sequelae with significant impact on quality of life: Weakness, paralysis, aphasia
5. Early detection, prevention, prophylaxis: Instituting aggressive treatment of infectious causes and hypertension may postpone or prevent development of this complication
6. Signs and symptoms
   a. Vary according to site of infarction or vessel affected
   b. Symptoms that should initiate investigations of cerebrovascular accident (CVA)
      (1) Sudden unilateral weakness in limb(s)
      (2) Difficulty finding words, speech arrest
      (3) Unilateral neglect of a limb
7. Diagnosis: Cerebral imaging
   a. CT (double dose)
   b. MRI with gadolinium
8. Treatment
   a. Diagnose and treat underlying cause, if infectious in origin
   b. Medical and nursing support during acute phase
   c. Refer for rehabilitation (physical therapy, occupational therapy, speech therapy) as indicated; rehabilitation improves quality of life even given the shortened life expectancy
9. Laboratory results and other indices to

monitor for disease progression and response to therapy
   a. Ongoing neurologic assessment
   b. Close observation for worsening clinical status and monitoring of thrombolytic therapy, if initiated
10. Patient education: Report even subtle changes in neurologic function (e.g., transient speech arrest, numbness, tingling) for evaluation

H. Delirium

1. Etiology and disease process
   a. Definition: An organic mental symptom with global cognitive impairment
   b. Most AIDS patients have one or more risk factors, potential etiologic agents
      (1) Mass lesions, tumors (e.g., CNS lymphoma)
      (2) Infectious agents: Toxoplasmosis, CMV, herpes zoster, bacterial meningitis, sepsis, progressive multifocal leukoencephalopathy
      (3) Hypoxia (e.g., pneumocystis pneumonia)
      (4) Vascular events
      (5) Medication: Histamine blockers (e.g., cimetidine); sedatives, anxiolytics, narcotics; steroids; antivirals; antituberculars
      (6) Metabolic disturbances
         (a) Hyponatremia
         (b) Syndrome of inappropriate secretion of antidiuretic hormone (SIADH)
         (c) Hypercalcemia, hypophosphatemia
      (7) Functional, environmental changes
         (a) Hearing loss (e.g., age, nephrotoxic drugs)
         (b) Visual changes (e.g., CMV retinitis)
         (c) Sleep deprivation
         (d) Social or physical isolation
         (e) Alcohol/drug use
2. Frequency and distribution
   a. Less common with HIV infection, more common with AIDS, especially when multiple risk factors present
   b. Varies with risk factors

3. Relationship to natural history of HIV disease: May occur with event precipitating diagnosis or any time during illness progression
4. Morbidity and mortality
   a. If untreated, may lead to or worsen dementia
   b. Source of injury to patient, safety concern
   c. Source of distress to patient/SO
5. Early detection, prevention, prophylaxis
   a. Understanding risk factors may allow for early intervention or prevention
   b. Early intervention can produce reversal of symptoms and prevent clinical deterioration
   c. Distinguish between delirium and dementia; delirium may be superimposed on dementia and depression
6. Signs and symptoms
   a. Key characteristics
      (1) Distractibility
      (2) Disorganized thinking
      (3) Misperception of environment or hallucinations
      (4) Change in level of consciousness and sleep-wake cycle (diurnal variations)
      (5) Abrupt onset (vs. dementia's slow onset)
   b. Mild delirium: Disoriented to time, anxious, jittery, unable to focus
   c. Moderate delirium: Disoriented to time, and place, sensory misperceptions, short-term memory loss, agitated, unable to follow directions
   d. Severe delirium: Disoriented to time, person, place; memory grossly impaired; unable to focus; agitated; combative; hallucinating or somnolent; comatose
7. Diagnosis: Look for underlying cause
   a. CT, MRI
   b. Blood culture
   c. LP
   d. Lab studies: ABG or pulse oximetry, electrolytes (including $CA+$, PO_4)
   e. Medication review
   f. Neurologic exam
   g. Environmental review

8. Treatment
   a. Treat underlying cause
      (1) Antibiotic, antiviral therapy
      (2) Electrolyte replacement
      (3) Discontinue or substitute unnecessary medications; keep medication regimen as simple as possible
      (4) Promote sleep hygiene, maintenance of social relationships
      (5) Chemotherapy, radiation for brain tumor
   b. Provide for safety needs
      (1) Constant companion
      (2) Remove sources of injury (e.g., sharp utensils, cluttered floors)
      (3) Anticipate needs
   c. Restructure environment to promote orientation, provide reassurance
      (1) Continuity of caregiver(s)
      (2) Maintain routine in ADL
      (3) Keep environment familiar
      (4) Reduce or control stimuli
      (5) Avoid confrontation; redirect activity
   d. Treatment with low-dose antipsychotic agents (e.g., haloperidol may help reduce agitation and promote comfort)
9. Laboratory results and other indices to monitor for disease progression and response to therapy
   a. Monitor severity and course of signs and symptoms
   b. Be alert for subtle changes in patient's behavior
   c. Vigilantly monitor for conditions that could exacerbate delirium (e.g., medication, environmental changes)
10. Patient education: See *Altered Mental Status: Delirium*, p. 200

I. Seizures

1. Etiology and disease process
   a. Mass lesions
      (1) Tumor
      (2) Abscess
      (3) Hematoma (e.g., subdural hematoma after a fall)
   b. Infectious processes
      (1) Bacterial meningitis
      (2) Viral meningitis
      (3) Parasitic infection (e.g., toxoplasmosis)
      (4) Progressive multifocal leukoencephalopathy
      (5) Fungal meningitis
   c. Cerebrovascular accident
      (1) Hemorrhage
      (2) Infarction
   d. Metabolic disturbances
      (1) Hyponatremia
      (2) Hypoglycemia
      (3) Vitamin deficiency
   e. Drugs
      (1) Antiviral agents
      (2) Antitubercular agents
      (3) Demerol
   f. Other causes
      (1) Drug/alcohol overdose
      (2) Lymphomatous meningitis
      (3) Scaring from recent or remote head injury
2. Frequency and distribution
   a. Varies according to presence and combination of etiologic processes
   b. 30% of AIDS patients have multiple neuropathologic processes present
3. Relationship to natural history of HIV disease: May occur at any time during course of illness, according to precipitating factors
4. Morbidity and mortality
   a. If treatment unsuccessful or unavailable, seizure activity may progress to status epilepticus, which has a reported mortality rate of 3%–20% (Adams & Victor, 1993)
   b. Repeated seizure activity may result in or cause the progression of neurologic dysfunction
   c. Complications of seizures (bone fracture, aspiration, pain, psychologic discomfort)
5. Signs and symptoms
   a. Focal motor seizures: Clonic movement (spasms or rigidity and relaxation) of the face, hands, arms, legs
   b. Jacksonian seizures
      (1) Clonic activity that spreads in an orderly fashion to adjacent areas
      (2) May become generalized
   c. Partial complex or temporal lobe seizures

(1) Attacks of unusual behaviors (e.g., lip-smacking, pill-rolling, grimacing), which the patient doesn't recall

(2) Auditory, olfactory hallucinations may occur

   d. Tonic-clonic (grand mal) seizures

(1) Sudden loss of consciousness with generalized tonic convulsions

(2) Later alternating with clonic convulsions

6. Diagnosis
   a. Observation/clinical exam
   b. EEG: Pinpoints epileptogenic focus

7. Treatment
   a. Early detection and prevention
     (1) Treat underlying disorders aggressively
     (2) If cerebral lesion present, prophylactic treatment with anticonvulsants may be indicated
   b. Acute
     (1) Protect patient
       (a) Loosen clothing
       (b) Remove furniture
       (c) Cushion head
     (2) Maintain airway
       (a) Position to side (tongue falls forward)
       (b) Suction oropharynx, if able
     (3) Administer antiseizure medication
       (a) Lorazepam, repeat q10–15min, or diazepam, repeat q10–15min until seizure stops
       (b) For long-term control, load with Dilantin in divided doses
       (c) Consider phenobarbital if seizures persist

   c. Postictal phase
     (1) Protect patient
       (a) Assist to bed/chair
       (b) Observe for recurrent activity
     (2) Maintain airway
       (a) Position to side until conscious
       (b) Administer supplemental oxygen prn
     (3) Reassure patient/family
   d. Maintenance
     (1) Administer anticonvulsant as ordered: Phenytoin, phenobarbital, carbamazepine, valproic acid
     (2) Treat underlying cause, when possible
       (a) Correct metabolic imbalance
       (b) Administer antimicrobial therapy
       (c) Evacuate hematoma
       (d) Review drug use
       (e) Treat underlying malignancy

8. Laboratory results and other indices to monitor for disease progression or response to therapy
   a. Serial neurologic exams; observation
   b. Monitor serum levels to ensure therapeutic range is maintained

9. Patient education
   a. Common side effects
   b. Therapy likely to be lifelong
   c. Importance of taking drugs as prescribed
   d. Use of Medic-Alert bracelet
   e. Discontinue driving, use of machinery

J. Neuromuscular Complications of HIV Disease

See *Myositis and Myopathy*, p. 194.

XI. CARDIAC COMPLICATIONS

A. Endocarditis

1. Etiology and disease process
   a. An inflammation of the heart, endothelium, and cardiac valves caused by bacterial, fungal, or viral infection
   b. The most common endocardial lesion reported in AIDS patients is nonbacterial thrombotic endocarditis (NBTE), also known as marantic endocarditis
   c. Usually associated with chronic wasting diseases, malignancies, and hypercoagulable states
2. Frequency and distribution: Variable; usually seen in IDUs; prevalence is increasing in southern Europe compared with North America
3. Relationship to natural history of HIV disease: Endocarditis in IDUs is common in patients with or without HIV disease
4. Morbidity and mortality
   a. Prognosis in patients with advanced HIV disease is poor: 40% mortality rate (10% in asymptomatic patients) (Bernard, 1993)
   b. The presentation of infective endocarditis similar in both HIV positive or negative risk
   c. Factors for acquisition: IV drug use often results in infectious endocarditis, although not found to be more prevalent in IDUs with AIDS
   d. Autopsies on cardiac-involved patients with histories of IV drug abuse: Active endocarditis 5% in AIDS, 87% in non-AIDS patients (Bondmass, 1994)
5. Early detection, prevention, prophylaxis
   a. Comprehensive cardiac assessment offered to patients who present with high index of suspicion (e.g., IDUs, previous history)
      (1) ECG, echocardiogram, chest x-ray
      (2) Labs: CBC with differential, blood cultures
   b. Prevention efforts directed toward lower incidence of IDU and subsequent needle sharing (e.g., needle-exchange programs)
   c. No effective prophylaxis

6. Signs and symptoms
   a. Fever, usually low grade
   b. Diaphoresis
   c. Chills
   d. Anorexia
   e. Weight loss
   f. Malaise
   g. Arthralgias
   h. S3 heart murmurs
   i. Splenomegaly
   j. Embolization
   k. Heart failure
7. Diagnosis
   a. Bacterial endocarditis should be presumed in HIV-positive IDUs presenting with fever and a regurgitant murmur or peripheral stigmata
   b. Anemia, hematuria, or proteinuria may be present
   c. Chest x-ray may reveal pulmonary infiltrates
   d. ECG in early infection may be normal
   e. Conduction defects (atrial fibrillations, flutter) may be present later in infection
   f. Echocardiogram may demonstrate vegetations or abscesses, valve involvement, and left ventricle involvement
   g. Differential diagnosis
      (1) Bacterial endocarditis, commonly caused by *Staphylococcus*; can also be caused by *S. pneumoniae* and *H. influenzae*
      (2) Fungal endocarditis often are the result of systemic spread from extra cardiac sources; pathogens include *Aspergillus, Candida,* and *C. neoformans*
8. Treatment
   a. Initiate empiric antibiotic therapy until specific pathogens are identified; duration of antibiotic therapy usually 4 weeks if valvular involvement or methicillin-resistant *S. aureus* (MRSA)
   b. Measuring serum bactericidal titer may be helpful when antibiotic regimen is unusual or when treatment appears to be failing; verify drug sensitivities
   c. Surgery is an option when severe valve

involvement (e.g., stenosis, regurgitation) is present, though persons with advanced symptomatic HIV disease are generally not good surgical candidates (Frater, 1990; Frater, Sisto, & Condit, 1989)

    d. Most endocardial complications in AIDS patients are treatable if diagnosed early

9. Laboratory results and other indices to monitor for disease progression and response to therapy
    a. Chest x-ray
    b. ECG
    c. Echocardiogram
    d. Antibiotic blood level titer; organism culture and drug sensitivities

10. Patient education
    a. Community/individual HIV health education/risk-reduction efforts to decrease injection drug use
    b. Identify IDUs who are at high risk for endocarditis and offer comprehensive cardiac screening
    c. Educate HIV healthcare providers, social service agencies, drug-treatment programs regarding the high incidence of endocarditis in the IDU population

B. Pericarditis

1. Etiology and disease process
    a. An inflammation of the pericardium
    b. May be due to bacterial, fungal, or viral infection; neoplasms; drug or radiation therapy

2. Frequency and distribution: Incidence of pericardial effusion: 4% for HIV-infected patients and 12% per year for patients with advanced HIV disease (Cheitlin, 1994)

3. Relationship to natural history of HIV disease
    a. Pericarditis is probably related to HIV disease either from direct involvement by HIV or weakened autoimmune defense mechanism
    b. Risk of pericarditis increases with the onset of advanced HIV disease

4. Morbidity and mortality
    a. Presence of pericardial effusion is a sign of poor prognosis; patients can have a 6-month mortality of 40% vs. 7% for patients without pericardial effusion (Heidenreich et al., 1993; Sande & Volberding, 1995)
    b. Most pericardial effusions are small, remain asymptomatic, and resolve spontaneously in up to 50% of cases
    c. Can result in cardiac tamponade

5. Early detection, prevention, prophylaxis: Cardiovascular assessment and history

6. Signs and symptoms
    a. Pain (sudden, severe, sharp) may radiate to back or shoulders, aggravated by deep inspiration or movement; may be relieved by leaning forward
    b. Pericardial friction rub, usually along lower left sternal border and apex
    c. Tachycardia, hypotension, and signs of reduced cardiac output (cerebral and renal hypoperfusion) may result if pericardial effusion is present and produces tamponade

7. Diagnosis
    a. ECG
      (1) ST-segment elevation in acute stage with return to baseline later
      (2) May have low-voltage QRS complexes in the presence of pericardial effusion
      (3) Atrial dysrhythmias may be present
    b. Chest x-ray
      (1) Cardiac silhouette will usually be enlarged with ≥250 ml of pericardial fluid present
      (2) Lung field should be clear
    c. Echocardiogram: Confirms presence of pericardial fluid (minimum 20 ml can be detected)
    d. MRI
      (1) Visualizes pericardium
      (2) Can define thickened pericardium to differentiate acute vs. chronic pericarditis
    e. Cardiac catheterization
      (1) Usually shows increased left and right atrial pressures with constrictive pericarditis
      (2) Diastolic pressure may be shown to equalize in all four chambers if tamponade is in progress

8. Treatment
   a. Asymptomatic small pericardial effu-
      sion needs no therapy
   b. A large effusion compressing the lungs
      or signs of tamponade indicates need for
      pericardiocentesis; may require surgery
      for pericardial window procedure
   c. Antimicrobial therapy
9. Laboratory results and other indices to
   monitor for disease progression and
   response to therapy
   a. Careful history and physical assessment
      are essential, along with knowledge of
      common cardiac involvement signs and
      symptoms
   b. Monitor closely for beginning signs and
      symptoms of tamponade, tachycardia,
      hypotension, dyspnea with clear lung
      field, distended neck veins at 30°, pres-
      ence of pulsus paradoxus, pallor,
      decreased urine output
   c. Chest x-ray
   d. ECG
   e. Echocardiogram
   f. Antibiotic blood titer
   g. Urine output.

XII. PULMONARY COMPLICATIONS

A. Infections

1. Etiology and disease process
   a. Pneumonia is an inflammation of the lung parenchyma
   b. May be caused by bacteria, fungi, parasites, mycobacteria, or viruses
   c. Certain pathogens more commonly cause disease in persons with HIV
      (1) Bacteria
         (a) Bacterial organisms that most commonly cause pneumonia are *Streptococcus pneumoniae, Staphylococcus aureus, Haemophilus influenzae*
         (b) Pneumonia from *Klebsiella pneumoniae, Pseudomonas aeruginosa, Escherichia coli*, and *Serratia marcescens* seen less commonly; however, the incidence of *Pseudomonas* pneumonia is thought to be increasing
         (c) Other bacteria that may cause pneumonia are *Legionella* species, *Chlamydia pneumoniae, Rhodococcus equi, Nocardia* species, *Moraxella catarrhalis, Mycoplasma pneumoniae, Neisseria meningitidis*, and *Actinomyces* species
         (d) Rarely, pulmonary disease may be caused by *Mycobacterium kansasii, M. gordonae, M. fortuitum*
      (2) Protozoa
         (a) *Pneumocystis carinii* is the protozoal organism that most commonly causes lung disease in HIV-positive patients
         (b) There is debate about whether *P. carinii* is a protozoa or a fungus
         (c) *T. gondii* may also invade the lungs
      (3) *Cryptococcus neoformans, Coccidioides immitis, Histoplasma capsulatum*, and *Aspergillus fumigatus* may cause lung disease in HIV-infected patients
      (4) Mycobacteria
         (a) *M. tuberculosis is* the most important in causing lung disease
         (b) *M. avium, M. intracellulare,* and perhaps other unclassified species may cause lung disease and are commonly termed *M. avium* complex (MAC)
      (5) Viruses: VZV and CMV are the most important viral organisms that may invade the lung
   d. Microorganisms reach the lungs via inhalation, aspiration, the blood stream, or (less commonly) from infection in site adjacent to lung
      (1) OIs originating from organisms that infected the patient earlier in life and are now reactivated (e.g., *P. carinii, C. immitis, H. capsulatum, M. tuberculosis*)
      (2) Community-acquired pneumonia is caused by bacterial organisms; presentation is similar in immunocompetent persons
      (3) Nosocomial pneumonia is usually caused by staphylococci or aerobic gram-negative rods, especially *P. aeruginosa*

2. Frequency and distribution
   a. Prevalence of pneumonia varies by geographic area
      (1) PCP rare in sub-Saharan Africa
      (2) TB common in Africa but affects only 4% of HIV-infected people in the U.S.; is the major OI worldwide (Stansell & Murray, 1994)
      (3) Coccidioidomycosis and histoplasmosis occur in endemic U.S. regions
   b. Bacterial pneumonia common; risk 5–80 times greater in HIV-infected people than in general population (Stansell & Murray, 1994)
   c. Viral pneumonia is relatively rare; CMV rarely causes pneumonitis (organism commonly present in pulmonary secretions but not thought to be cause of pulmonary disease)

3. Relationship to natural history of HIV disease
   a. Immunosuppression
      (1) Multiple alterations in normal respiratory tract defense mechanisms

occur as a result of HIV infection and predispose patient to pulmonary infection; extent of alterations varies with degree of immunosuppression

(a) Patients with normal CD4+ lymphocyte counts tend to have disease from organisms common to general population

(b) The more severe the immunosuppression, the less virulent the organism needs to be to cause disease

(c) TB and *S. pneumoniae* are more virulent and cause disease in patients with less immunosuppression; average CD4+ lymphocyte count of persons with TB is 326/µl (Stansell & Murray, 1994)

(2) HIV significantly increases likelihood that TB infection will progress to disease; *P. carinii* and MAC are less virulent than TB and tend to cause disease in patients with CD4+ lymphocyte counts <200/µl; incidence of bacterial pneumonia is 3 times higher for IDUs than for gay men in one large prospective cohort study (Hirschtick et al., 1995)

b. Many alterations in respiratory tract defense mechanisms occur as a result of HIV infection

(1) Decreased levels of IgA on surfaces of mucosa and impairment in killing of microorganisms by mononuclear cells predispose to infection with encapsulated bacteria

(2) Decreased concentration of salivary IgA increases likelihood of colonization of the oropharynx with microorganisms; IgA levels further reduced by *Candida* or HSV infection

(3) Alveolar macrophages likely to be reservoir for HIV; they are functionally impaired in HIV infection with reduced chemotaxis, altered phagocytosis, and altered generation of toxic compounds that kill microorganisms

(4) Natural killer cells do not function

in HIV disease, thus reducing host defenses against infection

(5) Reduced production of opsonizing antibodies in B-lymphocytes predisposes patients to bacterial pneumonia

(6) Response of polymorphonuclear leukocytes to infection is defective

(7) Antibody response to organisms that previously entered the body is altered; on reinfection with these organisms, there is therefore less phagocytosis and killing by neutrophils

(8) Other factors

(a) Colonization of airway with organisms such as *Candida* causes alterations in mucosal integrity and predisposes to colonization with pathogenic bacteria

(b) Smoking alters normal respiratory tract defense mechanisms and contributes to development of bronchitis and bacterial pneumonia; smokers with CD4+ lymphocyte counts <200/µl had a higher ratio of bacterial pneumonia than nonsmokers in a study of the pulmonary complications of HIV infection (Hirschtick et al., 1995)

4. Morbidity and mortality

a. Community-acquired pneumonia

(1) Generally, incidence of bacterial pneumonia exceeds that of PCP

(2) Treatment usually successful; in spite of this, 25%–50% of patients have recurrences

b. Nosocomial pneumonia

(1) High morbidity and mortality rates

(2) Generally, patients have severe immunosuppression and prior pulmonary infections that have resulted in airway damage or bronchiectasis

(3) Patients' airways often colonized with organisms that are difficult to eradicate

c. Multidrug-resistant TB (MDR-TB) emerged in 1990 as a public health issue; see *Mycobacterium Tuberculosis*, p. 55

(1) Several outbreaks were reported in hospitals and prisons in New York and Florida

(2) MDR-TB is defined as resistant to isoniazid and rifampin, the most important first-line drugs in TB treatment; it is not uncommon for patients to be resistant to ≥5 drugs; mortality from MDR-TB ranges from 70%–90%, with a median survival of <4 months from diagnosis to death

d. Fungal pathogens

(1) *Cryptococcus* causes approximately 5%–8% of OIs; pulmonary disease less common than meningitis; high risk or deterioration from cryptococcal pneumonia

(2) In one study (Fish et al., 1990), 40% of 77 patients infected with *C. immitis* had diffuse pulmonary disease, 26% had focal pulmonary disease; patients with diffuse pulmonary disease have a particularly poor prognosis, while those with localized infections of the lung may have the best prognosis

(3) *Aspergillus* (relatively uncommon in people with HIV disease)

(a) May present as one of three clinical syndromes: allergic bronchopulmonary aspergillosis, *A. mycetoma* or fungus ball, and invasive disease

(b) Usually occurs in patients with several coexisting OIs; the lung is the most common site of invasive aspergillosis

e. Protozoa

(1) *P. carinii* is the most important and prevalent parasite that causes pneumonia in patients with HIV

(a) Widespread use of chemoprophylaxis has reduced incidence of PCP to 46% of AIDS-defining diagnoses in 1991 from almost 66% earlier in the HIV epidemic

(b) Mortality from PCP remains significant in patients who develop acute respiratory failure, but improved therapy has reduced

rate from >80% to approximately 60% since 1986 (Stansell & Murray, 1994)

(2) Mortality rate from pulmonary toxoplasmosis is approximately 40%

(3) Pulmonary infiltrates occur in approximately 25% of patients infected with *H. capsulatum*

5. Early detection, prevention, prophylaxis

a. Bacterial pneumonia

(1) TMP-SMX reduced the risk of bacterial pneumonia by 32%–67% in one prospective study (Hirschtick et al., 1995)

(2) Pneumococcal vaccine advocated for patients early in HIV infection; delay immunization 4 weeks after starting AZT in patients with advanced disease

(3) TB: See *Bacterial Infections*, p. 55

b. MAC: Rifabutin is recommended prophylaxis in patients with CD4+ lymphocyte count <75/μl

c. PCP: See *Parasitic Infections*, p. 112

d. Fungal and viral pneumonia: No primary prophylaxis

e. Secondary prevention and prophylaxis

(1) Bacterial pneumonia: TMP-SMZ advocated if tolerated for patients with recurrent episodes

(2) TB and other mycobacteria: See *Bacterial Infections*, p. 55

(3) MAC: Patients with infection usually treated for duration of life

(4) PCP: Patients with prior history of PCP should also receive prophylaxis; regimens and dosages same as for primary prophylaxis

(5) Fungal pneumonia: Indefinite maintenance or suppressive therapy

(6) Viral pneumonia: No demonstrated value of maintenance therapy to prevent relapses of CMV pneumonia

6. Signs and symptoms

a. Bacterial pneumonia

(1) Similar in patients with and without HIV disease; generally, acute onset of fever, shaking, chills, cough productive of purulent sputum; duration of symptoms <3 days in 60% of patients

(2) Leukocytosis generally present with WBC count higher than patient's baseline, increased number of immature cells

(3) Hypoxia and hypocarbia common, depending on severity of pneumonia and presence of underlying lung disease

b. Mycobacterial pneumonia, MAC: See *Bacterial Infections,* p. 55

c. Protozoa: See *Parasitic Infections*, p. 112

(1) PCP may present with constitutional symptoms that persist for as long as 1 month, but pace of illness varies; commonly presents with fever, nonproductive cough, dyspnea on exertion

(2) Toxoplasma pneumonia generally incidental to encephalitis; cough and shortness of breath may be present

d. Fungi: See *Fungal Diseases,* p. 83

(1) Cough and shortness of breath

(2) Possible pleuritic chest pain

e. Viral pneumonia (see *Viral Infections*, p. 94): Necessary to rule out presence of disease from other organisms if viral pneumonia suspected; even if patient infected with viral organism in presence of another OI, symptoms generally resolve without antiviral therapy when the other nonviral OI is treated

7. Diagnosis

a. Bacterial pneumonia

(1) Frequently see focal consolidation on chest x-ray that may occur in multiple sites; bacteremia seen in 50%–80% of patients (Stansell & Murray, 1994)

(2) Initial Gram's stain, sputum/blood culture

b. Protozoal pneumonia

(1) PCP

(a) Generally see diffuse, symmetrical interstitial infiltrates on chest x-ray, although can present as focal infiltrate; pneumocystoceles may occur; few patients have a normal chest x-ray

(b) Pulmonary-diffusing capacity is usually <75% predicted when corrected for hemoglobin; the diffusing capacity may be useful in patient with normal chest x-ray

i) Some radiologists advocate performing a high resolution CT (HRCT) scan instead of a pulmonary-diffusing capacity if the patient has a normal chest x-ray

ii) In the patient with PCP the HRCT shows ground-glass abnormalities; if these are not present, it is highly unlikely the patient has PCP

(c) Elevated serum LDH present in 90% of cases, but is not specific

(d) Decreased arterial-oxygen tension or elevated arterial-alveolar oxygen gradient often present, but dependent on disease severity

(e) Diagnosis confirmed on sputum stain, bronchoalveolar lavage (BAL), or biopsy; presumptive diagnosis can be made on the basis of clinical findings

i) Induced sputum with inhalation of hypertonic saline aerosol increases sensitivity of sputum to as high as 77%

ii) Sensitivity of BAL: 86%–97%

(f) Transbronchial biopsy usually performed only if other procedures nondiagnostic

(g) Organism cannot be cultured; common stains used to identify cysts or trophozoites are methenamine sliver, Giemsa, toluidine blue 0, and immunofluorescent stain using monoclonal antibodies against cyst walls or trophozoites

(2) Toxoplasma pneumonia is difficult to diagnose; organism must be detected in BAL fluid or lung tissue specimen

c. Fungal pneumonia

(1) Cryptococcal pneumonia: Positive cryptococcal antigen in serum or pleural fluid; diagnosis confirmed

with culture of *C. neoformans* from sputum or BAL

(2) Coccidioidomycosis: Cultured from sputum, BAL, transbronchial biopsy (TBB), or identification of giant spherule on cytology

d. Mycobacterial pneumonia
 (1) Diagnosis established with culture of *M. tuberculosis*
 (2) Presence of AFB on smear of sputum, bronchoalveolar lavage fluid, transbronchial biopsy, pleural fluid or tissue is indication for empiric treatment until culture results are available
 (3) Atypical mycobacteria not distinguished on AFB smear; must be identified on culture
 (4) Patients suspected of having infection with atypical organisms may be treated empirically

e. Viral pneumonia is difficult to diagnose; requires pathognomonic cells with intranuclear or intracytoplasmic inclusion bodies, the demonstration of CMV antigen or DNA in lung tissue, or CMV on culture of lung secretions or tissue in absence of other pathogenic organisms

8. Treatment
 a. Bacterial pneumonia
  (1) Specific therapy for organism-causing pneumonia if identified on culture
  (2) Empiric antibiotic therapy based on clinical presentation and radiographic findings if organism not identified
  (3) TB: See *Mycobacterium tuberculosis*, p. 55
  (4) MAC: Treat with 2 drugs, usually a macrolide antibiotic and ethambutol
 b. for PCP, other pneumonias: See *Fungal Diseases*, p. 83, *Parasitic Infections*, p. 112

9. Laboratory results and other indices to monitor for disease progression and response to therapy
 a. Clinical status of patient primary indication of response to therapy or disease progression for any type of pneumonia
 b. Persistent fever, shortness of breath, hypoxemia, and lack of radiographic

improvement indicate lack of resolution of pneumonia or new process

c. More severely immunocompromised patient, or patient with underlying lung disease less likely to do well

d. Patients with PCP less likely to do well if presenting with significant degree of hypoxemia

e. Drug-susceptibility studies are very important in the management of TB

B. Pulmonary Neoplastic Complications

1. Etiology and disease process
 a. Kaposi's sarcoma (KS): Respiratory manifestations follow development of mucocutaneous lesions in 90%–95% of cases (Stansell & Murray, 1994)
 b. Non-Hodgkin's lymphoma (NHL): Respiratory system involvement less common than in KS

2. Frequency and distribution
 a. KS: Pulmonary involvement found in 50% of cases at autopsy, evident on clinical grounds in 33%; approximately two thirds of patients with pulmonary KS also have coexisting OI
 b. NHL: Pulmonary involvement less frequent than other system involvement and occurs in <25% of patients at time of diagnosis; pulmonary involvements seen more frequently at autopsy (Stansell & Murray, 1994)

3. Relationship to natural history of HIV disease: Intrathoracic KS usually late manifestation of HIV disease

4. Morbidity and mortality
 a. KS: Prognosis of patients with pulmonary KS is only a few months
 b. NHL: Poor response to chemotherapy or radiation

5. Signs and symptoms
 a. Pulmonary KS
  (1) May present with cough, hemoptysis, bronchospasm, hemorrhagic pleural effusions, and progressive dyspnea leading to respiratory failure
  (2) Radiographic abnormalities may occur in lung parenchyma with

nonuniform linear densities that follow septal lines, nodular lesions of varying sizes, pleural effusions, and hilar or mediastinal adenopathy

b. Pulmonary NHL
   (1) Depend on degree of intrathoracic involvement; may present with cough and shortness of breath; usually presents as disseminated disease with extranodal involvement; symptoms depend on location of involvement
   (2) May see approximately 25% of patients have diffuse, bilateral reticulonodular opacities, may see well-defined single nodule, or multiple nodules of varying sizes; pulmonary nodules generally grow rapidly

6. Diagnosis
   a. Pulmonary KS: Difficult to establish diagnosis on biopsy of airway or lung tissue; usually confirmed by appearance of lesions on bronchoscopy; see *Kaposi's Sarcoma*, p. 128, for staging
   b. Pulmonary NHL: Malignant lymphocytes on cytology or biopsy specimen
      (1) Usually diagnosed with needle aspiration of lymph node; isolated pulmonary disease may require bronchoscopy with biopsy
      (2) Generally see high-grade histology that responds poorly to treatment (see *Non-Hodgkin's Lymphoma*, p. 131, for staging)

7. Treatment
   a. Acute
      (1) Pulmonary KS
         (a) Treat coexisting OI if present
         (b) With CD4+ lymphocyte count <200/µl or history of OIs, systemic chemotherapy generally advocated with adriamycin, vincristine, and bleomycin, but usually only temporarily effective
         (c) Large lesions that obstruct airways may respond transiently to radiation
         (d) Sclerotherapy may or may not be effective for recurrent pleural effusions
      (2) Pulmonary NHL

         (a) Multiple cytotoxic drugs are prescribed for lymphoma
         (b) Radiation palliative for large obstructing lesions
   b. Maintenance
      (1) Oxygen may be necessary for hypoxemia; antibiotic therapy for intercurrent bacterial infections for pulmonary KS
      (2) Trial of inhaled bronchodilators or corticosteroids may be advocated
      (3) Continue acute treatment if patient continues to respond

8. Laboratory results and other indices to monitor for disease progression and response to therapy
   a. Clinical presentation for resolution or progression of pulmonary signs and symptoms
   b. Progression of pulmonary disease with chest x-ray findings (see *Non-Hodgkin's Lymphoma*, p. 130, for other labs to monitor systemic disease progression)
   c. ABG/O$_2$ saturation
   d. Intercurrent pulmonary infection common with pulmonary KS
      (1) Exacerbation of symptoms may reflect infection or progression of pulmonary KS
      (2) Postobstructive pneumonia possible if lesions obstruct airway
      (3) Response of cutaneous disease to therapy usually reflected in visceral disease as well

9. See also *Anxiety*, p. 245, *Dyspnea*, p. 208

C. Sinusitis

1. Etiology and disease process
   a. Agents can be bacterial, fungal, or viral
      (1) Bacterial: *S. pneumoniae, H. influenzae, P. aeruginosa*
      (2) Fungal: *Aspergillus* (most common), mucormycosis, other fungal agents identified as pathogens in PWA
      (3) Viral: Rhinovirus, parainfluenza, influenza
   b. Process
      (1) Viral upper respiratory infection (URI) causes increase in secretions,

decrease in ciliary action, mechanical obstruction

(2) Stagnant secretions provide medium for secondary infection

(3) Impaired immune function diminishes host response

2. Frequency and distribution
   a. All PWAs are at risk for viral URIs and subsequent secondary infections
   b. Viral agents are contagious through droplet spread and direct infection via contaminated objects
   c. Bacterial agents are generally normal flora of the upper respiratory tract
   d. Fungal agents are in environment, although marijuana and smokeless tobacco may be contaminated with aspergillus spores

3. Relationship to natural history of HIV disease
   a. Bacterial and viral sinusitis can occur any time in the HIV continuum
   b. Fungal sinusitis is most common in patients with CD4+ lymphocyte counts <50/µl

4. Morbidity and mortality
   a. Between one third and two thirds of PWAs will develop sinusitis at some point in their illness (Zurlo et al., 1992)
   b. Bacterial sinusitis is not life threatening per se, but complications such as sepsis or abscess can carry a high mortality rate
   c. Fungal sinusitis is associated with significant mortality

5. Early detection, prevention, prophylaxis
   a. Prevention
      (1) Smoking cessation; avoiding use of inhaled marijuana or smokeless tobacco
      (2) Use of decongestants prior to air travel to decrease congestion, stasis of secretions
   b. Eliminating/avoiding known allergens
   c. If using marijuana or smokeless tobacco, bake at 350°F for approximately 20 min to kill *Aspergillus* spores

6. Signs and symptoms
   a. Headache, nasal congestion, purulent rhinorrhea, cough (from post nasal drip)
   b. Tenderness over infected sinus, fever,

purulent post nasal drip, retracted tympana membrane, cobblestone appearance of posterior pharynx, boggy nasal membranes, purulent discharge from nasal turbinate

7. Diagnosis
   a. Tests/procedures
      (1) Physical exam
      (2) Radiologic imaging: Plain films to check for air fluid levels, CT to evaluate for thickened membranes, obvious infection or structural abnormalities
      (3) Antral puncture to obtain material for culture, usually after failure of empirical therapy
   b. Staging: Not uniform in definition
      (1) Acute: Associated with pain, fever, congestion, purulent rhinorrhea
      (2) Subacute: Resolution of pain, fever, but persisting purulent rhinorrhea
      (3) Chronic: Prolonged repeated acute infections lead to changes in mucosa, leading to overgrowth of bacteria (commonly anaerobes and gram-negative bacteria)
   c. Differential diagnosis
      (1) Muscle tension headache, cluster headache, migraine, trigeminal neuralgia
      (2) Dental abcess
      (3) Noninfectious rhinitis (vasomotor, allergic)

8. Treatment
   a. Acute: Treat the underlying infection
      (1) Antimicrobial agent depends on infectious agent and sensitivities
      (2) HIV-positive patients generally require a longer course of treatment for bacterial sinusitis
      (3) Antibiotics commonly used for other indications (e.g., TMP-SMX) may create resistance
      (4) Aspergillosis: Amphotericin B until improvement, then continue indefinitely
      (5) Correct structural abnormalities if present
      (6) Supportive measures for comfort: Analgesics, decongestants, antihista-

mines, steam inhalation, warm packs to face
b. Maintenance: If allergic component contributing to stasis of secretions or obstruction, nasal steroids may be used
9. Patient education
   a. Importance of completing full course of antibiotic, even if symptoms resolved
   b. Prolonged use of decongestants to be avoided as rebound may occur
   c. Persistent fever, facial swelling, and periorbital edema require immediate attention
   d. Ameliorating adverse effects of amphotericin-B

D. Inflammatory Airway Disorders

1. Etiology and disease process
   a. Acute bronchitis: inflammation of the airways
   b. Bronchiectasis: abnormal dilation of bronchi resulting from destruction of muscular and elastic components of the walls
   c. Acute bronchitis and bronchiectasis generally are caused by the same bacteria that cause pneumonia (see *Pulmonary Complications*, p. 151)
   d. *Aspergillus* species may be found if cause of bronchiectasis is allergic bronchopulmonary aspergillosis
   e. *Pseudomonas* and *E. coli* may be found in secretions of patients with bronchiectasis
2. Relationship to natural history of HIV disease
   a. Acute bronchitis occurs throughout course of HIV disease
   b. Acute bronchitis and bronchiectasis may be seen more frequently in patients with recurrent pulmonary OIs
   c. Smokers are at increased risk of bronchitis
3. Morbidity and mortality
   a. Incidence of bronchitis in patients with HIV disease: 9.96/100 person years compared to 4.93/100 person years in normal controls in one large prospective study (Wallace et al., 1993)
   b. Incidence of bronchiectasis not well described in patients with HIV disease
4. Early detection, prevention, prophylaxis
   a. Urge patients to stop smoking
   b. No primary or secondary prophylactic therapy; there may be lower incidence of bronchitis in patients on TMP-SMX prophylaxis for PCP; however, this has not been demonstrated in any prospective studies
   c. Appropriate treatment and prophylaxis of pulmonary OI may reduce incidence of bronchiectasis
5. Signs and symptoms
   a. Bronchitis
      (1) Cough, usually productive of purulent sputum, that persists for at least 48 hours
      (2) Fever, wheezing, and shortness of breath may also be present
   b. Bronchiectasis
      (1) Chronic cough productive of foul-smelling sputum
      (2) Also fever, weakness, weight loss
6. Diagnosis
   a. Generally, diagnosis of bronchitis and bronchiectasis is based on signs and symptoms and absence of infiltrate on chest x-ray suggestive of pneumonia
   b. In bronchitis, thickened bronchial walls and "tram tracking" frequently seen on chest x-ray in bronchitis; bronchiectasis shows the same features with varying degrees of bronchial dilation—may include cysts with air-fluid levels
   c. Sputum Gram's stain or culture may be performed; however, patients are frequently treated empirically
7. Treatment
   a. Broad-spectrum antibiotic generally prescribed: TMP-SMX × 10 days, azithromycin × 4 days, clarithromycin × 7–14 days, augmentin × 7–10 days
8. Patient education
   a. Teach patient the relationship between smoking and bronchitis
   b. Institute a smoking-cessation program as patient desires

E. Interstitial Pneumonitis

1. Etiology and disease process
   a. Lymphocytic (lymphoid) interstitial pneumonitis (LIP): Cause unknown, possible viral etiology (e.g., EBV and HIV acting together to produce disease)
   b. Nonspecific interstitial pneumonitis (NIP): Etiology unknown
   c. Pulmonary lymphoid hyperplasia (PLH): Etiology unknown
   d. Drug-induced: TMP-SMX and cytoxic drugs (especially bleomycin) may cause interstitial pneumonitis; process usually resolves when drug discontinued
2. Frequency and distribution
   a. Incidence of interstitial lung disease is *very* low in adults with HIV infection, in contrast to incidence in children (see *Clinical Management of Pediatric HIV Patients,* p. 375)
   b. LIP: Rare in adults
   c. NIP
      (1) Varying frequencies reported; dependent on number of lung biopsies performed
      (2) Diagnosis not always considered in workup
   d. PLH: Similar to LIP; may be part of same process
   e. Drug-induced pneumonitis: Frequency not known
3. Morbidity and mortality
   a. NIP: Usually stabilizes or resolves without therapy
   b. Drug-induced pneumonitis: Usually short survival, intercurrent infections frequent and complicate issue
4. Signs and symptoms
   a. NIP: Usually presents with fever, exertional dyspnea, and nonproductive cough
   b. Drug-induced pneumonitis: Generally presents with fever, rash, neutropenia
   c. LIP: See *Clinical Management of Pediatric HIV Patients,* p. 375
5. Diagnosis
   a. Histology
      (1) LIP and PLH: Diffuse infiltration of lung by lymphocytes, plasma cells, plasmacytoid lymphocytes, immunoblasts
      (2) NIP: Infiltration of mononuclear cells, predominantly lymphocytes and plasma cells, with edema and deposition of fibrin
   b. Tests/procedures
      (1) Chest x-ray
         (a) LIP and PLH: Chest x-ray for patients of all ages shows bilateral reticulonodular interstitial abnormalities generally seen in lower lung zones
         (b) NIP: Diffuse interstitial pattern generally seen on chest x-ray; pleural effusions may occur; a few patients may have alveolar infiltrates or nodules (may also be normal)
      (2) Lung tissue biopsy necessary for definitive diagnosis
   c. Differential diagnoses: Infectious etiologies or other causes of lung inflammation such as oxygen or radiation therapy must be ruled out in all cases
6. Treatment
   a. Acute
      (1) Acute LIP not treated with any specific therapy if mild and hypoxia not present
      (2) Steroids prescribed with biopsy-proven disease and PaO_2 <85 mm Hg
      (3) Antibiotics to treat intercurrent bacterial exacerbations and inhaled bronchodilators for any symptoms of obstruction
      (4) Antiretroviral therapy may be beneficial
      (5) Oxygen therapy for hypoxemia
      (6) Intubation and ventilation for acute respiratory failure
   b. Maintenance
      (1) Antiretroviral therapy generally advocated; courses of antibiotics, steroids, bronchodilators as necessary for exacerbations
      (2) Oxygen therapy for chronic hypoxemia
7. Laboratory results or other indices to monitor for disease progression and response to therapy
   a. Chest x-ray
   b. ABGs
   c. Pulse oximetry
   d. Symptom improvement.

XIII. DERMATOLOGIC COMPLICATIONS

A. Papulosquamous Disorders

1. Seborrheic Dermatitis

a. Etiology and disease process
   (1) Possible association or causative role of *Pitysrosporum ovale* or resident skin fungus/yeast
   (2) Unclear theories
      (a) Diminished T-cell function
      (b) Decreased numbers of Langerhans cells
      (c) Pyogenic infection often present
      (d) Role of alcohol, diet, stress questionable
      (e) May be hormonally dependent
      (f) Vitamin deficiency
b. Frequency and distribution: Up to 80% incidence in AIDS patients compared with 5% in general population
c. Relationship to natural history of HIV disease
   (1) Incidence increases as CD4+ lymphocyte count falls below 150/μl
   (2) May be a cutaneous marker for HIV
   (3) Most common cause of blepharitis in HIV
d. Signs and symptoms
   (1) Red, scaly eruption
   (2) White, yellowish-red, greasy, scaling macules and papules
   (3) Areas of high concentration of sebaceous glands (face, presternal area, body folds, scalp, eyebrows, nasolabial folds)
   (4) Gradual onset, chronic
   (5) Pruritus variable
   (6) Superficial inflammatory disease
   (7) May be made worse by some neuroleptic drugs (e.g., haloperidol)
e. Diagnosis
   (1) History and physical exam, response to therapy
   (2) Differential diagnoses: Psoriasis, dermatophytosis (fungal), candidiasis, etopic dermatitis, fosacea
f. Treatment
   (1) Scalp: Selenium sulfide shampoo, zinc pyrithione, topical triamcinolone acetate 0.1% solution, topical antifungals (e.g., ketoconazole 2% cream)
   (2) Face/body
      (a) Hydrocortisone acetate cream 1%–2.5% twice daily
      (b) Topical antifungals (e.g., ketoconazole 2% cream)
g. Patient education: Review features, prevention, treatment

2. Psoriasis

a. Etiology and disease process: A chronic scaling skin disorder with an unclear etiology
   (1) Activity of CD8 cytotoxic/suppressor T cells, perhaps in response to dysfunctional or infected Langerhans cells
   (2) May flare with stress, sunburn, streptococcal pharyngeal infections, medications, localized trauma
   (3) Inflammation plus alteration of the skin cell cycle
   (4) Probably a cluster of diseases
   (5) Skin turns over 4–5 times faster
   (6) Sometimes associated with arthritis; see *Musculoskeletal System Complications*, p. 191
b. Frequency and distribution: Up to 2% of HIV-infected population compared with 1% of general population
c. Relationship to natural history of HIV disease
   (1) About one third of cases represent exacerbations of known psoriasis, but most cases of psoriasis present after HIV infection is diagnosed (Obuch et al., 1992)
   (2) Patients with HIV-associated psoriasis (especially psoriatic arthritis) have a high prevalence of HLA-B27 or B7 CREG antigens, suggesting a genetic predisposition to the development of psoriasis with HIV infection (Wright et al., 1991)
d. Signs and symptoms: Same as non-HIV infected
   (1) Chronic, scaly plaques on elbows, knees, lumbosacral areas

(2) Discrete guttate (droplike) plaques
(3) Diffuse dermatitis with thickening
(4) Nail dystrophy (25% of the time)
(5) Bilateral, rarely symmetrical
e. Diagnosis
  (1) Clinical: Distribution, appearance, and response to therapy
  (2) Exclude secondary infection by culture and stains
  (3) Biopsy for definitive diagnosis
  (4) Consultation with dermatologist
  (5) Differential diagnosis: Seborrheic dermatitis, pityriasis rosea, eczema, lupus erythematosus
f. Treatment
  (1) Variable, dependent on stage of disease, site and extent, degree of disability
  (2) Topical corticosteroids
    (a) Fluorinated corticosteroids in ointment base applied after removing the scales by soaking in water
    (b) Occlusion with plastic wrap overnight enhances response to ointment
    (c) Prolonged application of fluorinated agents leads to atrophy and telangiectasia
    (d) May treat small plaques with intradermal injections of triamcinolone acetonide aqueous suspension
  (3) Other treatments: tars, salicylic acid, Denorex, Anthralin, ultraviolet light therapy
  (4) Systemic therapy
    (a) AZT use may lead to improvement; usually requires >1 g/day
    (b) Etretinate (Tegison)
g. Patient instructions
  (1) No scratching or rubbing
  (2) Teach self-care measures and provide instruction on medications

B. Hypersensitivity Disorders

1. Drug Reactions

a. Etiology and disease process: Unclear; possibly dose related, cumulative effect

b. Common classifications
  (1) Toxic erythema; most common maculopapular rash
    (a) Occurs in up to 60% treated with TMP-SMX
    (b) 10 times more frequent in patients with HIV than in non-HIV infected
    (c) Occurs in up to 75% treated with clindamycin
    (d) Occurs in up to 44% with amoxicillin-clavulanate
    (e) Maculopapular eruption
  (2) Erythema multiforme: Can progress to Stevens-Johnson syndrome (severe allergic reaction)
  (3) Eczematous
  (4) Exfoliative dermatitis and erythroderma
  (5) Fixed eruptions
  (6) Urticaria (hives)
c. Signs and symptoms
  (1) Bright erythema
  (2) May be severely itchy
  (3) May be associated with fever and constitutional complaints
  (4) Symmetric distribution
  (5) Begins and is more pronounced on the trunk
  (6) Most commonly from antibiotics, sulfonamides, barbiturates, dilantin
  (7) Usually occur 7–14 days after initiation of the drug
d. Diagnosis
  (1) Review medication history
  (2) Subsides after drug withdrawal
  (3) CBC may show new leukopenia, eosinophilia, agranulocytosis
e. Treatment
  (1) Discontinue suspected drug and all nonessential drugs
  (2) Watch closely for systemic manifestations (fever, anemia)
  (3) Treat systemic manifestations
  (4) Antihistamines
  (5) Increase fluid intake
  (6) Hospitalization may be required if the patient develops Stevens-Johnson syndrome
f. Patient education: Review medication risks and signs and symptoms

2. **Pruritic Eruptions**
   a. Etiology and disease process: Unclear
   b. Signs and symptoms
      (1) Rash may or may not be present
      (2) Excoriations from scratching may be present
      (3) May be follicular
      (4) May be associated with systemic disease, especially if itching present without rash (renal, hepatic, endocrinologic, hematologic)
      (5) May be localized to anal or genital area; consider infectious, parasitic, inflammatory, or psychogenic causes
   c. Diagnosis
      (1) Scraping for microscopic evaluation (scabies, mite eggs)
      (2) Response to therapy
      (3) Biopsy
      (4) Differential diagnosis
         (a) Scabies, contact dermatitis, drug reaction, syphilis, folliculitis, insect bites, fungal infections, atopic dermatitis, neurodermatitis
         (b) Consider eosinophilic folliculitis (EF) if the following are present
            i) Chronic waxing and waning course
            ii) Discrete, erythematous, urticarial, follicular papules
            iii) Present primarily on the trunk, face, head, neck, and proximal extremities, 90% above the nipple line
            iv) CD4+ lymphocyte count <250/µl
            v) Relative or absolute eosinophilia
   d. Treatment (specific for cause): Antibiotics, topical steroids, antifungals, parasiticidals

3. **Insect Bites/Scabies**
   a. Etiology and disease process
      (1) Fleas, mosquitos, spiders, other insects
      (2) Scabies mites
         (a) Highly contagious: Direct and indirect contact
         (b) Concentrated around web spaces of fingers, wrists
         (c) Frequently involves nipples, penis, axilla
         (d) Distinctive burrows
         (e) Pruritus may persist after successful treatment
   b. Signs and symptoms: Papular urticaria, vesicular, sometimes tense bulla; itching may be intense
   c. Diagnosis
      (1) Clinically characteristic
      (2) Skin scraping for microscopic evaluation of scabies, mite eggs
      (3) Skin biopsy
   d. Treatment
      (1) Oral antihistamines
      (2) Topical antipruritic agents
      (3) Insect protection
      (4) Scabies: Lindane (Kwell) or permethrin (Elimite) preferred when CD4+ lymphocyte count <200/µl
         (a) May require repeated treatments
         (b) Recently worn clothing and linens should be washed in hot water
         (c) Assess household, intimate contacts for signs and symptoms of infestation

4. **Photosensitivity Eruptions**
   a. Etiology and disease process
      (1) Pathogenesis unknown
      (2) Severity of reaction a result of the concentration of the photosensitizing substance and intensity of light
      (3) Common with TMP-SMX, tetracyclines, and dapsone
      (4) May occur with topical or ingested substances
      (5) Types of photosensitivity
         (a) Phototoxic: Markedly increased sunburn response within 2–6 hours
         (b) Photoallergic: Sunburn response to exposed areas in 24–48 hours
   b. Signs and symptoms
      (1) Papular or scaly pruritic eruption, may become exudative
      (2) May appear similar to contact dermatitis

(3) Largely restricted to sun-exposed areas

(4) Facial eruption may resemble seborrheic dermatitis except different distribution

c. Relationship to natural history of HIV disease

(1) Any stage of HIV infection

(2) One of the most treatable dermatoses

d. Diagnosis: By history and distribution

e. Treatment

(1) Sun protection: SPF 15, hats (especially summer and midday)

(2) Alternate medications if possible

(3) Mild topical steroids to areas of eruption

f. Patient education

(1) Increase sun protection

(2) Decrease sun exposure

(3) Alternate medications if possible

C. General Changes of the Skin, Nails, and Hair

Skin

1. **Hyperkeratosis** (any horny superficial growth on skin)

a. Etiology and disease process: May be an isolated finding or associated with another illness (e.g., psoriasis, cutaneous fungal infection, Reiter's syndrome, Kaposi's sarcoma)

b. Signs and symptoms

(1) Thickening of the skin, especially the palms and soles

(2) May be areas of pustulation within keratotic plaques

c. Treatment

(1) See *Psoriasis,* p. 160

(2) Keratolytic agents (e.g., Keralyt Gel) must be used cautiously to avoid skin irritation or dryness

2. **Xerosis** (pathologic dryness of skin)

a. Etiology and disease process

(1) Often associated with excessive bathing, hot water, deodorant soaps

(2) People with atopic diatheses and the elderly are predisposed

(3) Those with hay fever, asthma, or previous atopic dermatitis may be predisposed

b. Frequency

(1) More severe in winter

(2) Occurs in up to 20% of patients with HIV

(3) Often involves anterior lower legs and posterior arms

c. Morbidity and mortality

(1) The most common cause of itching with no visible rash

(2) The most common HIV-associated scaling dermatosis

d. Relationship to natural history of HIV disease

(1) CD4+ lymphocyte count usually <400/µl

(2) Tends to be more severe with HIV progression

e. Signs and symptoms

(1) Generalized dryness

(2) Branlike scaling, minimal erythema

(3) Decreased skin turgor

(4) Often severely pruritic, widespread

f. Diagnosis

(1) By history and physical exam

(2) Differential diagnosis: Scabies, fungal infections

g. Treatment

(1) Mild soaps (e.g., Dove), axilla and groin only

(2) Water only to body, except scalp/face

(3) Emollients (e.g., Eucerin Cream) with urea and lactic acid (e.g., Lachydrin)

(4) Antihistamines (e.g., diphenhydramine, hydroxyzine) usually not helpful; may be resistant to antihistamines

(5) Weak topical steroids in ointment base (e.g., 1% hydrocortisone)

h. Patient education

(1) Avoid excessive bathing, hot water, deodorant soaps

(2) Provide patient with written self-care instructions for prevention and care

3. **Hyperpigmentation**

a. Etiology and disease process

(1) Enhanced melanin production; may follow any skin inflammation
(2) May be associated with medications (e.g., AZT)
(3) May be associated with sun exposure
b. Frequency and distribution: Most common in dark-skinned people
c. Signs and symptoms
(1) May involve areas of the skin, oral mucosa, or nails
(2) Nevi and freckles may become darker
(3) May be an increased number of nevi and freckles
d. Treatment: Limit sun exposure, skin irritation

Nails

4. **Onychomycosis** (fungal infection of the nail)
a. Etiology and disease process: Fungal infections
b. Signs and symptoms: Lusterless, brittle, hypertrophic, friable nails
c. Diagnosis
(1) By appearance
(2) Microscopic evaluation with 15% potassium hydroxide usually not necessary
(3) Culture: False-negative rate 30%–50%
(4) Nail biopsy
(5) Differential diagnosis: Psoriasis
d. Treatment
(1) Topical therapy of no use in 95% of cases and not cost-effective; only Naftin gel works
(2) Toenails difficult to cure; fingernails curable
(3) Systemic antifungals
e. Patient education: Review features, prevention, and treatment strategies

5. **Pigmented Nail Bands**
a. Etiology and disease process: Probably melanin deposits
b. Signs and symptoms

(1) More common in dark-skinned people
(2) Azure (blue) lunae
(3) Associated with AZT therapy within 4–8 weeks after initiation, usually reversible
c. Treatment: None required

Hair

6. **Hair changes**
a. Etiology and disease process: Possibly due to medications or HIV itself
b. Signs and symptoms
(1) Begins at crown, progresses frontotemporally; may be noticeable to patient only
(2) Thin hair shafts, no inflammation
(3) Premature frontal recession of hairline
(4) Premature greying
c. Common classifications
(1) Elongation of the eyelashes
(a) May be associated with any severe illness
(b) Prolongation of the hair growth phase
(2) Alopecia areata (patchy hair loss with discrete bald areas)
(a) Probably autoimmune
(b) Possibly abnormality in T-lymphocytes
d. Treatment
(1) Reassurance
(2) Area injected with steroids

D. Infectious/Neoplastic Conditions

1. Bacterial infections (e.g., *S. aureus*): See *Bacterial Infections*, p. 55, *Syphilis*, p. 67
2. Viral infections (e.g., *Herpesvirus*): See *Viral Infections*, p. 94
3. Fungal infections (e.g., *Candida*): See *Fungal Diseases*, p. 83
4. Neoplastic infections (e.g., *Kaposi's sarcoma*): See *Malignancies*, p. 128
5. See also *Musculoskeletal System Complications*, p. 191, *Impaired/Risk for Impaired Skin Integrity*, p. 222.

XIV. HEMATOLOGIC COMPLICATIONS

A. Anemia

1. Etiology and disease process
   a. Deficiency in the quantity or quality of red blood cells needed to meet tissue oxygen demands
   b. Pathophysiology
      (1) Typically, anemias are normocytic and normochromic with a low reticulocyte response
      (2) Ineffective erythropoiesis is due to
         (a) Nutritional factors
            i) Decrease in B_{12} levels and a decrease in serum iron and iron binding capacity
            ii) Clinically significant complications are rare
         (b) Direct infection of erythroid precursors by HIV
         (c) Cytokine-induced suppression and inhibition of progenitor cells
         (d) Infiltration of bone marrow (e.g., lymphoma, *M. avium*)
         (e) Immunologic impairment
         (f) Drug side effects (e.g., AZT): See *AZT-Induced Anemia*, p. 166
2. Frequency and distribution
   a. 70%–90% of patients with AIDS; the most common hematologic complication associated with HIV infection
   b. 5%–16% of patients with persistent generalized lymphadenopathy (PGL) and patients with symptomatic HIV disease have anemia
   c. 8% of patients with asymptomatic HIV infection
3. Relationship to natural history of HIV disease: Incidence increases with progression of disease
4. Morbidity and mortality
   a. Anemia leads to diminished oxygen transport and increased cardiac workload, which can cause severe fatigue, exercise intolerance, restrictions in ADL, and interference with work
   b. Drug-induced anemia may cause patients to stop or switch antiretroviral therapy, leading to disease progression
5. Early detection, prevention, prophylaxis
   a. Monitor for signs and symptoms of anemia (CBC, Hgb, Hct)
   b. Monitor for drug side effects: AZT, ganciclovir, dapsone, pentamidine, pyrimethamine, TMP-SMX, amphotericin B
   c. Nutritional guidance: dietary sources of iron (red meats), iron and vitamin supplements
6. Signs and symptoms (often asymptomatic with mild anemia):
   a. Cardiac: Fatigue, dyspnea on exertion, dyspnea at rest (severe anemia), tachycardia, palpitations, systolic ejection murmur
   b. Neurologic: Headaches, dizziness, tinnitus, insomnia
   c. GI: Anorexia, nausea, constipation or diarrhea, stomatitis
   d. Pallor: Skin and nail beds, conjunctiva, oral mucosa
7. Diagnosis: Based on lab findings
   a. Complete blood count; RBC, Hgb, Hct; reticulocyte count
   b. Nutritional deficiencies: Serum B_{12} level, folate and iron levels
   c. If suspect GI blood loss, send stool for occult blood; GI endoscopy to determine source of bleeding if needed
   d. Review history for medications that cause anemia
8. Treatment
   a. Decision to treat should be based on symptomatology
   b. Treatment should be based on the cause of the anemia
      (1) Nutritional deficiency: Dietary and supplemental iron, folate, vitamin B_{12}
      (2) Medications
         (a) Switch therapy to alternate medication if possible, *or*
         (b) Modify dosage or temporarily withhold the drug
      (3) Transfusion support; nursing considerations include
         (a) Preparation
            i) Explain procedure and

teach patient to report signs of transfusion reaction

  ii) Obtain baseline vital signs, premedicate as needed

  (b) Verification (per agency protocol)

  i) Verify physician order for transfusion

  ii) Inspect blood component (packed RBCs) for ABO and Rh type against patient's ID with 2nd nurse

  iii) Check expiration date of blood product

  iv) Verify patient's identification

  (c) Administration

  i) Start transfusion slowly (5 ml for first 15 min); recheck vital signs at 15 min and then per agency's policy

  ii) Administer within 30 min after removal from blood refrigerator

  iii) Infuse over 2–3 hours; change filter q4h or per agency protocol

  iv) Never add medications or diluents other than 0.9% normal saline, per agency's policy

  v) Use universal precautions when handling blood products

  (4) Recombinant human erythropoietin

  (5) Treat infections and cancers that cause myelosuppression and transfuse if indicated

9. Laboratory results and other indices to monitor for disease progression and response to therapy

  a. Iron stores are decreased along with total iron binding capacity

  b. Monitor CBC for improvement

  c. May have abnormal Schilling test

  d. False serum ferritin elevation due to inflammation, malignancy, or liver injury

10. Patient education

  a. Knowledge about anemia

  b. Impact on lifestyle and role relationships

  c. Activity tolerance (see *Fatigue*, p. 209)

  (1) Alternate physical activity with frequent rest periods

  (2) Enhance sleep quality

  (a) Decrease environmental noise

  (b) Use body massage and relaxation tapes (see *Massage*, p. 343)

  (3) Seek assistance with ADL when needed

  d. Medication management

  (1) Correct dosing and timing of medications

  (2) Knowledge of and timely reporting of early side effects

B. AZT-Induced Anemia

1. Etiology and disease process: Myelosuppressive effect of AZT, which inhibits erythroid colony-forming units (CFU-E)

2. Frequency and distribution

  a. 70% of patients treated with AZT will have macrocytosis within 2–3 weeks after initiation of AZT therapy

  b. In patients who do not show macrocytosis, an early indicator of AZT-related myelosuppression is a fall in the reticulocyte count

3. Relationship to natural history of HIV disease: Patients with AIDS or more advanced HIV disease develop anemia from AZT more frequently than people with less advanced HIV disease

4. Morbidity and mortality: AZT-induced anemia may necessitate cessation of therapy, leading to disease progression

5. Early detection, prevention, prophylaxis

  a. Avoid or closely monitor simultaneous use of drugs that enhance myelosuppression (e.g., probenecid, ganciclovir, trimetrexate)

  b. No available prophylaxis

6. Signs and symptoms (see *Anemia*, p. 165)

7. Diagnosis: Based on lab findings and excluding other etiologies of anemia

  a. Decrease in RBCs, Hgb, Hct

b. Macrocytosis (in 70% of patients taking AZT)

c. Decrease in reticulocyte count

d. Increased mean corpuscular volume (MCV); significance unclear

e. The following lab values are predictive of myelosuppression

   (1) Low CD4+ lymphocyte count

   (2) Low B_{12} level (or low normal)

   (3) Low folic acid levels

   (4) Low RBC and neutrophil counts

8. Treatment

a. Lower AZT dose or switch to alternate marrow-sparing drugs

b. Temporarily withhold drug therapy

c. Administer recombinant human erythropoietin as ordered

   (1) Stimulates red cell production

   (2) Therapeutic effects

      (a) Increased reticulocyte count in 1–2 weeks

      (b) Increased sense of well-being

   (3) Side effects: Hypertension, seizures, encephalopathy

d. Transfuse as indicated

e. Oxygen therapy

9. Laboratory results and other indices to monitor for disease progression and response to therapy

a. Monitor CBC for changes

b. Response to treatment

   (1) Oxygenation status

   (2) Signs and symptoms of anemia

10. Patient education

a. Regular lab work for drug-induced anemia

b. Early recognition and reporting of medication side effects

c. Correct dosage and timing of medications

d. Dietary and vitamin supplements

e. Pace ADL to alleviate fatigue; see *Fatigue*, p. 209

C. Leukopenia

1. Etiology and disease process

a. A decrease in the total number of white cells (granulocytes and lymphocytes) to <3,000 cells/mm³

b. Origin is multifactorial

   (1) Coexisting infection

   (2) B-cell neoplasm (or other neoplasms)

   (3) Antibiotics

   (4) Cytotoxic drugs

2. Frequency and distribution: 75% of patients with AIDS

3. Relationship to natural history of HIV disease: Incidence increases with disease progression

4. Morbidity and mortality

a. Leukopenia impairs ability of the patient to fight infection; increases susceptibility to infectious organisms and life-threatening infections

b. Drug-induced leukopenia may be an indication for cessation of treatment and progression of life-threatening infections

5. Signs and symptoms (signs of infection may not be apparent with severe leukopenia)

a. Respiratory tract: Cough, sputum production

b. Urinary tract infection: Frequency, urgency, burning

c. Abnormal WBC count

d. Fever

e. Nonspecific pain, fatigue, tachycardia, tachypnea

6. Diagnosis

a. Blood work: CBC with WBC differential

   (1) Decrease in leukocyte counts

   (2) Atypical lymphocytes present

   (3) Vacuolated monocytes

b. Review medications for side effect of myelosuppression

7. Treatment

a. Administration of granulocyte macrophage colony stimulating factor (GM-CSF)

   (1) Stimulates proliferation and differentiation of hematopoietic progenitor cells

   (2) Therapeutic effect (increase in leukocyte counts)

   (3) Contraindications: Hypersensitivity to GM-CSF and yeast products

   (4) Precautions with pregnancy; children; renal, hepatic, cardiac, and lung diseases; pericardial and pleural effusions

(5) Possible drug interactions
  (a) Antineoplastic drugs
  (b) Corticosteroids
  (c) Lithium
b. Prophylactic antibiotics and antifungals
c. AZT
8. Laboratory results and other indices to monitor for disease progression and response to therapy
  a. Response to treatment with GM-CSF
    (1) Increase in leukocyte counts (granulocytes, monocytes, neutrophils)
    (2) Toxicity related to GM-CSF use: Fatigue, asthenia, mild thrombocytopenia, and erythema at injection site
    (3) Obtain baseline renal and hepatic studies
  b. Response to treatment with antimicrobial therapy: Resolution or prevention of infection
9. Patient education: See *Potential for Infection: Neutropenia,* p. 235

D. Thrombocytopenia

See *Potential for Bleeding: Thrombocytopenia,* p. 234

E. HIV-Related Idiopathic Thrombocytopenic Purpura

See p. 141

F. Thrombotic Thrombocytopenic Purpura

1. Etiology and disease process
  a. Pathophysiology: Immune complex damage to vascular endothelium
  b. A rare disorder characterized by clinical picture of
    (1) Microangiopathic hemolytic anemia
    (2) Thrombocytopenia
    (3) Renal abnormalities
    (4) Fluctuating neurologic signs
    (5) Fever
  c. Etiology unknown
2. Frequency and distribution
  a. Thrombotic thrombocytopenic purpura

(TTP) is rarely seen; however, there is an association with HIV infection (Stricker, 1991)
  b. TTP should be suspected in patients with HIV infection and thrombocytopenia of unknown origin (Chu et al., 1995)
3. Morbidity and mortality
  a. No data available on HIV-infected patients
  b. Prognosis
    (1) Depends on severity of symptoms
    (2) Improves with early recognition and prompt initiation of treatment
4. Signs and symptoms
  a. Fever
  b. Anemia, thrombocytopenia
  c. Dyspnea
  d. Transient neurologic signs
    (1) Headache, confusion
    (2) Slurred speech, aphasia
    (3) Apraxia
    (4) Motor weakness, numbness, tingling
5. Diagnosis
  a. Possible subtle clinical presentations in patients with HIV infection
    (1) Chronic low-grade hemolytic anemia
    (2) Mild renal impairment
    (3) Mild neurologic abnormalities
  b. Blood work
    (1) Decreased Hgb and Hct
    (2) Decreased platelet count
    (3) Elevated creatinine and BUN
    (4) Elevated LDH
    (5) Peripheral blood smear shows microangiopathic hemolytic anemia
    (6) Vascular endothelial cell markers indicate coexistence of hypercoagulable and hypofibrinolytic state
6. Treatment
  a. Plasmapheresis using fresh frozen plasma replacement (a procedure that separates plasma from whole blood to remove abnormal plasma constituents)
  b. Unproven treatments: Corticosteroids, antiplatelet drugs, IV IgG
7. Laboratory results and other indices to monitor for disease progression and response to therapy: Platelet count, Hgb and Hct, LDH.

XV. GASTROINTESTINAL SYSTEM COMPLICATIONS

A. Periodontal Disease

1. Etiology and disease process
   a. HIV-related gingivitis and periodontitis are characterized by rapid progression from mild inflammation to painful, spontaneously bleeding periodontitis over a short period
   b. Terminology to describe these oral lesions is evolving:
      (1) HIV-associated gingivitis (HIV-G), more recently called linear-gingival erythema
      (2) HIV-associated periodontitis (HIV-P), more recently called HIV-necrotizing ulcerative periodontitis (HIV-NUP)
   c. Multiple gram-negative pathogens involved: *Actinobacillus actinomycetem-comitans, Bacteroides gingivalis,* and *Wolinella recta*
      (1) In HIV-periodontal pathology, these organisms are probably joined by other, as yet unspeciated pathogens
      (2) The presence of these bacteria alone does not entirely explain the pathogenesis of this disease; other organisms (e.g., yeast) may elicit a hyper-immune phenomenon resulting in tissue destruction
2. Frequency and distribution
   a. There is a correlation between the incidence of HIV-NUP and stage of HIV illness; one study (Klein, Quart, & Small, 1991) indicated that 95% of all people with HIV-NUP had CD4+ lymphocyte counts <200/µl; the prevalence of HIV-NUP in PWAs is approximately 6%, with an increased incidence in homosexual/bisexual men in one study (Klein et al.) and in women in another (Glick, 1994)
   b. There is evidence of a decreased incidence of HIV-NUP in people taking TMP-SMX or dapsone for PCP prophylaxis
3. Relationship to natural history of HIV disease: HIV-NUP is associated with a decrease in CD4+ lymphocyte count

4. Morbidity and mortality
   a. HIV-NUP morbidity: Clinical presentation includes edema, erythema, fetid breath, deep pain, spontaneous bleeding, loss of soft and hard tissue, periodontal detachment, and bone loss
   b. Mortality is not directly related to HIV-NUP, but its occurrence is a poor prognostic indicator. The Glick (1994) study indicated a mortality rate of nearly 60% within 18 months of a HIV-NUP diagnosis.
   c. HIV-NUP could be a source of gram-negative sepsis
5. Early detection, prevention, prophylaxis
   a. Prophylaxis should be geared to general oral hygiene, but there are no standards
   b. People without symptoms should have a full dental exam q6mos
   c. People with symptomatic HIV disease, CD4+ lymphocyte count <200/µl or with oral pathology, reduced salivary flow, and taking multiple oral suspensions should be seen q3mos
6. Signs and symptoms
   a. Chief complaints: Reddening of the gums to severe oral pain
   b. Other: Bleeding during brushing
   c. In advanced cases: Spontaneous bleeding
      (1) Often occurs at night
      (2) Patients will complain of finding blood on the pillow or clots in the mouth
   d. Dental exam also reveals bone loss, loss of soft and hard tissue, and periodontal loss
7. Diagnosis
   a. HIV-NUP is a clinical diagnosis usually made by the dentist
      (1) Early disease is classified as linear-gingival erythema
      2) Advanced disease is referred to as HIV-NUP
   b. Histology
      (1) Histologic exam of HIV-NUP indicates extensive inflammatory infiltrate

(2) Linear-gingival erythema lacks a cellular inflammatory component

8. Treatment
   a. Scaling of affected teeth, with thorough debridement of infected tissue
   b. Antibacterial mouth rinse
      (1) Chlorhexidine gluconate 12% 2/day, or
      (2) Povidone-iodine, following by chlorhexidine gluconate 12% 2/day
   c. Systemic antibiotics for 4–5 days: Metronidazole, or tetracycline, or augmentin, or clindamycin
   d. Dental care
      (1) Treatment modified according to medical condition; ability to tolerate long or short visits will have an impact on overall treatment plan
      (2) Antibiotic prophylaxis is routine for people at risk for developing subacute bacterial endocarditis
         (a) May include those with a long IDU history
         (b) For patients with severe neutropenia (an absolute neutrophil count of <500/mm^3), the antibiotic must be bactericidal (e.g., penicillin, amoxicillin, cephalosporin) because bacteriostatic antibiotics may lead to bacterial overload after discontinuation

9. Laboratory results and other indices to monitor for disease progression and response to therapy: Serial dental exams, gum inspections, routine teeth cleaning

10. Patient education
    a. Daily oral care: Brush twice and floss daily
    b. Report any excessive bleeding or gum pain
    c. Refer to a dentist for evaluation
    d. Teaching oral care best done by a registered oral hygienist

B. Aphthous Ulcers

1. Etiology and disease process
   a. Erythematous ulcers that usually appear on soft palate, mouth, oropharynx, esophagus; the etiology is unclear
      (1) While many non-HIV-infected people have minor aphthous lesions (<6 mm in diameter), HIV-infected patients frequently present with giant aphthous ulcerations (several cm in diameter) (Tami & Lee, 1994)
      (2) These giant lesions are usually the result of smaller lesions coalescing into large ulcers (Tami & Lee, 1994)
   b. Recurrences are common

2. Relationship to natural history of HIV disease: Generally occurs with severe immunosuppression

3. Morbidity and mortality
   a. Cause of significant morbidity: Aphthous stomatitis, if unresponsive to treatment, causes severe odynophagia leading to anorexia, dehydration, malnutrition, and wasting (death may result)
   b. Morbidity
      (1) Difficulties with speech
      (2) Decreased quality of life, physical strength, and other clinical problems associated with malnutrition
   c. Secondary infection adds to the severe pain and constitutional symptoms accompanying this condition

4. Early detection, prevention, prophylaxis: Recurrent aphthous ulcers may require continuous steroid therapy

5. Signs and symptoms
   a. Patient first reports painful sores in mouth; begins as small, discrete, or grouped papules or vesicles that become necrotizing ulcerations; severe aphthous ulcers present with large necrotic ulcers of 2–4 cm
   b. Depending on extent and severity, may interfere with oral intake; weight loss and complaints of odynophagia, anorexia are common

6. Diagnosis
   a. No specific diagnostic procedures or tests; appearance, history, and responses to empiric therapy guide the diagnosis
   b. Rule out HSV first by the location of ulcer, viral culture, and empiric treatment with acyclovir
   c. Differential diagnosis: HSV, mucous patches of early syphilis, candidiasis, erythema multiforme, avitaminoses,

lymphoma, CMV, and other OIs (e.g., histoplasmosis)

7. Treatment

   a. Topical steroid elixir (swish and spit) for less severe aphthous ulcers

   b. More severe ulcers usually respond to short course of oral steroid therapy; intralesional steroid injections may be used

   c. There have been reports of aphthous ulcers that recur and increase in severity despite steroid therapy; may be completely unresponsive to treatment

   d. Clinical trials being conducted to test efficacy of thalidomide for recurrent aphthous ulcer

   e. Because lesions are often secondarily infected, a systemic antibiotic may be initiated

   f. If oral intake is compromised, treatment for malnutrition is initiated (e.g., nasal feeding tube, percutaneous gastroscopy [PEG] tube)

   g. See also *Stomatitis*, p. 238, *AIDS Wasting Syndrome*, p. 134, *Dehydration*, p. 204, *Dysphagia/Odynophagia*, p. 207, *Nutritional Deficit: Weight Loss, Anorexia*, p. 227

C. Oral Candidiasis

For a thorough review of candidiasis, see *Fungal Diseases*, p. 83

D. Oral Herpes

For a thorough review of herpes simplex virus, see *Viral Infections*, p. 96

E. Microbial-Related Esophagitis

1. **Candidiasis**

   a. For detailed information, see p. 83

   b. Signs and symptoms: Dysphagia, association with oral candidiasis

   c. Diagnosis

      (1) Endoscopy to visualize esophagus may be required to confirm diagnosis

      (2) Differential diagnosis: Herpes simplex, CMV, aphthous ulcers

2. **Herpes simplex**

   a. For detailed information, see *Herpes Simplex Virus*, p. 96

   b. Signs and symptoms: Dysphagia; if untreated, odynophagia and retrosternal pain

   c. Diagnosis

      (1) Endoscopy to visualize esophagus

      (2) Direct culture of ulcers

      (3) Differential diagnosis: Candidiasis, CMV, aphthous ulcers

3. **Cytomegalovirus**

   a. For detailed information, see p. 94

   b. Frequency and distribution: Approximately 5% of CMV disease is seen in the GI system

   c. Signs and symptoms: Severe odynophagia, substernal chest pain, dysphagia, fevers

   d. Diagnosis

      (1) Endoscopy to visualize esophagus reveals extensive, large, shallow ulcerations that may be multiple

      (2) Biopsy shows intranuclear inclusions in endothelial cells

      (3) Differential diagnosis: Candidiasis, HSV, aphthous ulcers

F. Gastroesophageal Reflux and Esophagitis

1. Etiology and disease process

   a. Reflux of gastric or intestinal contents into esophagus

   b. Esophageal mucosal damage occurs from repeated exposure to stomach or intestinal contents; occurs in patients who experience prolonged periods of recumbency so that the gastric contents settle near the gastroesophageal junction

2. Relationship to natural history of HIV disease: More common in debilitated persons with HIV disease

3. Morbidity and mortality: Causes gastric distress, may interfere with adequate nutritional intake

4. Early detection, prevention, prophylaxis: Debilitated and bedbound patients should

have head of bed elevated during and after meals
5. Signs and symptoms
   a. Reflux without esophagitis usually asymptomatic
   b. Heartburn is most common symptom
   c. Less frequently, anginalike or atypical chest pain
   d. Dysphagia is suggestive of pyloric stricture
6. Diagnosis
   a. In mild cases with a clear-cut history of reflux, a therapeutic trial of antacids or H2 blocking agents may establish diagnosis
   b. For nonresponsive cases, a barium swallow, esophagoscopy, and esophageal motility with pH monitoring
7. Treatment
   a. Keep head of bed elevated during and after meals
   b. Antacids and H2-blocking agents to neutralize acidity
   c. Maintenance: As above

G. Pill-Induced Esophagitis

1. Etiology and disease process
   a. Etiology: Ingestion of certain pills
   b. Pathophysiology: Esophageal mucosal damage presenting as redness, friability, bleeding, superficial linear ulcers, and exudates
2. Relationship to natural history of HIV disease
   a. Doxycycline, tetracycline, clindamycin account for >50% of cases
   b. Aspirin, potassium chloride, ferrous sulfate, quinidine, alprenolol, AZT, and various steroidal and nonsteroidal anti-inflammatories can cause other cases
3. Morbidity and mortality: Causes discomfort
4. Early detection, prevention, prophylaxis: Take medications (unless otherwise indicated) after meals; do not lie down for at least 30 min after taking medications
5. Signs and symptoms: Heartburn and (less commonly) anginalike chest pain or atypical chest pain
6. Diagnosis: Usually diagnosed through a review of clinical symptoms and the medication schedule; barium swallow, esophagoscopy, esophageal motility studies may be indicated
7. Treatment
   a. Acute
      (1) Antacids or H2-blocking agents
      (2) Discontinue offending medication if no relief with other treatment
   b. Maintenance: Continue antacids or H2-blocking agents if these offer relief while patient is on the offending medication, or discontinue the offending pill

H. Kaposi's Sarcoma

1. For a thorough review, see *Malignancies*, p. 128
2. Frequency and distribution
   a. GI tract most common extracutaneous site
   b. GI-tract lesions found in 40% of patients with KS diagnosis; on autopsy, up to 80% have lesions
3. Relationship to natural history of HIV disease: Patients with advanced HIV disease and GI KS have poorer prognosis than those without GI KS (theorized that the extent of GI involvement correlates with the severity of immunosuppression)
4. Morbidity and mortality: Although GI KS is generally asymptomatic, prognosis is poor
5. Signs and symptoms: Rarely causes symptoms; there are reports of GI bleeding from ulcerated lesions
6. Diagnosis
   a. Endoscopic visualization of KS lesions
   b. Biopsies frequently negative because lesions are submucosal
   c. More extensive GI workup includes esophagogastroduodenoscopy, sigmoidoscopy, and colonoscopy
   d. Differential diagnosis: CMV infection, especially in colon, may resemble hemorrhagic KS lesions

I. Non-Hodgkin's Lymphoma

1. For a thorough review, see *Malignancies*, p. 130

2. Frequency and distribution: GI tract is a common extranodal site of NHL
3. Signs and symptoms
   a. Depends on location and size; aggressive nature means patients rarely remain asymptomatic
   b. Luminal lesions cause diarrhea, pain, obstruction, bleeding, or perforation
   c. Hepatic disease causes dull pain, fevers, rising alkaline phosphatase
4. Diagnosis
   a. CT scan and ultrasound useful for hepatobiliary lesions
   b. Barium contrast studies or endoscopy for luminal tumors
   c. Biopsies are indicated to confirm the diagnosis when tumor is detectable by contrast studies

J. Enterocolitis and Malabsorption: Intestinal Pathogens

1. Etiology and disease process
   a. Microbial agents
      (1) Small intestine: *Cryptosporidium, Microsporidium [Enterocytozoon bieneusi], I. belli*, MAC, *Salmonella* and *Campylobacter* species, *Giardia*, HIV
      (2) Large intestine: CMV, *Cryptosporidium*, MAC, *Shigella* group D, *C. difficile, C. jejuni, H. capsulatum*, adenovirus, HSV
      (3) Unexplained or idiopathic diarrhea is frequently called "AIDS enteropathy"; a comprehensive patient evaluation, however, usually uncovers an infectious agent(s) as an etiology of the diarrhea
      (4) Other diarrheal illnesses can be caused by neoplasms, other bacteria (e.g., *Salmonella*), fungi (e.g., histoplasmosis), but protozoal disease causes most of the enterocolitis and small-intestine malabsorption diarrhea in AIDS patients
   b. Pathophysiology
      (1) *Microsporidium:* Protozoal infection that may cause villous atrophy and cell degeneration
      (2) MAC: Villous blunting and suffu-

sion of macrophages with mycobacteria
      (3) *C. difficile*: Bacterial pathogen
      (4) Adenovirus: Colonic mucosa appear normal or inflamed
      (5) HIV
         (a) Mild chronic inflammation of duodenal mucosa sometimes associated with partial villous atrophy
         (b) Reduced or normal levels of B12 with abnormal Shilling test
2. Frequency and distribution: At least half of all patients with HIV will develop diarrhea during course of disease; pathogen identifiable in 50%–80% of cases (Lew et al., 1995)
   a. *Microsporidium:* Estimated that 30%–50% of diarrhea results from this organism
   b. MAC: Some studies show MAC as the most commonly identified pathogen
   c. CMV: One of most common and potentially serious GI infections
   d. *C. difficile:* Common, particularly if antibiotics have been used
   e. Adenovirus: Conflicting reports regarding incidence; however, thought to be small
   f. HIV: Identified organism in GI tissue of up to 40% of patients with HIV disease; role in causing diarrhea unclear
3. Relationship to natural history of HIV disease
   a. All organisms tend to cause more severe infections with more suppressed immune system
   b. *C. difficile* is not correlated with immune function but with antibiotic use
4. Morbidity and mortality
   a. Depending on organism and severity of diarrhea, enterocolitis can lead to wasting and malnutrition, which has deleterious effects on the immune system, survival, and quality of life
   b. In one study (Lubeck et al., 1993), AIDS patients with chronic diarrhea had annual healthcare expenses that were 50% higher than for similar patients without diarrhea; these patients also reported significant work loss and a

greater need for assistance in the home

5. Early detection, prevention, prophylaxis
   a. Avoid waterborne microorganisms
   b. Prevent person-to-person acquisition of organisms via the fecal-oral route
   c. Chlorination has no impact on *Cryptosporidium*; if cryptosporidiosis is suspected, use ammonia for fecal spills, laundry, and bathroom cleaning
6. Signs and symptoms
   a. *Microsporidium*
      (1) Watery diarrhea, malabsorption, flatulence; fever not present unless cholangitis has developed
      (2) Nonbloody, nonmucoid diarrhea occurring sporadically throughout the day
      (3) Associated with gradual weight loss and impaired appetite
   b. MAC: Watery diarrhea, abdominal pain, malabsorption, weight loss, fever (with or without night sweats), anorexia
   c. CMV: Colitis evidenced by diarrhea, fever, and frequently by hematochezia and abdominal pain
   d. *C. difficile*
      (1) Diarrhea, usually watery and voluminous
      (2) Abdominal cramps and tenderness, fever, leukocytosis
      (3) Symptoms may vary
   e. Cryptosporidiosis: Profuse watery diarrhea, malabsorption, flatulence, nausea and vomiting
   f. Adenovirus: Chronic, watery, non-bloody, nonmucoid diarrhea with weight loss
   g. HIV: Chronic diarrhea, weight loss, malabsorption
7. Diagnosis
   a. Thorough history and physical examination, paying attention to travel history, medications that may cause diarrhea (e.g., ddI), dietary problems that may cause diarrhea (e.g., lactose intolerance), and illnesses (e.g., pancreatitis) that cause diarrhea
   b. Stool cultures × 3 for *Salmonella* species, *S. flexneri, C. jejuni,* and assayed for *C. difficile*
   c. Examine stool specimens for parasites and AFB using special stains
   d. Perform D-Xylose testing to confirm a suspected malabsorption
   e. If symptoms suggest small-bowel diarrhea, arrange for gastroenterologist to perform upper endoscopy with small-bowel biopsy of distal duodenum or proximal jejunum
   f. If symptoms suggest colitis
      (1) Some centers do flexible sigmoid-oscopy first and if results negative do colonoscopy next, as per gastro-enterologist
      (2) Multiple random biopsies of even normal appearing mucosa should be obtained
      (3) Appropriate cultures and stains performed
      (4) Examine biopsy specimens by electron microscopy for *Microsporidia* and adenovirus
      (5) HIV enteropathy diagnosed by excluding all other possible causes of diarrhea
8. Treatment
   a. Infections may not always respond to standard therapy and frequently require long-term suppressive maintenance regimens
      (1) *Microsporidium*: No standard treatment
         (a) Fluconazole and metronidazole have been tried with minimal success
         (b) Ongoing studies using albendazole appear promising
      (2) CMV: Ganciclovir or foscarnet
      (3) *C. difficile:* Oral vancomycin or metronidazole usually effective
      (4) Adenovirus: Symptomatic
      (5) HIV: Symptomatic, antiretroviral therapy
      (6) May require low-fat diet, ceasing medications that may cause diarrhea, use of antidiarrheal medications (e.g., kaolin and pectin, opium, belladonna alkaloids, loperamide), use of octeotride acetate, and supportive use of fluid replenishment, nutritional supplements, and rest

9. Laboratory results and other indices to monitor for disease progression and response to therapy: If specific organism is identified, then response to treatment for that organism determines disease progression and treatment response

10. Patient education: See *Diarrhea*, p. 205, *Nutritional Deficit: Weight Loss, Anorexia*, p. 227, *Dehydration*, p. 204, *AIDS Wasting Syndrome*, p. 134, *Infection Control*, p. 363; food and water safety in Table 10.3, p. 371; and the appropriate protozoal, bacterial, viral, and fungal diseases

K. Anorectal Disease: Nonmalignant

1. Etiology and disease process
   a. Bacteria: *C. trachomatis, Lymphogranuloma venereum, N. gonorrhoeae*
   b. Viruses: HSV, CMV
   c. Fungi: *C. albicans,*
   d. Protozoa: *E. histolytica*
   e. Miscellaneous: *Condyloma acuminatum* (anogenital warts)
      (1) Epithelial tumors resulting from infection of skin or mucous membranes with papillomavirus
      (2) *C. acuminatum* transmitted by close personal contact

2. Frequency and distribution: High incidence among homosexual male patients with HIV disease

3. Relationship to natural history of HIV disease
   a. Most anorectal infections not associated with late stage HIV disease, except for CMV and fungal or chronic perianal herpes infection lasting longer than 1 month
   b. Higher incidence among homosexual men

4. Morbidity and mortality: Cause of pain and discomfort

5. Signs and symptoms
   a. *C. trachomatis*: Mild rectal pain, mucus discharge, tenesmus, bleeding (occasionally)
   b. *L. venereum*
      (1) Initially present with anal ulcer or diarrhea, tenesmus, bloody or mucopurulent anal discharge associated with diffuse or discrete ulcerations in the rectosigmoid colon
      (2) Fever, other constitutional symptoms with inguinal and perirectal lymphadenopathy
      (3) Complications: Fistula in ano, perirectal abscesses; rectovaginal, rectovesical, and ischiorectal fistulas
   c. *N. gonorrhoeae*: Most patients asymptomatic; may have acute proctitis, manifested by anal pruritus, tenesmus, purulent discharge, or rectal bleeding
   d. HSV: Chronic, cutaneous perianal ulcers; painful
   e. CMV: Perianal ulcerations that resemble anogenital HSV ulcerations (most patients also have coexistent enteric CMV infection)
   f. *C. albicans*: Intense pruritus; may involve anal canal and spread over perineum
   g. *E. histolytica*: Ulcerative or condylomatous lesions that slowly enlarge over weeks to months; cause pain and bleeding
   h. *C. acuminatum*: Appear as solitary or multiple, round, or cauliflowerlike projections in anogenital region

6. Diagnosis
   a. *C. trachomatis*
      (1) Rectal culture or direct immunofluorescence test for *C. trachomatis*
      (2) Differential diagnosis: Gonococcal or HSV infection
   b. *L. venereum*
      (1) Rectal biopsy
      (2) Isolation of LGV serovar (culture positive in 30% of suspected cases)
      (3) Complement fixation test with elevated titers suggestive
      (4) High micro-immunofluorescent antibody titer to one of LGV immunotypes more sensitive and specific
      (5) Differential diagnosis: Syphilis, HSV, chancroid, non-LGV strains of *C. trachomatis*
   c. *N. gonorrhoeae*
      (1) Presumptive diagnosis if intracellular gram-negative diplococci

observed in leukocytes on Gram's stain smears

(2) Rectal specimens plated on modified Thayer-Martin medium (or equivalent) containing trimethoprim lactate

(3) Differential diagnosis: HSV, *C. trachomatis*

d. CMV

(1) Biopsy, light microscopic and electron microscopic examination of biopsy specimens, or virus isolation

(2) Exclude other causes of perianal ulcers, which may have multiple etiologic agents

e. *E. histolytica:* Presence of *E. histolytica* trophozoites in purulent exudate or on biopsy

f. *C. acuminatum*

(1) Usually diagnosed by history and physical exam

(2) Biopsy atypical lesions

7. Treatment

a. *C. trachomatis*

(1) Preferred: Doxycycline, azithromycin

(2) Alternatives: Ofloxacin, erythromycin ethylsuccinate, erythromycin base, sulfisoxazole

b. *L. venereum:* Doxycycline preferred; alternative—erythromycin, sulfisoxazole

c. *N. gonorrhoeae:* Ceftriaxone, ciprofloxacin, ofloxacin, cefixime, doxycycline

d. *E. histolytica:* Metronidazole plus iodoquinol, diloxanide fursate, or paromomycin

e. *C. acuminatum*

(1) Topically applied podophyllum preparations have resolution rate <50%; other treatments include cryosurgery, electrodesiccation surgical excision, and ablation with laser

(2) Failure of and recurrence with these treatments is common

f. Patient education: See *Anorectal Signs and Symptoms,* p. 201, and appropriate bacterial, fungal, and viral diseases

L. Hepatic Disease: Diffuse Hepatitis and Granulomatous

1. Etiology and disease process

a. Etiologic agents

(1) *M. avium, M. intracellulare,* CMV, *M. tuberculosis, Cryptococcus, P. carinii*

(2) Hepatitis C, B, D (see *Hepatitis Viruses A–E,* p. 98); bacillary peliosis hepatis (see *Bartonella,* p. 76)

(3) Lymphoma

(4) KS

(5) Drug induced: Associated with antibiotics; antidepressants; anti-inflammatory, antifungal, and antiviral agents

b. Pathophysiology

(1) *M. avium, M. intracellulare:* Poorly formed granulomas containing AFB within foamy histiocytes

(2) CMV: Viral inclusion in Kupffer's cells and occasionally in hepatocytes or sinusoidal endothelial cells

(3) *M. tuberculosis*: Well-formed granulomas, few AFB

(4) *Cryptococcus*

(a) Causes inflammatory response in liver that may be granulomatous

(b) Granulomas often poorly formed and consist of loose aggregates of macrophages surrounding microabscesses

(5) *P. carinii*: Similar to lung; foamy eosinophilic exudate containing cysts within hepatic sinusoids

(6) Bacillary peliosis hepatis

(a) Peliosis hepatis form randomly distributed lesions in liver parenchyma that are characterized by multiple, small, blood-filled cystic spaces

(b) In HIV disease the most frequent cause is two related bacteria, *B. quintana* and *B. henselae*

(7) Drug induced

(a) Variable morphologic pattern

(b) May have pattern indistinguishable from viral hepatitis or may simulate extrahepatic bile duct obstruction

(c) May also include bridging hepatic necrosis or hepatic granulomas

2. Frequency and distribution
   a. Most patients with HIV have clinical hepatomegaly and have abnormal transaminases or alkaline phosphatases; no correlation between elevations and disease
   b. OIs diagnosed in approximately one third of liver biopsies
   c. *M. avium, M. intracellulare, M. tuberculosis:* Mycobacterial disease is the most common infection of liver
   d. CMV: One of commonest organisms to infect liver
   e. Bacillary peliosis hepatis: Rare
   f. Lymphoma: Hepatic parenchymal lesions uncommon
   g. KS: Most common postmortem liver neoplasm
   h. Drug induced: Increasing in frequency as more drugs being used to maintain patients

3. Morbidity and mortality
   a. Bacillary peliosis hepatis: Can cause liver failure
   b. Drug induced: May cause symptoms or abnormal liver function tests

4. Early detection, prevention, prophylaxis: None, but when potentially hepatotoxic drugs are prescribed, evaluate liver enzymes periodically and discontinue the drug if enzymes start to rise

5. Signs and symptoms
   a. Bacillary peliosis hepatis: Fever, abdominal pain, cutaneous and lytic bone lesions
   b. Lymphoma: Dull pain in association with fevers and rising alkaline phosphatase
   c. KS: Aminotransferase elevations
   d. Drug induced: May be similar to those of acute hepatitis or asymptomatic with elevated liver enzymes

6. Diagnosis
   a. Bacillary peliosis hepatis
      (1) Liver biopsies demonstrate areas of myxoid stroma with granular purple material
      (2) Warthin-Starry stain or electron microscopy show clumps of organisms
      (3) Polymerase chain reaction, culturing on chocolate agar, or by using lysis centrifugation of blood cultures
   b. Lymphoma: CT scan, ultrasound
   c. KS: May be incidentally discovered at liver biopsy or postmortem
   d. Drug induced
      (1) Elimination of suspected drug with subsequent resolution of symptoms or return to normal of previously elevated enzymes
      (2) May be process of elimination

7. Treatment
   a. Bacillary peliosis hepatis: Erythromycin, tetracycline, and cephalosporin for >2 months
   b. Drug induced: Discontinue offending drug
   c. Maintenance: None

M. Sclerosing Cholangitis

1. Etiology and disease process
   a. Etiologic agents: *Cryptosporidium,* CMV
   b. Pathophysiology: Organisms cause a progressive, inflammatory, sclerosing, and obliterative process that affects extrahepatic and intrahepatic bile ducts

2. Frequency and distribution: Unknown

3. Relationship to natural history of HIV disease: Increased risk of hepatobiliary disease if cryptosporidial or cytomegaloviral disease present in other sites

4. Morbidity and mortality: Poor prognosis

5. Signs and symptoms
   a. Jaundice, pruritus, right upper quadrant abdominal pain
   b. With progression: Complete biliary obstruction, secondary biliary cirrhosis, hepatic failure, or portal hypertension with bleeding varices

6. Diagnosis
   a. Endoscopic retrograde cholangiopancreatogram (ERCP) shows thickened ducts with narrow, beaded lumina
   b. Microscopic analysis of ductal aspirate during ERCP may establish infectious cause

7. Treatment

a. CMV, *Cryptosporidium*: Treat as recommended
b. Cholestyramine to control symptoms of pruritus
c. Where complete or high-grade biliary obstruction has occurred, balloon dilatation or surgical intervention may be appropriate
d. Maintenance: As appropriate for etiology
8. Laboratory results and other indices to monitor for disease progression and response to therapy
    a. Improvement of symptoms
    b. Lowered bilirubin levels

N. Pancreatic Disease

1. Etiology and disease process
    a. Etiologic agents
        (1) OIs (CMV, *M. tuberculosis, M. avium, Cryptococcus*, HSV), medication toxicity, neoplasms
        (2) Medication (pentamidine, dideoxyinosine)
        (3) Glucose intolerance: Pentamidine
        (4) Peripancreatic mass: Neoplasms (lymphoma, KS), OIs
        (5) Pancreatic abscess: OIs
    b. Pathophysiology
        (1) Acute pancreatitis
            (a) Activated (endotoxins, exotoxins, viral infections act as activators) proteolytic enzymes digest pancreatic and peripancreatic tissues and activate other enzymes
            (b) Active enzymes digest cellular membranes and cause proteolysis, edema, interstitial hemorrhage, vascular damage, coagulation necrosis, fat necrosis, and parenchymal cell necrosis
            (c) Activation and release of bradykinin peptides and vasoactive substances believed to produce vasodilatation, increased vascular permeability, and edema
            (d) Cellular injury and death liberate activated enzymes
            (e) Cascade of events leads to acute necrotizing pancreatitis

(2) Glucose intolerance
    (a) IV pentamidine causes pancreatic B-cell toxicity resulting in acute hypoglycemia from increased insulin secretion
    (b) B-cell death may result and diabetes mellitus develop; see *Pentamidine-Induced Hypoglycemia and Diabetes*, p. 187
(3) Peripancreatic mass
    (a) Neoplasms tend to produce solid mass
    (b) Infections tend to produce heterogenous or fluid-filled mass
(4) Pancreatic abscess: Develops from severe acute pancreatitis
2. Frequency and distribution: On autopsy, pancreatic lesions in about 10% of patients
3. Relationship to natural history of HIV disease
    a. Pancreatic disease is linked to the presence of an OI or neoplasm, which generally occurs when the patient has a CD4+ lymphocyte count <200/µl
    b. Risk with medications at any point of HIV infection
4. Morbidity and mortality: Asymptomatic to potentially life-threatening
5. Early detection, prevention, prophylaxis
    a. Dideoxyinosine: While patient is taking medication, check amylase and lipase levels regularly; discontinue medication if they start to rise
    b. Pentamidine: Monitor blood sugars
6. Signs and symptoms
    a. Acute pancreatitis
        (1) Abdominal pain
            (a) Nausea and vomiting
            (b) Hyperamylasemia
            (c) Hyperlipasemia
            (d) Elevated amylase to creatinine clearance ratio
            (e) Elevated serum pancreatic isoamylase
        (2) Glucose intolerance: Signs and symptoms of hypo- and hyperglycemia
        (3) Peripancreatic mass: Neoplasm
        (4) Recent weight loss: Anorexia, jaundice

b. OIs: Fever, night sweats, rigors, malaise, and leukocytosis are common
7. Diagnosis
   a. Acute pancreatitis
     (1) Serum amylase and lipase determinations
     (2) Abdominal ultrasonography or CT demonstrates enlarged, edematous pancreas and heterogeneous peripancreatic tissue
   b. Glucose intolerance: Blood glucose monitoring
   c. Peripancreatic mass
     (1) CT identifies mass, peripancreatic adenopathy, invasion of adjacent vessels
     (2) Ultrasound may help differentiate fluid-filled from solid mass
     (3) Needle biopsy (with normal clotting parameters) obtains samples for histological analysis, culture for mycobacteria, fungi, and virus
   d. Pancreatic abscess: CT or ultrasonography may demonstrate a nonhomogeneous peripancreatic mass, fluid collection, air-fluid levels, displacement of adjacent viscera, bowel fixation, and peripancreatic lymphadenopathy
8. Treatment
   a. Acute pancreatitis
     (1) Goal is to "put pancreas to rest" by reducing pancreatic secretions
     (2) Analgesics for pain, IV fluids to maintain hydration, npo
     (3) Treat underlying cause of pancreatitis
     (4) Peripancreatic mass
       (a) Refer to treatment of KS and lymphoma
       (b) Treat OIs appropriately
     (5) Pancreatic abscess
       (a) May drain abscess by nonsurgical percutaneous catheter techniques, using CT guidance
       (b) Laparotomy with stump drainage and possible resection
   b. Maintenance: Depends upon etiology
9. Laboratory results and other indices to monitor for disease progression and response to therapy: Follow appropriate laboratory markers for return to normal levels, relief of symptoms after appropriate treatment
10. Patient education: See *Pain*, p. 229

O. Appendicitis

1. Etiology and disease process
   a. Etiologic agents: KS, *Cryptosporidium,* CMV, *M. avium, M. intracellulare*
   b. Pathophysiology: Luminal obstruction by enlarged lymphoid follicles associated with viral infection and tumors associated with neoplasm
2. Frequency and distribution: Uncommon, KS most common cause
3. Relationship to natural history of HIV disease: All causes of appendicitis associated with lower CD4+ lymphocyte counts
4. Morbidity and mortality: Without surgical removal of appendix rupture will ensue, resulting in peritonitis and possibly death
5. Signs and symptoms: Abdominal pain located in right lower quadrant, anorexia, nausea and vomiting
6. Diagnosis: By symptoms and characteristic pain; may have leukocytosis
7. Treatment: Appendectomy as soon as patient can be prepared
8. Laboratory results and other indices to monitor for disease progression and response to therapy: Improvement with surgery

P. Cholecystitis

1. Etiology and disease process
   a. Etiologic agents: CMV, *Cryptosporidium, Candida, Enterobacter*
   b. Pathophysiology
     (1) Acute inflammation of gallbladder wall following obstruction of cystic duct
     (2) Inflammatory response stimulated by etiologic agents
2. Frequency and distribution: Uncommon; CMV and *Cryptosporidium* most common causes
3. Morbidity and mortality: Causes pain; interferes with nutritional intake
4. Signs and symptoms
   a. Localized right upper quadrant pain

and tenderness, positive Murphy's sign
b. Pain may radiate to interscapular area, right scapula, or shoulder
c. Anorexia, nausea and vomiting may occur
5. Diagnosis: History is suggestive, radionuclide biliary scan and ultrasound may be confirmatory
6. Treatment: Surgery, pain medication
7. Laboratory results and other indices to monitor for disease progression and response to therapy: Treatment should resolve symptoms

Q. Generalized Peritonitis

1. Etiology and disease process
   a. Etiologic agents: KS, lymphoma, CMV, *Campylobacter fetus, N. brasiliensis, M. tuberculosis, Candida, C. neoformans, H. capsulatum*
   b. Pathophysiology: GI perforation from tumor or OIs; perforation leads to secondary bacterial contamination of peritoneum
2. Frequency and distribution: Unknown
3. Relationship to natural history of HIV disease: Related to etiologic organism
4. Morbidity and mortality
   a. Increased because of delay in diagnosis secondary to atypical presentation
   b. Poor wound healing, malnutrition, protein deficiency, poor general medical status, concurrent infections, suscepti-

bility to bacteria and OIs
5. Signs and symptoms
   a. Abdominal pain
   b. Pyrexia
   c. Tachycardia, tachypnea
   d. Hypotension
   e. Involuntary abdominal guarding, direct abdominal tenderness, rebound abdominal tenesmus, abdominal distention
   f. Patients with HIV infection may have altered symptoms
6. Diagnosis
   a. Abdominal x-ray with patient erect may show subdiaphragmatic air, bowel wall thickening, intestinal mucosal thumbprinting, indistinct colonic haustra, intramural intestinal air, air in portal vein
   b. CT and paracentesis when ascites present
   c. Differential diagnosis: Pancreatitis, colonic pseudo-obstruction, toxic megacolon, intraperitoneal abscess
7. Treatment
   a. Approximately 4% will require laparotomy
   b. Broad spectrum IV antibiotic therapy for secondary bacterial infection
   c. IV rehydration
8. Laboratory results and other indices to monitor for disease progression and response to therapy
   a. If surgery performed, monitor condition for improvement
   b. Without surgery, follow symptoms and laboratory parameters.

XVI. GYNECOLOGIC COMPLICATIONS

A. Cervical Cancer
See *Malignancies*, p. 128

B. Condylomata Acuminata

1. Specific etiologic agent and disease process
   a. Human papillomavirus (HPV) is a sex-ually transmitted infection that causes anogenital condylomata (warts); HPV is also associated with anogenital dyspla-sia in both men and women
   b. Anogenital warts are usually soft, moist, pink, or red lesions that cluster in the labia and vagina, on the cervix, or around the anus
2. Morbidity and mortality: Anogenital warts are difficult to treat effectively, particularly in more immunocompromised patients
3. Early detection, prevention, prophylaxis: The use of barrier precautions (condoms) may interrupt transmission
4. Signs and symptoms: Classic appearance of the lesions
5. Diagnosis
   a. Biopsy if lesions are atypical in appear-ance or if the warts prove to be very resistant to standard therapies
   b. Pap smear for cervical warts
   c. Differential diagnosis: Secondary syphilis
   d. All HIV-positive women diagnosed with condylomata acuminata should have a colposcopy
6. Treatment
   a. Trichloroacetic acid, if lesion is <2 cm; after treatment the tissue will slough and heal in 7 – 10 days; alternative agent is podophyllin resin
   b. Resistant vaginal or cervical lesions may be treated with 5-fluorouracil cream
   c. Persistent or recurrent lesions may require surgical excision, cryosurgery, or CO_2 laser surgery
   d. Treatment of large cervical condylomata in pregnant women is deferred until after delivery
7. Laboratory results and other indices to monitor for disease progression and response to therapy: Frequent anogenital exams to verify response to treatment
8. Patient education: Teach treatment regi-mens and application of medications as needed

C. Herpes Simplex
See *Viral Infections*, p. 96

D. Menstrual Irregularities

1. Etiology and disease process
   a. Few changes in the normal endocrine system are noted in early HIV disease
   b. The normal endocrine system is com-plex. The function of the normal men-strual cycle is conception, with the releasing of an egg (oocyte) from the ovary (approximately q23 – 39d) and the building of the lining of the uterus (endo-metrium) to support the implantation and growth of the fertilized egg. The female endocrine system (hypothala-mus, anterior pituitary gland, ovary, endometrium of the uterus) is a com-plex system of hormones (e.g., gonadotropin-releasing factor [GnRH], follicle-stimulating hormone [FSH], luteinizing hormone [LH], estradiol, and progesterone) that regulate the menstrual cycle. Menses occurs as a result of endometrial shedding under the influence of estrogen and proges-terone. Changes at any level of this complex and intertwined system can impact the menstrual cycle and cause dysfunction within the hypothalamic-pituitary-ovarian axis.
   c. Two recent studies (Ellerbrock et al., 1996; Shah et al., 1994) concluded that the hypothalamic-pituitary-ovarian axis remains intact and is not significantly altered by HIV disease
      (1) Both studies revealed that HIV-infected women have regular menses varying from 21 – 35 days
      (2) Neither study, however, had signifi-cant numbers of women with drasti-cally low CD4+ lymphocyte counts

to evaluate the severity of HIV disease impact on the normal menstrual cycle

d. There is currently no research to prove differences in the evaluation of menstrual irregularities (ovulatory and anovulatory) between HIV-infected and uninfected women

e. Common causes of vaginal bleeding in ovulatory women

  (1) Trauma (e.g., lacerations of the vulva, vagina, cervix as the result of surgery, accidents, foreign bodies in the vagina [e.g., tampons, retained condoms, contraceptive sponges, toilet paper]) emotional stress, sexual assault/rape, domestic violence occur in approximately 25% of American women and is probably higher in HIV-infected women (Campbell, 1992)

  (2) Anatomic abnormalities

    (a) Uterine fibroid tumors in HIV-infected women are generally more symptomatic for abnormal and heavier uterine bleeding; usually more common in women >40 years and in African-American women (Bayer & DeCherney, 1993); one study (Johnston et al., 1995) has raised the possibility of a link between actual infiltration of the endometrium and intermenstrual bleeding in HIV-infected women

    (b) Cervical stenosis following treatment for cervical disease

  (3) Inflammation

    (a) Allergic reactions to latex, creams, foams containing nonoxynol 9, and feminine hygiene products (Vagisil, perfumed douches) can create small vaginal tears and result in vaginal bleeding

    (b) Cervical herpetic lesions, especially those with secondary bacterial infections, and cervical disease can cause postcoital bleeding; HIV-infected women are more susceptible than uninfected women to cervical disease (Wright et al., 1994); postcoital bleeding secondary to herpes has been clinically observed both with and without genital herpes

    (c) Vaginal bleeding can occur secondary to vaginitis, STDs, and PID. Two studies (Cu-Uvin et al., 1995; Ellerbrock et al., 1995) showed no significant differences with respect to STD rates between HIV-infected and uninfected women.

  (4) Coagulopathy: Must be normal for menses to cease without complication

    (a) Rule out diseases such as Von Willebrand's, ITP, DIC, leukemia

    (b) Consider depressed platelet counts as a secondary cause or side effect from medications

  (5) Medications

    (a) The hypothalamic-pituitary-ovarian axis is often disrupted in substance-abusing (cocaine, crack, heroin, marijuana, narcotics) women, resulting in amenorrhea

    (b) Intermenstrual bleeding from contraceptive methods (e.g., IUDs, Depoprovera, Norplant)

    (c) HIV medications (e.g., AZT, INH, miconazole) have the potential to cause thrombocytopenia or leukopenia (see *Potential for Bleeding: Thrombocytopenia*, p. 234)

    (d) Prescription drugs (e.g., methadone, Dilantin)

    (e) Other medications

      i) Aspirin and NSAIDs (e.g., ibuprofen, naproxen sodium) used for dysmenorrhea. *Caution*: This type of medication can decrease platelet counts and should be used cautiously with CD4+ lymphocyte count <200/μl as patients may also be on other drugs with the potential for similar side effects.

ii) Some homemade remedies, tinctures, and herbal medications, especially when used in excess

f. Etiology of anovulatory menstrual irregularities: Generally indicative of an interruption in the hypothalamic-pituitary-ovarian-uterine axis, unlike ovulatory menstrual irregularities where the axis remains intake

(1) Pregnancy is the most common etiology of amenorrhea

(2) Anatomic abnormalities can be genetic; usually detected in adolescence

(3) Systemic disorders resulting from ovarian or adrenal dysfunction, ovarian or adrenal tumor, hyperthyroidism, hypothyroidism, hyperprolactinemia, Cushing's disease, renal or liver failure, perimenopausal state, or obesity; generally presents as amenorrhea or dysfunctional uterine bleeding

(4) Hypothalamic or pituitary dysfunction generally presents as amenorrhea and is often caused by tumors, pituitary insufficiency, Sheehan's syndrome, stress, extreme weight loss, malnutrition, chronic disease, anorexia nervosa, or Kallmann's syndrome; clinicians report from observation that AIDS patients with markedly low CD4+ lymphocyte counts and significant weight loss (with or without substance abuse) experience amenorrhea; however, well-controlled studies have not been done in this area

(5) Medications

(a) Excessive illicit drug and alcohol use

(b) HIV medications that potentially cause endocrine imbalance (e.g., foscarnet, IV pentamidine, rifampin, diflucan or ketoconazole, megace)

2. Relationship to natural history of HIV disease

a. No conclusive data at this time; however, it appears to be related to the severity of the HIV disease process itself; no significant changes until CD4+ lymphocyte count is drastically low

b. Some preliminary studies suggest that the endometrium may have an active role in HIV replication throughout some or all stages of HIV disease; this could be one explanation for intermenstrual bleeding and could potentially aid in HIV staging in women (Johnston et al., 1995)

c. One study (Greenblatt et al., 1995) reported a high association between occurrence of neurologic symptoms and menstrual irregularities; there was no association between menstrual irregularities and abnormal body/mass in that study

d. Significant episodic vaginal bleeding may occur secondary to HIV-associated thrombocytopenia

e. Endocrine hormones are pulsatile and require 24-hour monitoring; they are therefore intricate and costly to study, hence the paucity of studies

3. Morbidity and mortality

a. Irregular bleeding problems are generally more chronic, episodic, and profuse than in the normal population

b. HIV-positive women with Stage IV disease appear to experience amenorrhea, as is common in other debilitating diseases

4. Early detection, prevention, and prophylaxis

a. Primary prevention: Educate about normal menses, fertility concerns, and characteristics of abnormal bleeding; include a discussion about contraceptive methods and the woman's needs

b. Secondary prevention: Hormone management of perimenopausal symptoms or bleeding problems (specific to etiology) and resolution of specific etiologic problem as prolonged untreated uterine bleeding can result in anemia

5. Signs and symptoms

a. Ovulatory women

(1) Intermenstrual bleeding is the most

common symptom seen in HIV-infected women
   (2) Menorrhagia (excessive profuse or prolonged uterine bleeding)
   (3) Dysmenorrhea (pain with menses)
   (4) Dyspareunia (pain with sexual intercourse)
  b. Anovulating women
   (1) Metrorrhagia (irregular, acyclic uterine bleeding occurring frequently)
   (2) Menometrorrhagia (excessive bleeding occurring at irregular intervals)
   (3) Polymenorrhea (bleeding at regular intervals <21 days)
   (4) Oligomenorrhea (interval varies from 36 days to 6 months)
   (5) Amenorrhea (3–6 months of no bleeding)
6. Diagnosis
  a. Identify normal and abnormal bleeding patterns; distinguish between ovulatory and anovulatory cycles; rule out common causes of vaginal bleeding
  b. Medical history and general physical exam
  c. Medication history, especially changes in the past 2 months: new medications (when started, dosage), changes in doses, illicit substance abuse (what, frequency, route)
  d. Sexual history (include risk factors for STDs, number of partners present and past, prostitution, etc.)
  e. History of emotional stress (e.g., just lost a partner or child to HIV, family member ill or deceased recently, domestic unrest, disclosure issues, financial concerns, job-related stress, just moved)
  f. Tests/procedures
   (1) Lab tests
    (a) CBC with bleeding time, PT, PTT
    (b) CD4+ lymphocyte counts
    (c) Serum b-HCG assay to rule out pregnancy
    (d) FSH and LH levels to rule out anovulation
    (e) Anovulatory women: Renal, hepatic, thyroid, and endocrine workup
   (2) Pap smear, STD workup

   (3) Abdominal or vaginal sonogram to rule out anatomic abnormalities
   (4) Endometrial biopsy (especially in women >40) to rule out uterine cancer, endometrial polyps, endometrial hyperplasia
  g. Differential diagnosis: Necessary to differentiate between the multiple non-HIV causes and ovulatory and anovulatory menstrual cycles when evaluating endocrine dysfunction
7. Treatment
  a. Observation
  b. Acute: Treatment for uncontrolled bleeding might include surgical uterine interventions (D&C, laparoscopy, hysterectomy); it should also include additional histology and procedures to isolate the problem
8. Laboratory results and other indices to monitor for disease progression and response to therapy
  a. A menstrual calendar is frequently maintained as a diagnostic tool to measure response to therapy
  b. Anticipate menstrual disorders as CD4+ lymphocyte count falls

E. Pelvic Inflammatory Disease

1. Etiology and disease process
  a. Pelvic inflammatory disease (PID) is an infection that may involve one or more of the following: endometrium, pelvic veins, pelvic peritoneum, ovaries, and fallopian tubes
  b. Pathophysiology
   (1) Usually caused by *Chlamydia* or *Neisseria*
   (2) Other possible causes
    (a) Virus, parasite, or fungus emanating from the vagina and migrating through the vagina and cervix into the uterus
    (b) The organism(s) can enter uterine veins or the lymphatic system as they pass into the pelvis by the fallopian tubes
    (c) After infection, adhesions can develop and form strictures, which may result in sterility

(3) One of the most serious complications of PID is infertility
2. Frequency and distribution
   a. PID is common in the U.S.; approximately 10%–15% of U.S. women have had an episode of salpingitis (Chiasson & Wright, 1995)
   b. In HIV-infected women, evidence is growing that it may occur more frequently and may be more difficult to treat that in immunocompetent women (Chiasson & Wright, 1995)
3. Relationship to natural history of HIV disease: Not yet adequately documented
4. Morbidity and mortality: HIV-infected women require lengthier hospitalizations and more frequent surgery than HIV-negative women for abscess formation associated with PID; they also reported less tenderness and had a lower leukocyte count on hospital admission (Korn, Landers, Green, & Sweet, 1993)
5. Early detection, prevention, prophylaxis: Interuterine devices increase the risk of PID, and their use should be avoided in HIV-infected women
6. Signs and symptoms: May vary
   a. Subacute infection: Only nonspecific abdominal pain or no pain at all
   b. Some patients may experience severe abdominal pressure or pain, intermenstrual spotting, painful intercourse, malaise, nausea and vomiting, fever, chills, foul-smelling vaginal discharge

7. Diagnosis
   a. WBC
   b. Culture and gram stain of vaginal secretions
   c. Ultrasound
   d. Laparoscopy will confirm diagnosis of PID
   e. Therapeutic trial of antibiotics
8. Treatment
   a. Administration of parenteral antibiotics
   b. In some cases, hospitalization or surgical intervention are necessary
9. Laboratory results and other indices to monitor for disease progression and response to therapy: Symptoms that persist despite optimal treatment may indicate immune system dysfunction
10. Patient education
   a. Instruct patient in forms of birth control as needed; inform her of risk associated with interuterine devices
   b. Inform patient to monitor for recurrent disease
   c. Stress the important of frequent gynecologic services and care

F. Syphilis
See *Bacterial Infections*, p. 67

G. Vaginal Candidiasis
See *Fungal Diseases*, p. 83.

XVII. ENDOCRINE COMPLICATIONS

A. Hypogonadism in Men

1. Etiology and disease process
   a. Primary testicular failure: Low testosterone levels with elevated levels of luteinizing hormone (LH) and follicle-stimulating hormone (FSH)
   b. Functional disorder of the hypothalamus: Despite a normal gonadotropin response, there is low testicular function due to the lack of stimulating hormones from the hypothalamus
   c. Testicular infections: CMV (most common), *M. avium intracellulare,* toxoplasma
   d. Severe malnutrition and wasting syndrome
   e. Adverse effects from medications
      (1) Prolonged treatment with ganciclovir may be associated with suppression of testosterone
      (2) Ketoconazole has caused decreased testosterone secretion
      (3) Opiate use increases risk of developing hypogonadism
2. Frequency and distribution: Not known at this time
3. Relationship to natural history of HIV disease
   a. Incidence increases in advanced HIV disease
   b. High correlation with malnutrition and wasting syndrome
   c. Opiate use increases risk for hypogonadism
4. Morbidity and mortality
   a. A low serum testosterone level may be the most common endocrine abnormality in patients with HIV disease (Dobs, Dempsey, Landerson, & Polk, 1988)
   b. In a study of 70 men (Dobs et al., 1988), gonadal dysfunction was seen in 50% of the men with AIDS and 44% with symptomatic HIV infection
   c. Correlates with lower lymphocyte counts, greater weight loss, and worsened mortality
   d. In a study of 70 men, 55% of hypogonadal men died within first 12 months vs. 26% of men who were eugonadal (Dobs et al., 1988)
5. Early detection, prevention, prophylaxis
   a. Supplementation with androgens currently under consideration
   b. Hypogonadism is reversible when drug therapy with ketoconazole is discontinued
6. Signs and symptoms
   a. Decreased libido
   b. Impotence
   c. Decreased serum testosterone levels (normal 270 – 1,070 ng/dl)
   d. Decreased sperm counts
7. Diagnosis
   a. Patient history reveals complaints of impotence or decreased libido
   b. Histology: Inflammation, interstitial fibrosis
   c. Procedures/tests
      (1) Serum testosterone levels
      (2) LH and FSH levels
      (3) Gonadotrophic response to gonadotropin-releasing hormone (GnRH)
      (4) Sperm count
      (5) Thyroid function tests
   d. Differential diagnoses: Rule out malignancy, OIs
8. Treatment
   a. Testosterone replacement
   b. Improve nutritional status
   c. Avoid medications that decrease testosterone production
   d. Psychologic support for sexual dysfunction concerns, treatment for impotency
9. Laboratory results and other indices to monitor for disease progression and response to therapy: Serum testosterone levels, improved libido and penile erection fraction
10. Patient education
    a. Actions and side effects of medications
    b. Adequate nutrition
    c. Safer sex instructions

B. Pentamidine-Induced Hypoglycemia and Diabetes

1. Etiology and disease process
   a. Extensive pentamidine-induced pancreatic necrosis
   b. Extensive destruction of B cells results in an unphysiologic release of stored insulin with resulting hypoglycemia
   c. Later progression to diabetes mellitus with or without ketoacidosis
   d. Long tissue half-life of pentamidine can result in hypoglycemia days or weeks after discontinuing a therapeutic course of the drug (Stahl-Bayliss, Kalman, & Laskin, 1986; Waskin, Stohr-Green, Helmick, & Sattler, 1988)
2. Frequency and distribution
   a. Incidence of pentamidine-induced hypoglycemia in persons with advanced HIV disease is higher (14%–28%) than in the non-HIV infected (6.2%–9.1%) (Bouchard et al., 1982; Osei et al., 1984)
   b. Incidence of symptomatic hypoglycemia is more common in people with advanced HIV infection (25%) (Chernow et al., 1990) than in the non-HIV infected (12%)
3. Relationship to natural history of HIV disease
   a. Reason for increased sensitivity of patients with *advanced* HIV disease to pentamidine-induced hypoglycemia (Stahl-Baylis et al., 1986; Waskin et al., 1988) is unknown
   b. Predictors for the development of hypoglycemia
      (1) Presence of azotemia during therapy
      (2) Total dose and duration of pentamidine therapy
      (3) History of previous pentamidine therapy
4. Morbidity and mortality
   a. True incidence of pentamidine hypoglycemia may be greater, as present estimates have been based on in-hospital studies that may not account for reactions resulting from the drug's long half-life
   b. Drug-induced diabetes mellitus may develop with the extensive multiorgan system complications of diabetes (e.g., renal, eyesight)
   c. Mortality unknown
5. Early detection, prevention, prophylaxis
   a. Early recognition and management of pentamidine-induced hypoglycemia
   b. Frequent blood glucose monitoring during course of treatment
6. Signs and symptoms
   a. Low blood glucose levels
   b. Inappropriately elevated insulin levels
   c. Weakness, fatigue
   d. Restlessness, irritability, thirst
7. Diagnosis
   a. Hypoglycemia post pentamidine therapy
   b. Pancreatic necrosis
   c. Blood glucose level
   d. Differential diagnoses: Rule out OIs, malignancies of the pancreas, rule out megestrol acetate drug-induced diabetes mellitus
8. Treatment
   a. Acute
      (1) Discontinue pentamidine
      (2) Adjunctive therapy rarely necessary as symptoms usually resolve after withdrawal of the drug
      (3) Institute alternative therapy for PCP
   b. Maintenance
      (1) Alternative therapy for PCP prophylaxis
      (2) Treatment and management of diabetes mellitus if it occurs (e.g., insulin therapy)
9. Laboratory results and other indices to monitor for disease progression and response to therapy
   a. Blood glucose
   b. BUN
   c. Abnormal regulation of glucose in patients receiving pentamidine may also be associated with the development of pentamidine-associated nephrotoxicity
10. Patient education
   a. Hypoglycemia and diabetes-related instruction, including dietary changes, foot care, insulin instructions; refer to a diabetes treatment specialty team
   b. Arrange for a Medic-Alert bracelet or wallet card indicating if patient is hypo- or hyperglycemic

C. Thyroid Function Abnormalities

1. Etiology and disease process
   a. Primary thyroid dysfunction is rare in HIV/AIDS
   b. OIs associated with thyroid disease for HIV/AIDS patients: CMV, cryptococcus, *P. carinii*
      (1) Euthyroid sick syndrome is the most common cause of thyroid abnormality in HIV disease; it is associated with any chronic debilitating illness and manifested by the decreased peripheral conversion of thyroxine [T_4] to triiodothyronine [T_3]
      (2) Euthyroid sick syndrome: Indicates that the thyroid gland is normal but that systemic disease has altered thyroid hormone physiology
   c. Rifampin may precipitate hypothyroidism in people with limited thyroid reserve
2. Relationship to natural history of HIV disease: Thyroid function tests (TFTs) can be altered in early stages of HIV disease but is generally more common in advanced HIV disease
3. Morbidity and mortality: Low T_3 correlated with hypoalbuminemia is an accurate predictor of mortality in hospitalized patients with advanced HIV disease (Fried et al., 1980; Tang & Kaplan, 1989)
4. Signs and symptoms of hypothyroidism
   a. Fatigue
   b. Increased coarseness of hair
   c. Dry skin
   d. Loss of appetite
   e. Slow reaction time
5. Diagnosis
   a. Abnormal thyroid function studies
   b. Tests/procedures
      (1) Thyroxin (T_4) (normal 4.5–12 μg/dl)
      (2) Thyroid-stimulating hormone (TSH) (normal 0.4–4.8 IU/ml)
      (3) Triiodothyronine (T_3) (normal 250–390 ng/100 dl)
      (4) Reverse triiodothyronine rT_3 (normal 2.6–18.9 ng/dl)
      (5) Thyroxine-binding globulin (TBG) (normal 12–28 μg/ml)
   c. Differential diagnoses
      (1) Thyroid mass: Rule out KS, other malignancy
      (2) Hashimoto's thyroiditis
6. Treatment
   a. Thyroid hormonal replacement for primary thyroid deficiency
   b. Treatment of OIs and malignancies
   c. Hormonal replacement for euthyroid sick syndrome is not indicated—may even be detrimental
   d. Monitor patients on rifampin for signs and symptoms of hypothyroidism
7. Laboratory results and other indices to monitor for disease progression and response to therapy
   a. Elevated thyroxine-binding globulin and a progressive decline in rT_3 is associated with advancing HIV disease
   b. Low serum T_3 concentrations are associated with poor outcome in people with PCP
8. Patient education: Signs and symptoms of hypothyroidism (e.g., fatigue, increased coarseness of hair); report to the patient's healthcare provider

D. Adrenal Disease

1. Etiology and disease process
   a. Opportunistic pathogens that result in adrenalitis, inflammation, or necrosis
      (1) CMV (most common)
      (2) *C. neoformans*
      (3) Toxoplasma
      (4) *M. tuberculosis*
      (5) *M. avium intracellulare*
   b. Malignancies: KS, lymphoma
   c. Medications
      (1) Ketoconazole
         (a) Inhibits adrenal synthesis of cortisol and aldosterone
         (b) Blunts cortisol response to ACTH
      (2) Rifampin: Alters metabolism of glucocorticoids
2. Frequency and distribution: Glucocorticoid (cortisol) deficiency is relatively uncommon (>90% of the adrenal tissue must be destroyed before clinically significant cortisol deficiency occurs)
3. Relationship to natural history of HIV disease

a. Monitoring for adrenal insufficiency is warranted in people with an OI, KS, or on drug therapy with ketoconazole or rifampin, as these conditions and drugs are associated with adrenal destruction or insufficiency
   b. Relationship to HIV infection itself is unknown
4. Morbidity and mortality: Although post-mortems reveal adrenal gland involvement in substantial numbers of patients, most did not manifest symptoms commonly associated with adrenal insufficiency and were not suspected to have an adrenal disease process
5. Early detection, prevention, and prophylaxis
   a. Prophylaxis for OIs
   b. Secondary prevention and prophylaxis
      (1) Early diagnosis and treatment of OIs
      (2) Monitor patients receiving ketoconazole or rifampin for signs and symptoms of adrenal insufficiency
6. Signs and symptoms
   a. Hyponatremia
   b. Hyperkalemia; may occur in conjunction with pentamidine therapy
   c. Hypotension
   d. Fatigue or weakness
   e. Anorexia and weight loss
   f. Orthostasis
   g. Nausea and vomiting
   h. Hyperpigmentation, a usual sign, not found
7. Diagnosis: Decreased absolute cortisol level after ACTH stimulation
   a. Peak value of ≥20 μg/dl indicates normal adrenal reserve
   b. Peak value of ≥22 μg/dl indicates normal adrenal reserve recommended for people with advanced HIV disease (Membreno et al., 1987)
8. Treatment
   a. Acute (adrenal insufficiency)
      (1) Hydrocortisone
      (2) Fludrocortisone to provide adequate mineralocorticoid activity; more commonly needed to treat hyperkalemia in patients receiving pentamidine
      (3) Loading doses of hydrocortisone in

divided doses during periods of stress or severe infection
   b. Maintenance
      (1) After initiation of therapy, individualize treatment based on patient response
      (2) Avoid >30 mg of hydrocortisone/day to prevent worsening an already immunosuppressed condition
9. Laboratory results and other indices to monitor for disease progression and response to therapy
   a. Absolute cortisol level after ACTH stimulation
   b. Potassium level
   c. Sodium levels
10. Patient education
   a. Actions and side effects of medications
   b. Signs and symptoms of adrenal disease to report to their healthcare provider

E. Disorders of Water Balance and Posterior Pituitary

1. Etiology and disease process
   a. Hyponatremia results from stress or drug-induced syndrome of inappropriate antidiuretic hormone secretion (SIADH)
   b. SIADH results from excessive antidiuretic hormone secretion from the pituitary gland, even in the face of subnormal serum osmolarity
   c. Associated causes of SIADH thought to stimulate the pituitary gland
      (1) Active pulmonary disease
      (2) CNS infections
      (3) Opiate or barbiturate administration
2. Frequency and distribution
   a. Incidence of hyponatremia is highest in acutely ill hospitalized patients with an OI, especially pulmonary infections
   b. Incidence of hyponatremia is also high in stable outpatients (20%)
3. Relationship to natural history of HIV disease: Risk factors are pulmonary and CNS infections and the administration of opiates and barbiturates
4. Morbidity and mortality: Hyponatremia is seen in 31%–36% of patients with HIV disease, is associated with high (30%) in-hospital mortality (Vitting et al., 1990)

5. Early detection, prevention, and prophylaxis
   a. Prophylaxis for common pulmonary and CNS opportunistic infections
   b. Secondary prevention and prophylaxis: Early treatment of pulmonary and CNS infections
6. Signs and symptoms
   a. Fluid retention
   b. Dilutional hyponatremia
   c. Diminished GI function
   d. Alterations in level of consciousness, seizures; coma may be evidenced if serum sodium falls below 120 mEq/L
   e. Elevated blood pressure, full and rapid pulse
7. Diagnosis
   a. Tests/procedures
      (1) Daily intake and output, weights
      (2) Serum sodium concentrations <130 mEq/L
      (3) High urine osmolarity
      (4) Low serum osmolarity
      (5) Arginine vasopressin levels inappropriately high for the serum osmolarity
      (6) Measurable serum antidiuretic hormone (ADH)
   b. Neurologic exam, mental status
   c. Differential diagnoses: Rule out renal

salt wasting, adrenal insufficiency, iatrogenic hyponatremia due to hypotonic fluid therapy
8. Treatment
   a. Acute: Fluid restriction; patients unresponsive to fluid restriction may benefit from treatment with demeclocycline HCl
   b. Maintenance
      (1) Closely monitor fluid and electrolyte balance, cardiovascular or neurologic changes
      (2) Report weight gain at ≥2 lb
      (3) Treatment with trimethoprim may impair sodium conservation during saline replacement
9. Laboratory results and other indices to monitor for disease progression and response to therapy
   a. Blood chemistry (serum sodium levels)
   b. Urine osmolarity
   c. Serum osmolarity
   d. Arginine vasopressin level
10. Patient education
   a. Report any mental status changes, signs and symptoms of pulmonary changes to patient's healthcare provider
   b. Record daily weight; report a gain of ≥2 lb to the healthcare provider.

XVIII. MUSCULOSKELETAL SYSTEM COMPLICATIONS

A. General Information

1. Musculoskeletal disorders constitute one of the less well-known manifestations of HIV infection
2. Since 1986, the National Institute of Arthritis and Musculoskeletal and Skin Diseases (NIAMS) has studied the cutaneous and rheumatic manifestations of HIV infection and AIDS
3. Research has demonstrated that arthralgia commonly occurs in the HIV-infected; often associated with severely painful joints
   a. The most frequently observed type of arthritis seen in HIV infection is Reiter's syndrome
   b. Arthritis associated with HIV disease has been described as
      (1) Idiopathic—presumably those caused by HIV itself
      (2) Associated with rheumatic or autoimmune disease
      (3) Septic
      (4) Psoriatic arthritis, vasculitides
      (5) A Sjögren's-like syndrome
   c. Inflammatory muscle diseases include myositis, myopathy, and myopathy associated with AZT therapy
4. Musculoskeletal disease often accompanied by integumentary system involvement
   a. All forms of psoriasis
   b. Seborrhea and onychodystrophy with or without nail pitting
5. Increased life span of HIV-infected people has enabled diagnosis of more musculoskeletal complications

B. Arthritis

1. Etiology and disease process: The etiology of HIV-associated arthritis remains undefined
   a. Limited data available on synovial immunopathology
      (1) In some patients, changes of non-specific chronic synovial inflammation are present with high synovial fluid cell counts
      (2) In others, signs of inflammatory changes are minimal
   b. HIV appears to have a cytopathic effect on the joints; the possibility that HIV is arthrogenic is supported by animal studies of other lentiviruses
   c. It remains unclear whether HIV infection predisposes to arthritis, or whether viral or immune mechanisms associated with HIV disease play a role in the development of joint pathology
2. Frequency and distribution
   a. Arthritis in HIV disease has been reported among various racial groups in Africa, Europe, and the United States
   b. Studies conducted in Cleveland, New York, and Tampa have recorded a 15%–25% incidence of inflammatory arthritis in unselected HIV-positive people (Keat & Rowe, 1991)
   c. Many HIV disease centers have not reported arthritis as a clinical problem, which may reflect a low incidence or a lack of recognition by clinicians
3. Relationship to natural history of HIV disease
   a. Precipitating factors that may cause arthritis in HIV disease include (Itescu, 1991)
      (1) Enteric infections, manifested by diarrhea, caused by *Shigella, Campylobacter,* and *Yersinia*
      (2) Urethritis caused by *Chlamydia*
      (3) Other infectious diseases (e.g., oral candidiasis, perianal herpes simplex, herpes zoster)
   b. No consistent relationship to CD4+ lymphocyte counts
   c. Can occur at any stage of HIV disease, but by the time arthritis is diagnosed in the HIV-infected, circulating CD4+ lymphocytes can be depleted
4. Morbidity and mortality
   a. Insufficient epidemiologic data
   b. One hypothesis under continuing investigation: The development of arthritis in Reiter's syndrome may contribute to

enhanced viral replication and deterioration in HIV disease, resulting in an earlier diagnosis of AIDS (Keat & Rowe, 1991)

5. Signs and symptoms
   a. Reiter's syndrome was the first HIV-associated rheumatic disease identified
      (1) The classic triad—arthritis, urethritis, conjunctivitis—occurs in some HIV-infected patients, with all three features completely or partially present
      (2) The associated constitutional features of fever, weight loss, malaise, lymphadenopathy, and diarrhea are common and indistinguishable from symptomatic HIV disease
         (a) Arthritis is often seen with low CD4+ lymphocyte counts and an absolute increase in CD8 lymphocyte cells
         (b) In many patients lab evaluation will reveal HLA-B27
   b. Enthesopathy, a disorder of the muscular or tendinous attachment to the bone, most frequent site of inflammation involving ankle/foot
      (1) Ambulatory patients may demonstrate a broad-based ataxia, shifting their weight to the outer margins of the foot to minimize ankle pain (sometimes referred to as "AIDS foot")
      (2) Multidigit dactylitis common; usually painless
      (3) Knee involvement common; most often asymmetric
      (4) May also occur in shoulder, elbow, wrists
      (5) Periarticular muscle atrophy is possible
      (6) Can be a major cause of disability; in its severest form, patient may be restricted to a wheelchair
   c. Psoriatic arthritis has been diagnosed in HIV-infected patients
      (1) Most common sites of inflammation are ankles, feet, sacroiliac/spine
      (2) Psoriatic manifestations are multiple and include vulgaris, guttae, sebopsoriasis, pustular, and exfoliative forms
      (3) The course of disease can be aggressive, leading to joint destruction, mild and chronic, with intermittent joint involvement
   d. Acute symmetric polyarthritis (ASP) also identified as HIV-related
      (1) Involves small joints of the hands (similar to rheumatoid arthritis)
      (2) Onset is sudden and acute accompanied by symmetric ulnar deviation and swan-neck deformities
   e. AIDS-associated arthritis
      (1) A subacute oligoarthritis characterized by extreme disability and pain
      (2) Unlike other types of arthritis seen in HIV disease, is of short duration (1–6 weeks)
   f. Painful articular syndrome
      (1) Severe articular or bone pain that occurs in the knees, shoulders, or elbows
      (2) Characterized by its short duration (2–24 hours)
   g. Axial joint disease: Manifested by spinal pain, commonly in cervical and thoracolumbar regions
   h. An emerging area of spondyloarthritic disease, now under study, is the identification of avascular necrosis (AVN) of the bone in HIV-infected patients
      (1) Usual risk factors associated with AVN (corticosteroid therapy, trauma, regular alcohol consumption) are absent
      (2) Initial presentation usually pain; may occur concurrently with arthritides such as Reiter's syndrome

6. Diagnosis
   a. Radiographic studies may not reveal features of spondyloarthropathic disease
   b. Synovial fluid biopsies are variable; may reveal nothing more than nonspecific chronic synovitis
   c. Erythrocyte sedimentation rates and C-reactive protein are elevated in all arthritic patients with HIV disease
   d. Tests for autoantibodies, including rheumatoid factor and antinuclear antibodies, are negative

e. Tissue typing shows a strong link between HLA-B27 and Reiter's syndrome
f. Differential diagnosis
   (1) Rule out possible infection of the bone, joint, or muscle (perform synovial fluid culture)
   (2) Extra-articular signs and symptoms may suggest OIs with joint involvement
7. Treatment
   a. Phenylbutazone
      (1) Sulfasalazine
      (2) Prednisone
      (3) Depot steroids (corticosteroid injections) combined with joint immobilization using a splint
      (4) Myochrysine
      (5) Hydroxychloroquine sulfate
      (6) Etretinate
      (7) Cyclosporine A
   b. Issues related to treatment
      (1) Therapeutic response to steroids in HIV-infected patients varies; some patients respond well and tolerate corticosteroids; others have developed severe invasive candidiasis; corticosteroids may increase risk of CMV infection
      (2) Avoid other immunosuppressive agents (e.g., methotrexate, ultraviolet B light therapy for psoriatic disease); their use has been associated with sudden fulminant immunodeficiency and the appearance of KS and severe OIs
      (3) Physical therapy is an absolute requirement
8. Laboratory results and other indices to monitor for disease progression and response to therapy
   a. Monitoring disease progression and the patients response to treatment is a complex task; signs and symptoms such as those seen in Reiter's syndrome exactly duplicate those seen in progressive HIV illness
   b. Cytopenia may limit the use of certain medications (e.g., NSAIDs)
   c. The benefits versus the risks of corticosteroids must be carefully weighed

   (1) Evaluating response to therapy is primarily based on patient self-report, physical findings (e.g., ROM, ability to carry out ADL)
   (2) Equally important is the observation of possible comorbid conditions (e.g., weight loss), which may result from functional limitations and the inability to obtain food and prepare meals; evaluate the need for home care services
9. Patient education: See *Pain*, p. 229, *High Risk for Ineffective Management of Therapeutic Regimen*, p. 258, *Impaired Mobility*, p. 221, *Body Image Disturbance*, p. 247, *Nutritional Deficit: Weight Loss, Anorexia*, p. 227

C. Diffuse Infiltrative Lymphocytosis Syndrome

1. Etiology and disease process
   a. Diffuse infiltrative lymphocytosis syndrome (DILS), a Sjögren's-like disease, is presumed to be caused by HIV, resulting in an unusual host-immune response
   b. Characterized by circulating CD8 lymphocytosis, marked reversal of the CD_4:CD8 T-cell ratio, and CD8 lymphocytic salivary gland infiltration, which contrasts to the CD4 lymphocytic infiltration seen in classic Sjögren's syndrome
      (1) Classic, idiopathic Sjögren's syndrome is comprised of keratoconjunctivitis sicca, xerostomia, and polyarthritis
      (2) Additional manifestations that differentiate DILS seen in HIV-infected people from idiopathic Sjögren's
         (a) Massive parotid gland swelling
         (b) Large neck masses
         (c) Absence of arthritis
         (d) Xerophthalmia is less of a problem
         (e) Extraglandular visceral features are common
2. Frequency and distribution
   a. No data available
   b. Studies of HIV-infected people in the U.S. and Brazil report that DILS

predominately occurs in men, while idiopathic Sjögren's is usually diagnosed in middle-aged women

3. Relationship to natural history of HIV disease: The propensity for developing DILS is related to the increasing numbers of circulating CD8 cells and their infiltration of the parotid glands and organ systems

4. Morbidity and mortality
   a. Although morbidity due to extraglandular involvement often includes the reticuloendothelial, respiratory, GI, and neurologic systems, thus far the clinical course of DILS is reportedly mild, with no noted mortality
   b. It has been hypothesized that DILS may benefit HIV-infected patients by suppressing HIV progression—CD8 lymphocytes that are positive for CD 29 and other lymphocytes have been shown to suppress HIV viral replication

5. Signs and symptoms
   a. Glandular features
      (1) Moderate to massive bilateral parotid gland enlargement, salivary gland enlargement, xerostomia, xerophthalmia
      (2) Related symptoms include facial pain, recurrent sinusitis, and middle ear and oral cavity infections
      (3) Middle ear infections may have accompanying hearing loss
   b. Extraglandular involvement: Lymphadenopathy, pneumonitis, hepatitis, gastritis, cranial nerve VII palsy, meningitis, optic neuritis, bilateral motor neuropathy, and thymoma

6. Diagnosis
   a. Diagnosis is made by history, physical findings on examination, and negative autoimmune results
   b. Lymphocyte subset studies reveal high CD8+ lymphocyte counts and significant reversal of the CD4:CD8 ratio
   c. Culture and sensitivity studies to rule out treatable infections
   d. Differential diagnoses
      (1) Rule out bacterial sialoadenitis, viral infections such as mumps, EBV, direct infection due to HIV, tumors
      (2) Evaluation of xerophthalmia and

xerostomia to include careful drug history; these side effects associated with tricyclic antidepressants and antihistamines

7. Treatment
   a. Symptomatic therapy for related symptoms using artificial tears and artificial saliva
   b. AZT therapy is beneficial to most patients and will usually result in partial resolution of symptoms
   c. Immunosuppressive therapy using prednisone is restricted to progressive extraglandular, life-threatening involvement

8. Laboratory results and other indices to monitor for disease progression and response to therapy
   a. Xerostomia can lead to a high incidence of periodontal disease and cavities
   b. Xerophthalmia can lead to corneal ulcerations

9. Patient education
   a. For xerophthalmia: Teach proper use of contact lenses, to wear sunglasses when outside, and to carry artificial tears at all times
   b. For xerostomia: Teach use of artificial saliva; keep liquids at hand to sip on all the time
      (1) Avoid sugar as the inadequate salivary flow will lead to dental caries and oral cavity infections
      (2) Brush teeth after eating or rinse well with water
      (3) Avoid alcohol and tobacco as they may aggravate the condition
   c. Recommend turtleneck shirts, scarfs, and other dressing techniques to compensate for altered body image due to glandular enlargement in the neck
   d. See *Periodontal Disease*, p. 169, *Hearing Loss*, p. 217, *Body Image Disturbance*, p. 247

D. Myositis and Myopathy

1. Etiology and disease process
   a. Myositis and myopathy occur in HIV-infected patients as a result of the HIV-related inflammatory response or AZT therapy

b. HIV-induced myopathy does not appear to result from direct infection of the muscle by the virus, but rather from the immunopathologic process triggered by HIV, mediated by autoaggressive CD8+ lymphocytes

c. AZT-induced myopathy results from the depletion of mitochondrial DNA in both cardiac and skeletal muscles

2. Frequency and distribution
   a. At present, incidence of myositis and myopathy related to HIV has not been defined
   b. AZT-induced myopathy is estimated to occur in approximately 10% of patients; appears 6 months to 2 years after initiation of therapy

3. Relationship to natural history of HIV disease
   a. Myopathies can occur at various stages; not necessarily related to patient's immune status
   b. Drug-induced myopathy is seen shortly after the initiation of AZT therapy

4. Morbidity and mortality
   a. Ranges from mild to severe motor impairment that has a direct affect on the person's ability to perform ADL as well as on quality of life
   b. Mortality: No data available

5. Signs and symptoms: Diffuse, symmetric weakness with sparing of sensory and autonomic functions
   a. Initially, difficulty in squatting, walking up stairs
   b. Myalgia, and muscle tenderness
   c. Proximal weakness in the upper and lower extremities; in some cases, distal weakness may be observed
   d. Proximal weakness in proximal muscles, especially in the legs, of patients taking AZT (also known as "saggy butt syndrome")

6. Diagnosis

a. History, physical examination, electromyography, and muscle biopsy will usually confirm the diagnosis

b. MRI may be useful in identifying pathologic muscle

c. Creatinine kinase levels are frequently elevated

d. Differential diagnosis
   (1) Discontinuing AZT therapy may empirically assist in making the diagnosis
      (a) In most patients symptoms will disappear within 6–8 weeks
      (b) Persistent symptoms at that point indicate either HIV-induced myopathy or neuromuscular infection caused by e.g., herpes, CMV
   (2) Rule out myopathy, which usually shows a preservation of the tendon reflex and sensory function, from chronic inflammatory demyelinating polyneuropathy (CIDP), which does not

7. Treatment
   a. For patients on AZT, withdrawal of therapy and switching to ddI or ddC is recommended
   b. For patients who have not received AZT, initiation of therapy may prove beneficial
   c. Combination therapy with NSAIDs and analgesics
   d. In profound, disabling cases, prednisone may be initiated until improvement in muscle strength is noted; then tapered to alternate day dosing for several months

8. Laboratory results and other indices to monitor for disease progression and response to therapy
   a. Serum creatine kinase levels
   b. Muscle strength and associated complaints of tenderness and myalgia

9. Patient education: See *Impaired Mobility*, p. 221.

XIX. RENAL COMPLICATIONS

A. Fluid and Electrolyte Imbalance

1. Etiology and disease process
   a. Many of the complications result from infections or malignant disease due to immunocompromised status
   b. Most common cause of renal failure: Nephrotoxic drugs
   c. Much of the pathologic information on HIV-associated renal disease comes from autopsy
   d. Trimethoprim and other drugs have been associated with development of hypercalcemia in patients with advanced HIV disease
   e. The kidney is not a "target" organ for the replication or dissemination of HIV
   f. Severe immunosuppression is thought to play a role
2. Frequency and distribution
   a. Abnormal concentrations of serum electrolytes are common in PWAs
   b. The most common acid-base disturbances in AIDS patients are due to pulmonary infections resulting in progressive renal insufficiency
   c. 10% of patients have moderate to severe proteinuria
3. Morbidity and mortality
   a. Fluid and electrolyte imbalances are a common complication of AIDS
   b. Most can be reversed with adequate treatment
4. Signs and symptoms
   a. Hyponatremia is the most frequent abnormality, caused by
      (1) Hypovolemia: Results from loss of sodium-containing fluids from diarrhea and replacement with fluids that produce dilutional hyponatremia
      (2) SIADH secretion associated with pulmonary infections such as PCP (see *Disorders of Water Balance and Posterior Pituitary,* p. 189)
      (3) Abnormalities in adrenal steroid synthesis
   b. Hypokalemia

   (1) Results from excessive renal and extrarenal losses of potassium due to protracted vomiting or diarrhea
   (2) Renal potassium wasting from drugs such as amphotericin B, rifampin, pentamidine
   (3) Can be caused by infection
   (4) Renal insufficiency associated with acute or chronic renal parenchymal disease
   c. Hypercalcemia
      (1) Results from renal insufficiency associated with acute or chronic parenchymal disease
      (2) Can be a manifestation of mineralocorticoid deficiency from either Addison's disease or more selective defects in aldosterone biosynthesis
   d. Acid-base disturbances
      (1) Caused by pulmonary OIs; respiratory alkalosis is often the initial sign but as the pulmonary condition worsens and gas exchange is compromised, hypercapnia and respiratory acidosis will occur
      (2) Metabolic acidosis with a normal anion gap can occur in patients with renal tubular acidosis; it is caused by severe, protracted diarrhea with large losses of bicarbonate in the stool
5. Diagnosis
   a. Medical history from patients to include all medications patient is taking (include OTC meds), history of OIs
   b. Targeted physical
   c. Intake and output
   d. Labs
      (1) CBC
      (2) Chemistries; include mineral panel
      (3) Urinalysis
      (4) Urine sodium
      (5) Cortisol stimulation test
      (6) ABG
6. Treatment
   a. Hyponatremia associated with hypervolemia: Restore adequate sodium and intravascular volume
   b. Hyponatremia from SIADH: Fluid

restriction—results in a negative water balance and a rise in serum sodium

c. Hyponatremia from abnormalities in adrenal steroid synthesis: May benefit from glucocorticoid replacement

d. Hypercalcemia will often respond by treating the underlying cause of the imbalance, also loop diuretics and fludrocortisone to correct distal tubal defects

e. Acid-base disturbances are best corrected by treating the underlying condition and using bicarbonate to correct the acidosis

B. Acute Renal Failure

1. Etiology and disease process
   a. Acute tubular necrosis due to hypovolemia, sepsis, and toxic drugs
   b. Acute interstitial nephritis due to drug toxicity
   c. Renal interstitial edema due to massive proteinuria and hypoalbuminemia
   d. Tubular obstruction from hyperphosphatemia and hyperuricemia as a result of tumor lysis syndrome
   e. Hemolytic-uremic syndrome
   f. Postinfection immune complex glomerulonephritis
2. Frequency and distribution: Occurs in 20%–40% of PWAs who are critically ill with HIV-related malignancies or infections (Mazbar, Schoenfeld, & Humphreys, 1990; Valeri & Nevsky, 1991)
3. Morbidity and mortality
   a. Depends on underlying cause of renal failure
   b. Depends on the ability of the kidney to recover function
   c. Depends on successful treatment of the underlying cause of the renal failure
4. Relationship to natural history of HIV disease
   a. Both infections and malignancies are risk factors for developing renal failure
   b. Prior renal insufficiency is an additional risk factor
5. Signs and symptoms
   a. Hyperkalemia: Weakness, paresthesia, muscle cramps, bradycardia, ECG

changes, diarrhea, nausea
   b. Hyperphosphatemia: Oliguria, anuria
   c. Hypocalcemia: Muscle twitching, carpopedal spasm, tetany, laryngospasm, paresthesia, convulsions, hypotension, ECG changes
   d. Hypomagnesemia
   e. Hyperuricemia: Nausea, vomiting, diarrhea, lethargy, edema, flank pain, hematuria, azotemia, oliguria, anuria
   f. Both oliguric and nonoliguric forms of renal failure can be encountered
6. Diagnosis
   a. Extensive medical history and physical exam
   b. Drug history, to include OTC medications
   c. Labs
      (1) CBC
      (2) Complete chemistry panel
      (3) Mineral panel
      (4) Liver function tests
      (5) Serum creatinine, creatinine clearance
      (6) Uric acid
      (7) PT, PTT
      (8) ABG
      (9) Urinalysis, including osmolality
      (10) BUN
   d. ECG
   e. Intake and output
   f. Continuous monitoring of fluid status by weight, observation of edema, distended neck veins, shortness of breath or drop in urine output
7. Treatment
   a. Adequate hydration
   b. Supportive measures
   c. Aggressive treatment of the underlying cause of the renal failure
   d. Uric acid to prevent crystallization in the renal tubules
   e. Potassium and magnesium may need to be replaced
   f. Urine output to be maintained at 3 L/day
   g. Diuretics may be administered as adjunctive therapy
   h. Strict monitoring of intake and output is essential
   i. Electrolyte readjustments as needed
   j. Dialysis may be necessary

C. HIV-Associated Nephropathy

1. Etiology and disease process
   a. HIV-associated nephropathy (HIVAN) is pathologically distinct from other recognized forms of renal disease
   b. Seen in all stages of HIV/AIDS
   c. Nonspecific glomerulosclerosis and tubulopathy seen in PWAs
2. Frequency and distribution
   a. Prevalence is highest in the U.S. (cities most affected are New York, New Jersey, and Miami where progressive renal disease is seen in 5%–10% of HIV-infected patients) (Schoenfield & Feduska, 1990; Seney, Burns, & Silva, 1990)
   b. HIVAN occurs more frequently in African Americans, and men (Schoenfield & Feduska, 1990)
3. Morbidity and mortality
   a. Can be life threatening, resulting in end-stage renal disease
   b. A significantly shortened survival time has been seen in patients with HIVAN than in other AIDS patients
4. Relationship to natural history of HIV disease: Risk factors are related to race, gender, drug use
5. Signs and symptoms
   a. Proteinuria
   b. Progressive azotemia
   c. Normal blood pressure
   d. Enlarged kidneys on ultrasound
   e. Rapid progression to end-stage renal disease
6. Diagnosis
   a. Renal ultrasound
   b. Renal sonogram
   c. Laboratory testing
      (1) Chemistry panel
      (2) Creatinine
      (3) Creatinine clearance
      (4) Urinalysis
      (5) Kidney biopsy
7. Treatment
   a. Supportive; close clinical monitoring
   b. Dialysis may be necessary
8. Laboratory results and other indices to monitor for disease progression and response to therapy
   a. Vital signs
   b. Labs
   c. Intake and output.

Section 5

Management of Common Symptoms, Signs, and Other Responses to HIV Infection/AIDS

The focus of this section is management of the adult patient or the HIV-affected family. It outlines some of the most common physiologic and psychosocial responses to HIV/AIDS and specifies the nursing management. The material presented here is not intended to be interpreted as practice guidelines nor as standards of care. However, the nursing management strategies can serve as the basis for institutional development of such guidelines or standards.

The editors deliberately decided to combine physiologic and psychosocial responses in order to give equal importance to both. By its very nature this section could be considered as intensive symptom management or nursing care planning. We hope it will serve all these purposes.

Each condition contains a definition, etiologies, goals of care, assessment, and intervention strategies. In addition, *key points* serve as critical indicators or cues to immediate action or to specify complications or sequelae not addressed elsewhere. Nursing research or other findings are incorporated wherever relevant. Any overlap between this and other sections, particularly Section 4, is a deliberate effort to enhance the nursing management of the response. The focus of Section 4, however, is primarily *disease* management.

I. PHYSIOLOGIC SIGNS AND SYMPTOMS

A. Altered Mental Status: Delirium

1. Definition/Description
   a. A cluster of signs and symptoms, not an actual medical or nursing diagnosis
   b. Other terms used to describe delirium: Acute confusional state, confusion
   c. Characterized by
      (1) Acute change in level of consciousness (e.g., impaired alertness, attention, awareness)
      (2) Altered cognition (e.g., rambling speech, disjointed thought processes, faulty comprehension)
   d. Restlessness, illusions, and hallucinations may also be present
   e. Prevalence
      (1) Approximately 10% of hospitalized patients are admitted with or develop delirium
      (2) Elderly and most seriously ill at highest risk
      (3) Rate in people with HIV disease is unknown but believed to be significant
2. Etiology: Single or multiple simultaneous etiologies may be present
   a. Toxic
      (1) Medications (prescribed, OTC)
      (2) Alternative or complementary therapies
      (3) Drug or alcohol intoxication/withdrawal
   b. Metabolic: Electrolyte disturbances, endocrine disorders, hypoxia, fever, renal or liver insufficiency
   c. Infectious: May involve any system, may be present with or without fever
   d. Vascular: Congestive heart failure (CHF), CVA, anemia
   e. Neurologic: Encephalopathy, CNS lesion(s), seizures, postictal state
   f. Psychiatric: Severe depression, mania
3. Goals of Care
   a. To recognize underlying cause(s) swiftly; psychiatric evaluation indicated if no medical reason for the delirium identified
   b. To apply appropriate therapies to reverse or control symptoms
   c. To prevent injury to patient or others
4. *Key points*
   a. A sudden change in mental status warrants immediate nursing intervention with referral for emergency evaluation
   b. Newly introduced medications should be high on list of differential diagnoses
   c. Level of alertness may vary from agitation to lethargy, stupor, or coma
   d. Patients are generally drowsy and inattentive, require repeated explanations by caregivers/examiners
   e. Abrupt disturbances in sleep patterns or changes in level of activity should raise suspicions
   f. Early signs and symptoms of delirium may be inaccurately attributed to anxiety
5. Assessment
   a. Mental status exam
      (1) Orientation
      (2) Level of alertness/sedation
      (3) Attention or concentration
      (4) Thought processing
      (5) Perceptual alterations (e.g., visual, auditory, olfactory hallucinations; delusions)
      (6) Judgment, safety
   b. Interview caregiver and observe patient to assess
      (1) Functional status, including sleep patterns
      (2) Medications taken
      (3) Substance use
      (4) Other new signs and symptoms
      (5) Any history of similar delirium or precipitating event from caregiver
   c. Prepare patient/caregiver for the usual medical workup
      (1) CBC, chemistries, urinalysis, chest radiograph
      (2) As indicated, other tests such as ABGs, CT scan, toxic screens may be ordered
6. Interventions
   a. Provide safe and consistent environment; increase supervision of patient by family or staff as indicated

b. Institute appropriate treatment for causative condition; monitor patient's response, any adverse effects of treatment
c. Communicate in clear, simple terms to avoid misperceptions
d. Educate patient/family/significant other regarding
   (1) All care and diagnostic procedures to enlist patient's cooperation at the time procedure performed
   (2) Medications being given, anticipated effect
   (3) Reorient to person, place, time, situation; enlist family's help to do same and to bring in patient's watch, eye glasses, and hearing aid to minimize altered sensory input and disorientation
   (4) Delirium may be associated with acute and reversible medical problems
e. Consult with provider if patient is at risk for endangering self or others (see *Potential for Violence/Harm to Self or Others*, p. 265) to determine need for chemical/physical restraints
f. Ensure patient's ADL are met
g. Attempt to organize care to ensure patient's nighttime sleep is undisturbed with routine care activities that are not essential
h. Evaluate patient/caregiver resources for continuing care when hospitalization is no longer required
i. If patient does not sleep through the night, nighttime help or temporary placement may be necessary until patient's sleep/activity needs are reestablished or patient does not require 24-hour supervision
j. See *Delirium* p. 145

B. Anorectal Signs and Symptoms

1. Definition/Description
   a. Pain, bleeding, drainage, diarrhea, a mass, incontinence, itching, or lesions (Schecter, 1991)
   b. Proctalgia: Pain at the anus or in the rectum, the most common presenting complaint of HIV-infected patients with anorectal disease
   c. Anorectal disease in HIV-infected male homosexuals or bisexuals has been reported in as many as 30% of those with advanced disease (Wexner, Smithy, Milsom, & Dailey, 1986)
   d. Injecting drug users (IDUs) who have AIDS have a lower incidence of anorectal disease than male homosexuals or bisexuals with AIDS (Wolkimor, Barone, Hardy, & Cotton, 1990)
   e. In general, homosexual men who indulge in penetrative anal sex are thought to be at risk for anorectal disease
   f. Rectal symptoms can range from self-limiting to debilitating
2. Etiology: In people with HIV infection, conditions may or may not be related to their infection, associated with anal intercourse, or caused by neoplasia or OIs
   a. Pain
      (1) HSV (primary or reactivation)
      (2) VZV
      (3) Ulcerations/fissures
      (4) Neoplasm (lymphoma, KS, squamous cell carcinoma)
      (5) Pressure sores
      (6) Abscess formation
      (7) Abrasions, from scratching for relief of pruritus
      (8) Irritation from chronic diarrhea
      (9) Invasive diagnostic and therapeutic procedures
     (10) Hemorrhoids
     (11) Anal trauma
   b. Bleeding: Fissures, hemorrhoids, coloproctitis, malignancy
   c. Drainage
      (1) Gonococcal proctitis
      (2) Chlamydial proctitis
      (3) Mucosal prolapse
      (4) Lax anus
      (5) Prolapsed hemorrhoids
   d. Diarrhea (see p. 205)
   e. Mass
      (1) Anal condylomata
      (2) Squamous cell carcinoma
      (3) KS
      (4) Lymphoma

(5) Intraepithelial neoplasia
f. Fecal incontinence
   (1) Diarrhea due to multiple OIs
   (2) Dementia
   (3) Autonomic dysfunction
   (4) Proctitis
   (5) Inefficient continence mechanism
   (6) Fecal impaction with overflow (unusual cause)
g. Rectal itching
   (1) Infectious lesions (*Candida*, HSV, *Molluscum*)
   (2) Nonspecific rashes or dermatitis: drug rashes, lupuslike autoimmune phenomena
   (3) Increased serum bilirubin levels
   (4) Dry skin (xerosis)
   (5) Scabies
   (6) Folliculitis
   (7) Pinworm
h. Idiopathic or unknown etiology
3. Goal of Care: To control or decrease rectal symptoms
4. *Key points*
a. The anorectal junction is a complex area, both anatomically and physiologically (Borcich & Kotler, 1991)
   (1) The epithelial lining layers include skin, rectal mucosa, and transitional zone
   (2) Tissues underlying the skin and mucosa differ and are complicated by differing environments and immune defenses
   (3) The lining of the mucous membranes provides a weak physical barrier to penetration by viruses, bacteria, and other pathogens
b. HSV-1 and HSV-2 are clinically indistinguishable
   (1) Either type of virus is capable of infecting above or below the waist
   (2) All rectal lesions should be managed as herpes until etiology is identified
c. Early recognition and intervention of rectal symptoms may facilitate little to no disruption in ADL; delayed intervention may lead to uncontrolled pain, immobility, decreased nutritional intake, delayed healing, superimposed infections, emotional distress, social isolation

5. Assessment
a. Subjective data
   (1) Presenting symptoms/complaints
      (a) Onset
      (b) Frequency
      (c) Recurring pattern
      (d) Location
      (e) Duration
      (f) Aggravating factors
      (g) Alleviating factors, description of response
      (h) Behavioral response to pain
      (i) Response to analgesics and other treatments; ability and willingness to use alternative methods of pain control
   (2) Bowel habits
      (a) Frequency
      (b) Consistency
      (c) Color
      (d) Change in habits
      (e) Use of stool bulking agents, laxatives, or antidiarrheals
      (f) Enema use, frequency
   (3) Sexual practices
      (a) Anal insertive/receptive
      (b) Pain associated with anal intercourse
      (c) Condom/lubricant use
      (d) Insertive objects
b. Objective data
   (1) Inspect skin condition in anorectal area; pay particular attention to pressure points, skin folds, and perianal area
   (2) Spread buttocks and inspect the skin for
      (a) Rectal lesions: Assess for local erythema, red papules, vesicles, or pustules on mucosal surfaces and areas of broken skin. (*Note*: HSV lesions may coalesce into a large ulcerative area)
      (b) Local or disseminated erythema
      (c) Pattern and location of macules, vesicles, pustules, or crusting
      (d) Bleeding and location
      (e) Maceration
      (f) Hyperpigmentation
      (g) Pearly, umbilicated lesions

(h) Fine, white scaling without erythema

(i) Papules or nodules that may appear cauliflowerlike

6. Interventions

a. Administration of therapy

(1) Administer analgesic therapy, evaluate effectiveness

(2) Encourage use of alternative therapies to relieve discomfort, if appropriate (distraction, guided imagery, relaxation exercises)

(3) Provide topical measures to relieve pain or itching for HSV lesions

(a) Cool or warm saline soaks (tub and sitz baths are contraindicated)

(b) Apply Burrow's solution (aluminum acetate) soaks q4h to promote encrustation

(c) Apply refrigerated hydrogel dressings

(4) Administer antimicrobials (e.g., acyclovir) as ordered and monitor response

(5) Provide relief of pruritus (see *Impaired/Risk for Impaired Skin Integrity,* p. 222)

(6) Protect noninfected, nondraining, open wounds once HSV has been ruled out

(a) Apply hydrocolloid dressings

(b) Maintain moist wound therapy

(7) Protect irritated perianal skin with skin sealants

(8) Use fecal drainage device to collect watery, frequent stools in the patient too weak to toilet

b. Educate patient/family/significant other regarding primary episode vs. reactivation of HSV lesions

(1) Concepts of viral shedding and time frames

(2) Recognition of variables influencing recurrence (HSV)

(3) Modes of transmission, risk reduction, infection control measures (see Tables 10.2, *Universal Precautions,* p. 367, and 10.3, *Reducing the Risk of/ Preventing Exposure to Opportunistic Pathogens,* p. 371)

(4) Autoinoculation and means to reduce (e.g., meticulous hygiene, do not scratch)

(5) Symptom management and care techniques

(6) Medical diagnostic procedures, resultant nursing care

(7) Risk, benefits, and consequences of alternative therapies

(a) Vitamins A, B, and B complex supplements have been reported as "helpful" for HSV (Stein, 1992)

(b) Numerous nutrient supplements, including minerals, have been suggested to diminish the duration of herpetic symptoms (Olshevsky, Schlomo, Zwang, & Burger, 1989)

i) Amino acids have been a commonly used OTC for herpes prophylaxis and treatment

ii) L-lysine dietary supplements have been used for herpetic suppression, but the FDA has published information stating this treatment is not safe and effective

c. Counsel regarding support groups to assist in adaptation to living with chronic, unpredictable symptoms

d. See *Anorectal Disease,* p. 175

C. Cough

1. Definition/Description

a. Cough is a reflex triggered internally or resulting secondarily from environmental irritants

b. Prevalence in persons with HIV disease is not well-documented; however, in a study of HIV patients seeking emergency room care, 34% reported dyspnea or cough as their presenting complaint (Chang, Wong, Gold, & Armstrong, 1993)

c. Cough is a frequent and often disabling symptom in patients with pulmonary conditions

2. Etiology

a. Any pulmonary condition
b. Post bronchoscopy
c. Sinusitis
d. Aspiration
e. Esophageal reflux
f. Auditory canal irritation
g. Noxious substances
h. Exercise/activity
i. Cold air

3. Goals of Care
   a. To eliminate or treat the underlying cause of a chronic cough
   b. To minimize the discomfort associated with chronic cough

4. *Key points*
   a. Cough is a protective mechanism
   b. Immediate cough suppression may be necessary at times
   c. Complications from severe cough: Hemoptysis, pneumothorax, rib fracture, syncope, emesis

5. Assessment
   a. Subjective data
      (1) When did the cough begin?
      (2) Is the cough productive?
      (3) What is the character of the cough?
      (4) Is there a time of day when the cough is more bothersome?
      (5) Is there a relationship to position or posture?
      (6) Any accompanying signs/symptoms?
         (a) Hemoptysis
         (b) Shortness of breath
         (c) Wheezing
         (d) Chest tightness
         (e) Heartburn
         (f) Edema or orthopnea
         (g) Sinus pain
         (h) Headache
         (i) Postnasal drip
   b. Objective data: Complete pulmonary exam (see *Dyspnea*, p. 208)

6. Interventions
   a. Administer cough medications (antitussives, expectorants) on a scheduled basis rather than prn; schedule expectorants appropriately between, not with, meals
   b. Prevent stasis of secretions by encouraging deep breathing, ambulation, and postural drainage/percussion if necessary
   c. Maintain hydration and thin secretions by encouraging fluid intake of 2.5–3 L/day as tolerated
   d. Suction to remove secretions if cough is ineffective
   e. Position to prevent aspiration and reflux, such as elevating the head of the bed or using a wedge-shaped pillow for sleep
   f. Demonstrate splinting techniques to minimize the pain associated with coughing
   g. Offer throat-soothing remedies such as tea with honey and lemon, cough drops, warm saline gargle
   h. Avoid oxygen administration without adequate humidification
   i. Encourage to avoid activities or noxious substances that precipitate cough
   j. Encourage rest periods and energy conservation
   k. Evaluate patient's ability to
      (1) Identify effective cough remedies
      (2) Report changes in frequency/severity of cough
      (3) Demonstrate effective cough technique

D. Dehydration

1. Definition/Description
   a. Reduction of water content; occurs when water output exceeds intake
   b. High risk of dehydration for AIDS patients with diarrhea or fever

2. Etiology
   a. Water deprivation
   b. Excessive loss of water (diarrhea, vomiting, fever)
   c. Reduction in total quantity of electrolytes
   d. Adrenal or renal disease
   e. Infusion of hypertonic solutions

3. Goals of Care
   a. To restore homeostasis
   b. To prevent dehydration by assuring adequate fluid and electrolyte intake to patients at risk

4. *Key points*
   a. Immediate action is required if the

patient is experiencing intractable vomiting and diarrhea or fever
b. Left uncorrected, severe dehydration may lead to profound circulatory collapse and death
c. There is controversy about whether or not dehydration in the terminally ill is uncomfortable or requires extraordinary intervention such as IV fluids
d. Alters quality of life with corresponding weakness, lethargy, and altered mental status
5. Assessment
   a. Subjective data: Interview patient/caregiver to determine
      (1) Volume of diarrhea
      (2) Frequency and volume of emesis
      (3) Frequency of fever
      (4) Approximate fluid intake and urinary output for 24 hours
   b. Objective data
      (1) Physical signs of dehydration
         (a) Decreased skin turgor
         (b) Dry mucous membranes
         (c) Increased urine output
         (d) Increased heart rate
         (e) Weight loss
         (f) Elevated serum sodium
      (2) Presence of postural hypotension (a drop of 5–10 mm Hg either sitting or standing)
      (3) Mental status changes (lethargic, weak, confused, obtunded)
      (4) Laboratory data
         (a) Plasma sodium, potassium, BUN, creatinine
         (b) Urine sodium, urea, creatinine, osmolality
6. Interventions
   a. Maintain IV access and administer IV fluids as ordered, following principles of fluid rehydration
      (1) Replace volume with 0.9% saline if serum Na concentration is normal
      (2) Replace 2–3 L saline for moderate depletion
      (3) Correct electrolyte abnormalities as needed
   b. Encourage oral intake of at least 2–3 L fluid if tolerated, especially electrolyte-rich fluids

      (1) Sports drinks (e.g., Gatorade)
      (2) Oral rehydration salts mixed in water
      (3) A solution of 1 part oral rehydration salts and 1 part fruit nectar drink
   c. Monitor blood pressure, urine output, skin turgor, and weight to evaluate for fluid overload or congestive heart failure
   d. Monitor lab values
   e. Maintain skin integrity (see *Impaired/Risk for Impaired Skin Integrity,* p. 222)
   f. Evaluate safety needs, ability to meet ADL, need for supportive services

E. Diarrhea

1. Definition/Description
   a. An abnormal increase in daily stool weight (>300 g/24 hours) (Greenberger, 1986), stool liquidity, or stool frequency
   b. An estimated 50%–60% of AIDS patients experience diarrhea at some point in the course of their illness (Dworkin, Wormser, & Rosenthal, 1985)
   c. Alters quality of life significantly
   d. Immune deficiency renders all HIV-infected people at risk for developing diarrhea from food or water-borne pathogens or from OIs
2. Etiology
   a. OIs or malignancies
      (1) *Cryptosporidium, Microsporidium, I. belli*
      (2) Amebiasis, *Giardia*
      (3) *M. avium intracellulare* (MAC)
      (4) *Salmonella, Shigella, Campylobacter*
      (5) KS
   b. Other causes
      (1) Bacterial overgrowth such as *C. difficile* following antibiotic therapy
      (2) Villous atrophy due to malnutrition or repeated bowel infections
      (3) Contaminated nutrients (raw or undercooked meat, fish, poultry, or prolonged hang time of tube-feeding formula)
      (4) Low serum albumin level
      (5) Zinc deficiency or excess
      (6) Inadequate/absent digestive enzymes or bile salts (fat malabsorption)

(7) Lactose intolerance

(8) AIDS enteropathy

3. Goals of Care

  a. To identify treatable causative agents

  b. To control diarrhea with dietary changes and medications

  c. To prevent complications of diarrhea

4. *Key points*

  a. Large-volume watery diarrhea for a prolonged period requires a full workup for treatable causative agents

  b. The sequelae of untreated or failed treatment for diarrhea include

    (1) Dehydration, vascular collapse, death

    (2) Fluid and electrolyte imbalance

    (3) Progressive malnutrition

    (4) Skin breakdown

    (5) Safety concerns

    (6) Social isolation

    (7) Dependence in ADL

5. Assessment

  a. Subjective data

    (1) Pattern of diarrhea: Onset, duration, amount, frequency, appearance (e.g., foul-smelling/frothy stools usually suggest fat malabsorption)

    (2) Associated symptoms: Cramping, flatus, abdominal distention, tenesmus, blood in stool

    (3) Patient's ability to care for self

    (4) Nutritional intake, including food acquisition and preparation

    (5) Impact of diarrhea on lifestyle and quality of life

  b. Objective data

    (1) Signs of dehydration (see *Dehydration*, p. 204)

    (2) Compare patient's current weight with usual body weight

    (3) Alterations in tissue perfusion or significant loss of muscle mass

    (4) Skin integrity

6. Interventions

  a. Administer/maintain IV hydration, encourage oral rehydration

  b. Administer antimicrobials and monitor response

  c. Educate patient/caregiver regarding

    (1) Diagnostic workup

      (a) For proper stool-collection procedure, see *Cryptosporidiosis*, p. 122

      (b) See *Enterocolitis and Malabsorption*, p. 173

  (2) Dietary changes to alleviate diarrhea

    (a) High-protein, high-calorie foods that are low fat, lactose and caffeine free

    (b) Liquid nutrition supplements with medium chain triglycerides and predigested protein

    (c) Increased soluble fiber

    (d) Lactaid pills before ingesting dairy products (or substitute soy milk)

    (e) Consider pancreatic digestive enzymes or bile salts

    (f) Parenteral nutrition may be necessary for prolonged secretory diarrhea

  (3) Maximizing an antidiarrheal agent before deeming it a failure

    (a) Give antidiarrheals on a schedule rather than prn

    (b) Agents used to control diarrhea: Kaopectate, opioid preparations (tincture of opium, codeine, morphine), Lomotil, and octreotide acetate

  (4) Antimicrobial medications used to treat underlying cause: Schedule and side effects

  (5) Problems to report to primary care provider

  d. Maintain skin integrity

    (1) Offer sitz baths

    (2) Provide gentle perineal rinsing and drying with soft cloth or wipes after toileting

    (3) Apply fecal collecting appliance if stooling is watery, urgent, and patient unable to toilet

    (4) Use perineal hygiene cleansers and skin-protection products to maintain skin integrity

  e. Refer patient to a nutrition support service or registered dietitian

  f. Monitor response to dietary changes and pharmacologic interventions

  g. Counsel regarding hygiene products to protect clothing if fecal urgency is a problem

  h. See also *Anorectal Signs and Symptoms*, p. 201

F. Dysphagia/Odynophagia

1. Definition/Description
   a. Dysphagia: Difficulty transferring a solid or liquid bolus from the mouth to the stomach via the esophagus
      (1) The difficulty may occur at multiple levels
      (2) May be described as food "sticking" in the esophagus
   b. Odynophagia: Pain that occurs with swallowing
      (1) Pain, described as constricting or burning, can usually be differentiated from heartburn by the reflux of gastric acid into the stomach
      (2) The pain of odynophagia may be so intense that it leads to fear of food intake
   c. Prevalence of either symptom is unknown across the spectrum of HIV disease, but these symptoms are commonly reported by patients in clinical settings
2. Etiology
   a. Dysphagia
      (1) Usually a consequence of a neuromuscular disorder or an obstructing lesion of the pharynx or esophagus
      (2) Causative organisms/processes
         (a) *C. albicans*
         (b) Herpes simplex
         (c) *Cryptosporidium* (rare)
         (d) KS
         (e) Lymphoma
      (3) See *Gastrointestinal System Complications*, p. 169, for esophageal disorders
   b. Odynophagia
      (1) Usually associated with esophageal mucosal damage
      (2) Causative organisms: CMV, herpes simplex
      (3) Secondary to chemotherapy-induced mucositis
      (4) See also *Gastrointestinal System Complications*
3. Goals of Care
   a. To provide/advocate for aggressive symptomatic management while the underlying cause is being identified and treatment initiated
   b. To maintain nutritional homeostasis, particularly during the acute phase but also until resumption of adequate oral nutritional intake
4. *Key points*
   a. Immediate action is required if the patient cannot swallow own saliva
   b. Left untreated, severe odynophagia will lead to malnutrition with subsequent poor response to medical therapies and prolonged recovery time
   c. Although uncommon, complications of OIs of the esophagus include
      (1) Upper GI bleeding (from *Candida* esophagitis)
      (2) Esophageal perforation (from CMV)
      (3) Esophageal stricture (from chronic inflammation due to *Candida*, herpes simplex virus, CMV)
      (4) Dissemination of viral or fungal infections
   d. Patients complaining of dysphagia and with visible evidence of thrush (oral candidiasis) are often presumed to have esophageal candidiasis; they are initially treated empirically while awaiting further diagnostic workup
5. Assessment
   a. Subjective data
      (1) Differentiate between pain with swallowing or the sensation of food "sticking" at a certain point in the esophagus
      (2) Severity, location, and other descriptors of the discomfort
      (3) Food and fluid intake
      (4) Associated signs and symptoms (e.g., fever, fatigue, weight loss)
      (5) History of CMV disease, prior thrush
      (6) Adherence to or compliance with therapy
   b. Objective data: Visually inspect the tongue, pharynx, palate, gingiva, buccal surfaces for
      (1) Oral candidiasis
      (2) Thrush or ulcerative lesions
      (3) Oral hygiene status
6. Interventions
   a. Administer prescribed therapies; monitor response and adverse

reactions (see *Candidiasis*, p. 171, *Cytomegalovirus*, p. 94, *Herpes Simplex Virus*, p. 96, and *Gastrointestinal System Complications*, p. 169, for esophageal disorders)

b. Educate patient/family/significant other regarding
   (1) Diagnostic procedures planned
       (a) Prep required (e.g., npo, preprocedure medications given, IV access)
       (b) Specific sensory information about the procedure itself, if known
       (c) Postprocedure instructions if going home following conscious sedation
       (d) Pain management plan
   (2) Oral and dental hygiene
       (a) Brush teeth 3x/day before meals
       (b) Floss at bedtime
       (c) See dentist q6mos unless otherwise indicated
       (d) Routinely check mouth for thrush or other lesions; report new symptoms to primary care provider
   (3) Medication administration techniques (po, topical, IV); scheduling of medications; side effects to report to primary care provider; possibility of need for life-long maintenance therapy to prevent recurrence
   (4) Nutritional interventions for specific dysphagia symptoms (Task Force on Nutrition Support in AIDS, 1989)
       (a) Serve foods cold or at room temperature
       (b) Small amounts of fluid with meals eases swallowing
       (c) Offer foods of a uniform consistency to form a cohesive bolus
       (d) Avoid thin liquids (water, juice) and slippery foods (Jell-O, bologna) if aspiration is a concern, and foods that stick to the palate (peanut butter)
       (e) Encourage liquid nutrition supplements between meals
c. Consult with primary care provider regarding the need for

(1) Speech pathologist or ENT specialist to determine best food consistency or to retrain the patient how to swallow
(2) Nutritional support services for enteral or parenteral feedings
(3) Intermittent or continuous nasogastric or nasointestinal tube feeding
(4) Peripheral parenteral nutrition (PPN) as a short-term bridge until the patient can eat again

d. Refer to a registered dietitian
e. See also *Pain*, p. 229, *Stomatitis*, p. 238
f. Evaluate comfort level, ability to take prescribed therapies, and nutritional intake; modify plan as indicated

G. Dyspnea

1. Definition/Description
   a. Difficult, labored, uncomfortable breathing
      (1) Subjective phenomenon; involves both the patient's perception of and reaction to the sensation
      (2) Distressing symptom to both patient and family
   b. Frequently accompanies a number of cardiopulmonary and neuromuscular diseases
   c. Prevalence in HIV disease not well-documented; however, Chang et al. (1993) found dyspnea or cough accounted for 34% of the presenting complaints of HIV patients seeking care at an emergency department
2. Etiology
   a. Pulmonary infections/causative agents
      (1) PCP
      (2) Bacterial pneumonias (e.g., *Pneumococcus, H. influenzae, P. aeruginosa*)
      (3) MAC
      (4) *M. tuberculosis*
      (5) *H. capsulatum*
      (6) *C. neoformans*
      (7) *C. immitis*
      (8) CMV
      (9) *C. albicans*
      (10) *Cryptosporidium*
   b. Pulmonary malignancies: KS, lymphomas

c. Autoimmune diseases of HIV: lymphocytic interstitial pneumonitis, diffuse infiltrative lymphocytosis syndrome

d. Anemia

e. Pneumothorax, pleural effusion

f. Dying process

3. Goals of Care

a. To identify and eliminate, or at least control, the causative factors

b. To develop strategies to manage dyspnea to provide maximum independence

4. *Key points*

a. Dyspnea is an important cause of functional impairment and disability that adversely affects quality of life

b. Dyspnea is a symptom of pulmonary insufficiency that may progress to respiratory failure if action is not taken

c. Dyspnea is a subjective sensation that may not always correspond to physiologic parameters; a person may report severe dyspnea while ABGs indicate moderate hypoxemia

5. Assessment

a. Subjective data

(1) Patient's report of breathing difficulty

(2) Types of patient-rating tools

(a) Graphic rating scale: Ask patient to quantify the magnitude of dyspnea experienced on a scale of 1–5 (1 = no difficulty breathing, 5 = severe difficulty)

(b) Visual analog scale (Gift, 1989): Horizontal or vertical line with word descriptors or anchors at either end (patient places a mark on the line indicating the degree of dyspnea experienced)

(3) Ascertain relevant history of the symptom: Onset, duration, frequency of episodes, aggravating/relieving factors

b. Objective data

(1) General appearance and color

(2) Pulmonary exam: Rate, amplitude of respiration, rhythm, symmetry of breathing, use of accessory muscles, breath sounds

(3) Lab and diagnostic data: ABGs, chest x-ray

6. Interventions

a. Reassess respiratory status at appropriate frequency, including before and after respiratory treatments

b. Eliminate/modify underlying causes of dyspnea

c. Administer pharmacologic agents (e.g., oxygen, antibiotics, corticosteroids) and opioids (e.g., morphine) for palliation; evaluate effectiveness and monitor for side effects

d. Assess need for bronchial hygiene (e.g., aerosol treatments, postural drainage, percussion, suctioning)

e. Encourage adequate fluid intake to maintain hydration and help thin secretions, unless contraindicated

f. Position patient to maximize both comfort and ventilation (e.g., sitting upright with pillows under elbows, leaning on overbed table)

g. Pace activities and treatments to level of tolerance; encourage energy conservation

h. Assist with ADL, especially those that require use of the upper extremities (e.g., feeding, shaving); keep frequently used items within reach

i. Instruct to prolong exhalation phase of breathing using pursed-lip and diaphragmatic breathing techniques

j. Demonstrate relaxation/panic control strategies (e.g., visual imagery, meditation)

k. Counsel to avoid exposure to irritants such as cigarette smoke, flowers, perfume

l. Evaluate patient's ability to

(1) Participate in self-care activities such as energy conservation/pacing activities, correctly using metered dose inhalers or other medications

(2) Report changes in frequency/severity of dyspnea

(3) Identify contributing factors related to dyspnea

H. Fatigue

1. Definition/Description

a. A feeling of sustained tiredness, weariness, or exhaustion that may affect functional ability and quality of life

b. May occur at any point along the HIV spectrum; usually worsens as disease progresses

c. Chronic fatigue is considered a constitutional symptom of HIV infection

d. Persistent fatigue may increase both the physical and psychologic burden of being HIV positive

e. Although the exact prevalence is unknown, fatigue is a frequent symptom reported by many persons living with AIDS

2. Etiology

a. Multifactorial etiologies

(1) Increased resting energy requirements that can occur early in HIV infection (Schambelan & Grunfeld, 1995)

(2) Physiologic, psychologic, or pharmacologic factors acting alone or in conjunction with one another

b. Commonly associated factors

(1) Malnutrition

(2) Circulatory problems due to anemia or cardiac disease

(3) Respiratory problems due to infections or malignancies

(4) Fever

(5) Psychologic stress

(6) Excessive activity or an activity level exceeding the person's functional capacity

(7) Prolonged immobility

(8) Medication side effects

(9) Sleep disturbances

(10) Depression

3. Goals of Care

a. To identify contributing factors to fatigue

b. To maintain a safe physical and psychologic environment

c. To maintain or regain optimal functional ability

4. *Key points*

a. Fatigue causes both physical and psychologic stress; stress is known to decrease immune function (Calabrese, Kling, & Gold, 1987)

b. The many etiologies of fatigue complicate identification of appropriate nursing care; it is important to identify the

cause of fatigue (e.g., PCP) in order to intervene correctly

c. Fatigue may be so severe that it interferes with the person's ability to meet ADL, necessitating immediate intervention

d. Because fatigue impairs functional ability and potentially impairs quality of life, depression may also be present and relationships with significant others may be affected

5. Assessment

a. Subjective data

(1) Verbal and nonverbal indicators

(2) Changes in subjective expressions of fatigue

(3) Times of peak energy and exhaustion

(4) Extent

(a) Is the person fatigued at rest, after minimal or moderate activity?

(b) Are there daily changes in the level of activity?

(5) Psychologic consequences: Effects on relationships, socialization, mood

(6) Adequacy of sleep pattern

(7) Recreational drug use

(8) Nutritional intake

b. Objective data

(1) Vital signs

(2) Motor strength, endurance

(3) Pulmonary assessment

(4) Cardiac assessment

(5) Laboratory data, especially Hgb, Hct, electrolytes

6. Interventions

a. Evaluate responses to medical therapies

b. Monitor physiologic state, evolving signs or symptoms of an infection

c. Evaluate the safety of the person who is living alone or with insufficient help at home

d. Counsel about

(1) The importance of well-balanced, nutrient-dense diet (see *Dehydration,* p. 204, *Nutritional Deficit: Weight Loss, Anorexia,* p. 227)

(2) New onset fatigue or change in pattern may be associated with an undiagnosed OI and should be reported to primary care provider

(3) The importance of controlling other symptoms that may contribute to fatigue (e.g., *Diarrhea*, p. 205, *Fever and Night Sweats* (in the right column), *Pain*, p. 229)

(4) Fatigue may be side effect of some medications (e.g., tricyclic antidepressant, colony stimulating factors); assess need to balance this side effect with intended purpose of the medication

(5) Reorganizing activity/rest schedule and prioritizing activities to coincide with peak energy times and personal goals

(6) Benefits of a regular conditioning exercise program with aerobic component as tolerated

(7) Not using alcohol, recreational drugs (e.g., speed), or caffeine to counteract symptom

e. Provide opportunity for the patient to describe the impact of this symptom on his/her life
(1) Refer to peer support person or group counseling if patient agrees (see *Social Support*, p. 272)
(2) Discuss with primary care provider need for mental health referral if there is evidence of depression

f. Refer to community-based agencies to provide homemaking and chore support

g. In case of suspected medication side effect, consult with primary care provider or pharmacist for possible changes in scheduling or therapy changes if fatigue is not self-limiting

h. Discuss with patient experimental interventions or complimentary therapies (e.g., hyperbaric oxygen) the patient is using to manage this symptom (Reillo, 1993)

i. Evaluate need for referrals to
(1) Occupational therapy for energy conservation techniques
(2) Physical therapy for reconditioning and strengthening exercises
(3) Nutritionist for diet counseling and nutritional evaluation

j. See also *Impaired Mobility*, p. 221

I.   Fever and Night Sweats

1. Definition/Description
   a. Fever
   (1) Abnormally high body temperature that occurs in response to pyrogens; during fever, thermoregulatory function remains intact but thermostatic centers of the hypothalamus are readjusted to maintain temperature at a higher level by compensatory warming responses
   (2) One of the most common responses associated with HIV/AIDS
   (3) Fever heralds many of the OIs that accompany HIV infection
   (4) Febrile episodes may be noninfectious in origin
   (5) Elevation of body temperature during fever is symptomatic of the antigenic response and *not itself an illness*
   b. Hyperthermia: Also refers to abnormally high body temperature, but differs from fever in its dysfunction of normal cooling mechanisms
   (1) Loss of thermoregulatory ability allows temperature to rise to lethal levels
   (2) Hyperthermic patients require active cooling interventions to prevent irreversible brain damage
   c. Night sweats: A nonspecific term that refers to heavy sweating during sleep
   (1) Commonly associated with mycobacterial infections
   (2) Also occur in noninfectious conditions (e.g., anxiety, estrogen deficiency, endocrine disorders, tumors, cardiac dysrhythmias) and in apparently healthy people without fever
   d. Pyrogens: Biochemical messengers that readjust the hypothalamic thermostat to a higher range
   (1) Exogenous pyrogens (e.g., microorganisms) come from outside the body; do not act directly on the hypothalamic thermostat but trigger the release of fever mediators from cells within the body
   (2) Endogenous pyrogens (EP)
   (a) Produced within the body by

monocytes and macrophages
- (b) Mediate fever by increasing synthesis of hypothalamic prostaglandins of the E group (PGE), which adjust the thermostatic set point to a higher level
- e. Cytokines: Antigen-nonspecific glycoproteins that are rapidly synthesized in response to a stimulus
    - (1) Act as intercellular messengers to recruit a variety of host defenses
    - (2) Include interleukins, colony stimulating factors, interferon, transforming growth factor, tumor necrosis factor (TNF)
    - (3) Interleukins (IL-1 through IL-12) are cytokines that communicate between leukocytes
        - (a) This family of closely related molecules has been shown to be the fever-mediating factor (also known as EP)
        - (b) Interactions between IL-1, IL-6, and TNF are particularly known to heighten febrile responses of people infected with HIV
- f. Dynamics of thermoregulation during normal and febrile conditions
    - (1) Thermal balance: Humans normally maintain a fairly constant internal body temperature within a narrow limit called the *set point* (range ± 36.2°–37.8°C)
    - (2) Dynamic interplay between neurologic, biochemical, and behavioral processes helps to maintain thermal balance
        - (a) The preoptic hypothalamic region functions as a thermostat, although sensory information received from the viscera, muscle, and skin receptors is integrated with that from the brain
        - (b) Cooling of skin receptors can override stimuli from other sites
        - (c) Deviations, above or below the acceptable set-point range, trigger cooling or warming responses to restore thermal balance
    - (3) Skin temperature is both *influenced*

by and *responsible for* autonomic thermoregulatory responses
- (a) Efforts to cool the skin cause warming by triggering shivering and vasoconstriction
- (b) Interventions that promote vasodilation or vasoconstriction of cutaneous vessels can therefore facilitate or inhibit loss of body heat
- g. The febrile response
    - (1) Fever is an adaptive host response in the immunocompetent person
    - (2) Fever is a catabolic state that is maladaptive for the chronically ill with wasting, dehydration, anemia
    - (3) Acute phase responses
        - (a) In the immunocompetent, phagocytic cells migrate and release cytokines that recruit a variety of host defenses
        - (b) When T-cell and host immune functions are impaired by HIV infection, fever and inflammatory responses occur but without many of the other host effects
        - (c) TNF (also called *cachectin*), IL-1, and IL-6 promote catabolic wasting and suppress appetite
    - (4) Thermal consequences of fever refer to the increase in body heat
        - (a) PGE activates the hypothalamic thermostat to adjust the thermostatic set point to a higher level (see Figure 5.1)
        - (b) Body-warming mechanisms respond to neuroregulatory control in order to raise core temperature to the higher set-point level
            - i) Muscular friction of shivering and heightened cellular metabolism generates heat
            - ii) Vasoconstriction conserves heat by shunting circulation away from body surface
    - (5) Mild temperature elevations up to 39°C appear to have few detrimental effects
    - (6) Some immunoregulatory functions are enhanced by mild temperature

Figure 5.1   Febrile Episode

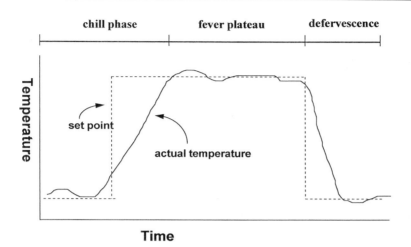

Hypothalamic set point responds to elevations in endogenous pyrogens by resetting at a higher level. Sensed discrepancies between existing and set point temperature levels elicit *chill phase*. Compensatory warming responses cause body temperatures to rise to higher levels in *plateau phase*. When endogenous pyrogen levels decline, set point readjusts to euthermic range. Compensatory cooling mechanisms promote heat loss during *defervescence phase* and return body temperatures to normal.

elevations up to 39°C, although this has not been documented in HIV infection; elevating body temperature to the febrile range has both positive and negative physiologic effects
   (a) Activates antiviral, antitumor, and antibacterial biochemicals
   (b) Reduces plasma iron, needed by many bacteria
   (c) Increases sweating and respiratory water loss, which promotes dehydration
(7) Fever runs a dynamic course with 3 distinct phases (see Figure 5.1)
   (a) Chill: Onset of the febrile episode evokes shivering, vasoconstriction, subjective feelings of cold, and rapid production of heat until core temperatures rise to the higher set-point range
   (b) Plateau: Once the higher set point is reached, core temperatures remain steady and warming defenses subside

   (c) Defervescence: The *crisis, flush,* or *break* in fever, caused by the falling EP level, allows set point to be lowered
     i) High core temperature evokes cooling responses
     ii) Subjectively, the person feels too hot
h. Metabolic costs of fever in HIV and AIDS
   (1) Fever increases metabolic rate and protein degradation
   (2) A recent study of people with HIV infection showed that current methods for calculating energy expenditure fail to fully estimate metabolic need (Anderson, Grady, & Ropka, 1994)
   (3) Fever imposes an added metabolic burden on patients who are anemic, dehydrated, and have poor nutritional intake
     (a) Cellular metabolism and oxygen consumption increase ± 10% with every added 1°C

(b) Shivering during febrile chills raises metabolic rate and oxygen consumption 3–5 times resting values

(c) Exertion of febrile shivering causes respiratory rate, heart rate, and blood pressure to increase to meet oxygen demands

(d) Catabolic effects of fever-producing biochemicals may actually hasten disease progression in AIDS by inducing anorexia, wasting, and dehydration

(4) During fever, less heat loss is required to elicit shivering and vasoconstriction, making the patient vulnerable to chilling even during plateau and defervescence phases

i. Dehydration is often both the cause and effect of fever

(1) The hydration status of the person with HIV infection may already be compromised by diarrhea or limited fluid intake

(2) Diaphoresis during fever causes both water and sodium loss

(3) The hypothalamic thermoregulatory center responds to sodium excess or water loss by elevating body temperature

2. Etiology

a. Pyrogens: infectious organisms, toxic drugs, chemical compounds, blood products, neoplastic cells, foreign bodies

b. Secondary to desiccation (water and sodium loss) and dehydration (pure water loss) related to diaphoresis, vomiting, diarrhea

c. Rarely the result of HIV infection alone

d. Commonly identified causes of fever in HIV disease: Respiratory, central nervous system, and urinary tract infections; abscesses, gingivitis, gastroenteritis, drug reactions, lymphoma

e. Drugs known to induce fever (Lee, 1995): TMP-SMX, atovaquone, amphotericin B (chills or rigors are secondary to fever), ddI, amoxicillin-clavulanic acid, dapsone, ceftazidine, ganciclovir

3. Goals of Care

a. To monitor the patient's response to these signs and their treatment

b. To promote comfort and adequate hydration

c. To prevent febrile shivering or aggressive chilling

4. *Key points*

a. Temperatures >40°C (104°F) carry risk of irreversible neural damage and loss of thermoregulatory function

b. In AIDS, the immunologic benefits of the febrile host response appear to be outweighed by negative catabolic effects

c. Patterns of fever or night sweats provide relatively few cues for diagnosis in PWAs

d. Tepid sponge baths, cooling fans, and alcohol baths are contraindicated because they promote shivering, energy expenditure, and patient discomfort; may actually raise body temperature

e. Aggressive cooling by ice packs or cooling blankets without supportive measures may promote febrile shivering, energy expenditure, and patient discomfort

f. Oral thermometers vary in accuracy by type, brand, and user technique; readings can also be influenced by smoking, talking, eating, or drinking hot or cold food and liquids, and by mouth breathing

(1) Digital thermometers have numbers that are easy to read and require only a few seconds to register; reliable manufacturers will guarantee level of instrument accuracy

(2) Sliding vs. simple placement of electronic thermometers under tongue can create significant difference in readings

(3) Mercury thermometers pose hazard for breakage that can harm the patient, are difficult to read, and require 3–7 min to register; accuracy varies with manufacturer and shelf life

g. Temperature indicator dots or stick-on strips are notoriously inaccurate and do not adhere well to skin of sweating febrile patient

h. Temperature varies widely between and within body regions, tissues, and organs; is higher in well perfused areas
   (1) If surface cooling and hypothermia are induced, skin and superficial tissues become poorly perfused
   (2) Changes in tissue perfusion during fever and cooling procedures widen existing discrepancies between rectal and central temperatures
   (3) Rectal temperatures tend to lag behind brain temperatures in dynamic thermal states (e.g., hypothermia, rapidly rising fever)
i. Choice of temperature site is important during dynamic hemodynamic changes associated with fever
   (1) The brain is the organ most at risk from elevated temperature, so monitoring sites that closely reflect brain temperature is ideal
   (2) Temperature measured from well-perfused sites near the brain more accurately reflect brain temperature
   (3) Oral thermometers, held sublingually with lips closed, reflect an offset of 0.5°C (1°F) lower than core temperatures but will effectively track fever with brain temperatures in conscious febrile patients
   (4) The tympanic membrane (TM) shares a portion of the same blood supply as the brain so that TM temperatures are close to those of the brain
   (5) TM thermometers vary in accuracy by type, brand, and user technique (use requires otoscopic technique)
       (a) Hand-held TM thermometers register temperatures in a few seconds
       (b) Indwelling TM thermistor ear-canal probes are generally bothersome to the conscious febrile patient
j. Antipyretic pharmacologic therapies
   (1) NSAIDs (e.g., aspirin, acetaminophen, indomethacin) are used for their antipyretic effects (promote heat loss, reduce temperature)
   (2) Precise sites of action are not known,

but salicylates appear to affect the regions of the brain where pyrogens influence neuronal function
   (3) Aspirin, indomethacin, and acetaminophen have no effect on EP production or activity, nor do they inhibit activity of preformed pyrogen, PGE
   (4) Evidence from research (Steffe et al., 1990) indicates that reducing fever with nonsteroidal antipyretics does not inhibit immune responses such as IL-1 synthesis, hepatic protein production, leucocytosis, or neutrophil lysozyme release
   (5) Decisions to restrict use of NSAIDs are more likely to be justified by their negative side effects than by any adverse effects on host defenses
   (6) Aspirin and acetaminophen have about the same antipyretic activity, but only aspirin offers analgesic effects to reduce fever-related discomfort
5. Assessment
   a. Body temperature
      (1) Body temperature and corresponding physiologic responses change rapidly during acute febrile illness
      (2) Routine methods with oral thermometers and twice daily intervals between temperature measurements are satisfactory for screening hospitalized patients without indications of fever
      (3) More frequent (e.g., q4h) measurement is needed with evidence of infection, tissue injury, inflammation; for patients receiving potentially pyrogenic agents such as blood; or if beginning treatment with antigenic drugs such as amphotericin B
   b. Hydration status
      (1) Suspect body water loss with sudden weight loss
      (2) Febrile patients are at risk for desiccation (isotonic dehydration) when both water and sodium are lost in profuse sweating
      (3) Dehydration (hypertonic dehydration) also occurs when only pure

water is lost from the airway or from renal dysfunction

   (a) Sodium excess normally leads to polyuria as kidneys respond to eliminate this electrolyte

   (b) Loss of water from polyuria and febrile sweating eventually leads to extracellular fluid volume deficit and hypovolemia

(4) Sensible water loss is seen in profuse sweating and the obligatory increase in urine output to eliminate metabolic wastes from fever catabolism

(5) Fever also increases insensible water loss from the airway and nonsweating sources by 10% for each 0.5°C increase in temperature

(6) Profound fluid loss leads to hypovolemia

   (a) Subjective symptoms of hypovolemia

      i) Weakness

      ii) Disorientation

      iii) Thirst (patients with sodium excess show a more severe thirst)

   (b) Objective physical signs of hypovolemia

      i) Rapid weight loss

      ii) Dry skin

      iii) "Sticky" mucous membranes

      iv) Loss of skin elasticity and turgor causing doughy texture (more pronounced when fluids and electrolytes are lost in isotonic proportions)

      v) Oliguria or anuria

      vi) Urinary specific gravity above 1.030

      vii) Slightly elevated hematocrit

      viii) Elevated serum sodium concentration

      ix) Lethargy; changes in personality and levels of consciousness

(7) Restoring fluids lost from sweating and the hypermetabolic state increases blood volume, restabilizes circulation to skin, and allows heat loss from the body surface

(8) Nonsteroidal antipyretics are used more often to promote comfort than to reduce body temperature

   (a) Antipyretics alone may be as effective as more aggressive means for patients not in imminent risk of hyperthermia

   (b) Where not contraindicated, antipyretics can be administered regularly around the clock rather than prn to people with chronic or frequent fevers to improve patient comfort

6. Interventions

  a. Manage temperature elevations

    (1) Administer pharmacologic therapies as ordered and monitor patient's response

    (2) Antipyretics may reduce restlessness and irritability caused by fever

  b. Implement supportive measures during aggressive cooling

    (1) If core temperatures continue to climb above levels of 40°C (104°F), thermoregulation may be deranged and therapeutic cooling measures are justifiable to prevent irreversible neurologic cellular damage

    (2) Cooling blanket: Rubberized hypothermia blankets, equipped with a motor that refrigerates and circulates a liquid coolant, promote conductive heat loss from the skin

      (a) Before applying the blanket, insulate extremities by wrapping with 3 layers of dry toweling (helps prevent shivering by reducing stimulus from nerve endings in skin of hands and feet, which are extremely sensitive to heat loss)

      (b) Know that diminished circulation to skin increases danger of skin breakdown or freeze burns

        i) Protect fingers, toes, and genitalia with gauze, towels, or other wraps

        ii) Place a sheet between the patient and the cooling blanket

(c) Conduct heat away from the body in the least abrupt manner possible to avoid shivering; lower temperature settings on the cooling blanket gradually so that body temperature is lowered no more rapidly than 0.5°C over 30 min

(d) Setting the temperatures of hypothermia blankets at 23.9°C will allow a smoother drop in body temperature, avoiding drift and eliciting fewer warming defenses

(e) Monitor core temperature continually during aggressive cooling to avoid hypothermia; turn off the cooling blanket when body temperature approaches desired level (within 0.5°C)

(f) If core temperature inadvertently falls to about 31°C, check for neurologic signs (confusion, stupor, exaggerated tendon reflex, hyperactivity); protect patient from injuring self; watch closely while stabilizing temperature with blanket controls

(g) Monitor blood pressure, heart rate for signs of hemodynamic instability that accompanies temperature drifts

(h) Premature ventricular beats can occur throughout cooling; if brain temperature drops below 28°C, be alert for atrial fibrillation and other dysrhythmias

c. Restore hydration
  (1) Do not give cold liquids to a febrile patient
    (a) Rapid ingestion can abruptly cool the body core at a time when the elevated set point is highly sensitive to cooling
    (b) Even when the febrile patient is no longer in the chill phase and feels hot, avoid cold drinks because the threshold for shivering is lowered
    (c) Frozen juice or flavored Popsicle sticks can be sucked or licked slowly and ingested gradually
    (d) Tepid or warm liquids can be tolerated in larger volumes than chilled ones
  (2) Semi- or jelled liquids may be tolerated and easier to swallow; encourage slow intake of Jell-O or other chilled foods
  (3) Maintain IV access and administer IV hydration fluids as ordered
  (4) Monitor electrolytes, intake and output, and orthostatic vital signs to evaluate patient's response to hydration efforts

d. Teach patient/caregiver how to manage ongoing fever
  (1) Use and read a thermometer in order to assess febrile episodes that occur at home
  (2) Encourage use of a fever diary to measure and write down temperature measurements when feeling ill, having night sweats, or losing fluids by diarrhea or vomiting
  (3) Talk through interventions in order to teach the principles of chill avoidance and shivering prevention
  (4) Provide a list of fluid alternatives and strategies for improving intake to encourage rehydration during fever

e. Monitor safety status (patient may become delirious with elevated fever)

J. Hearing Loss

1. Definition/Description: There are two types of hearing loss
  a. Conductive hearing loss: Caused by a defect in the middle or external ear
  b. Sensorineural hearing loss (SNHL): Results from inner ear or acoustic nerve (cranial nerve VIII) damage; occurs in 21%–49% of HIV-infected patients (Tami & Lee, 1994)
2. Etiology
  a. Disease related
    (1) Primary infection by HIV in either the CNS or peripheral auditory nerve
    (2) Infections affecting the external ear

(a) Otitis externa

(b) Pinna cellulitis

(c) Infections resulting in aural polyps (*P. carinii, M. tuberculosis*)

(3) Infections affecting the middle or outer ear

(a) Otitis media (acute otitis media [AOM], otitis media with effusion [OME])

(b) Acute bacterial mastoiditis

(c) Coalescing suppurative mastoiditis

(4) Infections affecting CNS and acoustic nerve

(a) CNS toxoplasmosis

(b) Cryptococcal meningitis

(c) Tuberculous meningitis

(d) Neurosyphilis

(5) Infections causing inflammation of the tympanic membrane (myringitis)

(6) Cancers: CNS lymphoma (affects CNS and acoustic nerve), KS (extends into tympanic membrane or middle ear)

b. Treatment related: Effects of ototoxic drugs (streptomycin, amikacin, vancomycin, gentamicin, azidothymidine, neurotoxic chemotherapeutic agents [e.g., vincristine], furosemide)

c. Lifestyle related: Impacted cerumen, chronic exposure to loud noises

d. Trauma related: Tympanic membrane perforation

3. Goals of Care

a. To prevent or detect early treatment-related hearing loss

b. To enhance patient adaptation to hearing loss

4. *Key points*

a. Conductive hearing loss, caused most frequently by infections of the middle and outer ear, will resolve with treatment

b. SNHL from ototoxic medications, neurologic infections, or cancers usually persists

(1) Degree of hearing loss is related to the extent of damage to the acoustic nerve

(2) Early detection and treatment of the cause of SNHL is vital to prevent further damage and total hearing loss

c. Potential sequelae of progressive hearing loss: vertigo, sensory loss, perceptual changes, altered communication, impaired safety, depression, social isolation, altered body image, learning difficulties in children

d. Persistent or recurrent pain or fever in the patient with AOM signals the need for either surgical drainage or a change in antimicrobial agent

5. Assessment

a. Subjective data

(1) Review of previous diseases, OIs, therapies affecting the ear

(2) Patterns of hearing loss—degree of loss, unilateral, bilateral

(3) Perceived significance of hearing loss to patient/significant other

(4) Impact on lifestyle, comfort, ADL

(5) Associated signs and symptoms (e.g., tinnitus, vertigo, speech impairment with early childhood onset)

(6) Use of any assistive devices to compensate (e.g., amplifier, hearing aid, TTY)

(7) Communication methods and efficacy

(8) Subjective reports of changes of hearing patterns

(9) Signs and symptoms of underlying infections, including CNS involvement

b. Objective data

(1) Ability to hear normal sounds

(a) Have patient cover one ear

(b) Hold a ticking watch or rub fingers together a few inches from other ear or stand about 2 ft behind and whisper a 2-digit number

(c) Repeat with other ear

(2) Complete neurologic exam, including sensory, motor, cognitive functions

6. Interventions

a. Communicate directly with patient rather than through family members

(2) Xerosis generalisata (generalized dry skin syndrome): Affects 30% of HIV-infected patients

(3) Seborrheic dermatitis: Affects hairy areas of the face, scalp, chest, back, and groin (40%–80% incidence)

(4) Psoriasis

(5) Ichthyosis

(6) Papular urticaria

e. Cutaneous bacterial infections

(1) *S. aureus* most common cause in HIV-infected patients; usually presents as folliculitis with or without pruritus on the trunk, groin, or face

(2) Less common presentations

(a) Bullous impetigo: Most common in hot, humid weather; usually found as superficial blisters or erosions in skinfold areas

i) Yellow crusting commonly occurs on open blisters

ii) Skin abscesses often occur as a result of subcutaneous drug injection

(b) Impetigo

(c) Ecthyma (ulcer)

(d) Cellulitis

f. Herpesvirus infections

(1) Oral, genital, or perirectal HSV infections common at all stages of HIV infection

(a) Reactivations are severe, prolonged, and refractory to medical treatment often causing erosions 10 cm in diameter in severely immunosuppressed patients

(b) Seen in 22% of AIDS patients (Goodman, Teplitz, & Wishner, 1987)

(2) Varicella zoster virus (shingles)

(a) May be seen before the onset of other HIV-related infections

(b) Causes dermatomal eruptions, which may be bullous, hemorrhagic, necrotic, and painful

(c) Healing time varies from 2–6 weeks depending on level of necrosis

g. Fungal and yeast infections

(1) Affect the skin most frequently in intertriginous (axilla, groin, scrotum) and inframammary areas; also may affect feet, nails, and scalp

(2) *Candida* lesions present as erythematous erosions in the depths of the skinfolds, sometimes with a white membrane covering the eroded surface

(3) Mildly burning pain and pruritus are common

(4) *Tinea* skin infections are pruritic and tend to occur most frequently in the groin and upper thighs

h. Kaposi's sarcoma

3. Goals of Care

a. To provide symptomatic and emotional relief

b. To remove exacerbating factors

c. To reduce risk of infection due to breaks in skin integrity

d. To promote healing and reduce recurrences of ulcerative lesions

4. *Key points*

a. Virtually 100% of HIV-infected patients will manifest some form of skin disorder over the course of their disease (Berger, 1990)

b. The risk of developing an alteration in skin integrity increases with disease progression; most skin disorders occur when CD4+ lymphocyte counts fall below 150/μl (Sadick, McNutt, & Kaplan, 1990).

c. Patients receiving sulfa drugs or anticonvulsants are at risk of developing severe hypersensitivity reactions (e.g., erythema multiforme, Stevens-Johnson syndrome, toxic epidermal necrolysis) that require urgent medical intervention

d. Institute appropriate infection-control procedures for institutionalized patients with Norwegian scabies, a potential source of hospital and hospice epidemics

e. Healing of ulcers in end-stage AIDS or in fungating KS lesions may not be a realistic goal

f. Skin ulcers are of concern because of the potential risk they pose to the HIV-infected patient for the development of life-threatening bacterial infections

g. Infectious skin disorders (caused by viruses, fungi, yeast, bacteria) predispose for the development of erosions and ulcers

h. Povidone-iodine and hydrogen peroxide inhibit epithelialization; used only on necrotic or dirty wounds where cleansing and debridement, not healing, are the immediate goals

5. Assessment
   a. Subjective data
      (1) History of hypersensitivity or exposure to drugs, food, insect bites, sun
      (2) History of symptoms
         (a) Dates of onset and progression of rash
         (b) Temporal relationships to changes in medication therapy
         (c) Associated symptoms (fever, pain, pruritus, relieving/aggravating factors)
      (3) Patient and caregiver's knowledge of skin care
      (4) Patient's lifestyle and living environment
   b. Objective data
      (1) Appearance/distribution of rash on face, trunk, groin, extremities, and within skinfold areas
      (2) Breaks in skin integrity
      (3) Cellulitis/exudates
      (4) Usual patterns of skin care (e.g., frequent bathing with deodorant soaps can be a precipitating factor)

6. Interventions
   a. Maintain hygiene without producing dry skin
      (1) Avoid deodorant (astringent) soaps
      (2) Use a supersaturated fatty acid soap for cleansing (e.g., Basis, Emulave, Dove)
      (3) Use tepid water to reduce risk of stimulating inflammatory reaction
      (4) Pat skin dry with towel without rubbing
      (5) Apply moisturizing cream after bathing and at bedtime
      (6) Avoid frequent or long showers or tub baths
      (7) Change position at least q2h
   b. Maintain environmental humidification

c. Promote comfort and prevent injury
   (1) Discourage scratching; explain scratch–itch cycle
   (2) Keep nails short and smooth to prevent injury
   (3) Keep bed unwrinkled and free of crumbs
   (4) Use old, soft sheets
   (5) Avoid overdressing and direct contact with sheepskins, foam pads, or other bed protectors that can promote diaphoresis or excessive skin warmth

d. Prevent development of secondary infection: If open lesions are present, avoid tub baths, use separate cloth to wash affected areas

e. For generalized pruritus
   (1) Emollient baths or compresses with Aveeno, baking soda, or a 50% solution of regular liquid starch and water
   (2) Allow emollient to air dry on skin (emollients are thought to keep moisture in skin)
   (3) Apply topical steroids after compresses/bath, if prescribed
   (4) Offer/educate on use of antipruritics (e.g., hydroxyzine, doxepin, astemizole, terfenadine), if prescribed

f. For seborrheic dermatitis
   (1) Scalp lesions
      (a) Regular use of dandruff shampoos (e.g., Selsun Blue, Head and Shoulders, Sebulex)
      (b) Nizoral shampoo effective but expensive
      (c) Topical steroid lotions
   (2) Face, trunk, and groin lesions: topical antifungal (ketoconazole, clotrimazole) and steroid creams

g. For biting insects
   (1) Block reaction to bite with antihistamines
   (2) Treat scabies in advanced AIDS patients with permethrin (Elimite) applications for 12 hours weekly for several weeks (Berger, 1995)

h. For photosensitivity reactions
   (1) Promote sun protection, sunscreens that block UVA and UVB

(2) Discontinue sensitizing medications
i. For herpesvirus infections
  (1) Use separate cloth for cleansing affected areas to prevent autoinoculation and dissemination
  (2) Mild cases: Wash lesions with soap and water
  (3) Severe cases: Apply saline compresses to debride necrotic tissue; follow with antibiotic ointment (e.g., Silvadene, bacitracin) to keep scabs soft and to prevent sticking to dressings; see also *Anorectal Signs and Symptoms*, p. 201
  (4) Perineal lesions: After each bowel movement cleanse anus gently with tepid water and pat dry
  (5) Encourage patient adherence to chronic suppressive antiviral regimens when prescribed
  (6) Administer analgesics (e.g., topical capsaicin cream [Zostrix]) to VZV lesions to reduce acute and chronic zoster pain
  (7) Monitor for development of bacterial superinfection
  (8) Avoid occlusive dressings (e.g., hydrocolloid, transparent) that promote a warm, moist environment and prevent drying or crusting of lesions
j. For bacterial infections
  (1) Staphylococcal infections
    (a) Wash infected area with antibacterial agent (Hibiclens, Betadine, benzoyl peroxide) to remove crusty, dry lesions and reduce bacterial surface concentration
    (b) Wash regularly with antibacterial soaps to prevent recurrence, followed by vigorous lubrication to prevent dry skin
  (2) Chronic ulcerations with macerated skin secondary to *P. aeruginosa:* Topical acetic acid gauze soaks tid followed by Burrow's solution gauze soaks, followed by silvadene-gauze packing dressing
k. For fungal infections
  (1) Treat dry, moist *Candida* erosions with saline compresses
  (2) Apply topical antifungals and administer systemic antifungal therapy as prescribed
l. For Kaposi's sarcoma
  (1) Leave dry and unbroken lesions open to air with no particular treatment
  (2) For draining ulcers
    (a) Cleanse with soap and water, pat dry
    (b) Apply topical antibiotic ointment and nonadhering dressing
    (c) Avoid semipermeable membrane dressings (e.g., Tegaderm, Op-site)
m. Monitor patient response to all prescribed medications
7. Patient education
  a. Causes of pruritus and methods to avoid causative factions
  b. Interventions (both pharmacologic and nonpharmacologic) that relieve symptoms
  c. Use of imagery or distraction at night when pruritus is usually worse

N. Nausea and Vomiting

1. Definition/Description
  a. Nausea: An unpleasant feeling unique to each patient; results when specific environmental triggers create an urge to expel gastric contents
  b. Vomiting: The act of releasing gastric contents forcefully through the mouth
  c. Delayed-onset nausea and vomiting occur between 24 and 48 hours after cytotoxic therapy
  d. Anticipatory nausea and vomiting is triggered by external and internal cues unique to each person with a significant psychoemotional component
2. Etiology
  a. OIs, malignancy in GI tract
  b. Mechanical obstruction
  c. Altered metabolism or organ malfunction
  d. Pharmacotherapy related
    (1) Specific medications and combinations of medications used to treat or prevent OIs

(a) PCP therapy: TMP-SMX, clindamycin, dapsone
(b) Antifungal therapy:
Amphotericin B, flucytosine (5
FC), ketoconazole, fluconazole,
itraconazole
(c) MAC therapy: Ciprofloxacin,
ofloxacin, clofazimine, clarithromycin
(d) Antiviral: Acyclovir
(2) Antineoplastic therapy to treat lymphomas, KS (known to stimulate the
chemoreceptor trigger zone and the
true vomiting center): Bleomycin,
cyclophosphamide, doxorubicin,
etoposide, ifosfamide, methotrexate,
vinblastine, vincristine
(3) Antiretroviral therapy: AZT, ddC
(4) The known and unknown use of
unproven or "quack" treatments for
AIDS/HIV
e. Radiotherapy related
f. CNS disease
3. Goals of Care
a. To control nausea and vomiting to
patient's satisfaction
b. To support nutritional needs while the
etiology is diagnosed and treated
4. *Key points*
a. Uncontrolled nausea and vomiting can
adversely affect quality of life or willingness to complete therapies
b. Inadequately prevented or controlled
chemotherapy-related nausea and vomiting may induce a learned behavioral
response in which environmental cues
(e.g., an infusion-center room, an aroma
associated with the treatment experience) stimulate nausea and vomiting
c. As with other problems that require
pharmacologic intervention to control
moderate or severely distressing symptoms, routine or around-the-clock
(rather than prn) dosing of antiemetics
is required to prevent nausea and
vomiting
5. Assessment
a. Subjective data
(1) Factors that contribute to nausea
and vomiting
(2) Description of the events surround-

ing the onset of symptoms (e.g.,
association with chemotherapy
treatment, after administration of
specific medication such as TMP-
SMX to treat PCP)
(3) Patient's perception of effectiveness
of present antiemetic regimen
(4) Description of the emesis—when it
occurs, frequency, how resolved
(5) Susceptibility to motion sickness or
other factors that may contribute to
anticipatory nausea and vomiting
(6) Patient/family/significant others'
concerns about nausea and vomiting or its management at home
(7) Impact of nausea and vomiting on
ADL, quality of life, or patient's willingness to continue treatment
(8) Ability to obtain necessary services
to meet illness and treatment
demands
(9) Adequacy and safety of living environment
(10) Support system (see also *Social
Support*, p. 272)
b. Objective data
(1) Weight, intake and output
(2) Electrolytes, renal function, liver
enzymes
(3) Current medication regimen
(4) Stage of HIV disease (include history of OIs, AIDS-related malignan-
· cies, wasting syndrome)
(5) Functional status
6. Interventions
a. Monitor and reassess regularly
(1) Weight
(2) Orthostatic vital signs
(3) Frequency of emetic episodes/day
(4) Persistence of nausea sensation
(5) Food/fluid intake
(6) Side effects of antiemetics, especially
extrapyramidal signs (e.g., involuntary movements, gait disturbances,
abnormal posture, muscle rigidity)
b. Modify chemotherapy treatment
environment to promote calm and
relaxation
(1) Minimize sights, odors, sounds that
serve as triggering stimuli
(2) Ventilate room adequately

(3) Dim lights
(4) Play calming music or relaxation tapes
(5) Avoid overhead paging or use of intercom
(6) Provide comfortable seating or positioning
c. Administer antiemetics regularly to prevent severe nausea and vomiting or the memory of same
d. Advocate for reevaluation of antiemetic regimen (drug, dose, frequency) if emetic episodes are not controlled to patient's satisfaction or if patient's intake is inadequate
e. Coach patient in relaxation techniques to assist in managing distress or anxiety associated with nausea and vomiting
f. Educate patient/family/significant other on
(1) Antiemetic therapy and its side effects; when to obtain prescription refills
(2) The importance of using antiemetic therapy around the clock, usually 30 min before meals, during periods of nausea and vomiting
(3) Keeping food/fluid diary if symptomatic to monitor nutritional intake
(4) Signs and symptoms of dehydration (see p. 204)
(5) Need to report effectiveness of strategies to control nausea and vomiting
(6) Relaxation techniques to be used when experiencing nausea
(7) Importance of maintaining adequate fluid intake (2–3 L/day)
(a) Electrolyte-rich fluids (Gatorade, Pedialyte)
(b) Drink beverages between, not with, meals
(8) Eat 5–6 small meals/day to counteract early satiety and improve daily caloric intake
(9) Avoid greasy, high-fat foods
(10) Serve food at room temperature to decrease aromas
g. Obtain prescription for antiemetic therapy to take at home
h. Administer IV hydration fluids as ordered

i. Consult with the pharmacist as to the optimum time to take antibiotics, antivirals, antifungals
j. Consult with social services if need for Meals-on-Wheels or assistance in the home for food preparation, shopping
k. Consult with dietitian for assistance in meal planning and additional nutritional counseling
l. Perform or assist patient to perform thorough oral care on rising, after meals, and at bedtime
m. Evaluate effectiveness of strategies to control nausea and vomiting
n. Evaluate patient/caregiver ability to
(1) Administer antiemetic medications
(2) Meet nutritional needs at home
(3) Recognize when to contact healthcare professional

O. Nutritional Deficit: Weight Loss, Anorexia

1. Definition/Description
a. Wasting syndrome is the AIDS-defining diagnosis in approximately 20% of reported cases; ultimately affects nearly all people with AIDS (Hellerstein, 1992)
b. Anorexia is a pervasive problem in HIV disease; chronic anorexia significantly alters quality of life
2. Etiology
a. Inadequate intake
(1) Physical causes
(a) Dysphagia/odynophagia
(b) Malabsorption/diarrhea
(c) Nausea and vomiting
(d) Altered mental status
(e) Weakness, fatigue, malaise
(f) Early satiety
(g) Altered taste or smell due to disease process or treatments
(h) Megadosing of vitamins instead of eating
(2) Social causes
(a) Lack of funds
(b) No stove or refrigerator
(c) No caregiver to shop for or prepare meals
(d) Social isolation
(e) Lack of meal-delivery program

(f) Lack of culturally appropriate meal program

(3) Psychologic causes
  (a) Depression
  (b) Food aversions
  (c) Anticipatory nausea and vomiting
  (d) Fear of exacerbating nausea, vomiting, diarrhea
  (e) Altered mental status

(4) Increased nutrient needs
  (a) Fever
  (b) Infection
  (c) Drug reactions
  (d) Dyspnea
  (e) Medications (steroids)
  (f) Hypermetabolism
  (g) Malignancy

b. Altered metabolism: See *AIDS Wasting Syndrome*, p. 134

c. Malabsorption/diarrhea: See *AIDS Wasting Syndrome*

d. Medications that induce anorexia: ddC, pyrimethamine, metronidazole, ciprofloxacin, interferon-alpha (Wilkes, 1995)

3. Goals of Care
  a. To control or reduce symptoms exacerbating weight loss
  b. To prevent nutritional compromise from decreased oral intake
  c. To prevent, stop, or reverse weight loss early in the disease process whenever possible and as clinically appropriate

4. *Key points*
  a. Malnutrition has many adverse effects
    (1) Physiologic: Weight loss, delayed recovery from infections, impaired pulmonary and cardiac function, altered structure and function of the gut, weakness or fatigue
    (2) Immunologic: Impaired cell-mediated immunity, decreased IgA secretion, decreased macrophage activity
    (3) Psychologic: Loss of body image and role status
    (4) Financial: increased length of hospitalization, repeated infections requiring therapy
  b. The magnitude of wasting predicts timing of death, which generally occurs when patients are at 66% of their ideal

body weight, 54% of body cell mass (Kotler, Tierney, Wang, & Pierson, 1989)

c. Cytotoxic doses of medications and radiation may be close to lethal if the patient is cachectic

5. Assessment
  a. Subjective data
    (1) Appetite, especially if weight loss has occurred
    (2) Access to food
      (a) Is there a meal-delivery program or significant other who can shop for and prepare meals?
      (b) Availability of a refrigerator or stove
    (3) Meaning of food or weight loss
    (4) 24-hour diet recall (food and fluid)
    (5) Concurrent signs and symptoms (e.g., nausea, diarrhea, pain)
    (6) Medication regimen, including timing of medications relative to meals
    (7) Changes in taste or smell
    (8) Difficulty chewing or swallowing
  b. Objective data
    (1) Overall appearance
    (2) Mouth: Condition of mucous membranes; presence of thrush, KS lesions, dentition
    (3) GI: Abdominal pain, distention
    (4) Neuro: Ability to swallow
    (5) Musculoskeletal: Muscle wasting, tone, strength
    (6) Laboratory data
      (a) Albumin 3.4−4.7 g/dl (normal range); low serum is a late indicator of protein loss
      (b) 24-hour urine urea nitrogen 5−6 (normal range) indicates positive nitrogen balance
    (7) Serial measurement of weight
    (8) Other measurements of lean body mass as available, such as anthropometric measures (skinfold thickness) and bioelectrical impedance analysis (BIA)

6. Interventions
  a. Control symptoms
    (1) Once weight loss is identified, advocate for a thorough evaluation to diagnose and treat etiologies
    (2) Refer to registered dietitian for a full

nutrition assessment and recommendation, including enteral or parenteral nutrition

(3) Serve small, frequent meals on small plates, so the patient does not become discouraged or overwhelmed

(4) Offer liquid nutrition supplements between meals

(5) Encourage eating in the company of others, in a pleasant atmosphere

(6) Promote nutrient-dense foods and nutritional supplements (e.g., yogurt, cheese, peanut butter, bagels with cream cheese, tuna sandwiches, instant breakfast drinks, milk shakes, liquid supplements, nutrition bars)

(7) Fresh air and activity may increase appetite

(8) Discuss with primary care provider the use of appetite stimulants (e.g., Megace, Marinol)

b. Prevent nutritional compromise

(1) Teach patient/family/significant other the importance of nutritional homeostasis (increased energy, improved quality of life, longevity)

(2) Maintain or improve nutritional status if patient has normal gut function

(a) Consume 3–6 meals per day and take 1 multivitamin daily

(b) Drink liquid nutrition supplements 2–3 times daily

(c) Take appetite stimulants as prescribed

(d) Do low-level exercise

(e) In the presence of an active infection, more aggressive nutritional interventions (e.g., tube feeding, PPN) may be indicated to meet energy needs

(f) For patient with abnormal gut function, see *Enterocolitis and Malabsorption*, p. 173, *Diarrhea*, p. 205

c. Monitor response to interventions monthly until patient is stable

d. For food and water safety, see Table 10.3, *Reducing the Risk of/Preventing Exposure to Opportunistic Pathogens*, p. 371

P. Pain

1. Definition/Description

a. An unpleasant sensory and emotional experience associated with actual or potential tissue damage, or as described in terms of such damage (IASP, 1979)

b. Pain is whatever the experiencing person says it is (McCaffery, 1979)

c. Classifications of pain

(1) Acute: Short-term pain related directly to tissue injury, which resolves with tissue healing as in acute pancreatitis, postoperative pain

(2) Chronic benign: Multifactorial pain that exists after tissue healing, may be persistent or episodic as in tension headaches, low back pain

(3) Chronic HIV-related: Multidimensional pain related to HIV pathology

d. Prevalence

(1) HIV-positive: In a study of 191 HIV-positive men, 28% of people with asymptomatic HIV disease were found to have HIV-related pain (Singer et al., 1993)

(2) AIDS

(a) Prevalence estimates vary from 53%–97% (Schofferman, 1988; Singh, Fermie, & Peters, 1992)

(b) No difference in prevalence of pain related to injecting drug use (Anand, Carmosino, & Glatt, 1994; Hoyt, Nokes, Newshan, Stalts, & Thorn, 1994; Newshan & Wainapel, 1993)

(c) Pain increases with disease progression (Loveless, Bell, & Coodley, 1993)

2. Etiology

a. Gastrointestinal

(1) Oropharynx/esophagus

(a) Fungal infections (e.g., candidiasis, histoplasmosis)

(b) Aphthous ulcerations

(c) Intraoral KS

(d) Dental abscess

(e) Necrotizing gingivitis

(f) Herpes simplex

(g) CMV ulcers

(h) Streptococcal infection
(i) Gastric reflux disorder
(2) Abdomen: May present in a variety of ways (crampy, diffusely sore, focal sharpness)
  (a) CMV colitis/ileitis
  (b) Intestinal infections (e.g., *Cryptosporidium, Shigella, Salmonella, Campylobacter,* MAC, *G. lamblia, I. belli, E. histolytica, Cryptococcus, C. difficile*)
  (c) HIV enteropathy/colitis
  (d) Lymphoma
  (e) KS
  (f) Pelvic inflammatory disease
  (g) Cholecystitis related to gallstones, *Cryptosporidium,* MAC, KS, lymphoma, *Campylobacter,* CMV
  (h) Pancreatitis related to IV pentamidine, ddI, ddC, CMV, alcohol, toxoplasmosis
(3) Anorectum: Perirectal abscess or fistula, herpes simplex ulcers, anorectal carcinoma, hemorrhoids, foreign object, proctitis related to herpes, CMV, *C. trachomatis, N. gonorrhoeae*
b. Genitourinary: HSV, epididymitis, cystitis, bartholinitis
c. Neurologic
(1) Headaches
  (a) CNS toxoplasmosis
  (b) Meningitis related to *Cryptococcus, Syphilis histoplasmosis, M. tuberculosis*
  (c) Aseptic meningitis
  (d) CNS nocardia
  (e) Herpes encephalopathy
  (f) Progressive multifocal leukoencephalopathy
  (g) Sinus infections
  (h) Medication related
(2) Neuropathy
  (a) Progressive sensory inflammatory polyneuropathy
    i) Can be related to HIV, CMV, or medications (e.g., ddI, ddC, d4T, INH)
    ii) Characterized by numbness, sensory loss, edema, burning sensation

  (b) Chronic inflammatory demyelinating polyneuropathy: Thought to be related to HIV or CMV; characterized by sensory loss, weakness
  (c) Mononeuritis complex
  (d) CMV polyradiculopathy
(3) Spinal: Spinal/epidural abscess, spinal MAC, lymphoma
d. Dermatologic: Herpes zoster, post-herpetic neuralgia, bacterial abscess, bulky cutaneous KS
e. Musculoskeletal
(1) Arthropathy
  (a) HIV-related arthralgia
  (b) Psoriatic-related arthritis
  (c) Reactive (e.g., Reiter's syndrome)
  (d) Nonspecific arthralgias
  (e) Avascular necrosis due to steroids or trauma
  (f) MAC related
(2) Myopathy: Polymyositis
  (a) Characterized by muscle weakness, elevated creatine kinase, myalgia, cramping
  (b) May be related to AZT, HIV, microsporidia, INH, use of crack/heroin/alcohol
f. Cardiac: Pericarditis, endocarditis
g. Other (e.g., postoperative, Stevens-Johnson syndrome, burns, trauma, otitis media, procedure-related [chest tubes, bone marrow aspirate, lumbar puncture])
3. Goal of Care: To control pain so that patient may achieve the optimal level of comfort and functioning with the fewest medication-related side effects
4. *Key points*
a. Pain is a subjective experience that may or may not be associated with physiologic indicators
b. Sequelae of undermanaged pain
(1) Physical effects: Difficulty sleeping, poor appetite, decreased mobility, shallow breathing
(2) Psychologic effects: Anxiety/fear, depression, reduced quality of life, difficulty concentrating, suicidal ideation

(3) Social effects: Impaired relationships, increased stress on friends/
caregivers
(4) Spiritual effects: Human suffering
c. Assessment of pain and response to
treatment is an ongoing process
d. The right dose of strong opiates is whatever it takes to relieve the pain with
fewest side effects
(1) Avoid polyopiates
(2) For persistent pain, use around-the-
clock rather than prn dosing to prevent pain
(3) Oral/rectal routes are preferable to
parenteral to provide steady-state
levels of the opiate
(4) Remember to use equianalgesic
doses when switching routes
(5) Common opioid side effects:
Drowsiness, constipation
(6) Do not apply topical preparations to
broken or irritated skin; do not use
with heating pad
e. Anesthetic/neurosurgical interventions
rarely used in HIV-related pain; generally reserved for pain unresponsive to
opiate therapy
5. Assessment: Pain is a subjective phenomenon; patient self-report is the most reliable
indicator
a. Onset and duration
b. Location
c. Character of pain (e.g., burning, sharp,
dull)
d. Intensity
e. Exacerbating and relieving factors
f. Response to current and past treatments
g. Cultural responses to pain
h. Meaning of pain to patient
i. History of chemical dependence
j. Assessment tools
(1) Numerical scale: 0–10 or 0–5 scale
(0 = no pain, 10 or 5 = most intense
pain)
(2) Verbal scale (none, small, mild,
moderate, large, severe)
(3) Pediatric faces pain scale (useful
when verbal skills are inadequate)
6. Interventions
a. Always treat the underlying etiology of
the pain

b. Individualize each patient's pain
regimen
c. Choose the least invasive route of
administration first
d. Evaluate the response to the plan continually; change the drug, interval, dose,
route, modality, and treat side effects as
needed
e. Effective pain relief can be accomplished by preventing pain
f. Because most nurses do not prescribe
analgesics, pain management requires
interdisciplinary collaboration
g. Nurses play a key role in advocating for
adequate pain management based primarily on their assessment of the
patient's pain and their observations of
the patient's response to pharmacologic
and nonpharmacologic therapies
h. WHO 4-step analgesic ladder
(1) Step 1: Nonopiates
(a) Acetaminophen
i) No effect on platelet
function or renal status
ii) May not provide
antiinflammatory effect
iii) Avoid in cases of hepatic
insufficiency
iv) Maximum dose 4 g/day
(b) Nonsteroidal antiinflammatory
drugs (NSAIDs)
i) If sufficient analgesia is not
obtained with one NSAID,
switch to another in a
different class
ii) Salsalate and tolmetin
produce less inhibition of
platelet aggregation than
other NSAIDs
iii) Always administer with
food
iv) People with low albumin
are more susceptible to
toxic effects from NSAIDs
v) Advantages of NSAIDs
a) Potent antiinflammatory
and antiprostaglandin
activity
b) Useful with throbbing,
aching pain
vi) Disadvantages of NSAIDs

a) Ceiling dose effect (above a certain dose analgesia ceases and only toxic effects occur)
b) Most will affect platelet function
c) Most cause gastric irritation
d) Cannot be used with renal insufficiency
e) Maximum dose aspirin 10 g/day
f) Use with caution in people with asthma

(2) Step 2: Mild opiates or combination opiate/nonopiate (e.g., acetaminophen with codeine, oxycodone with ASA or acetaminophen)
  (a) Use all opiates with caution in people with asthma, increased ICP, and hepatic failure
  (b) Some patients will require a bowel regimen to avoid constipation; however, this is not typically a problem in PWAs
  (c) Maximum dose of combination agents is usually limited to toxicity or ceiling doses of the nonopiate
  (d) Propoxyphene HCl (Darvon), propoxyphene HCl with acetaminophen (Darvocet), and propoxyphene HCl with aspirin and caffeine (Darvon compound) are not recommended due to poor analgesic effect as well as possible accumulation of neurotoxic metabolite, norpropoxyphene
  (e) Meperidine (Demerol) not recommended po due to poor analgesic effect as well as possible accumulation of neurotoxic metabolite, normeperidine

(3) Step 3: Adjuvants (compounds that may either enhance the effect of the opiate or have independent analgesic activity)
  (a) May be added at any step of analgesic ladder
  (b) NSAIDs: Will both provide addi-

tive effect to opiate analgesia and increase duration of effect
  (c) Corticosteroids
    i) Useful in treating aphthous ulcers and reducing cerebral edema
    ii) Generally used with caution in people with cavitary infections, bullous lung disease, renal insufficiency, thrombocytopenia
    iii) Side effects: Gastric bleeding, candidiasis
  (d) Antidepressants (e.g., amitriptyline, doxepin, smynamine, desipramine); can boost efficacy of opiates
    i) Provide independent analgesia for neuropathy and post-herpetic neuralgia
    ii) Side effects: Dry mouth, urinary retention, drowsiness
  (e) Anticonvulsants (e.g., phenytoin, clonazepam, carbamazepine) can be helpful in neuropathic and post-herpetic pain
  (f) Antihistamines (e.g., hydroxyzine) provides additive analgesia as well as antiemetic and anxiolytic effect
  (g) Oral anesthetic (e.g., mexiletine) can be useful for neuropathic pain

(4) Step 4: Strong opiates
  (a) Morphine sulfate
    i) Short-acting (available as liquid, pill, suppository, parenteral): Length of action 4 hours
    ii) Long-acting pill: Length of action 8–12 hours
      a) Do not crush or break to preserve protective coating
      b) Encourage high fluid intake to activate release of morphine
      c) May not be absorbed or released in the presence of malabsorption syndrome

iii) Equianalgesic dose: 10 mg
IM/SC = 20–30 mg po
(b) Hydromorphone: Available in
pill, suppository, liquid,
injectable forms
i) Usual length of action 3–4
hours
ii) Equianalgesic dose: 2 mg
IM/SC = 4 mg po
(c) Levorphanol: Available in pill or
injectable form
i) Long elimination half-life
of 12–16 hours
ii) Can accumulate with
repetitive dosing
iii) Usual length of action 6–8
hours
iv) Equianalgesic dose: 2 mg
IM/SC = 4 mg po
(d) Dolophine (Methadone):
Available in pill, liquid,
injectable forms
i) Long elimination half-life
of 24–36 hours
ii) Accumulates with
repetitive dosing; monitor
closely for sedation
iii) Usual length of action 6–8
hours
iv) Equianalgesic dose: 10 mg
IM/SC = 20 mg po
(e) Meperidine (Demerol)
i) Not recommended; only
exception may be for
short-term relief of acute
pain
ii) Oral form not
recommended
iii) Usual length of action 2–3
hours
iv) Toxic metabolite of
normeperidine can
accumulate at doses >300
mg/day; can lead to
tremors, restlessness,
seizures
v) Demerol 100 mg IM =
morphine sulfate 10 mg IM
(f) Fentanyl transdermal patch
(Duragesic)
i) Not for acute pain

ii) During initial application,
use short-acting opiate
until efficacy of patch is
established
iii) Place only on intact,
nonirritated skin
iv) Fever will increase release
of fentanyl, so monitor for
sedation as well as
decreased duration of
analgesia
v) Patch may be worn
continuously for 72 hours,
but increased metabolic
rate of some AIDS patients
results in shorter duration
of analgesia
i. Topical preparations
(1) Lidocaine HCl: Available as topical
ointment as well as viscous solution
for painful mouth sores
(2) Benzocaine: Available as spray, ointment, or drops for ear pain
(3) Menthol (e.g., mineral ice): Useful
with joint pain
(4) Capsaicin
(a) Useful for joint pain, neuropathy,
and post-herpetic neuralgia
(b) Must be used consistently before
analgesia obtained
(c) May cause initial burning, which
resolves with use
(5) Lidocaine/prilocaine mixture
(EMLA): Useful for very localized
anesthesia (e.g., to prevent pain
from injections)
j. Nonpharmacologic interventions: See
Wellness Strategies, p. 327
(1) Music, TV, distraction, humor (p. 353)
(2) Heat/ice
(3) Massage/vibration (p. 343)
(4) Therapeutic touch (p. 329)
(5) Acupuncture (p. 333)
(6) Imagery
(7) Relaxation techniques
(8) Biofeedback
(9) Transcutaneous electrical nerve
stimulation (TENS)
(10) Prayer
(11) Movement therapy, yoga (p. 341),
stretching, exercise

(12) Hypnosis
(13) Ultrasound
k. Radiation therapy
  (1) May be used for bulky KS lesions
  (2) May be used to alleviate pain caused by other neoplastic disease (e.g., lymphoma, cervical cancer)
7. Special population: Chemically dependent (CD)
  a. *Key points*
    (1) Apply same principles of pain management as with non-CD patients
    (2) CD people may have higher opiate tolerance, requiring higher opiate doses than non-CD people
    (3) Acting out and noncompliance are frequent responses to poor pain management
    (4) Address abuse behaviors that occur
    (5) Be attuned to your own prejudices and possible biases against drug users
  b. Methadone maintenance
    (1) Methadone used for maintenance does not provide analgesia
    (2) People on methadone maintenance need additional opiates for pain control
    (3) Dilantin and rifampin can increase metabolism of methadone
      (a) Observe patients for early symptoms of withdrawal (e.g., agitation, abdominal pain)
      (b) The dose of methadone may need to be increased or split
  c. Definitions
    (1) *Tolerance*: A pharmacologic effect in which, with repeated administration, increasing doses of a substance are needed to provide the same effect
    (2) *Physical dependence*: A pharmacologic effect characterized by withdrawal symptoms on abrupt discontinuation of the substance
    (3) *Addiction*: A complex set of behaviors characterized by the compulsive use of a drug, frequent intoxication, abandonment of social or occupational activities because of the use of the drug, and continued use of the

drug despite adverse effects
  d. Abuse behaviors
    (1) Frequent alleged loss or theft of opiate prescriptions
    (2) Refusal to undergo diagnostic tests, only wanting pain medications
    (3) Missing clinic appointments but coming in for opiate prescriptions
    (4) Excessive negotiation around pain medications
    (5) Borrowing or stealing others' pain medications
    (6) Positive urine toxicology for nonprescribed substance
  e. Possible interventions for abuse behaviors
    (1) Enlist aid of substance-abuse counselor
    (2) Directly address issue with patient
    (3) Contract with patient regarding prescriptions (e.g., limit prescriptions to a 1-week supply with no refills if it is lost/stolen
    (4) Escort patient to pharmacy to get prescription filled
    (5) Be consistent; do not engage in power struggles
8. Ethical considerations
  a. Placebo: 2 out of 3 people will respond favorably to a placebo
    (1) Placebo use cannot differentiate between "true" and "fake" pain
    (2) Placebo use is unethical without patient consent
  b. Inadequate attempts to manage pain
    (1) Bias against drug users
    (2) Acceptance of pain by healthcare providers
    (3) Failure to call in consults and pain experts
  c. Inappropriate use of analgesics
    (1) Use of pain medicine to reward or punish
    (2) Withholding pain medicine to coerce behavior or compliance

Q. Potential for Bleeding: Thrombocytopenia

1. Definition/Description
  a. Platelet count <l00,000/mm^3

(1) <100,000/mm³: Clinically significant
(2) <50,000/mm³: Mild injury may result in bleeding
(3) <20,000/mm³: Patient is at serious risk for a major bleeding episode that may occur spontaneously

b. Platelets are responsible for homeostasis; a decrease in platelets increases the risk of bleeding

2. Etiology
   a. Platelet-associated immunoglobulin: Circulating immune complexes block the ability of the spleen to remove antibody-coated platelets from the circulation or lead to destruction through clearance via the reticuloendothelial system
   b. Medication therapy (e.g., AZT, ganciclovir)
   c. Vascular injury caused by immune complexes, or an endotoxin may cause thrombotic thrombocytopenic purpura (TTP)
   d. Infiltrative disease of the bone marrow
      (1) Fungal (*Coccidioides, Cryptococcus, Histoplasma*)
      (2) Mycobacterial (MAI, *M. tuberculosis*)
   e. Progressive disease increases risk of thrombocytopenia

3. Goal of care: To prevent severe bleeding

4. *Key points*
   a. Critical indicators of thrombocytopenia
      (1) Sudden drop in hematocrit
      (2) Presence of petechiae and ecchymoses
      (3) Prolonged bleeding from venipunctures, minor cuts
      (4) Frank bleeding from any body orifice
      (5) Occult blood in excreta

5. Assessment
   a. Subjective data: Pattern of fatigue, report of blood in urine or stool, tendency to bruise
   b. Objective data
      (1) Lab values: Hgb, Hct, platelet count
      (2) Check for presence of occult blood in excreta or frank bleeding

6. Interventions
   a. Assess routinely for petechiae, ecchymoses, and obvious bleeding from

mucous membranes, rectum
   b. Administer red cell or platelet transfusions as indicated
   c. Monitor laboratory response to therapy
   d. Educate patient/caregiver to
      (1) Avoid penetrative anal or vaginal intercourse
      (2) Avoid vaginal or anal suppositories, vaginal douching, rectal enemas
      (3) Use caution if unable to avoid handling sharp objects
      (4) Avoid skin popping or shooting illicit drugs into veins
      (5) Apply pressure to any bleeding cuts
      (6) Report any signs of mental status changes, acute pain, or any injury to primary care provider
   e. Monitor for other safety concerns and modify environment if possible

R. Potential for Infection: Neutropenia

1. Definition/Description
   a. Normal neutrophil count is 1,830–7,250 cells/mm³ (Gallin, 1994)
   b. World Health Organization (WHO) classification of neutropenia
      (1) Grade I, 1,500–1,000 cells/mm³
      (2) Grade II, 750–1,000 cells/mm³
      (3) Grade II, 500–750 cells/mm³
      (4) Grade IV, <500 cells/mm³)
   c. Neutrophils provide first line of defense against bacterial invaders; a decreasing count correlates with increasing risk of bacterial infection
   d. Neutropenia occurs in a significant number of patients with AIDS, independent of drug therapy (Hambleton, 1995); prevalence increases with progressing disease

2. Etiology
   a. Most common cause: Ineffective granulopoiesis
   b. Drug induced
      (1) AZT: More likely to cause neutropenia as disease progresses, longer duration of therapy may also increase risk, may require dosage reduction or switch to other antivirals (ddI, ddC)

(2) Cancer chemotherapy drugs
   (a) Overall, neutropenia is the most common complication of these drugs
   (b) The nadir represents the lowest drop in neutrophil counts as a result of chemotherapy; can usually be predicted based on the single drug or combination of drugs used
(3) Other potentially myelosuppressive drugs: Flucytosine, trimethoprim, trimetrexate, ganciclovir, sulfonamides, pyrimethamine
   c. Neoplastic infiltration of the bone marrow (usually due to lymphoma)
   d. Infectious infiltrative disease of the bone marrow (e.g., MAC, coccidioidomycosis, histoplasmosis)
3. Goals of Care
   a. To control neutropenia and prevent severe grade that increases risk of infection
   b. To prevent neutropenia
4. *Key points*
   a. Fever with neutropenia may indicate active infection
   b. Prolonged neutropenia increases risk of infection
   c. Severity of neutropenia grade correlates to risk of infection (Grade IV neutropenia has higher risk of infection than Grade I)
5. Assessment: Objective data
   a. Fever (often the only sign of infection in neutropenic patients)
   b. Absolute neutrophil count (ANC) <1,500/mm^3 is diagnostic of neutropenia
6. Interventions
   a. Educate patient/family/significant other regarding
      (1) Risk factors for neutropenia (AZT, ganciclovir, chemotherapy)
      (2) Self-administration of colony stimulating factor (e.g., G-CSF to prevent or ameliorate neutropenia)
      (3) Strategies for prevention/early detection of infection
         (a) Use meticulous hand washing and other hygiene practices
         (b) Avoid adults and children with acute URI or GI symptoms or fever
         (c) Cook foods well
            i) Wash all fresh fruits and vegetables
            ii) Boil water if in an area at risk for water-borne organisms
         (d) Quit smoking
         (e) Take meticulous care of and monitor any invasive device (e.g., central venous access device [see Appendix E, p. 424]) for signs and symptoms of infection
         (f) Monitor temperature
         (g) Report any fever, new onset cough, sinus congestion, sputum production, GI symptoms, new rash or skin lesion, urinary tract symptoms to primary care provider
   b. Modify environment as needed
      (1) Limit exposure to symptomatic people
      (2) Initiate food and water safety precautions (see Table 10.3, *Reducing the Risk of/Preventing Exposure to Opportunistic Pathogens*, p. 371)
      (3) Ensure adequate heat, ventilation
   c. Administer antimicrobials as ordered and monitor response
   d. Monitor ANC counts at chemotherapy drug nadirs on ongoing basis as indicated

S. Potential for Injury: Falls

1. Definition/Description
   a. Falls are a common problem for people with advanced HIV disease, particularly for the hospitalized
   b. Serious morbidity and mortality as a consequence of a fall is less common in people with HIV disease than in the hospitalized or community-residing elderly
2. Etiology
   a. Orthostasis due to: Hypovolemia, adrenal insufficiency
   b. Urinary or fecal urgency

c. Peripheral neuropathy
d. Confusion or impaired judgment due to delirium, dementia
e. Medication side effects
  (1) Orthostasis: Tricyclic antidepressants (e.g., amitriptyline)
  (2) Confusional state
     (a) Sedatives-hypnotics (e.g., benzodiazepines) used in conjunction with other agents to provide conscious sedation for diagnostic/therapeutic procedures
     (b) Opioids
     (c) Steroids
  (3) Extrapyramidal tract signs: Phenothiazines
f. Impaired mobility
g. Seizures
3. Goals of Care
a. To prevent falls
b. In case of a fall, to minimize serious injury to a patient
4. *Key points*
a. Repeated falls in a person living alone in the community and the risk of serious injury may require investigation into need for additional supportive services in the home or possible placement in a residential facility
b. Respect for the principle of patient autonomy in a competent person with HIV disease who falls and who refuses more restrictive measures (e.g., physical restraints) may lead to repeated falls if
  (1) Additional supervision not available
  (2) The underlying cause of the falls cannot be corrected
c. No standardized screening tool is currently available to predict the risk for falling in a person with HIV disease
5. Assessment
a. Subjective data
  (1) History of falls (in particular, recent falls)
  (2) Presence of urinary urgency, fecal urgency, lower extremity paresthesias
  (3) Use/nonuse of assistive device to walk
  (4) Medication review
     (a) Newly prescribed agents

(b) Dose increases in suspect medications
(c) Patient/caregiver administration of suspect medications
b. Objective data
  (1) Cognitive exam: short-term memory, judgment, orientation
  (2) Motor exam: lower and upper extremity strength, gait
  (3) Orthostatic vital signs
6. Interventions
a. Identify people at risk for falls
b. Notify all care team members of the patient's risk for falling in order to promote additional support and surveillance
c. Implement environmental adaptations to remove possible hazards and promote safety
  (1) Pad sharp or hard corners of tables, beds, sofas
  (2) Keep walkways uncluttered; remove throw rugs
  (3) Provide adequate nonglare lighting
  (4) Provide/keep bedside commode, bedpan, or urinal and other essential items nearby
  (5) Keep hospital bed in low position and side rails up generally
  (6) Ensure patient has a method to call for help (e.g., call light, bell, intercom)
  (7) Rearrange room or place bed/chair to increase opportunities to observe patient directly
d. If patient has a new onset of falls or other possible neurologic findings, report to primary care provider for appropriate evaluation
e. Counsel patient regarding
  (1) Changing position slowly and avoiding prolonged standing/sitting with legs dependent
  (2) Asking and waiting for help
  (3) Keeping important or essential items nearby
  (4) Strengthening exercises for lower extremities
  (5) Monitoring side effects of medications that may increase the risk of falling

f. Refer to physical therapist for gait evaluation, reconditioning exercises, evaluation for assistive device

g. Consult with pharmacist/primary care provider regarding potential contributing medications, particularly for patients on polypharmacy

h. Advocate for the evaluation and symptomatic relief of contributing symptoms

i. Remind all caregivers that informed, competent patients have the right to refuse protective interventions

j. Evaluate
   (1) Frequency of patient falls despite interventions
   (2) Adverse outcomes resulting from a fall
   (3) Based on evaluation, provide increased support or supervision
       (a) Increased home health aide visits/hours; mobilize patient's support system to stagger visits to provide more supervision
       (b) Close observation while hospitalized
       (c) Monitoring devices (e.g., alarms, intercom) to alert caregivers that patient is attempting to get up
   (4) Possible placement in the community if patient is a danger to self
   (5) For patient living alone, devise an emergency response plan for neighbor/friend to call at a certain time of day and send help if no response. Ensure patient has access to phone if at all possible.

k. See also *Impaired Mobility*, p. 221, *High Risk for Ineffective Management of Therapeutic Regimen*, p. 258

T. Stomatitis

1. Definition/Description
   a. Inflammation of the mucous membranes that comprise the oral cavity
      (1) May extend down through the esophagus (esophagitis)
      (2) May further include the mucous membranes that line the GI tract (mucositis)
   b. Can create pain and lingering discom-

fort; if dysphagia/odynophagia is present, has the potential to impair nutritional intake

2. Etiology
   a. Infections invading the oral cavity/mucous membranes
      (1) Bacterial: HIV-related gingivitis, necrotizing stomatitis, HIV-related periodontitis
      (2) Viral: Herpes simplex, hairy leukoplakia
      (3) Fungal: *C. albicans*, histoplasmosis
      (4) Other: Aphthous ulcers
   b. Kaposi's sarcoma
      (1) Primary involvement of the mucous membranes of the GI tract
      (2) Invasive KS extending to one or more areas of the oral cavity/GI tract
   c. Chemical-related tissue injury
      (1) Results in ulcerations that appear 5–7 days after cytotoxic treatment
      (2) Chemotherapy agents, either as single agent or in combination, to treat AIDS-associated malignancies and known to induce stomatitis: Doxorubicin, bleomycin, etoposide, cyclophosphamide, vincristine, vinblastine, methotrexate
   d. Radiation therapy of the head and neck, chest, abdominal region
   e. Malnutrition, dehydration, and poor dental condition may also be factors in the development of stomatitis
   f. Smoking, alcohol use

3. Goals of Care
   a. To control pain and discomfort
   b. To maintain adequate hydration and nutritional status
   c. To promote healing through oral hygiene measures

4. *Key points*
   a. Impaired salivary gland function puts the myelosuppressed patient at risk for local and systemic infection; it causes a lack of the immune components in the saliva needed to coat the mucous membranes lining the GI tract
   b. Invasion of the oral cavity/mucous membranes by infectious agents may lead to
      (1) Alterations in taste

    (2) Changes in physical characteristics of the basal layers of mucous membranes

    (3) Altered motility of the GI tract

5. Assessment

  a. Subjective data

    (1) Current medications

    (2) Factors intensifying/relieving oral pain

    (3) Frequency and description of oral hygiene

    (4) Frequency and event(s) leading to consultation with a dental professional; dental history

    (5) Diet, smoking, use of alcohol and other drugs

    (6) Effect of stomatitis on ability to perform ADL and self-concept

  b. Objective data

    (1) Severity rating of stomatitis

      (a) Grade 1: Slight discomfort in the mouth with white areas on gums

      (b) Grade 2: Moderate erythema, pain, and slightly recessed ulcerations, white patches

      (c) Grade 3: Severe erythema and pain, bleeding, deep ulcerations, white patches; patient unable to eat, drink, swallow

    (2) Treatment regimen (past and present)

    (3) Stage of HIV disease

    (4) Present nutritional status

      (a) Current weight, recent weight loss

      (b) Signs of dehydration

      (c) Nutritional laboratory values

      (d) See *Dehydration*, p. 204, *Nutritional Deficit: Weight Loss, Anorexia*, p. 227

    (5) Change in appearance, frequency, and consistency of stool and saliva

    (6) Speech pattern

6. Interventions

  a. Relieve pain and discomfort

    (1) Encourage fluid intake (e.g., 2–3 L/day); liquids should be room temperature or slightly cool and nonacidic

    (2) Encourage consistent oral hygiene with soft toothbrush, sponge swab, or approved oral rinse ≥5 times/day

    (3) Reassess pain and effectiveness of prescribed analgesics on a regular basis

    (4) If patient unable to speak, provide alternate means of communication (e.g., paper and pens, erasable board and marker); avoid open-ended questions

    (5) Use topical anesthetics or topical protective lubricants

  b. Prevent dehydration and malnutrition

    (1) Monitor intake and output

    (2) Provide menus or diet instructions for soft, bland diet using high-calorie, high-protein foods/fluids

    (3) Assess ability of patient or caregiver to plan/manage dietary changes necessary to minimize complications of stomatitis

    (4) Encourage adequate (2–3 L/day) fluid intake

  c. Promote healing and education

    (1) Educate patient/caregiver on

      (a) Healthy nutrition

      (b) Ways to promote good oral hygiene

      (c) Potential complications, how to treat them, and when to call the healthcare professional

    (2) Counsel patient to cut down or eliminate smoking and alcohol intake, if possible

    (3) Encourage routine dental care (especially important before initiation of chemotherapy or radiation therapy, which may induce stomatitis)

    (4) Reinforce verbally and provide written information to patient/family/significant other on when to notify the healthcare professional of complications

      (a) Weight changes

      (b) Increased oral pain or dysphagia

      (c) Inability to perform oral hygiene regimen

      (d) Inability to maintain fluid/food intake

      (e) Inability to swallow saliva

      (f) Fever or other new signs and symptoms

d. Evaluate
  (1) Patient's satisfaction with pain management
  (2) Adequacy of nutritional intake
  (3) Ability of patient/caregiver to manage care needs (e.g., oral regimen, dietary needs, follow-up appointments)
e. See also *Dehydration*, p. 204, *Dysphagia/Odynophagia*, p. 207, *Pain*, p. 229

U. Vaginal Symptoms

1. Definition/Description
  a. Symptoms of itching, burning, discharge, odor; embarrassment may cause women to need prompting before reporting these symptoms
  b. Prevalence: Not known, but believed to be widespread
  c. Risk factors: History of diabetes, use of antibiotics (superinfection), birth control pills, pregnancy
2. Etiology
  a. Sexually transmitted diseases (STDs) (e.g., gonorrhea, chlamydia, herpes, trichomonas)
  b. Vaginal candidiasis (superinfection of normal flora)
  c. Secondary to sexual excitement or sexual intercourse; prior to and during menstrual period; following use of foam, jelly, or cream for birth/infection control
  d. Chemical irritation or allergy secondary to factors such as douches, deodorants, latex
  e. Sexual abuse
  f. See *Vaginal Candidiasis*, p. 185, *Gynecologic Complications*, p. 181
3. Goal of Care: To control symptom(s), with resulting improvement in physical comfort
4. *Key points*
  a. Vaginal candidiasis may occur at any CD4+ lymphocyte count; often a chronic problem
  b. Because HIV is a sexually transmitted disease, case finding for other STDs is essential and needs to be repeated periodically
  c. Most women with vaginal/cervical chlamydia have no symptoms, but this infection can progress to pelvic inflammatory disease

5. Assessment
  a. Subjective data
    (1) Ascertain the nature of the discharge (color, odor, amount, duration, physical discomfort)
    (2) Explore the events associated with the occurrence of discharge (e.g., sexual intercourse, use of sex toys, masturbation, time around menstrual period, rigorous or unwanted sexual activity)
    (3) Inquire about
      (a) Pap smear (frequency, results)
      (b) Contraceptive method (e.g., IUD, sponge)
      (c) History of and treatment for other STD (e.g., chlamydia)
      (d) Allergy to latex
      (e) Satisfaction with sexual relationships
    (4) Determine whether woman is using alternative therapies (e.g., acidophilus to restore normal flora, L-lysine for herpes)
  b. Objective data
    (1) Color, amount, consistency, odor of discharge
    (2) Erythema of labia
    (3) Excoriation of labia, vaginal canal; ulceration
6. Interventions
  a. Consider need for culturing vaginal discharge and urine for culture and sensitivity
  b. Discuss self-help strategies
    (1) Wear cotton underpants
    (2) Avoid tight-fitting clothing
    (3) Avoid spreading anal secretions to vaginal area both during sex and after toileting
    (4) Avoid commercial douching and feminine hygiene products
    (5) Minimize sugar, sweets, and refined foods in diet
    (6) Kill yeast on underpants by boiling, bleaching, ironing or, if damp, microwaving for 5 min
  c. Instruct woman who is allergic to latex

that male sexual partner should wear latex condom and then a natural-skin condom; avoid colored condoms; consider female condom

d. Instruct to have Pap smear twice during the first year, annually when the initial smears are normal, and every 6 months if history of problems (AHCPR, 1994)

e. Discuss prescriptive therapies with primary care provider for specific causative organism (see Appendix B, *Common Medications Used in Treating the Patient with HIV/AIDS*, p. 401)

f. Teach how to insert vaginal suppository or applicator; observe a return demonstration

g. Advise that systemic medications for thrush or herpes may control vaginal symptoms

h. Counsel patient about her right to a safe and satisfying sexual relationship

   (1) Refer to support services for battered or raped women if sexual or physical abuse is suspected

   (2) Notify any legal authorities as required by statutes

i. Advise woman to use ice pack to control vaginal burning; vinegar or betadine douche is prescribed to control vaginal odor/discharge not controlled by regular bathing and antimicrobials

V. Visual Loss

1. Definition/Description

   a. Ocular impairment from an OI may be a primary or secondary involvement

   b. HIV-related visual loss, although relatively infrequent, except in advanced HIV disease, may be severe and life altering

2. Etiology

   a. CMV retinitis (see also *Viral Infections*, p. 94)

      (1) Prevalence is 5%–30% in people with AIDS; however, evidence of clinical visual impairment may only be present in 10% (Drew, Buhles, & Erlich, 1995)

      (2) Progression of CMV may continue in spite of appropriate treatment

   b. Toxoplasmosis

   c. Noninfectious microangiopathy may produce "cotton-wool spots" (usually asymptomatic)

   d. Conjunctival, eyelid, or orbital involvement from KS or lymphoma

   e. Neuro-ophthalmic lesions (e.g., syphilitic optic neuritis)

   f. Anticholinergic effects of certain medications may cause blurred vision

3. Goals of Care

   a. To detect vision changes early

   b. To promote patient's safety and autonomy

   c. To support patient's adaptation to visual impairment or loss

4. *Key points*

   a. Patients with CD4+ lymphocyte counts <50/µl are especially at risk for CMV ocular impairment (Drew et al., 1995); untreated sight-threatening CMV disease is progressive, permanent, and irreversible

   b. Treatment for ocular OIs may be life long; in the case of CMV retinitis, it may require central venous access devices and daily IV infusions

   c. The burden of threatened/actual visual loss relates to

      (1) Fear of impact from this disability on personal autonomy and independent community living

      (2) The demands of long-term IV therapy, care required, and the risks associated with venous access devices (plus potential drug interactions of ganciclovir with antiretrovirals [particularly AZT] causing severe neutropenia)

5. Assessment

   a. Subjective data

      (1) Impact of visual loss on mood, self-concept, relationships

      (2) Reported symptoms: decreased visual acuity, floaters, blurred vision

      (3) Date of last ophthalmic/fundoscopic examination

      (4) Ability to manage ADL

      (5) Availability of supportive services, family, friends

   b. Objective data

(1) Unilateral visual field loss: Impairment usually begins unilaterally but bilateral involvement is common, especially if left untreated
(2) Decreased acuity during
   (a) Eye chart test
   (b) Routine activities (e.g., reading a newspaper); determine literacy level before diagnosing a loss of visual acuity based on ability to read print
(3) Peripheral or central vision loss noted on testing visual field
(4) Observed photosensitivity

6. Interventions
  a. For AIDS-related ocular OIs or malignancies
    (1) Administer, or instruct re administration of, prescribed medications, schedule, and side effects
    (2) Manage/instruct re management of venous access devices (e.g., flushing, site/dressing changes)
    (3) See *Cytomegalovirus*, p. 94, Appendix B, *Common Medications Used in Treating the Patient with HIV/AIDS*, p. 401, Appendix E, *CVADs*, p. 424
  b. Provide symptomatic relief using appropriate pain-control techniques (e.g., cool compresses, eye drops, avoiding bright lights)
  c. Educate the patient/family/significant other

(1) Report new or worsening ocular symptoms to primary care provider as soon as possible
(2) Have regular fundoscopic exams, especially when CD4+ lymphocyte count is <50/μl or known to be CMV-antibody positive
(3) Possible role of medications in contributing to visual symptoms
  d. For medication side effects impairing vision, clarify with the primary care provider if alternative treatments possible
  e. Refer to services for visually impaired/blind for assistance modifying home environment to maintain safety and promote independence (e..g., magnifying glass, books on tape, individual counseling/support groups; in some instances, occupational therapy may provide additional assistance with adaptive devices and home modifications for visual impairment)
  f. Remind caregivers not to move furniture or rearrange patient's belongings without the patient's consent in order to avoid disorientation, injury
  g. Allow for verbalization of feelings (from both HIV-positive person and significant other) regarding visual impairment/loss
  h. Facilitate necessary community referrals as needed to maintain a safe and adequate environment (e.g., Meals on Wheels, home health).

II. PSYCHOSOCIAL RESPONSES

A. Alterations in Family Functioning

1. Definition/Description
   a. Family functions serve the needs of both individual family members and of society (Friedman, 1992; Johnson, 1992)
      (1) Affective function (to meet the psychosocial needs of family members)
      (2) Socialization and social placement function (to socialize children to become productive members of society; to transmit culture from one generation to another)
      (3) Personal security and acceptance (to provide a home with stability that permits family members to grow and develop)
      (4) Ensuring continuity of companionship (to provide sympathetic companionship and encouragement to one another)
      (5) Giving satisfaction and a sense of purpose (to provide activities so that family members can enjoy life with each other)
      (6) Imposing controls and a sense of what is right (to learn rules, rights, obligations, and responsibilities of being a member of society)
      (7) Healthcare function (to provide physical necessities such as food, clothing, shelter, and health care)
   b. Alterations in family functioning arise when families are unable to perform these functions, thus threatening the integrity of the family unit and the ability of the family to fulfill societal obligations
   c. Signs and symptoms: Family's inability to
      (1) Adapt constructively to crisis or stress
      (2) Communicate openly among family members
      (3) Perform the activities associated with the functions already listed
      (4) Seek or accept help appropriately

   d. Prevalence not known
   e. Risk factors
      (1) Probably similar to those for family caregiver burden, but not definitively known
      (2) Critical points in HIV disease: Diagnosis of HIV or AIDS, first hospitalization, first OI, new symptoms, recurrences/relapses, awareness of terminal phase
      (3) See etiology of *Family Caregiver Burden/Strain,* p. 251
2. Etiology
   a. HIV infection presenting as a major life transition that is out of sequence with what is expected
   b. Increasing dependence of PWAs, coupled with increasing responsibility of family caregiver for care of PWAs, requires shifts in who performs which functions within the family
   c. Disruption in family routines (e.g., home care routines, visits from home health workers)
   d. Emotional responses of family members to course of HIV (often viewed as being on a roller coaster, not knowing what is going to happen next)
   e. Financial constraints due to medical treatments, medications
   f. Hospitalizations for acute episodes
   g. Changes in family roles
3. Goals of Care
   a. To recognize a family in crisis that needs respite intervention
   b. To support the family's adaptation to living with a life-threatening illness of one of its family members in a manner that seems appropriate for the particular family
   c. To identify resources that will support the family and individual members of the family to manage the demands of the loved one's illness
4. *Key points*
   a. Given the range of family constellations represented by people with HIV infection, a broad definition of family must be used to include both family of origin

and family of choice, whether related biologically or legally, or not
  (1) Conflicts may arise (e.g., between family of origin and family of choice)
  (2) Families members may be struggling with reconnecting with estranged PWAs from conflicts related to lifestyle choices and history of drug abuse
  b. The nurse's role is that of health educator, facilitator of problem solving, and resource linker
    (1) Take care not to take over unwittingly the family's problems and solve them for the family (Balzer, 1992)
    (2) Consider contracting and empowering as means to assist families in promoting health (Loveland-Cherry, 1992)
5. Assessment
  a. Definition of family from patient's perspective (Otto, 1973)
    (1) Family strengths
    (2) Effective communication
    (3) Ability to provide support and encouragement
    (4) Capacity to maintain community relationships
    (5) Ability to perform family roles flexibly
    (6) Ability for self-help and to accept outside help
    (7) Mutual respect for individuality of family members
    (8) Ability to use a crisis as a means of growth
    (9) Concerns for family unity, loyalty, cooperation
  b. Role performance (identifying which family members perform the functions listed above)
  c. The Friedman (1992) Family Assessment Model
  d. For other scales to assess family functioning see Danielson, Hamel-Bissell, & Winstead-Fry (1993)
6. Interventions
  a. Convey acceptance of family by attending to nonverbal cues (e.g., maintaining eye contact, nodding head while person speaks), conveying interest in helping them, and in displaying genuineness, respect, empathy, self-disclosure (Danielson et al., 1993; Janis, 1983)
  b. Discuss effects of PWA's illness on family's ability to perform functions
  c. Assist with problem solving to realign family roles and develop strategies to perform necessary functions
    (1) Identify problem
    (2) Appraise challenges associated with change
    (3) Identify/weigh alternatives, deliberating about commitment, adhering despite negative feedback
  d. Discuss the nature of the "sick role" as it affects obligations and responsibilities of the sick person during times of illness
  e. Acknowledge strengths of family (e.g., "You seem to communicate easily with one another.")
  f. Acknowledge the negative emotions family members may be feeling such as guilt, anger, resentment, blame; encourage verbalization and assist in resolving these emotions
  g. Respect privacy of individual family members
  h. Counsel family about conflict resolution
  i. Facilitate open communication among family members
  j. Counsel family members about HIV testing and safer sex; refer for testing, if appropriate
  k. Initiate family care conferences when appropriate
  l. Refer to family counselor or family therapist
  m. Provide crisis intervention, if indicated
  n. See *Family Caregiver Burden/Strain*, p. 251
  o. Interventions related to death and loss
    (1) Assist family in acknowledging a wide array of losses they may have experienced such as a future together, financial security, possible death of a loved one, a life as they have known it (Brown & Powell-Cope, 1993; Powell-Cope, 1995)
    (2) Discuss the impact of AIDS on having to face one's own mortality

(3) Provide grief counseling, including anticipatory grief counseling, stages of grief, grieving as a "normal" process

(4) Refer to psychiatric/mental health professional, clergy as indicated

(5) See also *Grief and Loss*, p. 253, *Spiritual Distress*, p. 273

p. Assist family to garner support (Powell-Cope & Brown, 1992)

(1) Help family members to disclose to others their involvement with AIDS, based on others' need to know, by staging information and by checking out others about how they are likely to respond

(2) Suggest that by telling others of their association with AIDS they will not only be exposing themselves to possible discrimination, isolation, and negative judgments but will also be creating opportunities to receive support

(3) Discuss possible benefits of becoming politically active in fighting against AIDS, of engaging in activist activities

(4) See *Social Isolation*, p. 269, *Stigma*, p. 274

q. See discussion of multigenerational infected families, p. 394

B. Anxiety

1. Definition/Description

a. A diffuse, uncomfortable feeling of dread or apprehension; ranges from mild to severe

(1) Mild: Can increase energy, alertness, concentration, motivation

(2) Severe: Can be disabling

(3) Panic: Most severe form

(a) Patient is terrified, with a sense of doom

(b) Attention is narrowed, learning is impossible

(c) Significant sympathetic nervous system response

(d) Patient may be psychologically and physically immobilized

b. Prevalence

(1) Common in adults

(2) Patients with serious illness will experience anxiety

(3) Common in HIV-positive patients

(a) Serious illness coupled with social stressors

(b) Uncertainty about future (dementia, physical disability, pain)

c. Risk factors in HIV

(1) Changes in health status: Seroconversion, AIDS diagnosis, acute illness, medication changes

(2) Life changes: Illness or death of friends, change in financial or insurance status, change in healthcare provider, significant anniversaries

2. Etiology

a. Internal conflict

(1) Inability to reconcile internal drives with behavior; basic impulses are frustrated by disease

(2) Anticipated disapproval by important others (family/friends, caregivers, employer)

b. Threat to self (physical, social, psychologic, spiritual)

(1) Threat of disability, disfigurement, pain, death

(2) Threat of stigmatization (see *Stigma*, p. 274)

(a) Related to HIV status or life choices

(b) Potential loss of healthcare benefits; medication

(3) Threat to life role and ability to complete life tasks and goals

(a) Impaired ability to function in role as partner, lover, parent, employee, friend

(b) Impaired ability to complete developmental tasks and goals of adulthood

(4) Inability to reconcile disease and death with spiritual beliefs; questions regarding meaning of life in general and patient's own life in particular

(5) Threats may be real or perceived

c. Effect of drugs

(1) Medications used in HIV treatment (AZT, NSAIDs)

(2) A common effect of street drugs

(3) Seen in alcohol and drug withdrawal

(4) Made worse by caffeine

3. Goals of Care

a. To reduce patient's level of discomfort

b. To help patient identify source of anxiety

c. To assist patient to develop alternative ways of coping

4. *Key points*

a. Assessment must be ongoing

(1) Anxiety tends to recur

(2) Levels tend to fluctuate

(3) Signs and symptoms may not accurately reflect level of anxiety; patient's verbal report is often best indicator of subjective severity

b. Respond immediately to patient in great physical or psychologic distress; potential complications can negatively affect health status

(1) May render patient unable to learn about illness or follow treatment

(2) May exacerbate medical conditions such as dyspnea; some studies show a relationship between anxiety and immunosuppression

(3) Panic may result if anxiety not relieved; unrelieved panic can lead to suicide

5. Assessment

a. History

(1) Current health status and medications

(2) Previous episodes of anxiety: Precipitants and effective interventions

(3) Losses

(4) Financial concerns, relationships

(5) Support systems, including social functioning; meaning of these to patient

b. Physical signs

(1) Sympathetic nervous system response (e.g., increased heart rate, increased blood pressure, constricted pupils)

(2) Somatic complaints (shortness of breath, palpitations)

(3) Worried facial expression

(4) Increased motor activity

(5) Tremors or twitching

(6) Hand wringing

c. Physical symptoms: Muscle tension, tingling hands or feet, restlessness, GI disturbance, chest pain, palpitations, confusion, headache, shortness of breath

d. Psychologic or behavioral symptoms

(1) Worry, rumination

(2) Unexplainable feeling of discomfort (may be described as feeling of impending doom)

(3) Irritability

(4) Preoccupation

e. Changes in level of distress: Elicit what exacerbates or ameliorates symptoms

6. Interventions

a. Administer/monitor effects of anxiolytic medications

(1) Short-acting agents prn for episodic anxiety (lorazepam is effective and well-tolerated by HIV patients)

(2) Longer-acting agents for more pervasive or chronic anxiety (clonazepam q4h is effective and safe)

(3) Monitor and educate about side effects

(a) Sedation: Can interfere with ADL, be a cause of falls

(b) Interaction with other drugs and alcohol: Cumulative effect with other CNS depressants, neutralized by stimulants

(c) Potential withdrawal problems if abruptly discontinued

b. Counseling and education

(1) Understanding the cause often helps patients feel less anxious

(a) Teach patient to identify feelings related to anxiety (e.g., nervousness, dread, restlessness)

(b) Explore situation just before negative feeling began (include environmental stimuli, activity, thoughts, emotions)

(2) Explain how needs will be met if disability or pain becomes severe; involve family, friends, healthcare providers

(3) Help to identify and practice alter-

native strategies to manage anxiety (relaxation, deep breathing, and stress reduction can be helpful)
  (4) See *Massage*, p. 343, *Meditation*, p. 355, *Yoga*, p. 341
 c. Supportive therapy
  (1) Individual professional or peer counseling provides an accepting and nurturing environment
   (a) A safe place to discuss fears and difficult issues (e.g., feelings of guilt related to lifestyle, interpersonal relationships; suicidal thoughts)
   (b) Talking about concerns can aid in resolution or make concerns seem more manageable
   (c) See *Individual Psychotherapy*, p. 345
  (2) Group therapy decreases feeling of being alone or different; see *Social Support*, p. 272
 d. Family/friends education and support
  (1) Knowledge of cause and effects of anxiety helps them support patient
  (2) Involvement of family and friends may itself reduce anxiety
  (3) As disease progresses family and friends may become more anxious (see *Alterations in Family Functioning*, p. 243, *Family Caregiver Burden/ Strain*, p. 251)
 e. Consider cultural variations in expression of anxiety
  (1) Involve bicultural staff if possible
  (2) Listen carefully to content of patient's speech; signs and symptoms may be different from those you expect
  (3) Use language and interventions that are culturally appropriate and meaningful to patient

C. Body Image Disturbance

1. Definition/Description
 a. Body image: A standard or frame of reference that individuals use when relating to themselves and their physical and social environment (Bramble, 1991, p. 218)
 b. Body image disturbance: "Disruption in the way one perceives one's body image" (NANDA, 1994, p. 72)
 c. The emphasis in our culture on physical and functional perfection can leave the patient threatened by illness or disability with a sense of frustration, despair, or anger
 d. Changes in body image are common in debilitating illnesses and particularly with AIDS
 e. Variables influencing body image are body boundaries, cultural influences, internal and external influences, interaction with others, and chronicity (Bramble, 1991)
 f. Coping with disturbances in body image can be as complex as the variables influencing it
2. Etiology: KS lesions, premature aging with chronic disease, alopecia, wasting, edema (local and truncal), social isolation, neuropathies (functional losses), adaptive devices (e.g., canes, walkers, hearing aids), urinary catheters, central venous catheters
3. Goals of Care
 a. To help the patient identify positive self-concept statements
 b. To help the patient demonstrate functional adaptive behaviors
4. *Key points*
 a. Crisis points in the continuum of the disease or treatment effects can produce intense psychosocial reactions; recognition of psychopathology and, particularly, suicide risk necessitate urgent referral
 b. Gay men with HIV disease may be at particularly high risk for severe body image disturbances because of the culture's value on the perfect body
5. Assessment
 a. Current distress
  (1) What aspect of the illness is most distressing and bothersome?
  (2) How has this illness or its treatment affected the way the patient perceives his/her body?
  (3) Objective variables
   (a) Actual change in structure or function

(b) Not looking at body part
(c) Change in social environment
(d) Hiding or overexposing body part
(4) Subjective variable (NANDA, 1994, p. 73): Patient report of
  (a) Change in lifestyle
  (b) Fear of rejection or reaction by others
  (c) Focus on past strength, function, or appearance
  (d) Negative feelings about body
  (e) Feelings of helplessness, hopelessness, or powerlessness
  (f) Preoccupation with change or loss
  (g) Personalization of part or loss by name
  (h) Depersonalization of part or loss by impersonal pronouns
  (i) Refusal to verify actual change

b. Coping
  (1) Previous and current coping mechanisms and their effectiveness
  (2) Perceived ability to adapt to changes
  (3) Past experiences with illness or hospitalizations and previous alterations in body image (Flaskerud, 1995)

c. Psychosocial history: Interpersonal relationships, education, career, use of nonprescribed drugs and alcohol, previous psychiatric care, developmental stage

d. Social support
  (1) Available sources of support (family, spouse, partner, friends, groups)
  (2) Individual's social identity
  (3) Cultural or subcultural groups patient belongs to
  (4) Possibilities for support within social identity

e. Individual identity: Sources of self-esteem, valued achievements, future goals

f. Grief and loss (see *Grief and Loss*, p. 253)

6. Interventions
a. Collaborate with mental health professionals regarding care
b. Use anxiety-reducing techniques to assist in adapting self-concept
c. Encourage verbalization of thoughts and feelings

(1) Be honest
(2) Point out and limit self-negation statements
(3) Do not support denial; focus on reality and adaptation, realistic goals
(4) Be aware of own nonverbal communication and behavior
(5) Encourage patient to try to note differences in situations and events
(6) Build on coping mechanisms
(7) Refer to community and social support resources
(8) Encourage assertive behavior
(9) Involve family/significant other in discussion and problem-solving activities as appropriate
(10) Encourage grieving over loss of body image
(11) Encourage use of available resources (prosthetic/assistive devices, cosmetic resources, occupational/physical therapy)

d. Educate patient, family/significant other regarding physiologic and psychologic changes patient may experience

e. See also *Stigma*, p. 274

D. Depression

1. Definition/Description
a. Mood characterized by sadness, apathy, social withdrawal, anhedonia, and lowered self-esteem
b. Can be physiologic or reactive
  (1) Physiologic: Usually insidious onset, often a previous personal or family history, responds well to antidepressants
  (2) Reactive: Sudden onset, with clear precipitating event (usually a loss); usually responds to medications, often to supportive therapy

c. Prevalence
  (1) Approximately 5% in general population (Wilson & Kneisl, 1996)
  (2) Between 4% and 14% of HIV patients affected (Folkman, Chesney, Pollack, & Coates, 1993)
  (3) Common in patients with severe medical illness (Perry, 1990)

d. Risk factors
   (1) Previous history of depression
      (a) May indicate a physiologic pre-disposition or a coping style of depressive reactions
      (b) Overwhelming stress in addition to HIV disease itself
      (c) Family history of depression or suicide
   (2) Any loss significant to patient
      (a) Illness or death of friend
      (b) Loss of status (employment, valued role)
      (c) Loss of family members (alienation, inability to care for children)
      (d) Change in health status (sero-conversion, acute illness, increased disability leading to greater dependence, final states of illness)
2. Etiology
   a. Physiologic
      (1) Imbalance of neurotransmitters nor-epinephrine, serotonin
      (2) Exacerbated by external stimuli
      (3) Caused by some medications used to treat HIV disease (e.g., AZT, corticosteroids, dapsone, NSAIDs)
   b. Reactive
      (1) Response to external stimuli (real or perceived event)
      (2) Serious illness is a common cause
      (3) Survivor guilt
         (a) Continuing living after partner, lover, or friends have died
         (b) Often complicated by anger, ambivalence (see *Guilt*, p. 255)
3. Goals of Care
   a. To reduce patient's feelings of sadness and hopelessness
   b. To help the patient learn a more effective coping style
      (1) Increased hope, optimism, power lead to more active involvement in treatment
      (2) Some studies connect a fighting attitude with improved immune response
      (3) Patient can have relationships, continue with life work as long as physically possible

4. *Key points*
   a. Differential may be difficult
      (1) Vegetative signs of depression (fatigue, weight loss, slowed or agitated movement) mimic HIV disease
      (2) May be confused with dementia (poor concentration, impaired memory, apathy or agitation, social withdrawal); with CD4+ lymphocyte count >200/μl dementia is less likely; see *AIDS Dementia Complex*, p. 138
      (3) May overlap, mimic, confuse, or exacerbate any medical condition; assess for depression whenever clinical picture changes
   b. May be viewed as appropriate response to serious illness; intervention/treatment is important because quality of life may be significantly improved
      (1) Increases interest and involvement in treatment
      (2) Enhances ability to complete life business
      (3) Improved mood can positively affect health
   c. As mood improves, suicidality may increase (more energy is available to act)
   d. Self-medication with alcohol or drugs possible; many substance users have preexisting underlying depressions
5. Assessment
   a. Mental status
      (1) Appearance: Lack of self-care may be evident, posture and facial expression may have depressed appearance, poor eye contact
      (2) Mood and affect: Depressed or irritable, sad or blunted affect
      (3) Cognition: Poor attention and concentration may result in impaired learning ability and short-term memory; may be confused
      (4) Thought processes: Themes of guilt, self-deprecation, worthlessness are common
      (5) Perceptions may be distorted: May perceive everything bad as his/her fault; in severe depression

hallucinations or delusions, congruent with depressed mood, are possible

(6) Suicidality
  (a) Assess for ideation, plans, lethality of method, ability to carry out plan
  (b) Degree of depression is significant; suicide occurs in middle range of depression when patient still feels hopeless but can mobilize energy to act

b. Signs: Sad, downcast facial expression; slumped posture; slowed movement
c. Symptoms: Sadness, feeling empty, hopelessness, sleep or appetite disturbance, lack of pleasure in activities previously enjoyed, fatigue or lack of energy
d. Neuropsychiatric testing can be valuable in diagnosis

6. Interventions
  a. Provide support
    (1) Staff who are emotionally available (sit, listen, empathize) can help decrease sense of loss, promote feeling of being accepted and cared for
    (2) Individual or group support, professional or peer facilitated, can decrease feelings of isolation
    (3) Grief counseling: See *Grief and Loss,* p. 253
  b. Monitor and counsel regarding effects, side effects of medications and ways to manage them
    (1) Tricyclics
      (a) Require 3–6 weeks to be effective
      (b) Significant anticholinergic side effects
        i) Cumulative with other anticholinergic meds
        ii) May cause confusion in HIV patients, especially if some cognitive impairment already present
        iii) Major reason for patients to discontinue medication
          a) Educate regarding dry mouth, blurred vision, constipation

  b) Anticholinergic effects decrease over time

(2) Selective serotonin reuptake inhibitors (SSRIs)
  (a) Fewer anticholinergic effects
  (b) Some potential side effects (decreased appetite, insomnia) may negatively affect HIV disease
  (c) Relative safe in overdose
  (d) Some side effects may be intolerable (e.g., initial stimulatory effect, chronic sexual dysfunction)

(3) Bupropion
  (a) Less sedating than tricyclics
  (b) Less simulating that SSRIs
  (c) May lower seizure threshold

(4) Stimulants
  (a) Rapid effect
  (b) May allow severely depressed patient to increase energy to cope with illness, participate in treatment
  (c) If mood not improved in 3–6 weeks, consider another medication

c. Institute behavioral therapy: Develop a plan for patient to resume some activity and receive reward when activity completed
  (1) Choose an activity patient previously enjoyed and a reward that is meaningful to patient
  (2) Increase patient's involvement in planning as condition allows

d. Consider cultural variations in expression of depressed feelings
  (1) Culturally appropriate affects range from open, demonstrative expressions to stoicism
  (2) The expression of depression is not a reliable indicator of the degree of feeling

e. Provide education and support to significant others
  (1) Understanding depression can help them support patient by being nurturing and encouraging independence
  (2) Dealing with illness and impending death of loved person can cause sadness, anger, ambivalence

(a) Support groups decrease feeling of isolation, help in working out feelings and problem solving (see *Support Groups*, p. 348)

(b) If depression is significant, more intensive intervention may be indicated; refer to psychotherapy or for medication (see *Individual Psychotherapy*, p. 345)

E. Family Caregiver Burden/ Strain

1. Definition/Description
   a. No consistent, agreed-upon definition of caregiver burden
   b. The terms *burden* and *strain* are used interchangeably to describe the impact of caregiving
   c. Burden is a subjective state reflecting the amount of inconvenience and discomfort experienced by caregivers as they carry out tasks to assist impaired or ill relatives
   d. Signs and symptoms
      (1) Depression, demoralization; family conflict
      (2) Feeling stressed, worried
      (3) Not enough resources to provide the care needed (NANDA, 1994, p. 44)
   e. Prevalence unknown, but expected to increase as more people are affected with HIV, the trend toward home care continues, family members assume more responsibility for care
   f. Risk factors
      (1) Illness characteristics
         (a) Severe illness
         (b) Changes in preexisting patient behaviors or manifestation of new symptoms
         (c) Suddenness of illness onset
      (2) Caregiver variables
         (a) Sex: Women tend to show higher levels of distress than men
         (b) Role relationship: Parents of young children may be particularly vulnerable
         (c) Age
         (d) Socioeconomic status
      (3) Other life stressors (e.g., poor health

of caregiver or other family members, as in multiinfected family living with HIV)
         (a) Prior psychologic adjustment
         (b) Relationship cohesiveness
      (4) Other
         (a) Relationship communication skills
         (b) Family developmental stage
         (c) Social support (see p. 272)

2. Etiology
   a. Unrelenting nature of caring for a person with a debilitating condition
   b. The vast array and large number of service organizations and providers with whom the caregiver must interact
   c. Financial constraints
   d. Isolation from friends, family, community
   e. Fear of contagion
   f. Multiple losses (e.g., possible death of a loved one, a lifestyle, a future)
   g. Changing relationship between ill person and caregiver
   h. Pervasive uncertainty about the meaning of symptoms, the future of caregiving, and strategies to provide the best care for the loved one

3. Goals of Care
   a. To enhance the quality of life for both caregiver and ill person
   b. To prevent illness, disability, psychiatric and physical morbidity of the caregiver

4. *Key points*
   a. To date, there has been no research to evaluate strategies to prevent or to treat caregiver burden in AIDS family caregivers and few descriptive studies examining its prevalence or characteristics; many recommendations presented here are extrapolated either from descriptive studies of AIDS family caregivers or from the caregiving literature in populations with other chronic illnesses (e.g., cancer, dementia), but even these studies report conflicting results
      (1) AIDS family caregiving may resemble caregiving for patients with cancer

(2) The stigma of AIDS may cause differences and result in isolation; also, the AIDS caregiver may be HIV-positive and therefore confronting many of the same issues

(3) Women with HIV who are caring for children with HIV may be at high risk for role strain as they focus more on their child's care while having to cope with their own health problems and declining health

b. The major burden for AIDS family caregivers arises from the enormous demands of providing care

  (1) Burden may be aggravated by conflicts between different families (e.g., between family of origin and family of choice) about how to care for PWA

  (2) Burden may be increased for parent and sibling caregivers who have negative attitudes toward homosexuality if PWA is gay, or toward substance abuse if PWA is currently abusing or had abused

c. Although primarily used in research, several evaluation instruments that assess caregiver burden may be useful in clinical situations (Vilaliano, Russo, Young, Becker, & Maiuro, 1991; Vilaliano, Young, & Russo, 1991)

5. Assessment

a. Risk factors and etiologies

b. Caregivers' subjective perception of tasks they perform

  (1) How easy or difficult is each task?

  (2) To what extent does caregiving cause strain with regard to work, finances, and emotional and physical status, social life?

  (3) Resultant depression, anxiety, and changes in caregiver's health status

6. Interventions

a. Work in partnership with the PWA and caregiver to provide appropriate care

  (1) Validate importance of caregiver's role, commitment to PWA, and knowledge base related to caregiving

  (2) Discuss strategies caregiver can use to interact with healthcare providers to secure high quality care for the loved one

b. Teach universal precautions and basic nursing skills as necessary (e.g., skin care, personal hygiene, medication administration); provide necessary written materials

c. When family expresses readiness, suggest readings about other families who have struggled with AIDS (see Selected References on facing page)

d. Assist caregivers to find meaning in their caregiving experiences by asking, "What does caregiving mean to you?" "What has caregiving been like for you?"

e. Explore caregiver's strengths and weaknesses

f. Discuss goals of caregiving as perceived by the caregiver (e.g., quality vs. quantity of care, any conflict with the ill person's goals)

g. Refer to community services (family caregiver courses, counseling, support groups, respite care services, home care) as needed

h. Discuss feelings associated with possibility of deciding to institutionalize the ill person or to end family caregiving role; assist in problem solving

i. Provide information about disease process, expected course of illness, diagnostic tests, medical treatments, and symptom management as appropriate with interpretation of new symptoms and manifestations of illness, particularly changes in PWA's mental status

j. Facilitate problem solving related to treatment decisions

k. Refer for case management services to assist in coordinating care

l. Discuss coping strategies: Taking one day at a time, letting go of what is not important, putting the future on hold, cherishing special moments and time spent with loved ones

m. Discuss importance of the caregiver's taking care of self through health-promotion activities, particularly if the caregiver is also HIV-positive

  (1) Stress-reduction techniques

(2) Proper nutrition, adequate rest/ sleep

(3) Maintaining activity and exercise patterns; taking time-out periods

(4) Avoiding substance use/abuse

n. Assist in mobilizing resources, friends, and family to help in caregiving activities; role play asking for help

o. Assist parent and sibling caregivers to understand choices and lifestyles of gay family members and to understand gay relationships, particularly in the context of a chronic, life-threatening illness

p. Discuss, in conjunction with the PWA, healthcare durable power of attorney and living will; refer for legal assistance if indicated

q. Discuss uncertainty related to caregiving, its sources, manifestations, and ways to manage or to accept it

r. Discuss how the family caregiver can promote the PWA's sense of autonomy and independence

s. Encourage caregiver to discuss relationship difficulties with PWA to resolve feelings of burden and resentment; encourage caregiver to ask the PWA for things he/she is able to give (e.g., thank you, words of appreciation)

t. Facilitate caregiver's ability to provide care when PWA is hospitalized

u. See *Alterations in Family Functioning*, p. 243

7. Selected References for Family Members

Brown, M., & Powell-Cope, G. (1992). *Caring for a loved one with AIDS: The experiences of families.* Seattle, WA: University of Washington Press. (*A guide for family caregivers based on a study of the experiences of AIDS family caregivers*)

Eidson, T. (Ed.). (1993). *The AIDS caregiver's handbook* (rev. ed.). New York: St Martin's Press. (*A comprehensive guide for caregivers*)

Centers for Disease Control. (Undated). *Caring for someone with AIDS.* Washington, DC: U.S. Department of Health and Human Services, Public Health Services. (*Information pamphlet for friends and family members who care for a person with AIDS at home*)

Glaser, E., & Palmer, L. (1992). *In the absence of angels.* New York: Berkeley Publishing. (*An account of a woman's family and their fight against AIDS in herself and her two children*)

Moffatt, B., Spiegel, J., Parrish, S., & Helquist, M. (1987). *AIDS: A self-care manual.* Los Angeles: AIDS Project Los Angeles. (*Covers a wide range of issues of concern for caregivers including testing, medical treatment, psychosocial issues, resources*)

Monette, P. (1988). *Borrowed time: An AIDS memoir.* New York: Avon Books. (*A powerful account of a man caring for his lover*)

Shelby, R. (1992). *If a partner has AIDS.* New York: Harrington Press. (*Described as a guide to clinical intervention for relationships in crisis, but also useful to lay readers who want to understand more about the psychosocial experiences of AIDS*)

F. Grief and Loss

1. Definition/Description

a. Loss

(1) The experience of parting with a valued object, person, belief, or relationship

(2) A loss necessitates a reorganization of one or more aspects of a person's life

(3) Losses vary in significance: May be minor or major

b. Grief

(1) A person's reaction to a loss; has emotional, cognitive, physical, behavioral components

(2) The grieving process helps a person break ties with who or what is lost and adapt to life after the loss

c. Mourning

(1) The process of participating in socially and culturally dictated behaviors after a loss

(2) Does not necessarily indicate the presence of grief

d. Factors influencing grief response

(1) Individual characteristics: Age, personality, usual coping pattern, previous experiences with loss, physical

and mental health, spiritual/religious beliefs, concurrent stressors
   (2) Illness/death circumstances: Amount of forewarning; degree of pain, disfigurement, or mental deterioration
   (3) Social support, economic status
  e. Anticipatory grief: Precedes the loss, helps prepare for the impending loss; if prolonged, may impair resolution of grief
  f. Phases of grief: Shock, protest, disorganization, reorganization
  g. Dysfunctional grief: Prolonged grieving, exaggeration of grief manifestations, absence of grief
2. Etiology: Loss of significant other, body part or function, significant object (e.g., home, car, lifestyle, health insurance)
3. Goals of Care
  a. To facilitate progress of patient/family/significant other through the grieving process
  b. To identify people at risk for dysfunctional grief
4. Key points
  a. Indications a person is coping adaptively with the loss include: Talking about the loss, finding meaning in life or, if dying, in death; developing effective coping strategies, maintaining physical health
  b. HIV-infected persons and their caregivers experience numerous losses throughout the disease process
  c. Signs and symptoms of normal grief (e.g., fatigue, weight loss, difficulty concentrating) in the HIV-infected patient or family member may be misinterpreted as evidence of disease progression
  d. The risk of suicide in the HIV bereaved is higher than in the general population
  e. Grief associated with HIV infection is often complicated by: Stigma, fear of contagion, disclosure issues, discrimination, multiple losses, uncertainty
5. Assessment
  a. The individual experiencing grief and loss: Manifestations of normal grieving

   (1) Emotional: Denial, sadness, anger, guilt, relief, loneliness
   (2) Physical: Sleep disturbances, appetite problems, chest pain, weight loss, fatigue
   (3) Cognitive: Difficulty making decisions, preoccupation with thoughts of what was lost, loss of interest, life perceived as meaningless
   (4) Behavioral: Accident prone, neglect of appearance, increased use of alcohol or drugs, poor health habits
   (5) Social: Withdrawn
   (6) Almost all responses are normal during early phase of grief
      (a) Many remain intense for 6–9 months
      (b) Should decrease in intensity over time
  b. The family experiencing grief and loss
   (1) Family resources: Physical/financial, emotional
   (2) Family stressors: HIV/AIDS-related stressors, concurrent stressors or problems
   (3) Family function: Adaptability, cohesion, roles
   (4) Stage of family development
   (5) Children's grief responses
      (a) Effect of developmental age on grief
      (b) Differences in children's grief from adults
  c. Needs of grieving children
   (1) Openness
   (2) Talk at the child's level of understanding
   (3) Assurance the child will be taken care of
  d. Special concerns related to children
   (1) How and when to disclose HIV status
   (2) Children's ability to maintain confidentiality
   (3) Potential discrimination against children
6. Interventions
  a. During anticipatory grief
   (1) Mobilize support systems
   (2) Connect with a hospice program
   (3) Encourage spiritual/religious practices

(4) Suggest alternative healing strategies (e.g., self-hypnosis, visualization, biofeedback)

(5) Encourage expression of thoughts, feelings; listen and be supportive

(6) Support all behavior and responses as long as they are not destructive to self or others

b. During the shock phase of grief

(1) Protect bereaved from physical harm

(2) Provide physical care if needed

(3) Encourage expression of diverse thoughts and emotions

(4) Help person to mobilize own support system

(5) Remind person to use coping behaviors proven effective in the past

(6) Encourage to participate in mourning rituals

(7) Support all nondestructive behaviors and responses

c. During protest phase of grief

(1) Provide guidance about the grieving process

(2) Refer for financial and legal assistance prn

(3) Remind to maintain physical health
   (a) Discourage use of alcohol, drugs, and caffeine
   (b) Promote appropriate sleep and exercise habits

(4) Continue to encourage expression of thoughts and feelings

(5) Provide opportunities for reminiscence about who or what was lost

(6) Encourage involvement in spiritual/religious activities

(7) Provide role models who have successfully coped with a similar loss

(8) Introduce new coping behaviors

d. During disorganization phase

(1) Continue interventions begun in shock phase

(2) Refer to self-help groups or group/individual counseling; see *Individual Psychotherapy*, p. 345, *Support Groups*, p. 348

(3) Counsel regarding avoiding making major lifestyle decisions (e.g., selling home, quitting job, moving out of the country)

e. During reorganization phase

(1) Encourage new or renewed interests: Refer to career counseling, educational programs, social activity programs

(2) Foster development of a realistic memory of the deceased

f. For people who manifest dysfunctional/maladaptive (self-destructive) behavior, refer to appropriate mental health services

G. Guilt

1. Definition/Description

a. Self-blame for some error, omission, or imperfection; any symbol of the error may trigger a torrent of guilty, negative thoughts (e.g., "If only I had been a better son, my mother would not have died.")

b. To reduce distress, patients may avoid situations that trigger guilt and later fail to recognize what precipitates self-accusatory thoughts

c. Perceptions of guilt may be based on reality or fantasy (e.g., "If I had been sober, I would not have infected my lover.")

d. Types

(1) Self-accusations for acts committed or omissions (e.g., "I should have used protection" or "I should not have survived."); guilty people often ignore the limits of their control or ability to prevent outcomes

(2) Survivor, anticipatory, altruistic, real or imagined guilt (e.g., "I never told my father I loved him, so he died unhappy."); guilt may arise out of altruism and an exaggerated sense of responsibility for the happiness and well-being of others

(3) Attached to behaviors (e.g., burdening loved ones, exposing others to illness, surviving illness or trauma when others did not)

(4) Separation guilt: The belief that one is harming loved ones by leaving them

2. Etiology

a. Internal locus of control: People with an internal locus of control tend to blame themselves instead of others for poor outcomes

b. Stigma: People with HIV infection and their caregivers may feel guilty because they are associated with a stigmatized disease (see *Stigma*, p. 274)

c. Guilt may arise when one's behavior is associated with increasing risk of disease (e.g., people with HIV disease may be blamed for their sexual/drug-use history)

d. Survivor guilt: People believe they have received a benefit or were spared at the expense of others

e. Guilt may be associated with religious or early family patterns that inculcated shame, guilt, or excessive responsibility

3. Goal of Care: To help the patient explore feelings of guilt and to reduce associated distress

4. *Key points*

a. Guilty feelings often influence decision making and indecisiveness (e.g., "I don't want to live with my parents; I need to live with my lover but can't deprive my parents by leaving.")

b. HIV/AIDS encourages guilt

c. Guilt becomes pathologic and requires treatment when it

  (1) Interferes with life activities or relationships

  (2) Promotes excessive use of alcohol or drugs

  (3) Triggers severe depression/suicidal ideas

d. Pathologic guilt is often associated with complicated bereavement (e.g., the bereaved who gives up his/her life and takes on the life of the deceased or keeps everything as a shrine to the deceased)

e. Some people are often reluctant to give up guilt

  (1) Guilt may have benefits

  (2) Many people may be accustomed to functioning with some degree of guilt that provides motivation or compels action but does not lead to immobility

5. Assessment

a. Explore type of guilt and related behaviors (e.g., patient discounts good feelings or accomplishments), risk factors and etiology (e.g., child abuse, early childhood trauma, alcoholism or depression, pessimism, internalization)

b. Differentiate if guilt is recent, temporary, a relatively permanent burden, or if it is related to overstepping moral principles

c. Determine potential consequences if guilt continues or includes survivor guilt; evaluate for depression

d. Determine patterns of self-criticism (e.g., belief that problems are due to some disgraceful deficiency in the self that may lead to unrealistic self-blame)

  (1) Is patient aware of pervasiveness of self-criticism or self-blame and able to consider alternate, external causes of the problem

  (2) Ask "If I made your mistakes, would you despise me?" If the patient is more tolerant of others than self, self-criticism may be exaggerated.

e. Assess patient's ability to ask rational questions in response to deprecatory self-blaming, guilty thoughts; can the patient consider different actions are not guaranteed to alter outcome (e.g., Jim felt guilty—that his lover's death was his fault because he didn't hospitalize him sooner. Yet his lover, Fred, was always stubborn and refused hospitalization. Fred had his way regardless of nudging.)

6. Interventions

a. Label and examine guilt feelings

  (1) Ask the patient to keep and discuss a diary or log of precipitants, thoughts, feelings associated with guilt

  (2) The log helps patient focus on a specific problem related to guilt (e.g., survivor guilt) and examine precipitants (e.g., excess work; unrealistic expectations; exaggerated difficulties)

b. Build a trusting relationship

(1) Accept patient's feelings; evaluate patient's ability to observe, describe, and label the sequelae of guilt (e.g., guilt leads you to avoid your family and delay resolving these relationships so you blame yourself more)

(2) Accept patients who prefer to keep guilt private; if they do not elect to share with you, encourage to have at least one other person (e.g., counselor, chaplain) to confide in

(3) Can the patient examine the costs/benefits of guilt feelings (e.g., "I wonder if the guilt keeps you from encountering rejection or support")?

(4) Reduce factors that potentiate guilt, when possible

  (a) Excessive anticipation of personal power or control over external circumstances, excess responsibility, low self-esteem, irrational ideas

  (b) Predisposition to feel guilt or shame when things were not perfect or mistakes were made

  (c) Unrealistic perception of limits of personal control or realistic perception that one's error led to serious negative consequences for others

c. Educate/encourage patient to

(1) Examine, test, and describe reality

  (a) Patients need to change "should" to "could"

  (b) Test the associations between guilt and feelings of being a failure

(2) Challenge irrational or unrealistic expectations by suggesting that some of these expectations may be impossible to accomplish; if the person feels guilty for not being perfect or not always meeting others' needs, suggest that these goals are impossible for everyone else also

(3) List thoughts and feelings associated with guilt; discuss options and conclusions for each item (e.g., "You feel guilty you didn't resolve difficulties with your sister and tell her you loved her before she died. What did you conclude? Perhaps she knew you loved her?")

(4) Introduce the concept of forgiveness instead of excessive punishment for a mistake; patients can list their offenses to others, offer apologies, and make amends to those who have been offended or harmed

(5) Introduce concept of a trial and the ideas that the patient has

  (a) Tried him/herself and been found guilty and forever sentenced to punishment

  (b) Been deprived of due process or even presumed innocence

(6) Identify religious practices (e.g., confession, prayer) or alternate spiritual practices (e.g., laying on of hands, talismans) to relieve guilt; refer to pastoral counselors, chaplains, psychiatric liaison nurses or psychosocial counselors; see *Therapeutic Touch*, p. 329

(7) Consider psychologic practices involving use of the mind (e.g., distraction, imagery, attitude change practices, visualization, hypnosis) that can also be used to alleviate guilt

d. Educate family about the precipitants of guilt and ways to reduce pessimism; encourage consideration of alternative, external explanations for problems

e. Use humor cautiously to help patient manage guilt; when patient accepts excess responsibility for things beyond his/her control, suggest with humor that it must be difficult when others expect the patient to have power or magic to control the weather or sunrise; see *Humor*, p. 353

f. Advocate that patient's informed decisions regarding going for further treatment are respected and such decisions are not guilt-inducing experiences about letting family or providers down

g. Evaluate and intervene to help family provide understanding and support when family conflict increases patient's guilt

h. Avoid strategies that encourage guilt

such as telling patients what they "should" do

   i. Help patient set goals that are realistic and reflective of the patient's, not others', wishes/expectations

H. High Risk for Ineffective Management of Therapeutic Regimen

1. Definition/Description
   a. A nursing diagnosis to use when there is the potential or probability that a patient will not be able to self-manage own treatment regimen effectively
   b. NANDA (1994) definition: "A pattern of regulating and integrating into daily living a program for treatment of illness and the sequelae of illness that is unsatisfactory for meeting specific health" (p. 56)
2. Etiology
   a. OIs that result in functional, cognitive, or sensory deficits
   b. Care environment lacking necessary resources to manage the illness or to allow the patient to remain safe at home
   c. Psychosocial factors, e.g.
      (1) Lack or loss of income, insurance, family/caregiver support
      (2) Lack of available community resources
      (3) Depression or coping difficulties that interfere with patient's self-care or decision-making abilities
      (4) Substance use interfering with adherence to self-care activities
      (5) Denial interfering with adherence to treatment or self-care activities
3. Goals of Care
   a. To coordinate services that match the patient's needs with goals and wishes over time
   b. To develop a care regimen that patient is able and willing to follow
4. *Key points*
   a. The complications and treatment demands of HIV disease make requirements for a therapeutic regimen extremely complex and seemingly never ending

   b. Other life events (e.g., role responsibilities, housing) may affect the patient's ability to manage (or adhere to) the therapeutic regimen
   c. Nurses need to be knowledgeable about and sensitive to day-to-day implications of treatments on patients' lives and the availability of supportive services
   d. Depending on patient's status, family/caregiver support, care environment, and community resources, different aspects of assessment and intervention will apply
   e. Competent patients may make less-than-optimal care decisions; unless their decisions compromise the safety of others or their decision-making capacity is impaired, there may be no direct intervention the nurse can take to change or control these situations
5. Assessment: Assess strengths and deficits in each area to answer, "Can the patient's care, safety, and treatment needs be met by the family/caregivers with the resources available in the care environment and community?"
   a. Functional ability; ADL, recent falls, sensory functions (vision, hearing), speech/communication, language, literacy
   b. Cognitive functioning: Adequacy of short- and long-term memory, ability to concentrate, decision-making/problem-solving abilities, orientation
   c. Mental health: Affect/mood, usual coping strategies and effectiveness; self-esteem; history of mental illness/treatment; substance use; culture, lifestyle, spiritual beliefs/behaviors
   d. Patient's beliefs/wishes related to current situation
      (1) Perceptions/meanings associated with HIV status
      (2) Belief in importance of adhering to prescribed regimen
      (3) Perceived adequacy of social support
      (4) Meaning of quality of life
      (5) Short- and long-term goals related to treatment and care
   e. Family/caregiver support

(1) Parenting, other caregiving responsibilities
(2) See *Family Caregiver Burden/Strain,* p. 251, *Social Support,* p. 272
  f. Care environment
(1) Housing (homeless, temporary shelter, permanent housing)
(2) Safety (e.g., steps in home, structural defects, violence in home/housing or community)
(3) Access to and adequacy of basic needs (e.g., running water, heat, condition of toilet, telephone, refrigerator)
  g. Illness and treatment demands
(1) Current medical problems
(2) Medication regimen
(3) Chronic or distressing symptoms
(4) Other treatments, including complementary ones; see *Wellness Strategies,* p. 237
  h. Community resources: Services, eligibility requirements, state and local regulations guiding HIV care
6. Interventions
  a. Patient: Given the complexity of supporting patient's care in the community, all interventions must be negotiated with the patient and family. More than with other aspects of care, reassessment and coordination with other discplines/services are essential.
(1) Work with patient to establish short- and long-term goals concerning living situation options, healthcare regimen, etc.
(2) Work with family/caregiver and patient to set up a regimen to meet these goals; include as much self-care and decision making as possible
(3) Educate patient in a manner that is culturally appropriate regarding
    (a) Possible course of HIV disease and management of possible opportunistic event
    (b) Importance of adherence to treatment to ensure maximum benefit
(4) Refer to social worker or lawyer for assistance with DPOA or guardian-

ship as indicated, living will, last will and testament
(5) Collaborate with primary care provider/others to simplify regimen whenever possible (e.g.. eliminate medications no longer necessary or marginally effective)
(6) If you are concerned about the patient's decision-making capacity, consult with the primary care provider on need for psychiatric consultation for competency evaluation or possible neuropsychologic testing
(7) Refer for mental health or substance-abuse assistance as indicated
(8) Consult with social worker/dietitian/case manager to evaluate patient eligibility for special programs/services according to need (e.g., pharmacy providing overnight drug delivery, Medicaid program coverage of nutritional supplements)
(9) Promote patient's understanding of actual or potential effects of denial, substance abuse, or lack of adequate support in home on patient's ability to maintain therapeutic regimen
(10) Collaborate with primary care provider for maximal symptom control
  b. Family/caregivers
(1) Obtain patient's consent to involve family in care before implementing any of the remaining interventions
(2) Facilitate family/caregivers meeting to communicate patient wishes, evaluate adequacy of supports, delegate care tasks, etc.
(3) Educate on HIV transmission precautions in the home and specific care tasks required (e.g., medication administration, proper body mechanics for patient transfers)
(4) Counsel on anticipating care requirements of patient and how to integrate the necessary caregiving activities into daily life
(5) Refer for personal care services, chore provisions grant, or buddy

services when indicated and as available

(6) Arrange for patient day-care services in instances when primary caregiver is employed or other supports are lacking or insufficient

(7) Refer to caregiver respite program when indicated and as available

c. Care environment
   (1) Arrange for home health nursing services for skilled care needs and evaluation of care adequacy in home
   (2) Facilitate arrangement for outpatient, ambulatory, or home administration of medical therapies when possible and appropriate
   (3) Evaluate safety of care environment; modify environment to decrease risk of injury
   (4) Arrange delivery of medical equipment to care environment congruent with patient needs (e.g., wheelchair, bedside commode, hospital bed)
   (5) Consult social worker to arrange for placement at a skilled nursing facility, hospice, residential living program, physical rehabilitation program, substance-abuse program or other facility consistent with patient's wishes or short- and long-term goals
   (6) Consult social worker for utilities shut off or lack of heat, electricity, telephone, refrigerator

d. Community
   (1) Advocate for provision of needed services at local or state level (e.g., day care, respite care, skilled nursing facilities accepting patients with HIV disease)
   (2) Public/agency education to diminish fear and ignorance leading to prohibition of services for HIV patients
   (3) Refer patients to legal assistance for discrimination complaints or barriers to appropriate access to services because of HIV status or lifestyle issues
   (4) Collaborate with other people and agencies supportive of appropriate

service provisions to people with HIV disease to focus on service gaps or communitywide issues and problems

(5) Lobby at local, state, and national levels for public policies and laws supportive of fair service provision for people with HIV disease

I. Hopelessness

1. Definition/Description
   a. A subjective state in which an individual sees limited or no alternatives or personal choices available and is unable to mobilize energy on own behalf (NANDA, 1994)
      (1) May be specific to a particular situation or may reflect a general perspective on life
      (2) May be limited to a brief period, or become so enduring it resembles a trait rather than an emotional state
      (3) The feeling of discouragement, combined with a belief that nothing can improve, promotes inactivity so alternative approaches are often not considered or attempted
   b. Can be experienced at different levels of intensity
      (1) At a low level hopelessness may not always progress to a more severe level, but progression is always a possibility
      (2) Inadequate tangible resources (e.g., shelter, food, health care, transportation) or distressing symptoms can quickly escalate feelings of hopelessness

2. Etiology
   a. Depression is most often associated with hopelessness
      (1) Often severe, continues until the depression is successfully treated
      (2) Low self-esteem or a past history of depression or hopelessness predispose a person to feeling hopeless
      (3) Hopelessness, by itself, is not sufficient for a diagnosis of depression
   b. Persistent and severe hopelessness often leads to suicide

c. Recurrent crises, multiple losses, chemical dependency, and other psychiatric problems: Many people with HIV/AIDS have experienced multiple losses that may reduce resistance to hopelessness via recurrent episodes of grief and a reduced network of close friends

d. Being stigmatized (e.g., from HIV/AIDS, homosexuality, drug use) may prompt some to fight back while others may feel the odds are too great and succumb to feelings of hopelessness; see *Stigma*, p. 274

3. Goals of Care

  a. To guide the patient toward feelings of hopefulness

  b. To help the patient initiate strategies to prevent recurrence of hopelessness

4. *Key points*

  a. The nurse must take immediate action when the patient endangers personal safety or threatens existing resources

    (1) The most immediate threat to personal safety is suicidal behavior associated with the triad of depression, helplessness, and hopelessness

      (a) 80% of depressions usually respond well to treatment

      (b) Hopelessness and depression are painful experiences

    (2) If untreated, suicidal thoughts can progress to suicide attempts and premature death; indicators of a severe threat of suicide include a well-formulated plan, lethal method, access and means to carry out plan

  b. Family and friends may respond to the hopeless person's increasing isolation, irritability, or sense of pessimism by distancing themselves from negative interactions. Taking action promptly may prevent social relationships from deteriorating at a time when the person most needs access to supportive friends and family.

  c. When social resources have always been scarce, the hopeless person will probably not have enough interest or energy to become involved in new groups or activities. A vicious cycle of withdrawal, diminishing resources, and intensification of hopelessness can develop if action does not interrupt this cycle.

  d. Hopefulness is not unrealistic even during terminal illness; hopefulness does not represent denial of the patient's current situation

5. Assessment

  a. Severity of hopelessness, most often revealed by a person's verbalizations or behaviors

    (1) Mild

      (a) "No point in my planning on an education now."

      (b) "It doesn't matter if I try that new treatment or not, they are all the same—poison of one kind or another."

      (c) "Why tell my family? They've never cared what happens to me before—why would they care now?"

      (d) Mild social withdrawal

      (e) Increased fatigue

      (f) Decreased motivation

      (g) Inconsistency in following treatment, diet, that formerly were followed

      (h) Increase in unhealthy behaviors (e.g., drinking, smoking, unsafe sexual practices, using street drugs)

    (2) Severe

      (a) "There is no future for me."

      (b) "I've given up. There's nothing for me now. I don't even go through the motions any more—just sitting here waiting to die."

      (c) "Nothing will help. The federal government is playing politics and the drug companies are just after money. There won't be a cure."

      (d) Apathy, lack of interest or ambition

      (e) Rejection of social overtures made by others

      (f) Pessimism, indecisiveness

      (g) Lack of assuming responsibility for self

(h) Rejection of medications and therapies that formerly had been important

(i) Deterioration of personal environment and appearance

b. Internal resources

(1) How has the person confronted and managed personal and health problems in the past: Diverse problem-solving strategies or reliance on one or two approaches? Effectiveness?

(2) Does the person portray the future as holding something good for him/herself?

(3) What feelings does the person experience?

(4) Recent changes in the person's spiritual beliefs?

(5) How does the person see the world today and tomorrow (bleak and empty, or good and meaningful)? Are perspectives distorted through overgeneralizations, personalization, concreteness, negativeness?

c. Medical and personal history: Is there

(1) A history of depression? of reliance on drugs or alcohol during times of stress?

(2) Continuing family discord from previous strain or breaks in family relationships?

6. Interventions

a. Provide support to the patient and supportive others (the most important nursing intervention)

(1) Establish a safe climate and encourage to express feelings

(2) Listen actively and accept the feelings expressed

(3) Monitor the person's sense and perspective of the future

(4) Help differentiate realistic from unrealistic goals

(a) Guide the person in establishing plans to meet goals

(b) Help to formulate contingencies in case one approach is not effective

(5) Help the person recall strategies that have been effective in the past when s/he overcame feelings of hope-lessness; adapt those strategies for use now

b. Provide information about HIV/AIDS as person needs and wants

c. Rehearse the patient for anticipated difficult encounters

d. Provide comfort and relief from stressful emotions via massage, meditation, guided imagery, distractions (e.g., watching videos, particularly comedies)—may help the person reengage emotions toward a safe object; see *Wellness Strategies*, p. 327

e. Refer to support groups, often the most effective therapeutic experiences for people in stressful situations (see *Support Groups*, p. 348)

f. Be alert to indications of progressive hopelessness (e.g., changes in self-care from healthy to unhealthy behavior patterns); monitor for risk behavior such as alcohol/drug use, previous suicide attempts; see *Potential for Violence/Harm to Self or Others*, p. 265

g. Refer to spiritual counselors/clergy to explore existential suffering or spiritual conflicts

J. Mania and Psychosis

1. Definition/Description

a. States in which the patient has a decreased ability to recognize reality, relate to others, and generally deal with the demands of life

(1) Thinking and behavior are disorganized, often bizarre

(2) There is a noticeable decline in functioning compared to premorbid abilities

b. Mania is an elevated mood accompanied by increased motor activity, rapid speech, decreased need for rest, and emotional lability

(1) May include altered perceptions: Delusions, hallucinations, disorganized speech or behavior

(2) Impaired judgment may lead to harmful behavior (e.g., indiscriminate sexual activity, impulsive deci-

sions, overspending, alcohol or drug use)

    (3) Usually feels good; patients are often reluctant to accept treatment; may be a psychologic defense against depression

  c. Psychosis is an alteration in thinking, perception, or affect

    (1) Patients may experience hallucinations (auditory, visual, or olfactory), which can be pleasant, neutral, or frightening

    (2) Delusions are common; paranoid delusions may be frightening

  d. Prevalence

    (1) Mania in a person without a history of bipolar disease usually occurs late in HIV disease

    (2) Exact rate of HIV infection in patients with mania or psychosis is unknown

  e. Risk factors: Preexisting major mental illness, lifelong maladaptive coping patterns, organic brain changes

2. Etiology: Both mania and psychosis may stem from neurochemical changes, may be psychodynamically influenced, may be side effects of medications (e.g., AZT, NSAIDs), may be related to other organic causes (e.g., CNS lesions, infection)

3. Goals of Care

  a. To maintain the safety both of the patient and others in the environment

  b. To decrease the manic or psychotic symptoms so the patient has increased behavioral control

4. *Key points*

  a. Mania and depression are extremes of a bipolar disorder

  b. Patient has poor control of his/her behavior; safety is an issue

  c. Patient may feel out of control and frightened

  d. Issues of safe sex and drug use must be addressed (patients may have poor judgment or be vulnerable to others)

5. Assessment

  a. Mental status examination

    (1) Appearance

      (a) In manic episode, person may dress oddly, wear bizarre or excessive makeup and accessories, or may look tired

      (b) During a psychotic episode, poor self-care may be evident; person may appear to be preoccupied with internal stimuli

        i) A person hearing voices will appear to listen, respond verbally or with body language

        ii) People with paranoid delusions may be hyperalert, constantly scanning the milieu

    (2) Mood

      (a) Manic mood is generally expansive; person may be labile; elation may change suddenly to anger

      (b) In psychosis, mood is usually bland; person may become irritable or angry if feeling threatened; mood and affect may be incongruent; person may laugh while describing horrifying hallucinations

    (3) Thinking

      (a) In mania, rapid associations or flight of ideas may be present; delusions (particularly of grandeur or persecution), illusions, distortions are common; hallucinations are less common

      (b) Psychotic thinking is characterized by disorganized or incoherent thoughts or by a paucity of thinking

    (4) Attention and concentration

      (a) In a manic state, patient is easily distracted

      (b) Psychotic patient may be preoccupied with internal stimuli and unable to focus on reality

    (5) Judgment may be gravely impaired in both mania and psychosis (patient is unable to recognize potentially dangerous situations or behavior)

  b. Signs and symptoms

    (1) Mania: Inflated self-esteem, increased energy, racing thoughts,

expansive mood, rapid or pressured speech, flight of ideas, rapid movements, sleeplessness

    (2) Psychosis: Delusions, illusions, hallucinations, disorganized or incoherent speech, grossly disorganized behavior, negative symptoms (flat affect, isolation, minimal or no speech)

6. Interventions

  a. Administer/monitor effects of medications

    (1) Mood stabilizers

      (a) Slow (several days) response time; benzodiazepines provide more immediate control

      (b) Lithium is effective but not completely safe in HIV-positive patients (has a high risk of toxicity due to potential fluid imbalance in HIV patients)

      (c) Valproic acid is generally effective and safe

    (2) Neuroleptics

      (a) Fairly rapid onset of action on florid psychotic symptoms; IM administration is faster acting, but may be very threatening or frightening to patient

      (b) Extrapyramidal tract signs can be severe in HIV

      (c) HIV-positive patients at risk for neuroleptic malignant syndrome (NMS)

        i) A life-threatening hypersensitivity reaction

        ii) Signs and symptoms include fever, muscle rigidity, elevated CPK, altered consciousness, tachycardia, leukocytosis

      (d) Midpotency neuroleptics offer best balance between EPS and anticholinergic effects; perphenazine is usually effective and well-tolerated by HIV-positive patients

      (e) Benzodiazepines can help and work synergistically with neuroleptics, allowing lower doses

  b. Maintain calm, safe environment

    (1) Manic patients do better in a low-stimulus environment

      (a) Low light and noise levels

      (b) Limited contact with others

      (c) Staff with calm demeanor are therapeutic

      (d) Physical exercise can safely expend energy

    (2) Psychotic patients need to feel safe

      (a) May be experiencing paranoid delusions or hallucinations

      (b) A calm response to frightening symptoms is therapeutic: Reorient and reassure; speak clearly, simply, quietly; state expectations clearly; consistency among staff is reassuring to patient

    (3) Establish a relationship with patient

      (a) A trusted staff person can create a feeling of safety

      (b) Accept and respect the person while helping to manage the psychosis; even the very psychotic are aware of how they are treated, and may describe it after acute episode resolves

      (c) It is not therapeutic to challenge psychotic thoughts that are very real to the patient

      (d) Explore fears and safety needs; patient may be able to say exactly what he or she needs to feels safe

      (e) Work as closely with family/support system as patient will allow

        i) Provides continuity of care and the consistency patient needs

        ii) Helps patient feel cared for

  c. Recognize culture-specific aspects of behavior

    (1) Involve family, friends, bicultural staff in obtaining history and planning interventions

    (2) Psychotic symptoms are usually symbolic of important issues and are culturally influenced

  d. Educate and support family/significant other

(1) Behavior that is out of control or bizarre evokes strong, often negative, feelings; education can help others to understand the process of the illness and be able to accept and support the patient

(2) Support groups can help to decrease isolation, increase problem solving (family or friends may blame themselves, others, or the patient)

K. Potential for Violence/Harm to Self or Others Related to Suicidality or Assaultive Behavior

1. Definition/Description
   a. Assaultive behavior: Destructive or violent aggression directed at others (people or objects in the environment)
   b. Suicide: Self-destructive behaviors that may be active/passive, acute/chronic, conscious/unconscious and that result in a person causing his/her death; further characterized by the nature of the action/intention
      (1) Attempt: An act intended to result in death; a "successful" attempt results in death
      (2) Gesture: An act intended to be an attempt but that results in minimal self-harm (e.g., overdose with very few pills ingested; superficial cuts to wrist/groin/ankle)
      (3) Threat: Verbal statement of intent to commit suicide (e.g., "I'm going to kill myself.")
      (4) Ideation: Thoughts about intent to attempt suicide
   c. Many patients infected with HIV experience neuropsychiatric complications
      (1) Complications become more profound as HIV disease progresses
      (2) Patient may have initial presenting symptomatology that makes the real etiology confusing
   d. It is never safe to assume that violence, whether self-harm (suicide) or intent to harm others (assaultive behavior), stems solely from a psychologic etiology;

investigation must include all possibilities to determine the behavior, treat it appropriately, and provide relief from the symptom
   e. Fear, loss of control, hopelessness, and isolation may contribute to overwhelming despair and to the possibility of harm, either self- or other-directed, in people with HIV disease

2. Etiology
   a. Assaultive behavior
      (1) Infection of the brain
      (2) Metabolic abnormalities related to pentamidine, sepsis, impaired liver function, diabetes/endocrine disorders, chemical dependency, seizure disorder
      (3) Organic impairment of the brain: Delirium, dementia, alcohol related
      (4) Hypoxia: Secondary to pneumonia, chemical-induced (e.g., cocaine, alcohol, heroin, hallucinogens/amphetamines)
      (5) Vitamin deficiencies (B_{12}, B_1, folate)
      (6) Personality disorders: Antisocial, borderline
      (7) Psychosis
      (8) Medication toxicity (e.g., corticosteroids)
      (9) History of impulse behavior (e.g., reckless driving, destruction of property, history of violence directed at others)
   b. Suicidality
      (1) Stigma
      (2) Untreated/inadequate symptom management
      (3) Poor quality of life due to multiple losses
      (4) Inadequate social support system
      (5) Chemical dependency
      (6) Denial as central and only defense mechanism
      (7) Personality traits; aggression, impulsivity, depression, hopelessness, borderline, antisocial
      (8) Psychiatric history: Schizophrenia, familial history (depression, anxiety, chemical dependency, organic mental disorders)
      (9) Spiritual distress

(10) Rational suicide (controversial):
Criteria
    (a) Realistic assessment of situation
    (b) Mental processes not impaired
       by psychologic illness or severe
       emotional distress
    (c) Motivation for committing sui-
       cide is understandable to the
       majority of uninvolved
       observers
(11) CNS involvement
(12) Progression of HIV disease/substan-
tial decrease in CD4+ lymphocyte
count

3. Goals of Care
  a. To prevent episodes of self- or other-
    directed violent behavior
  b. Should violence occur, to control symp-
    toms and promote safety

4. *Key points*
  a. A person who participates in the treat-
    ment plan (e.g., takes medications as
    prescribed, keeps healthcare provider
    appointments) and has established an
    alliance with staff has a *low* risk of vio-
    lent behavior toward others or self
  b. A person with a history of violence is
    considered at *high* risk for subsequent
    violent behavior toward others; when in
    doubt, err on the side of safety and
    intervene expeditiously and as policy
    dictates
  c. Asking about suicide will not cause
    patients to become suicidal; most
    patients are relieved to talk about suici-
    dal thoughts and appreciate the concern
    (this discussion can help alleviate isola-
    tion and hopelessness and create a path
    for education and advocacy)
  d. A person with transient, vague
    thoughts or ideas about suicide but no
    actual plan is considered a *low* suicide
    risk
  e. Frequent thoughts about suicide and
    occasional ideas about a plan is consid-
    ered a *moderate* suicidal risk
  f. A person with frequent/constant
    thoughts or preoccupation with suicide
    and with a specific plan should be con-
    sidered a *high* suicide risk
  g. A person with a history of suicide

attempts *or* who knew someone who
had a "successful" suicide should be
considered at *high* risk for suicide

5. Assessment
  a. Assaultive behavior
    (1) Chief complaint
    (2) Present and past illnesses
       (a) Medications (prescribed vs.
          unprescribed)
       (b) Laboratory findings
    (3) Medication toxicities
    (4) Mental status examination:
       Orientation, memory, judgment
    (5) Vital signs
    (6) Chemical dependency history
    (7) Neuropsychiatric history
    (8) History of violent behavior (how,
       what, when, why, where)
    (9) Relationships, social history
    (10) Behavior, appearance
       (a) Pacing, agitated
       (b) Argumentative, critical, uncoop-
          erative
       (c) Overreaction to external stimuli
          (e.g., noise)
       (d) Angry facial expression and
          body language
       (e) Verbally threatening others (e.g.,
          "Get out of my face." "When I
          get out of here I'm going to kill
          you.")
       (f) Tense
       (g) Grabbing potential weapons and
          attempting to use
       (h) Physical threats (may signify dis-
          appointment or rejection):
          Raising fist, pointing finger in
          face
  b. Suicidality
    (1) Chief complaint
       (a) Verbal: Direct ("I wish I were
          dead."); indirect ("You won't see
          me after your days off.")
       (b) Nonverbal: Hoarding medica-
          tions (especially controlled sub-
          stances), taking utensils off food
          tray
    (2) Present and past illnesses
       (a) Medications (prescribed vs. non-
          prescribed)
       (b) Laboratory findings

(3) Mental status assessment

(4) Medication toxicities

(5) History of chemical dependency

(6) Neuropsychiatric history: Hallucinations, depression, dementia

(7) Symptomatology: Pain, fatigue, GI complaints

(8) Suicide attempts (how, what, when, why, where)

(9) Spiritual distress

(10) Behavior, appearance

    (a) Drawing up a will, giving away personal possessions, agitation, poor grooming

    (b) Refusing medications

(11) Relationship history: Social isolation, recent loss of significant other

(12) Social history: Employment status

(13) Mood/emotions: Hopelessness (sees no future), helplessness, self-esteem, guilt, shame, self-blame

(14) Ask: "Are you planning to kill yourself?" "When are you planning to do it?" "How will you do it?"

c. If a violent episode occurs, investigate the etiology once the patient is symptomatically stable

6. Interventions

a. Refer to psychiatric clinician

b. Monitor response to prescribed medications (neuroleptics, antidepressants)

c. Change the environment as necessary: Move to single room or change roommate, remove actual/potential weapons, move closer to flow of traffic

d. Symptom management; explore issues of quality of life

e. Educate person on current treatment plan; involve in decision making

f. Make a pact with the patient

g. Suggest alternatives to cope with current situation; offer nonsuicidal, nonviolent choices when realistic

h. Give positive reinforcement for exhibiting positive alternative coping skills

i. Ensure staff consistency to avoid splitting and manipulation via treatment plan

j. Provide counseling and support

(1) Establish support and trust of patient/significant other

(2) Refer to support groups as appropriate

(3) Grieving process: See *Grief and Loss*, p. 253

(4) Spiritual support: See *Spiritual Distress*, p. 273

L. Powerlessness

1. Definition/Description

a. Powerlessness: A person's perception that s/he lacks autonomy and is unable to enact his/her will, control another's will, or exert control over situations, events, or life; can be actual or potential

b. Usually refers to the perception that one lacks choices, influence, or freedom to make choices even within their own restrictions

(1) May translate to a sense of impotence and a sense of waiting for whatever life hands out

(2) When the situation requires a number of resources greater than those available (e.g., health insurance benefits), power may be reduced; the patient's realistic assessment of such limited power may produce a sense of powerlessness

c. A sense of power is often associated with actively making choices

d. Powerlessness may be experienced episodically in relation to a specific event (e.g., becoming HIV positive) or may be an ongoing and pervasive experience and world view

e. Powerlessness is *experienced* as feelings of helplessness, discouragement, insignificance; *manifested* by indecision, passivity, dependency, social isolation, and functioning within a restricted range of choices

f. Risk factors that may increase a sense of powerlessness

(1) Past history of emotional distress or major depression

(2) Cultural or lifestyle characteristics

(3) Personality characteristic (e.g., poor self-esteem; change in role identity, diminished sense of personal value

secondary to illness; inability to break a problem into manageable parts)

    (4) Situational characteristics (e.g., healthcare settings do not value the patient as an active participant in own health care)

2. Etiology

  a. Poor ego formation may be implicated psychodynamically in the roots of powerlessness

  b. Interruptions in personal development that occur because of family disruption, major childhood illnesses, etc., may compromise development of a strong sense of self, leaving the person vulnerable to powerless responses during stressful situations

  c. AIDS-related dementia (ARD) offers a scenario of reduced ability to process information and participate effectively in decision making; as ARD progresses, so will powerlessness

3. Goals of Care

  a. To ensure maximal empowerment for the patient, allowing him/her to function as autonomously as possible in healthcare decisions

  b. To provide adequate information regarding disease process, progress, treatment options

4. *Key points*

  a. Patients who feel powerless may fail to act in their own best interest and suffer the consequences in their health status

  b. Empowerment is the process of preventing and correcting powerlessness

  c. When nurses ensure that patients and their families are partners in their care, the power in the nurse-patient relationship is more likely to be distributed evenly between the patient and nurse

5. Assessment: Signs and symptoms

  a. Passivity

  b. Decreased motivation and energy to follow through on treatments

  c. Decreased interest in information formerly viewed as relevant to make informed decisions about choices (the person who used to question nurses about procedures and treatments may

accept changes in approaches with few, if any, comments)

  d. Viewing the healthcare professional as all knowing and powerful

  e. Occasional angry outbursts and expressions of feeling left out or alienated

  f. Indicators of depression and poor self-esteem

  g. Forgetfulness, episodic confusion, or inability to process information to understand consequences of choices

6. Interventions

  a. Build a relationship with the patient to establish an environment where feelings can be expressed, problems explored, self-esteem increased

    (1) Be culturally sensitive to issues of gender, sexual identity, and developmental age

    (2) Use therapeutic communication strategies such as providing empathy, clarification, open-ended questions, feedback; reflecting content and feelings; summarizing

    (3) Help the patient to identify aspects of the situation that s/he can influence

  b. Help patient to participate in healthcare decisions and to function autonomously

    (1) Consider whether the decision choices offered patients are realistic or unrealistic, meaningful or trivial

    (2) Provide information relevant to the situation (e.g., medical treatment, nutrition, community resources, stress management strategies) even if the patient has not requested it

    (3) Use several media (verbal, written, videos) to enhance the patient's potential to use the information; suggest practical applications

  c. If the patient is powerless to act for self

    (1) Represent the patient's perspective when known

    (2) If the patient's wishes are not known, delay action until the patient is able to speak for him/herself

  d. Strengthen patient's physical or social environments by appropriate referrals

(1) Rehabilitation services if mobility problems emerge

(2) Optometric evaluations to enhance vision so patients can continue with activities that are meaningful to them

(3) Support groups (see p. 348) and social activities where patient can meet others with shared interests

(4) See *Grief and Loss*, p. 253, *High Risk for Ineffective Management of Therapeutic Regimen*, p. 258

e. Be alert for behavior changes that signal intensification in feelings of powerlessness

7. Ethical Considerations

a. Ensuring maximal empowerment includes the patient's right to choose a course of action when the consequences are judged as harmful, futile, or neutral; as long as the patient's choice of level and type of involvement in decision making is protected, powerlessness will not be enhanced

b. If it can be anticipated when the patient's ability to act for self is compromised, work with the patient to elicit information about who is the best person to function as the patient's advocate. The Patient Self-Determination Act of 1990 (PSDA) requires nurses in many types of agencies to ask patients about advance directives (living will, do not resuscitate, medical power of attorney).

M. Social Isolation

1. Definition/Description

a. Erikson (1978) identified intimacy vs. isolation as the primary developmental conflict of the young adult

(1) The young adult needs to resolve the intimacy/isolation conflict adequately in order to develop the capacity for commitment to interpersonal relationships, work, and love

(2) Failure to resolve intimacy/isolation conflict will leave the young adult vulnerable to inadequate interpersonal relationships in adult phases;

Erikson believed that prejudice could be linked to inadequate resolution of the intimacy/isolation conflict

b. Carpenito (1993) defined social isolation as being unable to have contacts with others (individuals or groups) with whom we have either a desire or need for contact

c. Isolation involves feelings of separation and loneliness, in addition to impersonal relationships

(1) Durkheim's (1897/1951) concept of alienation, or anomie, includes social isolation; discrimination or prejudice against an individual or group fosters social isolation

(2) Durkheim linked alienation with suicide for men and believed that a man's suicide risk would increase if he were alienated and lacked ties with and social status within his community

d. Adolescents may be especially vulnerable when they try to negotiate intimate relationships because of few role models, personal inexperience, and reliance on peer approval. Gay adolescents are especially prone to feelings of loneliness and isolation because they perceive themselves as different and because they encounter homophobia and internalized homophobia.

e. Intimacy is the quality of a relationship that can be associated with long-standing friends, nuclear family, lovers

(1) Intimate relationships involve trust, closeness, comfortableness, high levels of self-disclosure, and centrality

(a) Capacity for intimacy may be affected by age, sex, and culture

i) Societal disapproval of the type of relationship (homosexual couples, cohabiting, unmarried heterosexual couples) adds barriers to maintaining intimacy

ii) Stigma, such as associated with homosexuality, limits opportunity for satisfactory social interactions for people in the stigmatized groups

(b) Intimate relationships also can be a source of distress and suffering when

   i) One person observes a loved one's unrelieved suffering

   ii) One believes that s/he is the cause of a loved one's discomfort, pain, or illness

(2) Sexual relationships may or may not be included as intimate relationships, although sexual activity is often considered an intimate behavior

(a) Individuals have intimate relationships with others without including sexual activity

(b) Conversely, individuals may have sexual activity as a part of casual, even anonymous relationships

(c) Sexual activity can be an integral and enriching aspect of an intimate relationship

(d) Because sexual activity has often been a vehicle for HIV transmission, added strain may surround sexual interactions for couples because of fear or guilt about infecting a partner, or because of changes in intimate behaviors associated with safer sex precautions

f. Feelings associated with isolation occur when intimate relationships end, through separation or death

(1) Feelings associated with grief can occur in response to the loss of an intimate relationship (see *Grief and Loss*, p. 253)

(2) Many people with HIV/AIDS have lost friends and family (lovers, children, siblings) to AIDS

(3) Some people withdraw from friends because they feel they cannot endure more losses; they would rather not invest in social relationships in order to avoid potential pain

g. Social isolation may occur as illness advances so that progressive symptoms interfere with usual social activities, or leave little energy for relating to others

h. People may report feeling socially isolated when they perceive their social support resources are not meeting their needs

(1) The perception of adequate social support may occur without having anyone available who is described as intimate

(2) The perception of inadequate social support may occur despite having many acquaintances and being involved in many social activities

(3) See *Social Support,* p. 272

2. Etiology

a. Major distress and trauma when the person is attempting to master developmental tasks of attachment

b. Childhood abuse, dysfunctional families, and parental losses during childhood provide obstacles for learning attachment behaviors with others

c. Grief typically produces isolation, usually temporary

d. Social isolation can result when illness or associated symptoms interfere with ability to participate in social activities

3. Goal of Care: To help patient decrease feelings of isolation and maintain satisfying social relationships

4. *Key points*

a. Severe social isolation involves no intimate relationships and few social relationships or activities apart from interactions with healthcare providers

b. Depression and suicide often include social isolation as a key symptom

c. If severe social isolation represents a change in interpersonal relationships for the patient, the nurse should assess for depression, suicide potential, unresolved grief, guilt

(1) Consider referring the patient to a mental health specialist for assessment and any necessary treatment

(2) Severe isolation can become dangerous if the person is too ill to meet own needs and does not have social resources to help

(3) Severe isolation may compromise the patient's ability to receive the help needed; high technologic home and hospice care often depend on the patient's having others available to help monitor machines and treatments

d. The gay adolescent may experience ostracism from peers and show this rejection through engaging in unsafe behaviors that include unprotected sexual encounters, alcohol and drug use, and acting out conflict in other antisocial behaviors

5. Assessment
   a. Interpersonal relationships
      (1) Number, types, and quality of relationships (see *Social Support*, p. ••); a broad, general question might be, "I wonder if you would tell me about the men and women you are close to and about those relationships?"
      (2) Include current and past attachment status, sexual history, pets, leisure activities, and work history; pets may also be important links to feelings of connectedness and meaning
   b. New or more intense symptoms that now interfere with the patient's ability to socialize (e.g., shortness of breath, dyspnea, fatigue, pain, diarrhea and fecal incontinence, nausea and vomiting, problems with mobility or cognition, feeling depressed); see *Body Image Disturbance*, p. ••
   c. Sexual history: Changes in patient's sexual desire, activities, performance, satisfaction
   d. Factors that increase vulnerability for social isolation: Emotional problems, child abuse, dysfunctional family of origin, unresolved grief over losses
   e. Personal history of emotional problems that may recur in times of high personal stress (e.g., depression, substance abuse, schizophrenia)
   f. Changes that reflect increased social isolation evident in social activities, social and intimate relationships, verbalizations

6. Interventions
   a. Counseling strategies/approaches
      (1) Implement therapeutic communication strategies (empathy, clarifying, providing information, open-ended questions, feedback, reflecting content, exploring feelings, summarizing)
      (2) Counsel adolescents about intimate relationships: Assess relationships, identify goals, anticipate barriers, establish action strategies
      (3) Use strategies, including role play, to help patients overcome hesitations to seek out new affiliations where they can be involved in community activities and with other people
      (4) Help patients anticipate or work through grief tasks (e.g., managing affect, balancing activity and rest, finding meaning, realigning relationships) when trying to deal with impending or recent deaths of lovers, other family members, close friends
   b. Refer patients and their families for assessment and treatment of episodic or recurrent problems (e.g., dysfunctional grief, depression, substance abuse, schizophrenia) associated with social isolation
   c. Refer to support groups, compatible community groups, to reduce a sense of social isolation
   d. Modify the physical environment if necessary to improve patient's ability to participate in social activities and maintain social relationships
      (1) Place a pencil, pad, and paper beside the telephone; move patient to a first-floor apartment to conserve energy
      (2) Help patient modify style of dressing to distract attention from the physical problem (e.g., KS, skin rash, weight loss) that makes him/her uncomfortable in public
   e. Modify the patient's social environment
      (1) Request that patient have a volunteer (e.g., buddy) or help patient identify who can help with specific

tasks (e.g., shopping, child care)
(2) Explore with patient how s/he is
    meeting spiritual needs; arrange for
    chaplains, rabbis, ministers to visit,
    if the patient agrees
(3) Encourage family members or
    friends to write letters and cards to
    the patient who is homebound
f. Evaluate whether nursing and medical
   care regimens have become so complex
   that the time, energy, and concentration
   they require prevent the patient from
   focusing on social interactions; see *High
   Risk for Ineffectivement Management of
   Therapeutic Regimen*, p. 258
g. For long-standing social isolation
   (1) Refer for assessment to psychiatric
       liaison nurse, psychologist, psychia-
       trist, psychiatric social worker to
       determine if supportive therapy
       would be beneficial
   (2) If the patient has no motivation to
       reduce social isolation, initiate direct
       interventions to ensure the patient
       has sufficient social relationships for
       personal safety and health mainte-
       nance
h. See *Wellness Strategies* for further discussion of support groups (p. 348) and
   individual psychotherapy (p. 345)

N. Social Support

1. Definition/Description
   a. Emotional, informational, tangible help
      that may have health-sustaining and
      stress-reducing functions
   b. Also defined as the actual or perceived
      interpersonal relationship, or network
      of interpersonal relationships, in which
      the people involved provide a sense of
      security, social integration, nurturance, a
      sense of worth, reliable alliance, and
      guidance
   c. A resource that enables people to per-
      ceive situations as less threatening,
      enhancing reassurance and security, and
      promoting adaptive coping
   d. Serves as a buffer to the adverse health
      effects of stress

e. Linked to better health and well-being,
   lower level of depression, and higher
   levels of self-esteem and enhanced
   coping
f. Promotes a sense of belonging, a positive
   affect, and feelings of personal efficacy
g. Inadequate or insufficient social support
   may lead to unmet expectations,
   increased stress and depression

2. Etiology of Inadequate Social Support
   a. Poverty
   b. Unstable housing
   c. Overextended use of family/friend
      assistance and resources
   d. History of disruptive relationships
   e. Lengthy progressive illness
   f. Concurrent illness or deaths in network
   g. Geographically or emotionally distant
      family of origin
   h. Stigma associated with illness or
      lifestyle

3. Goals of Care
   a. To mobilize/enhance the patient's social
      support system
   b. To identify people at risk for poor
      health outcomes because of inadequate
      social support

4. *Key points*
   a. PWAs often lose many of their sources
      of social support early in the disease
      process
   b. As a result of the stigma associated with
      the disease and the secrecy surrounding
      the diagnosis, PWAs and their partners
      may be unable to draw on their usual
      social network or community resources
      for support

5. Assessment
   a. Number of people in social network
   b. Reciprocity (equal exchange between
      two persons), density (degree to which
      members of the network interact with
      each other), closeness
   c. Communication skills
   d. Complete the social support grid (see
      Figure 5.2) with the patient, to become
      aware of deficiencies in support

6. Interventions
   a. Assist patient to mobilize social sup-
      ports
      (1) Focus on factors that contribute to

Figure 5.2   Assessment of Social Support

Name, Address, Phone Number	Relationship Relative, Friend, Neighbor, Work Associate	Emotional Closeness High, Medium, Low	Perceived Willingness to Help High, Medium, Low	Types of Support Possible Emotional, Informational, Instrumental	Perceived Ability to Help High, Medium, Low
Jane Doe 123 Friend St. 348-6769	Friend	High	High	Informational	Low

the perception of support (e.g., closeness of the person, reciprocity of support exchanged)
(2) Assess patient's verbal and nonverbal skills in mobilizing support
(3) Teach communication skills, if indicated
(4) Role play more effective ways of communicating with others
(5) Deal with guilt (see p. 255)
(6) Encourage expression of appreciation for help received
b. Assist families, friends, and other supporters to facilitate social support at various stages of illness
(1) Prepare for the patient's illness and behavior
(2) Counsel about appropriate help
(3) Provide chances to discuss the problems
(4) Teach how to manage and control the anxiety inherent in their interactions with the patient/family in need
(5) Facilitate communication among the various participants
(6) Support them in their efforts
(7) Play the role of coordinator and mediator

O. Spiritual Distress

1. Definition/Description
   a. Spirituality: The capacity to make meaning through a sense of relatedness (intrapersonally, interpersonally, transpersonally), "to dimensions that transcend the self in such a way that empowers and does not devalue the individual" (Reed, 1992, p. 350)
   b. Spiritual distress: The dissonance experienced by an individual—physically, emotionally, or existentially—that impacts the person's ability to feel related and connected to self, others, or one's God
   c. Transcendence: The capacity to see beyond one's immediate circumstances and to realize that one is participating in something that goes beyond the self
2. Etiology

a. Religion of origin
b. Guilt/shame, hopelessness/despair
c. Uncertainty,
d. Fear of suffering, eternal punishment
e. Lack of forgiveness of self or others
f. Powerlessness
g. Meaninglessness/lack of purpose
h. Suffering (physical, emotional, spiritual/existential)
3. Goal of Care: To provide opportunities for the patient to explore spiritual aspects of his/her life situation
4. *Key points*
   a. Nurses need to be open to and nonjudgmental toward beliefs that differ from their own
   b. People with life-threatening illness have the capacity to have a transcendent experience
   c. Spiritual distress may exhibit as physical and emotional symptoms
5. Assessment
   a. Religion of origin, current religious involvement
   b. Indications of spiritual distress (separation from religious or cultural ties, challenged belief or value system)
   c. Spiritual beliefs and values, past and present
      (1) How do you conceive of your God or of something beyond yourself?
      (2) Can you tell me about religious and spiritual experiences you had as a child? Are they still relevant?
      (3) What does having HIV mean to you?
   d. Social support: Family of origin, family of choice
   e. Pastoral support
   f. Cultural beliefs and values
6. Interventions
   a. Being with/being there
   b. Remain nonjudgmental, listen actively
   c. Help the person to find meaning, make sense; ask
      (1) Can you tell me about the meaningful people and events in your life?
      (2) What has been the purpose of your life?
      (3) How can you continue to see a purpose in light of your current situation?

d. Involve appropriate others (family, friends, pastoral support, volunteer[s]) to assist in exploring religious beliefs and to reframe distressing beliefs through conversation, in care planning and case conferences
e. Instill hope
   (1) Explore meanings of hope and assist person in knowing hope can be more than being well or being cured
   (2) Find out if the person feels hopeless and what might be the source; see *Hopelessness*, p. 260
f. Help turn guilt into gratitude
   (1) Help identify specifics of what is triggering guilt and ways to resolve or be more at peace with them
   (2) Ask what patient can feel grateful about
   (3) Remind patient that feelings of guilt and gratitude can be experienced at the same time
   (4) See *Guilt*, p. 255
g. Read from religious and spiritual sources as patient desires
h. Use prayer when appropriate
i. Encourage quiet time for reflection (e.g., journaling, meditation); see *Dreamwork*, p. 350, *Meditation*, p. 355
j. Facilitate patient's participation in meaningful spiritual/religious practices or rituals (e.g., lighting candles, attending religious or cultural services, saying rosary)

P. Stigma

1. Definition/Description
   a. A trait, attribute, or characteristic that society defines as highly undesirable (Goffman, 1963)
   b. Possession of such a trait may result in
      (1) Changes in social identity
      (2) Less acceptance in social interactions
      (3) Denial or limitations of opportunities
      (4) Feelings of shame and self-loathing if the person shares society's evaluation of what the trait means or symbolizes about the person

c. Stigmatizing traits
   (1) Stigma of the body (physical deformities)
   (2) Stigma of character (evidence of a moral flaw such as dishonesty or weak will)
   (3) Tribal stigma (race, religion, nationality)
   (4) The intensity of the stigma response may be influenced by how much the trait is concealed, how it changes over time, its disruptiveness to interactions and issues of origin, responsibility, and peril (Jones et al., 1984)
d. A trait that carries a stigma does not necessarily produce a stigmatizing response; it is the inability to predict how others will respond that creates anxiety for the person with stigma
e. Some stigma are readily apparent while others are concealable
   (1) People with readily apparent stigma are unable to pass in most situations but may use strategies aimed at reducing tension
   (2) People with concealable stigma may be able to "pass" as normal and must cope with
      (a) Their own internal knowledge of not meeting expectations
      (b) Hearing brutally candid remarks about "the kind of person" who shares their trait
      (c) Pragmatic decisions not to disclose (e.g., HIV serostatus, sexual orientation) and to pass in order not to risk restrictions on opportunities (Schneider & Conrad, 1980)
   (3) Decisions about disclosure vs. concealment depend on a number of factors including the particular relationship involved
f. HIV-related stigma
   (1) Stigma perceived by the person who is seropositive: Awareness of actual or potential
      (a) Social disqualification
      (b) Denial or limitation of opportunity (e.g., housing, jobs)
      (c) Negative changes in social identity when others learn of the person's HIV serostatus
   (2) Possible consequences and reactions
      (a) Altered self-concept, with possible impact on self-esteem (Chung & Magraw, 1992; Siegel & Krauss, 1991)
      (b) Increased anxiety and depression (Crandall & Coleman, 1992)
      (c) Emotional reactions toward those stigmatizing the person and toward oneself (Laryea & Gien, 1993)
      (d) Use of management techniques to avoid or minimize enacted or actual rather than potential stigma (Bennett, 1990; Weitz, 1990)
         i) Information control such as passing, selective disclosure, attempts to predict the reactions of others (testing the waters)
         ii) Avoidance or withdrawal (e.g., curtailing scope of daily activities, reluctance to enter new social situations, changing/narrowing social network)
         iii) Tension-reduction maneuvers (once others know the person has HIV)
            a) Covering (to minimize obtrusiveness)
            b) Jokes/humor to try to put others at ease
            c) Overt acknowledgment to dispel ambiguity
      (e) Challenges to the definition of HIV infection as a stigma through activism or education
g. Prevalence
   (1) Surveys of both the general public (Herek & Capitanio, 1993) and healthcare workers (Scherer, Haughey, Wu, & Kuhn, 1992) demonstrated stigmatizing attitudes toward PWAs
   (2) Rejection is a pervasive theme (McCain & Gramling, 1992)
      (a) Subtle distancing or outright ostracism and discrimination in

housing and employment
(Bennett, 1990)
(b) Family member(s) may cease
contact after learning of the HIV
infection (Weitz, 1990)
h. Relative risk of experiencing HIV-
related stigma: May vary according to
(1) Geographical area (urban/subur-
ban/rural, by country)
(2) Degree of expected physical con-
tact/closeness/intimacy
(3) Imputed mode of transmission
(4) Possession of other stigmatizing
traits
(5) Characteristics of the person with
HIV or the other person (sex, level
of knowledge about HIV, cultural
background)
(6) Presence of visible physical changes
suggestive of having HIV (stigma
cues)
2. Etiology
a. Stigma is found in most cultures; the
traits selected reflect prevailing cultural
values (Freidson, 1970)
(1) In U.S. society, health is an important precondition for most valued
achievements (e.g., higher education, career, financial independence)
(2) Illnesses severe or long enough to
interfere with those achievements
may generate stigma
b. The course that stigma takes for people
with HIV remains a matter for specula-
tion as longitudinal studies of stigma in
the context of HIV are not currently
available; it is possible that
(1) People with HIV can remain
unaware of HIV-related stigma
indefinitely
(2) People with HIV may be aware of
stigma and of its potential consequences, and therefore successfully
conceal their HIV status for a prolonged period
(3) People with HIV tell one or a few
people when they first learn they
have HIV; the negative consequences may teach them to become
much more cautious about revealing
their HIV status for some time

(4) People with HIV may be more vulnerable to feelings of stigma when
first learning they have HIV, and
again on initial appearance of symptoms
(5) Good disclosure experiences would
be expected to decrease feelings of
stigma
(6) There are likely to be times when
other aspects of managing HIV
infection take priority over stigma
(7) Many people with HIV come to
reject the idea of society stigmatizing
them, and choose to pursue an
activist path; this may occur at any
point in a person's experience with
HIV
3. Goals of Care
a. To help the person experiencing stigma
to minimize its effects
b. To prevent stigma when possible
through education, training, and feedback for families and staff
4. *Key points*
a. The inability to predict reliably how
others will respond once a person's HIV
infection is known makes interactions
anxiety-provoking for people with HIV
b. The degree to which having HIV is concealable and the degree to which disclo-
sures have been made will influence the
person's experience of stigma
c. The potential for stigmatization may
negatively affect willingness to be tested
for HIV; it may also affect patients' willingness to adhere to therapy, especially
if interactions with healthcare providers
evoke stigmatizing reactions
5. Assessment
a. Internal psychologic sequelae of HIV-
related stigma: Depression, anxiety,
withdrawal, suicidal thoughts, anger
b. External sequelae of HIV-related stigma
(1) Discrimination in job/housing/
health care/insurance
(2) Social isolation
(3) Less satisfying relationships because
of lack of self-disclosure
(4) Loss of relationships that might
have provided tangible material
support

(5) Physical violence
c. Ask directly about
   (1) Relationships
   (2) Upsetting or unpleasant incidents, including physical or verbal assaults
   (3) Problems at home or on the job
   (4) Changes in living situation since diagnosis
   (5) Who is close to the person? Have they been told? If so, how did it go? If not told, why not?
   (6) The reason the patient thinks others responded as they did to her/him (crucial markers of stigma)
6. Interventions
  a. Provide counseling
   (1) Anticipatory counseling about issues of disclosure and possible discrimination and stigma should occur in conjunction with HIV testing (see *HIV Counseling and Testing,* p. 37), and in initial and ongoing evaluation of the patient in treatment settings
   (2) Tailor counseling individually
     (a) Recognize the ongoing tension between wanting to disclose (to feel more authentic and less isolated, to decrease need for constant self-monitoring) and fear of rejection and discrimination
     (b) Discuss ways to test the water with others (e.g., asking "How did you feel when you heard [someone famous] had HIV?")
     (c) Explore whether the patient has had previous experience with stigma (e.g., related to sexual orientation or other traits)
       i) How were those experiences managed?
       ii) What part of that experience can be applied to managing HIV stigma?
  b. Educate patient/family/significant other on
   (1) Actual risk of transmission and safety of household members; see Table 10.2, *Universal Precautions,* p. 367
   (2) What stigma is and how it operates
  c. Provide referrals to
   (1) Ongoing individual counseling
   (2) Support groups (see p. 348), which may offer practical suggestions for managing or avoiding stigma as well as opportunities to interact socially without the threat of HIV-related stigma
   (3) Supplemental services (e.g., legal referral resources, housing, job placement, volunteer assistance) as needed
  d. See also *Anxiety,* p. 245, *Guilt,* p. 255.

Section 6

Issues in Special Populations

The goals for this section are (1) to identify similarities and differences in how certain populations or communities have been affected by HIV/AIDS in relation to prevention, access to care/treatment or research, and treatment outcomes; (2) to describe approaches or interventions directed both to the individual patient and to the community; and (3) to identify specific community or population-focused resources.

What will be clear to most readers is that most people are members of multiple communities or groups. Therefore, no one affiliation can explain how a particular individual or community is responding to illness and its consequences.

Inherent in this section is the recognition and awareness of how the concept of diversity underscores this epidemic—not just the biologic diversity of the virus or other microorganisms, but how diversity affects the relationships, beliefs, values, and experiences of the individuals and communities affected by HIV/AIDS as well.

A. Adolescents

1. Definition/Description of the Population
   a. For clinical purposes, adolescence extends from ages 12 to 21 years
   b. Legally, adolescents are minors (under the age of majority) until age 18 in 47 states, and until age 19 in Alabama, Nebraska, and Wyoming
   c. A *mature minor,* covered by mature minor doctrine, can understand benefits and risks of treatment and is able to give informed consent
   d. An *emancipated minor* is married, serving in the armed forces, or living apart from parents and managing own financial affairs
   e. A *medically emancipated* minor is, in addition, above a specified age, minor parent or runaway, and deemed able to provide informed consent and to seek care for condition that, if left untreated, could jeopardize health of self or others (e.g., consent for pregnancy-related care, including contraceptive services; diagnosis and treatment of STDs, including HIV); substance-abuse treatment
   f. Demographics
      (1) According to a recent report (AHPA, 1996), 1 in 4 new HIV infections occurs in those under age 20
      (2) Through June 1995, 2,184 cases of AIDS (1,437 male, 747 female) were diagnosed in adolescents aged 13–19 at time of diagnosis (CDC, 1995c)
      (3) Through June 1995, 17,745 cases of AIDS (13,599 male, 4,146 female) were diagnosed in adolescents/ young adults aged 20–24 years (CDC, 1995c)
      (4) Approximately 20% of all AIDS cases are diagnosed in adults aged 20–29; given the 8- to 10-year clinical asymptomatic period, many were infected as teenagers
      (5) Geographic variation: Higher rates in urban centers, especially in the Northeast and South (Lindegren, Hanson, Miller, Bryers, & Onorata, 1994)
      (6) African-American and Hispanic adolescents and young adults (both male and female) are disproportionately represented in reported AIDS cases compared to their representation in the U.S. population
      (7) AIDS is a leading cause of death among 15- to 24-year-olds
   g. Common problems
      (1) Adolescence is time of growth and experimentation, stage of striving for independence and autonomy, a time of feeling curious and invulnerable; all these factors may lead to sexual and drug-related risk behaviors that increase exposure to HIV
      (2) Adolescents generally are concrete thinkers, especially under age 18, and therefore unlikely to think of long-term consequences of their actions
      (3) Denial is a strong defense mechanism; peer group is major directive of behavior
      (4) Majority of adolescents are unaware of their HIV status and may transmit virus unwittingly
2. Specific Issues
   a. Transmission/risk behaviors
      (1) Through June 1995, the HIV exposure categories associated with the highest number of cumulative AIDS cases reported to the CDC (1995c) were
         (a) Males
            i) 13–19 years old: Hemophilia/coagulation disorder, 43%; men who have sex with men, 33%
            ii) 30–24 years old: Men who have sex with men, 63%; IDUs, 13%
         (b) Females
            i) 13–19 years old: Heterosexual contact, 53%; risk not reported or identified, 22%; IDUs, 16%
            ii) 20–24 years old: Heterosexual contact, 50%; IDUs, 33%; risk not reported or identified, 14%

(2) In early puberty, physiologic immaturity of female cervical transformation zone increases vulnerability

(3) Adolescents at highest risk: School dropouts, transient/homeless youth, incarcerated youth

(4) Perception of need: Most adolescents do not personalize risk/threat of HIV infection

(5) Barriers to proposed or existing prevention programs

   (a) Parents, community organization, and school systems often refuse to support HIV/AIDS educational offerings

   (b) Local, state, and federal governments have blocked reaching adolescents through the media

   (c) Many adolescents at highest risk are the most difficult to reach (e.g., homeless or runaway youth, school dropouts, incarcerated youth)

   (d) Many adolescents know about transmission, but fewer know how to prevent infection or lack the skills to practice safer behaviors

   (e) In some instances, exposure has been linked to rites of passage (group norm)

(6) Confidentiality is essential to ensure use of testing and treatment facilities; adolescents have same rights as adults to confidentiality

(7) Proposed home collection kit for HIV antibody testing has greatest value to at-risk adolescents for early diagnosis

b. Access to care/treatment or research protocols: Barriers include

(1) Most care provided to adolescents is by those with no training in adolescent health

(2) Very few facilities exist for the treatment of adolescents with alcohol and substance-abuse problems

(3) Health care is not a top priority for most adolescents; many deny any threat to health

(4) Lack of available services that are convenient, appropriate, and attractive to youth

(5) Lack of unified support community

(6) There has been little adolescent-specific biomedical and behavioral research (AHPA, 1996)

c. Treatment outcomes

(1) Little is known about the natural history of HIV infection in adolescents compared to children or adults (e.g., what proportion will become symptomatic early after infection or remain asymptomatic for many years)

(2) Before the 1993 AIDS case definition revisions, AIDS-defining illnesses were similar for adolescents and adults; in order of frequency: PCP (41%), *Candida esophagitis* (22%), AIDS wasting syndrome (19%), MAC (9%), extrapulmonary cryptococcus (9%), chronic HSV (8%), HIV encephalopathy (6%), toxoplasmosis of the brain (5%), cryptosporidiosis (4%) (Lindegren et al., 1994)

(3) Adherence to a medical regimen may be especially difficult for disenfranchised adolescents or those with alcohol or other substance-abuse problems

3. Specific Approaches

a. Individual

(1) Build and maintain a trusting relationship based on authenticity and confidentiality

(2) Assess risk of STDs, unwanted pregnancy, alcohol and drug use, accidents, incidents of abuse/violence

(3) Use peers as educators/counselors: Teens are more receptive to input and suggestions from respected peers than from authoritarian adults

(4) Provide information to increase knowledge

   (a) Address common misperceptions (e.g., HIV can be transmitted only if sick)

   (b) Build communication and negotiation skills

b. Community/group

(1) HIV-prevention programs most successful if appropriate adolescents

(e.g., by age, race, culture) are involved in planning and presenting programs

(2) Prevention programs need to be implemented and sustained/reinforced preferably before practice of risky behavior (during or before early teens or by 7th grade)

(3) Include information on sexual practices

 (a) 86% of males and 75% of females are sexually active by age 20

 (b) Average age at first intercourse is 15 years; most sexual intercourse is spontaneous rather than planned

 (c) <50% of adolescents use condoms consistently; multiple partners are common

 (d) Once young women initiate sexual intercourse, they usually continue sexual activity

(4) Include information on drug use

 (a) 90% of high school seniors have tried alcohol, 40% have tried marijuana, and 9% have tried cocaine (DiClemente, 1992)

 (b) Alcohol and recreational drugs impair judgment, promote high-risk behaviors

 (c) First-time IDU frequently occurs under influence of either drugs or alcohol

 (d) Gender gap in drug use is declining

(5) Youths in high-risk situations for whom prevention programs are essential

 (a) Those with coagulation disorders

 (b) Runaway or rejected

 (c) Homeless, incarcerated, school dropouts

 (d) Gay, lesbian, or bisexual; survivors of sexual abuse

 (e) Racial and ethnic minorities

 (f) Young women and youth in rural communities

(6) For comprehensive HIV-prevention programs include information on

 (a) Exploring values and attitudes

 (b) Skills building

 (c) Access to services (medical, social, legal)

4. Specific Resources

 • Metro TeenAIDS
  1804 T Street NW
  Washington, DC 20009
  P.O. Box 15577
  Washington, DC 20003-5577
  Phones (800) 558-2437 (Resource Directory, toll-free, English); (202) 986-4310 (main);
  Fax (202) 986-0109
  [*Promotes, coordinates, supports, and conducts education, prevention, and referral programs to reduce the rate of HIV infection in youth and serves the needs of those already infected. The Resource Directory provides referrals to HIV-antibody counseling and testing sites as well as to adolescent HIV-related services.*]

 • STANDUP FOR KIDS (National Office)
  P.O. Box 461292
  Aurora, CO 80046-1292
  Phones (800) 365-4KID (toll-free, English); (303) 699-4KID (main)
  [*Provides support services, condom distribution, counseling, and education to street and homeless adolescents, and to adolescents employed in the sex industry.*]

 • National Organization on Adolescent Pregnancy, Parenting, and Prevention, Inc.
  4421-A East West Highway
  Bethesda, MD 20814
  (301) 914-0378
  [*An organization that consists of a network of individuals and groups focused on adolescent pregnancy, care, and prevention issues, including the issue of AIDS.*]

 • National Commission on Correctional Health Care (NCCHC)
  2105 N. Southport #200
  Chicago, IL 60614
  Phone (312) 528-0818 (main)
  Fax (312) 528-4915
  [*Provides educational services to incarcerated adolescents and adults and develops resource materials that address comprehensive health education within correctional environments.*]

- Hispanic Designers, Incorporated (HDI)
  National Hispanic Education and
    Communications Projects
  1000 16th Street NW #401
  Washington, DC 20036
  Phone (202) 452-8750 (main)
  Fax (202) 452-0086
  [*A communications and social marketing
  organization specializing in Spanish- and
  English-language education and information programs targeted to the Hispanic community. HDI is particularly concerned
  about reaching Hispanic adolescents in the
  12–17 age group, and women of all ages.*]

- Advocates for Youth
  1025 Vermont Avenue NW #210
  Washington, DC 20005
  Phone (202) 347-5700 (main)
  Fax (202) 347-2263
  [*Works to increase the opportunities for and
  abilities of youth to make health decisions
  about sexuality. The National Adolescent
  AIDS and HIV Prevention Initiative works
  primarily with organizations to assist them
  with the development of HIV/AIDS education programs appropriate for the youth
  with whom they work.*]

B. The African-American Community

1. Definition/Description of the Population
   a. The majority of African Americans are descendants of West Africans transported to America as slaves, beginning in the 1600s
   b. According to the U.S. Census Bureau, in 1990 there were approximately 30 million African Americans, comprising 12% of the U.S. population
   c. Americans of African descent have had the HIV epidemic superimposed on preexisting consequences of almost 400 years of social injustice
   d. Racism, poverty, discrimination, and social barriers have had disastrous effects on their overall health
      (1) U.S. morbidity and mortality rates reflect the disproportionate number of premature deaths, preventable diseases, and violent crimes affecting African Americans
      (2) In proportion to their presence in the U.S. population, African Americans are overrepresented in chronic and acute illnesses, homicides, AIDS, and TB
   e. Many African Americans have a mistrust of public health officials and agencies, physicians, nurses, and other health and social service workers based on complicated sociocultural history and mistreatment; many African Americans have encountered healthcare workers as authority figures and not as advocates and partners in care
   f. Cultural assimilation, assumed in the past to be part of the process of Americanization, has not happened for many ethnic groups; this is especially true for African Americans
   g. Though accounting for 12% of the population, African Americans comprised 33% of all AIDS cases reported to the CDC through February 1994 (National AIDS Clearinghouse, 1995)
   h. Women accounted for 18% of all reported U.S. AIDS cases in 1994; three fourths of women with AIDS are black or Hispanic; rates of AIDS in black women are 16 times higher, in Hispanic women 7 times higher than in white women (National AIDS Clearinghouse, 1995)
2. Specific Issues
   a. Transmission/Risk Behavior/Prevention
      (1) Multiple barriers exist in the African-American community: Insufficient funding, lack of culturally relevant education materials, denial of the epidemic, distrust of hospital and healthcare workers, myths and beliefs about the transmission and origins of HIV
      (2) African Americans are less likely than other groups to have health insurance and correspondingly less likely to benefit from early intervention and preventive treatments

(3) African Americans are no more bio-logically susceptible to HIV than any other people

b. Access to care/treatment or research protocols

  (1) For African Americans who are HIV seropositive, the infection is just another warp in a complex weave in an environment of addiction, illness, poverty, unemployment, crime, violence, malnutrition, teen pregnancy, illiteracy, and overall survival issues

  (2) HIV is often not the most important or urgent problem a patient faces day to day

    (a) Even if a person is symptomatic or is diagnosed with AIDS, the needs of children and partner and concerns about finances, shelter, and safety may take priority

    (b) Poverty is closely tied to African-American women and AIDS

    (c) Even if care is accessible the barriers for poor women may be intangible but real and insurmountable without astute advocacy, intervention programs, and outreach workers who are dedicated, patient, persistent, and often HIV positive themselves

  (3) Researchers have difficulty recruiting African Americans into clinical trials: Suspicions may be well founded and rooted in recent historical events such as the Tuskegee Study (where black men were knowingly not treated for syphilis) and the disclosure of forced sterilization of black welfare mothers in the South; it is uncertain to what degree findings in other populations at risk for HIV/AIDS can be generalized to African Americans

c. Treatment outcomes

  (1) The shorter life expectancy of African Americans with HIV has been shown to be more attributable to lack of access to early intervention and expert medical care than to biologic or sociodemographic factors

(Chiasson, Keraly, & Moore, 1995)

  (2) The prevalence of G6PD enzyme deficiency may limit drugs that can be used for PCP prophylaxis

3. Specific Approaches

a. Individual

  (1) Appreciate the role racism has played and continues to play in the lives of the African-American patient

  (2) Meet the patient half way in order to work together as equals and to help the patient identify important factors affecting his/her life

  (3) Whatever nurses' ethnic origin, they must understand and accept their own values in order to approach practice with an open mind, an open heart, a thirst for inquiry, and commitment to understanding

  (4) Do a cultural assessment to include

    (a) Beliefs, values, biases, taboos

    (b) Customs, traditions, language

    (c) Relationships with family and community

  (5) Build interventions on the awareness that for some patients the importance of the individual may not take priority over the family/larger extended family network, as it usually is in Western medicine

b. Community

  (1) Appreciate the richness, strengths, and challenges of diversity

  (2) Be willing to work with indigenous leaders who are trusted and respected

  (3) Acknowledge the role religion plays in the African-American culture

    (a) The "Black Church" (as it is often dubbed) exerts a powerful force in most African-American families; it influences the attitudes that congregants develop to those in their lives with AIDS/HIV

    (b) African Americans have traditionally drawn on their spiritual strength in times of pain or trouble

  (4) Recognize the class and ethnic/racial disparity among nursing staff

members; work to bridge the cultural and social gaps; team building by the staff can be key to success whether the patient is cared for in home, clinic, or hospital

(5) Interventions, practices, and programs that have been shown to work in African-American communities

(a) Peer outreach support groups for African-American gay men, adolescents, women, and teens

(b) Community advisory boards (if they are not tools of tokenism, are diverse, and share in decision making)

(c) Support groups for people affected and infected by HIV/AIDS (caregivers, partners, family, co-workers)

(d) Focus groups in communities, businesses, clinics, houses of worship

(e) Drop-in centers where HIV-positive people can find information and support

(f) Drug treatment centers when slots are available on demand

(g) Risk and harm-reduction models, if they have community support and a strong educational and nonjudgmental foundation

(h) Retreat programs where HIV-positive adults and families can experience healing in the context of community living for 3- to 4-day stretches

4. Specific Resources

- AIDS National Interfaith Network
  110 Maryland Avenue NE #504
  Washington, DC 20002
  Phone (202) 546-0807
  Fax (202) 546-5103
  [*Contact: Deborah Campbell. Religious network, pastoral care, advocacy.*]

- American Civil Liberties Union, National Office
  122 Maryland Avenue SE
  Washington, DC 20002
  Phone (202) 544-1681
  Fax (202) 546-0738
  [*Contact: Alexander Robertson. Legal assistance service, litigation support service, policy analysis.*]

- Blacks Educating Blacks About Sexual Health Issues (BEBASHI)
  1233 Locust Street
  Philadelphia, PA 19107
  Phone (215) 546-4140
  Fax (215) 546-6107
  [*Contact: Gary Bell. HIV testing, outreach education, case management.*]

- National Black Women's Health Project
  1237 Gordon St SW
  Atlanta, GA 30310
  (404) 758-9590
  [Education, outreach, policy analysis.]

- National AIDS Minority Information and Education Program
  Howard University
  2139 Georgia Avenue NW #2139
  Washington, DC: 20001
  Phone (202) 865-3720
  Fax (202) 865-3799
  [*Director: Dr. Peggy Valentine. HIV education specifically targeting African Americans.*]

- National Minority AIDS Council
  1931 13th Street NW
  Washington, DC 20009
  Phone (202) 483-6622
  Fax (202) 483-1135
  [*Contact: Paul Karvata. Model of education and leadership, advocacy, minority sensitive program.*]

- National Urban League
  500 East 62nd St, 10th Floor
  New York, NY 10021
  Phone (212) 310-9238
  Fax (212) 593-8250
  [*Contact: Anne Hill. Advocacy, education, outreach at the local level only.*]

C. The Deaf Community

1. Definition/Description of the Population
   a. The deaf community (nearly one million Americans) considers itself a minority population with unique culture, language, beliefs, perspectives, and social norms
      (1) The deaf culture is often misunderstood by outsiders who fail to appreciate the richness of American Sign Language (ASL)
      (2) ASL bonds the community and symbolizes its pride
   b. Impact of HIV/AIDS
      (1) Exact numbers of deaf people infected with HIV or diagnosed with AIDS is unknown as CDC does not consider deafness to be reportable demographic information; only Texas and Maryland currently report/record deaf PWAs
      (2) Denial of AIDS makes it difficult to survey the community to determine seroprevalence
      (3) Anecdotal evidence suggests dramatically high HIV seroprevalence rates in urban gay deaf communities; in Houston, 27% of deaf people tested were HIV positive (*Fact sheet on HIV/AIDS*, 1993)
   c. Common problems
      (1) Marginalization and isolation due to real and perceived communication barriers
      (2) Limited or nonexistent family planning, mental health, or substance abuse resources; 94% of AIDS service organizations surveyed provided no services for deaf patients (Dimming the lights, 1994)
      (3) Healthcare worker myths about the deaf/hearing impaired
         (a) Hearing impairment equals intellectual impairment
         (b) The deaf cannot learn like hearing people
         (c) Simply putting education in writing will break the communication barrier
         (d) Anyone who knows some sign language can act as an interpreter
      (4) 90% of the deaf (Dolnick, 1993) were born to hearing parents who may not accept their child's deafness, respect the deaf culture, learn their child's sign language; are likely to hide or deny child's deafness
      (5) Distrust of the healthcare system and feeling that things are done to them and not for them
      (6) Small, tightly knit community in which confidentiality is often lost, leading to denial and secrecy
      (7) Deaf people may exhibit poor self-esteem, lack of fluency in English, poor social and negotiation skills, and impulsivity
2. Specific Issues
   a. Prevention
      (1) HIV prevention vocabulary not understood by many of the deaf
      (2) The deaf learn better by peer discussion than by interpreted lectures
      (3) What education was available to the community was in large part reactive, not proactive—too little, too late
   b. Access to care/treatment or research protocols
      (1) Many deaf people have only a rudimentary understanding of anatomy/physiology, disease, medicine
      (2) In general, there is a lack of interpreters, TTYs, and user-friendly services for the deaf
      (3) There is an overall lack of understanding in the deaf community about the complexities of the healthcare system (Van Biema, 1994)
      (4) Low employment rates for the deaf translate to little private insurance coverage or chance of owning own transportation (*Fact sheet on HIV/AIDS*, 1993)
      (5) Attitudes, beliefs, or values that affect access to care
         (a) Distrust of the hearing world, especially authority figures

(b) Lack of empowerment to demand interpreting services

(c) Culture often accepts anecdotal mythology from peers as truth

c. Treatment outcomes

(1) The deaf are often diagnosed with HIV when symptomatic and die sooner than hearing counterparts due to lack of knowledge and comprehension of disease, support systems

(2) May not understand the concept of taking medicine before getting sick (prophylaxis)

(3) May not understand the distinctions between medicines (assuming all antibiotics can be used interchangeably, may stop taking medications when feeling better)

3. Specific Approaches

a. Individual

(1) Assure accurate, acceptable, and consistent interpreting services

(a) Interpreters must be professionals with variety of language skill levels available (e.g., minimal language, ASL, signed English skills)

(b) Use deaf counselors whenever possible

(2) Encourage questions and expression of fears and emotions

(3) Offer guidance in navigating the healthcare system

(4) Empower individuals to take responsibility for actions and understand consequences of personal decisions

(5) Role play negotiating safer sex

(6) Don't assume individual understanding of the vocabulary; explain all terminology and validate by encouraging deaf person to explain to counselor

(7) Small group discussions will accomplish more than individual counseling

b. Community

(1) Provide appropriate interpreting services at all levels of prevention and care provision

(2) Involve deaf persons at high risk in all levels of prevention planning

(3) Examine deaf culture to identify beliefs, perspectives, needs

(4) Develop a culturally appropriate approach to providing services

(5) Recruit, educate, and hire deaf peer counselors to provide established services and perform outreach activities and community education

(6) Develop targeted services for, e.g., deaf gays, deaf women, deaf IDUs, deaf African Americans

4. Specific Resources

- National Coalition on Deaf Community and HIV, Inc.
  c/o UCSF Center on Deafness
  3333 California Street #10
  San Francisco, CA 94118
  (415) 476-4980

- AIDS Education/Services for the Deaf (AESD), a project of the Greater Los Angeles Council on Deafness (GLAD)
  2222 Laverna Avenue
  Los Angeles, CA 90041
  TTY/voice (213) 550-4250
  Fax (213) 550-4255

- Deaf AIDS Project in Michigan
  c/o United Community Services
  (313) 226-9400

- National Coalition on Deafness and HIV/AIDS
  TTY (703) 960-8883
  or contact Steve Collins
  Chairman, Gallaudet University
  TTY/voice (202) 651-5199

- Deaf AIDS Action
  Box 2925
  Washington, DC 20013
  TTY (800) PWA-DEAF
  TTY (202) 546-9768

- CDC National AIDS Clearinghouse
  TTY (800) 243-7012

D. The Gay Male Community

1. Definition/Description of the Population
   a. Gay identity involves more than simple sexual responses and behaviors
      (1) The emotional, affectional, and spiritual investment in relationships colors the individual's perception of sexual orientation
      (2) There are many people who define themselves as gay or bisexual despite never having had a sexual encounter with another person of the same sex
      (3) Many men who have sexual experiences with other men do not think of themselves as gay or bisexual
      (4) *Men who have sex with men* (MSM) is currently used in statistical reporting of HIV exposure category rather than *gay* or *bisexual*. While the label MSM is preferred by some, many in the gay community consider it insensitive and offensive as it connotes merely physical interactions rather than relationships.
   b. Gay men were the first group in the U.S. to have AIDS, and thus have the longest experience with AIDS
   c. Gay men are not a homogeneous group. They may be white, African American, Hispanic; impoverished, blue collar, middle or upper class; adolescent or elderly; Baptist, Jewish, or Catholic; they may be IDUs, hemophiliacs, or have received blood transfusions.
   d. Impact of AIDS on the gay community
      (1) Gay men are the group with the largest number of AIDS cases
      (2) Nearly 60% of all those diagnosed with AIDS have been MSM
      (3) HIV seroprevalence estimates in U.S. gay communities range from 10%–70% (average in large urban centers is 50%) (Curran et al., 1988)
      (4) Seroconversion rates for gay men are estimated at 30 times that of the U.S. population average (Bartlett, 1994a)
   e. Common problems
      (1) Social stigma associated with homosexuality
      (2) Public disdain, harassment, even violence directed to gays ("gay bashing")
      (3) Sexual behaviors that are illegal in most of the U.S.
      (4) Desire to hide sexual behavior and affectional orientation from others
      (5) Need to hide sexual orientation to preserve employment, family, social relationships, religious affiliations
      (6) Entrance and orientation to gay culture often clandestine, guilt laden, and occasionally dangerous
      (7) Reliable information about gay community and culture often difficult to locate
      (8) Healthcare workers maintain social stereotypes, prejudices, and disdain of gay men; programs to educate and adjust attitudes are limited
      (9) Mental healthcare professionals often uneducated and insensitive to gay issues and psychologic/sociologic needs, especially related to the coming-out process; few mental health providers are equipped to counsel about multiple losses, grief, and bereavement overload for gay men experiencing tremendous losses of lovers, friends, and acquaintances to AIDS
      (10) Sensitive and accurate information about sexual practices is difficult to locate
      (11) Rate of alcoholism is high in gay community; amphetamine use is common in some members of the community
2. Specific Issues
   a. Prevention
      (1) Gay men developed successful behavior-change programs early in the epidemic, but programs were designed for short-term rather than lifelong behavior change
      (2) Healthcare professionals remain uncomfortable with gay sexuality and largely unaware of the complex sexual, emotional, and personal issues affecting prevention

(3) Prevention efforts largely included printed brochures, advertisements, and posters rather than one-to-one communication, group discussion, and skill-building activities; efforts for gay man were initiated when a large percentage of the population was already infected with HIV, which contributed to the perception of failure in individuals' attempts to change their behaviors

(4) Mandatory name reporting for HIV testing (required by law in most states) is incongruent with need to hide sexuality from society

(5) Difficult to target prevention messages for MSM if not self-identified as gay, bisexual, or connected with gay community

(6) As the epidemic continues, gay men suffer untold levels of death, grief, and bereavement, the effects of which are often unnoticed, invalidated, and ignored

(7) After the first decade of AIDS, gay men are beginning to present with recently acquired HIV infections, demonstrating failure of prevention programs to address relapse and ways to sustain lifelong behavior changes

b. Access to care/treatment or research protocols

(1) Gay men historically have been eager and willing participants in clinical trials; as a group they tended to exhibit high levels of compliance, flexibility, and scientific knowledge and provided researchers with important feedback

(2) After years of disappointments, gay men may not respond enthusiastically to new research protocols for fear of getting their hopes up too high

(3) Most medical research has failed to include quality-of-life measures; many research participants or subjects have felt treated as convenient guinea pigs, a sentiment that is particularly prevalent in communities

that have been historically exploited by unethical research practices (e.g., African Americans in the Tuskegee experiment); research sites that have researched gay men over years should acknowledge publicly their contribution to the current state of knowledge

c. Treatment outcomes: Depending on socioeconomic status, psychosocial characteristics, and support systems, gay men fare better than their counterparts with AIDS in quality of life, if not in longevity

3. Specific Approaches

a. Individual

(1) Validate individual's experience with AIDS, grief, and loss as personally and socially important

(2) Reassure HIV-negative men that survivor reactions and death anxieties are to be expected

(3) Employ gay men as outreach workers, clinicians, and counselors

(4) Use HIV-positive gay men to present to and motivate HIV-positive men; and use HIV-negative gay men to present to and motivate HIV-negative gay men

(5) Provide education, networking, counseling, and support for gay men coming out of the closet to reduce internalized homophobia and increase self-esteem

b. Community

(1) Homophobia must be identified, exposed, and publicly denounced; provide education and training for clinicians and staff

(2) Reevaluate safer sex messages for subtle sexual or moral judgments or messages that are culturally insensitive or inappropriate

(3) Prevention messages must acknowledge gay men not just as individuals, but as social beings with complex family, group, and community roles and relationships

(4) Foster a sense of "gay community," not just "HIV community," in high seroprevalence areas

(5) Provide discussion and bereavement groups for both HIV-negative
and -positive men to reduce grief
and bereavement overload

(6) Use the gay media (newspapers,
radio, TV) regularly to educate and
reach the community to build trust
and familiarity

(7) Work with gay community-based
organizations, if available

4. Specific Resources

- Association of Nurses in AIDS Care
(ANAC)
1555 Connecticut Avenue NW #200
Washington, DC 20036-1103
(202) 462-1038

- Gay Mens Health Crisis (GMHC)
129 West 20th Street
New York, NY 10011
(212) 807-7035

- National AIDS Information
Clearinghouse
P.O. Box 6003
Rockville, MD 20849-6003
(800) 458-5231

- PWA Coalition
31 West 26th Street
New York, NY 10010
(202) 532-0290

- San Francisco AIDS Foundation
Box 6182
San Francisco, CA 94101
(415) 863-AIDS

- University of California at San Francisco
(UCSF)
AIDS Health Project
Box 0884
San Francisco, CA 94143
(415) 476-6430

- HIV/AIDS Treatment Information Service
(800) 874-2572

E. People with Hemophilia

1. Definition/Description of the Population
   a. Hemophilia is a sex-linked genetic disorder characterized by an absence or
   deficiency of a plasma-clotting protein;
   because of inheritance patterns, most
   people with hemophilia are male
   b. Two types of hemophilia
   (1) Hemophilia A (classic hemophilia)
   caused by deficiency of clotting protein factor VIII; four times more
   prevalent than type B
   (2) Hemophilia B (Christmas disease)
   caused by deficiency of clotting protein factor IX
   c. Hemophilia is characterized by the
   severity of clotting disorder (normal factor level approximately 100%)
   (1) Severe: <1% of measurable clotting
   factor level
   (2) Moderate: 1%–5% measurable clotting factor level
   (3) Mild: >5% measurable clotting factor level
   d. U.S. incidence: 1 in 7,500 live male
   births; there are approximately 20,000
   people with hemophilia in the U.S.
   e. In the late 1970s and early 1980s, people
   with hemophilia were exposed to HIV
   through infusions of plasma-derived
   factor concentrates used to treat hemorrhages
   f. In 1982, CDC reported the first case of
   AIDS in a person with hemophilia
   (CDC, 1982)
   g. Through December 1995, 4,334 people
   with inherited bleeding disorder have
   been diagnosed with AIDS (CDC,
   1995d)
   h. It is estimated that 50% of those infused
   with clotting factors between 1978 and
   1985 became HIV seropositive, and that
   70% of those with severe hemophilia
   became HIV seropositive (Augustyniak
   et al., 1990)
   (1) Some HIV-infected people with
   hemophilia subsequently transmitted the virus to their sexual partners
   (a) Between 15% and 30% of the
   sexual partners of people with
   hemophilia became HIV
   seropositive
   (b) Vertical transmission has also
   occurred
   (2) CDC reported two cases of HIV

transmission occurring from one HIV-infected person with hemophilia to another person residing in the same household

    (a) One case occurred through IV or percutaneous exposure from home infusion (CDC, 1992a)

    (b) In the second case, the mechanism of exposure is from unrecognized or unreported incident of blood contact (CDC, 1993a)

  i. Viral inactivation of all factor concentrates began in 1984; since 1987, through surveillance methods no new HIV infections have been identified from factor infusions that have been virally inactivated and donor screened (Fricke et al., 1992)

  j. The natural history of HIV infection in people with hemophilia is both similar and dissimilar to other groups affected by HIV infection (Ragni et al., 1991)

    (1) KS is rare among people with hemophilia as an AIDS-defining illness

    (2) People with hemophilia are more likely to experience bleeding if they develop immune thrombocytopenia purpura because of their underlying bleeding disorder

    (3) Septic arthritis may develop in joints previously damaged by hemarthrosis

    (4) Lymphomas may present as pseudohematomas

  k. As with other people who have a chronic illness, people with hemophilia do not want to be identified by a disease (i.e., "hemophiliacs") but rather as people with a disease

2. Specific Issues

  a. Transmission/Risk Behavior/Prevention

    (1) Sexual partners of HIV-seropositive people with hemophilia are at risk for HIV infection and need to cope with changing their sexual practices and learning safer sex

    (2) Peer support and networking groups (e.g., Women's Outreach Network of the National Hemophilia Foundation [NHF]

[WONN], Men's Advocacy Network of the NHF [MANN]) were established to provide peer education and support and to prevent the spread of HIV among family members and sexual partners

  b. Access to care/treatment or research protocols

    (1) During the early 1980s people with hemophilia lived in constant fear of their HIV infection becoming known and being associated with a high-risk group; stigma presented a significant barrier to care

    (2) In the 1980s, people with hemophilia frequently lacked access to clinical trials because of geographic location of research sites or exclusion from particular trials because of elevated liver function tests associated with complications of hemophilia, particularly hepatitis

    (3) NHF has been recognized as an "AIDS Clinical Trial Unit (ACTU) without walls" to coordinate and monitor NIAID research protocols at hemophilia treatment centers (Kramer et al., 1990)

    (4) NHF also advocates for modification of inclusion criteria for research protocols so as not to exclude people with hemophilia

    (5) Most people with hemophilia are already connected to a hemophilia treatment center for their bleeding disorder; thus they could also have access to HIV care coordination and clinical trials

  c. Treatment outcomes

    (1) Complications of hemophilia (hemarthrosis, underlying bleeding disorder) may affect treatment for HIV (e.g., painful arthropathy is commonly treated with ibuprofen; however, the combination of AZT and ibuprofen may cause bleeding) (Ragni et al., 1988)

    (2) HIV therapies that may cause thrombocytopenia may be contradicted or need to be monitored more cautiously

3. Specific Approaches
   a. Individual
      (1) Counsel about universal precautions, including the handling and disposal of infusion products and equipment
      (2) Refer patient to local hemophilia support groups and services
      (3) Teach and reinforce safer sex practices
   b. Community
      (1) Promote hemophilia support services and programs, including peer programs
      (2) Participate in public policy discussions about access to hemophilia and HIV care, treatment, and advocacy in schools and other public institutions or in community-based organizations that provide services to people with HIV infection
4. Specific Resources

   • Hemophilia and AIDS/HIV Network for the Dissemination of Information (HANDI)
     110 Greene Street #303
     New York, NY 10012
     (800) 42-HANDI

   • National AIDS Information Clearing House (NAIC)
     P.O. Box 6003
     Rockville, MD 20850
     (800) 458-5231

   • National Association for People with AIDS (NAPWA)
     2025 1st Street #415
     Washington, DC 20006
     (202) 429-2856

   • AIDS Clinical Trials Information Service
     P.O. Box 6421
     Rockville, MD 20850
     (800) TRIALS-A

   • NHF Publications: For ordering information, contact the National Hemophilia Foundation at (212) 219-8180, or HANDI at (800) 42-HANDI
     HIV Disease in People with Hemophilia: Your Questions Answered
     What Women Need to Know About HIV Infection, AIDS and Hemophilia

Hemophilia, HIV and Safer Sex: The Choice Is Here
Living with HIV—Talking With Your Child
Living with HIV—For Adolescents With Hemophilia
Living with HIV—For Adults With Bleeding Disorders
Get Real!!! And Be Safe
Coping with Loss

F. The Hispanic Community

1. Definition/Description of the Population
   a. The Hispanic community is the fastest growing ethnic group in the U.S.
      (1) There are more than 22 million Hispanics in the U.S.; in spite of undercounting, this represents approximately a 40% increase since 1980 (National Council of La Raza, 1992)
         (a) Rapid increase in population results primarily from increased fertility, not immigration
         (b) The increase in the Hispanic population is likely to continue for some time given that the community is young
         (c) The population boom will take place in areas with the highest rates of HIV seroprevalence
      (2) HIV/AIDS has had a disproportionate impact on Hispanics, who comprise only 8.4% of the U.S. population but make up 16.2% of all AIDS cases (CDC, 1994a; Selik, Castro, & Pappaioanou, 1988); the increased relative risk holds true across both sexes and nearly all age groups
      (3) Rates for AIDS cases among Hispanics vary by birthplace and U.S. region (Selik, Castro, & Pappaioanou, 1989)
         (a) For instance, Mexican-born Hispanics residing in the South and West have the lowest rates, Puerto Rican-born Hispanics in the Northeast have the highest rates

(b) In Puerto Rico, as well as among Puerto Ricans residing on the U.S. mainland, more than half of those diagnosed with AIDS have reported injecting drug use (Colon, Sahai, Robles, & Matos, 1995; Selik et al., 1989)

(c) U.S.-born Hispanics carry the second highest relative risk, followed by Cuban-born Hispanics

(d) Mexican-born Hispanics tend to have a relative risk lower than whites

(4) Serologic surveys among the specific populations listed consistently exhibit higher rates of HIV infection among Hispanics than their white counterparts

(a) IDUs

(b) Men who have sex with men (MSM)

(c) Military recruits

(d) Women/pregnant women

(e) Female prostitutes

(f) STD-clinic patients

(g) Blood donors

(h) Prisoners (McKay & De Palma, 1991)

(5) Two trends are notable as one moves away from the Northeast: The relative risk for most subgroups diminishes but remains higher than non-Hispanics; MSM becomes the most common mode of infection

(6) Research has demonstrated persistence of a race effect, even after controlling for differences in high-risk drug-use behaviors (Feigal et al., 1991), suggesting that drug use explains only part of the racial/ethnic disparity

(7) Relatively few studies have explored the contribution of other HIV risk factors (e.g., socioeconomic status, sexual behaviors, STDs) to its prevalence among non-IDUs in Hispanic groups

(8) Economically, Hispanics have a lower socioeconomic status than non-Hispanics (COSSMHO, 1991; National Council of La Raza, 1992)

(a) 28% of Hispanics live below the poverty level

(b) 23% of Hispanic households are headed by single women with a medium income under $12,000

(c) 25% of Hispanic couples with children live in poverty

(d) Interestingly, of Hispanic families eligible for public assistance, only 29% are enrolled

(9) From a health perspective, Hispanics experience an increase morbidity/mortality and the predictable decreased access to health care associated with poverty

(10) As a group, Hispanics are far more likely to be uninsured than non-Hispanics; many work in service and manufacturing industries sectors where, in addition to low wages, a traditional absence of healthcare benefits has served to deny Hispanics access to health care

(11) Despite their lower incomes, Hispanics spend proportionally more of their disposable income than other Americans on health care

2. Specific Issues

a. Prevention

(1) Cultural and socioeconomic factors that vary from person to person, subgroup to subgroup, complicate efforts to prevent the spread of HIV/AIDS in the Hispanic community

(2) Barriers to successful HIV/AIDS education and prevention efforts among Hispanics

(a) Lack of awareness by Hispanics about the magnitude of the AIDS problem within their community

(b) Hispanics' level of knowledge varies directly with income, level of education, and degree of acculturation (Easterbrook et al., 1993; National Council of La Raza, 1992)

(c) A false perception by many Hispanics that AIDS is a gay, white, male disease

(d) Difficulty in providing prevention efforts in a nonthreatening environment, particularly for undocumented residents

(e) Cultural considerations, including the social stigma associated with high-risk behavior such as homosexual/bisexual activity, drug use, prostitution, promiscuous sexual behavior

(f) The traditional opposition of the Catholic Church (to which about 80% of Hispanics belong, at least nominally) to sex outside marriage, MSM, and artificial birth control, which complicates prevention efforts that stress the use of condoms

(g) Language, class, and cultural barriers (e.g., gender roles) present difficulties in reaching at-risk Hispanics through mass media, especially mainstream media

(h) The diversity of the population: Materials or approaches effective with one age, nationality, or regional group may be ineffective with other subpopulations

(i) Limited access for many Hispanics to health care and to health education and prevention programs

(j) Limited research on sexual attitudes and behavior among Hispanics, particularly relating to bisexuality

(k) Limited research on IDU behavior among Hispanics

(l) For the undocumented, fear of being reported to the Immigration and Naturalization Service and subsequent deportation pose significant barriers to seeking care

b. Access to care/treatment or research protocols
  (1) Limited by financial, language, and cultural barriers and the lack of healthcare workers who are members of the Hispanic community
  (2) In some states illegal residents are provided only emergency Medicaid benefits for hospital and lifesaving treatment; many chronic therapies and services may not be covered benefits
  (3) Many HIV-infected immigrants who are not legal residents avoid care if they are hoping to obtain permanent residency; evidence of HIV infection disqualifies them from legal residency
  (4) Family members may not be available as caregivers for undocumented residents; home care may not be an option when long-term care is needed
  (5) Limited education on the meaning of a clinical trial, random sampling, the nature of blinding, and the concept of a placebo and a fear of disclosure may limit participation in clinical trials (may be especially true for the undocumented)

c. Treatment outcomes
  (1) Hispanics with AIDS have had shorter survival periods than other groups (COSSMHO, 1991)
  (2) Hispanics also are more likely to die from non-HIV-related infections (e.g., syphilis, TB, meningitis, pneumonia, endocarditis) (COSSMHO, 1991)

3. Specific Approaches/Interventions
  a. Individual
    (1) Appreciate that threat of deportation and seeing healthcare professional as an authority figure may prevent the patient from being immediately forthcoming about all information about his/her health status because of fear of reprisals
    (2) Given the diversity of the Hispanic population, materials or interventions with one age, nationality, or regional group may be ineffective with other subpopulations
  b. Community
    (1) Work with Hispanic community-based organizations and Hispanic researchers
    (2) Advocate for healthcare services for

those in need regardless of payment, residency status

4. Specific Resources

- National Coalition of Hispanic Health and Human Services Organizations (COSSMHO)
  1501 16th Street NW
  Washington, DC 20036
  Phone (202) 387-5000
  Fax (202 797-4353
  [*COSSMHO is the sole organization focusing on the health, mental health, and human services needs of the diverse Hispanic communities. COSSMHO's membership has grown to more than 1,000 front-line providers and organizations. The organization fulfills its mission by working with community-based organizations; universities; federal, state, and local governments; foundations; and corporations. As the action forum for the Hispanic community, COSSMHO provides consumer education and outreach, training programs, technical assistance, model community-based programs, policy analysis, research, advocacy, infrastructure support and development, and development and adaptation of materials.*]

- National Council of La Raza (NCLR)
  810 1st Street NE #300
  Washington, DC 20002
  Phone (202) 289-1380
  Fax (202) 289-8173
  [*NCLR, the largest constituency-based national Hispanic organization, exists to improve life opportunities for the more than 22 million Americans of Hispanic descent. In addition to its Washington, DC headquarters, NCLR maintains field offices in Los Angeles, Phoenix, Chicago, and McAllen, TX. NCLR has four missions: applied research, policy analysis, and advocacy on behalf of the entire Hispanic community; capacity-building assistance to support and strengthen Hispanic community-based organizations; public infomation designed to provide accurate information and positive images of Hispanics; and special innovative, catalytic, and international projects.*]

G. HIV-Positive Nurses

1. Definition/Description of the Population
   a. Of the 304,651 AIDS cases in the U.S. reported to CDC through 1994 (CDC, 1995a) for whom occupational information was known, 14,591 (4.8%) had been employed in health care; 3,256 were nurses
   b. Most of these healthcare workers were infected from nonoccupational exposure to HIV; see Table 10.1, p. 365, for nurses who have occupationally acquired HIV infection
2. Specific Issues
   a. Access to care/treatment or research protocols
      (1) Physical concerns
         (a) Dealing with HIV-related fatigue while at work
         (b) Pushing too hard to prove one is healthy and can perform job responsibilities
         (c) Limiting exposure to OIs in the workplace (see "Work issues," below)
      (2) Psychosocial concerns
         (a) Overidentifying with own HIV, patients' physical and psychosocial issues
         (b) Need to be attentive to issues of grief overload, including loss of roles and changes in body image
         (c) Balancing the amount of HIV/AIDS work and volunteering
         (d) Allowing self to be the patient, not the nurse, with healthcare providers involved in own care
         (e) Adjusting to having friends and colleagues who are now one's caregivers
         (f) Allowing self to be a receiver rather than solely a giver of care
         (g) Working with own state nurses association and ANAC chapter
         (h) Learning to know how and what to ask for regarding own needs
      (3) Work issues
         (a) Deciding whom to tell (e.g., supervisor/manager, employee health, co-worker, infection control nurse)

i) May be helpful to practice first, talking it through with someone not at your place of employment
ii) Why tell? (scheduling flexibility; avoiding OIs)
iii) Whom can you trust?
(b) Working to develop practice guidelines to protect nurses from infections in patients
(c) Dealing with co-workers: Nonacceptance of HIV status; helplessness, knowing how to help; overprotectiveness
(d) Becoming familiar with Americans with Disabilities Act (ADA) and employer compliance
(e) Determining continued ability to work (e.g., fatigue, mental slowing)
(4) Financial/legal concerns
(a) Deciding when to go on disability (earlier vs. later in course of illness); changing from full- to part-time employment may affect insurance premiums and coverage by employers for health, life, and disability insurances
(b) Confidentiality issues if employed at the same place where one received health care
(c) Insurance issues
i) Preexisting condition clauses on new policies
ii) How to pay premiums when no longer working
(d) Requirements to report HIV status in one's state
i) Know what they are
ii) Bring a support person with you to any formal meetings regarding reporting
iii) Note any practice restrictions
b. Treatment outcomes: Necessary to deal with specific issues described above (e.g., effects of work-related stress on health status, risk of work-related OI exposure)

3. Specific Approaches
a. Individual
(1) Nurses caring for or working with an HIV-positive colleague
(a) Be aware of your own feelings of discomfort
i) If you feel any awkwardness and it seems appropriate to talk about this, acknowledge this with your colleague
ii) Failure to recognize your own feelings may lead to isolation of or withdrawal from your colleague
iii) Sometimes saying, "I don't know what to say or do; how can I help?" may be very supportive or helpful
iv) Get support for yourself
(b) Respect the right of your colleague not to talk about his or her health status or not to want support; your colleague needs to be the one to decide when and from whom to get support
(c) If your colleague is also your patient, be particularly cautious in protecting confidentiality (e.g., access to medical records, disclosure of clinical information, informal conversations on the elevator or in meal area)
(d) Be supportive without being overprotective
(e) Make reasonable accommodations when making work assignments
(2) Nursing manager supervising a HIV-positive nurse
(a) Be aware of the implications of the ADA and the need for reasonable accommodations
(b) Refer HIV-positive or other staff members to employee assistance if appropriate and available
(c) Know that job expectations and performance need to be fair and equitable for all employees; difficulties may arise if other co-workers feel they are not treated

in the same manner as their HIV-positive colleague

b. Community
   (1) Encourage involvement with HIV-positive healthcare workers for support and information
   (2) Refer to resources listed below

4. Specific Resources
   a. *For support and information*
      - ANAC HIV+ Nurse Committee
        1555 Connecticut Avenue NW #200
        Washington, DC 20036-1103
        (202) 462-1038
      - American Nurses Association
        600 Maryland Avenue SW #100W
        Washington, DC 20024-2571
        (202) 651-7000
      - Your state nurses association
      - Disability Rights Education and Defense Fund hotline
        (800) 466-4232
      - Equal Employment Opportunity Commission
        Americans with Disabilities Act information hotline
        (800) 669-3362
   b. *Legal assistance*
      - Medical Expertise Retention Program
        (415) 864-0408
   c. *Financial assistance*
      - Nurses House
        (212) 989-9393
      - Ryan White Funds (check with state health or human services department)

H. Homeless People

1. Definition/Description of the Population
   a. The Stuart B. McKinney Homeless Assistance Act (1988) defines the homeless as an individual or family
      (1) Who lacks a fixed, regular, and adequate nighttime residence
      (2) Who has a primary nighttime residence that is
         (a) A supervised, publicly or privately operated shelter
         (b) Public or private place not designed for or ordinarily used as a regular sleeping accommodation for human beings
         (c) Designed to provide temp-orary living such as welfare hotels, congregate shelters, transitional housing for the mentally ill
      (3) Whose shelter resources are limited to living temporarily with friends or relatives
   b. Health and social well-being risks among homeless: Diverse factors contribute to homelessness
      (1) Unemployment/underemployment, lack of affordable housing, and the failure of the social safety net
      (2) Indigence following overwhelming medical cost for care of physical disabilities or chronic illness
      (3) Abusive/neglectful home environments that force women, children, and adolescents onto the streets without shelter or social support
      (4) Problems related to drug use or mental illness
         (a) Drug, alcohol, and mental health problems that may arise in response to harsh and stressful conditions associated with homelessness, or
         (b) Homelessness exacerbates preexisting problems
      (5) Illegal immigrant status: Tend to be a hidden population among the homeless, living in substandard, crowded housing
   c. Common problems
      (1) Health problems (e.g., respiratory, foot, skin, parasitic intestinal infections; periodontal disease; infestations; TB)
      (2) Violence
         (a) High incidence of trauma-related injuries
         (b) Medications often stolen or lost

(3) No or limited access to hygiene facilities (toilets, bathrooms, shower, laundry); clothing often inadequate as protection in inclement weather

(4) Poor diet: Inadequate caloric and nutrient intake reduces resistance to illness and ability to heal

(5) Discriminatory treatment by health/service providers related to poor hygiene, dirty and infested clothing, substance use and behavior issues; alienates already marginalized people and reduces likelihood they will seek care

2. Specific Issues
  a. Transmission/risk behavior/prevention
    (1) The longer a person is homeless the greater the likelihood s/he will fall into one or more high-risk behaviors
      (a) Needle sharing among IDUs
      (b) Impaired judgment and decreased sexual inhibitions related to ETOH/drug use
      (c) Sex in exchange for drugs/money/food; sex solicitors will often pay more if condoms are not used
      (d) Despair/hopelessness
    (2) Homeless women are frequently victimized by rape or abuse at a disproportionately high rate; sex (consensual and nonconsensual) often takes place under unsafe and unclean conditions
    (3) An estimated 30%–40% of the homeless suffer some degree of mental illness; they are easily victimized, unlikely to receive appropriate treatment, and often self-medicate psychiatric symptoms with street drugs
    (4) Poor and infrequent access to health care may delay diagnosis and increase transmission rates
  b. Access to care/treatment or research protocols: Barriers include
    (1) Majority of homeless people have no form of health insurance (even Medicaid or Medicare) or ability to pay for care

    (2) Inability to navigate through the difficult and confusing healthcare system without assistance
    (3) Inability to tolerate long waits for care due to substance use, mental illness, risk of losing belongings or place in food or shelter lines
    (4) Lack of knowledge of where to go for care
    (5) Lack of transportation (or means to pay for it)
    (6) Negative experiences with discriminatory and insensitive treatment by care providers
    (7) Fear of arrest, deportation
    (8) Chaotic lifestyles may limit ability to adhere to research protocols
  c. Treatment outcomes
    (1) Barriers to care negatively affect outcomes to care and treatment
    (2) Inappropriate plans of care do not take into consideration a person's beliefs, living situation, ability to follow regimen
    (3) Other factors may affect outcomes
      (a) Delays in diagnosis and treatment of HIV and OI because of failure or resistance to seek care
      (b) Lack of consistent care
      (c) Poor adherence with medication schedules due to chaotic lifestyle; patients often do not fill prescriptions that necessitate travel, waiting time
      (d) Mental status changes (e.g., dementia, psychiatric disorders), substance abuse, lack of knowledge, fear
      (e) Multiple use of antibiotic/antifungal therapy with intermittent compliance can result in resistant strains of infection

3. Specific Approaches
  a. Individual
    (1) Establish trust through open, direct, nonjudgmental exploration of individual's beliefs, risk factors, and perceived needs and barriers to care
      (a) Use mutual goal setting approach to care and treatment

(b) Relationship may take time to develop; complete history may not emerge for weeks/months due to mistrust; be patient
(c) Listen carefully to what patients are trying to say, ask direct questions to clarify
(d) Assess social service, legal, and daily living needs; be aware that shelter, food, money, drugs/alcohol needs often take priority over health care; be prepared to assist with meeting basic needs first
(2) Assess financial support and eligibility for financial benefits: General Assistance, SSI, and AFDC can help get homeless people off the street, but there may be little left over for food or other essentials
(3) Base interventions on realistic picture of individual's lifestyle, daily needs, and functional capabilities
(a) Homeless people often do not keep calendars or wear watches; drop-in hours are more appropriate than strictly scheduled appointments
(b) Use multidisciplinary team approach to insure all patient's needs are being addressed
(c) Provide consistent patient advocacy through nursing case management
b. Community
(1) Explore the perceptions and reported needs of homeless people in the community to identify geographic location, social and community support, and available resources
(2) Use culturally representative outreach workers to gain entrance and trust in the community and to provide consistent presence, care, and messages within the community
(3) Advocate for one-stop healthcare and social service centers or mobile vans where patients can get housing, legal, financial, and healthcare (including mental health) needs met

(a) Expand use of community-based clinic and home care/public health nursing to increase accessibility to health care
(b) Provide appropriate, comprehensive mental health services and treatment centers to expand care options
(4) Work with public officials around fair housing issues in order to decrease behaviors that may put the person at risk for HIV infection/transmission
(5) Advocate for the establishment/legalization of needle-exchange programs

4. Specific Resources
a. *Local coalitions on homelessness*
- Community health centers, especially those in communities/neighborhoods where homelessness is common
- National HIV and AIDS Information Service (800) 342-2437
- Medicare/Medicaid Eligibility Information (800) 772-1213
- CDC (800) 227-8922

b. *Housing and shelter hotlines*
- U.S. Department of Housing and Urban Development (800) 669-9770
- Local Social Services Department

I. The Incarcerated

1. Definition/Description of the Population
a. Incarcerated refers to inmates in federal prisons, state prisons, and county/city jail systems; prisoners within jail systems are either being detained prior to trial or serving short sentences
b. In 1994, there were more than one million inmates in prison systems and more than 500,000 in jail systems (Bureau of Justice Statistics, 1995a)

c. Over the past 5 years, the U.S. has experienced increases in prison populations, increasing cases of HIV infection/AIDS within prisoners, and continuing HIV infections among inmates who are IDUs (Bureau of Justice Statistics, 1995b)

   (1) These trends contribute to the widely held perception that inmates living with HIV/AIDS are the epidemic's most underserved and disadvantaged group

   (2) The incarcerated live in treacherous settings that present enormous public health hazards and challenges (e.g., MDR-TB outbreaks)

d. It is estimated that <3% of all the incarcerated are HIV infected (both male and female) (Bureau of Justice Statistics, 1995b)

   (1) The distribution of infected inmates is uneven; it parallels HIV seroprevalence in the general community

   (2) Current trends in drug enforcement have resulted in increased numbers of inmates with established HIV/AIDS diagnoses entering prison and jail systems; many of these infections/cases are undetected

   (3) In some regions HIV seroprevalence rates among female inmates are actually higher than those among males

e. Common characteristics of female inmates

   (1) Often members of disadvantaged economic and racial/ethnic groups

   (2) HIV-infected female inmates are often serving sentences for drug-related crimes or prostitution

   (3) Injecting drug use or having sex with an IDU partner is the most common HIV risk behavior

   (4) Often have dependent children

   (5) Frequently have been involved in abusive relationships (Stevens et al., 1995)

f. Common characteristics of male inmates

   (1) Often are members of disadvantaged and vulnerable groups

   (2) Multiple incarcerations

   (3) Previous convictions for violent crimes, therefore serving long sentences

   (4) Had symptomatic HIV infection when entering the correctional system; become even sicker while incarcerated

   (5) Denied having sex with other men; more willing to report IDU

g. African Americans are disproportionately represented among the incarcerated and account for most AIDS-related deaths within correctional systems

h. Many inmates with HIV infection are not clinically identified as being infected or being ill while incarcerated; some inmates who know of their HIV infection or suspect they may be infected avoid medical care and being stigmatized as HIV positive

i. Other health-related concerns of inmates

   (1) TB, hepatitis, STDs

   (2) Depression; inmates within maximum security prison systems are often found to have severe personality and thought disorders

   (3) Predetention behaviors that compromise health status (e.g., IDU, homelessness, poverty, poor self-care skills, decreased motivation to seek care, nonadherence to treatment if care has been received)

2. Specific Issues

a. Transmission/Risk Behavior/Prevention

   (1) There are rare reports of inmates transmitting HIV infection to correctional officers (Jonsen & Stryker, 1983)

   (2) HIV infection transmission among inmates is estimated to be low (Jonsen & Stryker, 1983)

   (3) Few correctional systems allow distribution of condoms and dental dams to inmates

   (4) No correctional facility allows drug paraphernalia for injecting, although these are known to be available

   (5) The major strategies for controlling communicable disease within cor-

rectional systems are screening, control, and security

(6) HIV and STD preventive educational information is available within all correctional systems

(7) HIV testing of inmates
  (a) No clear CDC recommendations
  (b) Some states perform mandatory testing of inmates on entry to the system
  (c) All federal inmates are tested on release
  (d) Some counties and states permit mandatory testing in cases of possible exposure to correctional staff
  (e) Some inmates are tested by court order or are automatically tested following commission of certain crimes
  (f) Within some jail systems, anonymous testing is available through the local health department
  (g) Within all correctional systems voluntary testing under the order of a physician is available; however, this is at some potential risk to the inmate

(8) Pre- and posttest counseling
  (a) For medical testing, HIV counseling is available throughout all correctional systems
  (b) With mass or mandatory testing of inmates it is often difficult to provide both pre- and posttest counseling
  (c) Sometimes provided by non-healthcare providers

(9) Confidentiality/disclosure
  (a) Infected inmates whose serostatus is known to others are often subjected to physical and emotional harm and intense discrimination because of homophobia and racism
  (b) Because of the efficiency of the rumor mill it is often difficult to maintain confidentiality
  (c) Some states require disclosure of inmates' HIV serostatus to correctional administrators

  (d) In some states, efforts are underway to limit taxpayer funding of adequate medical care to infected inmates
  (e) Some state prison systems enforce blanket segregation policies for infected inmates (infected inmates are segregated from the general prison population)

b. Access to care/treatment or research protocols
  (1) The incarcerated are not eligible for Medicaid or Medicare benefits
  (2) Budgetary constraints, limited staffing, and few HIV/AIDS medical specialists within correctional systems can present barriers to adequate HIV medical care
  (3) The quality of HIV care in correctional systems differs widely; localities with higher community HIV seroprevalence are more likely to have HIV-experienced HCPs
  (4) Access to antiretroviral therapies and prophylactic regimens is generally available to inmates when indicated; however, access to mental health and drug rehabilitation services is often quite restricted
  (5) Since federal regulations were enacted in 1983 to protect inmates against research abuse, strict requirements have resulted in inmates being essentially excluded from clinical trials
    (a) Obtaining informed consent and assuring confidentiality for research studies are believed to be extremely difficult in most correctional systems
    (b) Inmates who are people of color may be distrustful of researchers, given past practices of abuse (e.g., the Tuskegee experiment) and avoid participating for fear of being treated as a guinea pig
    (c) Some propose that inmates be excluded in Phase I studies (Rold, 1995) but be eligible for participation in Phase II and Phase III trials (Dubler & Sidel, 1991)

c. Treatment outcomes
   (1) For inmates who come from unstable environments, incarceration with its limited access to drugs and alcohol may actually result in better treatment outcomes (Eichold, 1995)
   (2) There are reports that some patients experience few OIs (Eichold, 1995)
   (3) Under special circumstances, symptomatic prisoners are paroled back to society; female inmates with children are more likely than males to be paroled
3. Specific Approaches
   a. Approaches/interventions tailored for infected prisoners will need to match a correctional system's objectives of control, security, and punishment
   b. Individual
   (1) Counsel inmates individually about ways to reduce the risk of HIV transmission (see *Preventing the Transmission of HIV Infection*, p. ●●●) and allow time for questions
   (2) Inmates scheduled for release will require referrals and linkages with medical and social services; whenever possible, results from PPD screening and immunization records and copies of medical records should be provided
   (3) For inmates who are parents, it is important to involve other family members in planning for dependent children
   (4) For inmates who are dual or triple diagnosed (HIV, psychiatric illness, substance abuse), health or substance abuse services are provided
   (5) For those with extensive polysubstance abuse profiles, the recognition and treatment of depression are critical for drug rehabilitation
   (6) Individual coaching with a matter-of-fact and future-oriented approach may be more effective for counseling than a group approach
   (7) Avoid labeling and stigmatizing infected inmates
   (8) Educate inmates about preventive health behaviors and provide information that enhances decision making
   (9) Educate infected inmates regarding infection control measures to prevent exposure to other opportunistic pathogens (see Tables 10.2, p. 367 and 10.3, p. 371)
   c. Community: Identify and enlist advocacy resources (see following)

4. Specific Resources

   • American Correctional Health Service Association
   P.O. Box 2307
   Dayton, OH 43401
   (513) 223-9630
   [*Membership organization for health professionals working within correctional settings; publishes an AIDS update bulletin.*]

   • Correctional HIV Consortium
   3463 State Street #204
   Santa Barbara, CA 93105
   (805) 568-1400
   [*Nonprofit, national organization concerned with the incarcerated and with release issues confronting inmates; publishes a newsletter for infected inmates (Kite) and a professional's newsletter (Progress Notes).*]

   • National Association of Persons with AIDS
   1413 K Street NW #200
   Washington, DC 20005
   (202) 898-0414
   [*Advocacy for all people living with HIV/AIDS including those within jails or prisons.*]

   • American Civil Liberties Union (ACLU)'s National Prison Project
   1875 Connecticut Avenue NW #410
   Washington, DC 20009
   (202) 234-4830
   [*Medical care advocacy for the incarcerated.*]

   • National Commission on Correctional Health
   2105 N. Southport
   Chicago, IL 60614-4017
   (312) 428-0818
   [*Monitors and sets forth medical standards of care for all inmates.*]

- American Nurses Association
  (800) 637-0323
  [*Published "Scope and standards of nursing
  practices in correctional settings" (1993).*]

J. Rural Communities

1. Definition/Description of the Population
   a. Rural vs. nonmetropolitan designation
      (1) Either designation comprises
          20%–30% of nation
      (2) Rural area: <99 but >6 people per
          square mile
      (3) Frontier area: <6 people per square
          mile
      (4) Nonmetropolitan area: <50,000 resi-
          dents
   b. Rural life
      (1) Occupations: Most rural residents
          are not involved in agriculture;
          recent increases in white-collar and
          information-technology occupa-
          tions; increasing occupational
          diversity
      (2) Large proportion of other special
          populations (e.g., Native Americans,
          Alaskan natives, seasonal migrant
          workers, prison populations)
   c. Distribution of rural HIV/AIDS
      (1) CDC began reporting the prevalence
          of AIDS in nonmetropolitan areas in
          1991
      (2) Berry (1993) reported nonmetropoli-
          tan cases from 1991–1992
          (a) Rose at a higher percentage
              increase than any other residen-
              tial category
          (b) Had a higher rate of change in
              percentage of total cases than the
              rate of change in metropolitan
              areas with a population size
              between 50,000 to 500,000, and
          (c) Were equal to the increased rate
              of change in percentage of total
              cases in the largest metropolitan
              areas
      (3) Rural areas reveal first- and second-
          wave patterns of the epidemic
      (4) More recent data (Graham,
          Forrester, Wyson, Rosenthal, &

James, 1995) reveal a trend of more
in-migration ("coming home") of
people with HIV/AIDS than out-
migration and dramatically elevated
rates in rural black women
   d. Common problems among rural popu-
      lations
      (1) High rates of poverty, especially
          among the elderly
      (2) >50% of the nation's medically
          underinsured
      (3) Higher infant and maternal morbid-
          ity and mortality rates than in urban
          areas
      (4) Closer proximity to prison popula-
          tions
      (5) Low literacy levels
      (6) Transportation challenges
2. Specific Issues
   a. Prevention
      (1) Schools do not usually teach stu-
          dents healthy sexual behaviors
      (2) Limited access to purchase condoms
      (3) Drug and alcohol abuse dramati-
          cally increasing, especially among
          children and teenagers
      (4) Reluctance among medical
          providers to admit that infected
          populations can still remain sexually
          active and reproduce
   b. Access to care/treatment or research
      protocols
      (1) Effects of distance
          (a) Long travel distances to medical
              centers
          (b) Emergency services often deliv-
              ered by EMTs rather than para-
              medics
          (c) Life flight to treatment centers
              delays care
          (d) Home health or hospice nurses
              can be far away
      (2) Shortage of local HCPs for local care
          (a) Limited resources
          (b) Prevalent paternalism (e.g.,
              reluctance to teach infected preg-
              nant mothers about ACTG 076
              and seroconversion rates of
              infants)
          (c) Less experience with diagnosis
              and treatment

(d) Fewer professional networks to help patients and families

(e) Fewer integrated case management systems

(3) HIV counseling and testing services often part of circuit rider system, offered only intermittently

(4) HIV task forces support for current and long-term planning often depend on funds as a satellite site of larger urban task force; small pool of working members, limited local philanthropy

c. Treatment outcomes: HIV outcome data not available for people in rural areas

3. Specific Approaches

a. Individual/family

(1) Be culturally sensitive

(2) Assess and intervene to solve problems where nurses can offer real help

(a) Social isolation and fewer helpers to draw upon

(b) Financial strain from cost of illness and inability to work

(c) Daily needs such as bathing, eating, or driving to appointments that are far away

(d) Intermittent or long-distance access to emergency services and medical care

(3) Increased frequency of contact through outreach from experts who use telephone callbacks and telephone education and support systems

b. Community

(1) Build professional–community partnerships for prevention activities

(a) Involve community members in discussing and planning prevention activities among both uninfected and infected

(b) Prioritize risk assessment of different age groups and seropositive age groups (e.g., women of childbearing age)

(c) Form cooperative networks with schools and work sites

(d) Align with state health department prevention plans: School health programs, young adult prevention strategies, media campaigns geared to rural facts, situations

(2) Build professional-community partnerships for services to diagnosed population and families

(a) Educate community groups about needs of HIV/AIDS population in local area

(b) Appeal to local churches for family support services

(c) Consult with urban and state task forces about local needs

(d) Identify resources and obtain funding for services and support with the help of local business leaders and professionals

(e) Ease interactions with local authority systems, such as police

(f) Build alliances with other rural HIV/AIDS workers and organizations

4. Specific Resources

a. *Federal level*

- Department of Health and Human Services
Office of Rural Health Policy
5600 Fishers Lane
Rockville, MD 20857
(301) 443-0835

- Indian Health Services
5600 Fishers Lane
Rockville, MD 20857
(301) 443-1180

- Rural Information Center Health Services (RICHS)
National Agricultural Library
10301 Baltimore Blvd
Beltsville, MD 20705-2351
(800) 633-7701

b. *Other*

- State office of rural health, or statewide Rural Health Institute (call state capitol)

- National Rural Health Association
301 E. Armour Blvd, #420
Kansas City, MO 64111

K. Sex Industry Workers

1. Definition/Description of the Population
   a. Sex industry workers are people who exchange sexual services for money or drugs
      (1) Sex work includes prostitution, pornography, performance; not all forms of sex work are illegal
      (2) Men, women, and transgendered persons (both homo- and heterosexual) can be sex workers
      (3) Sex workers work in a broad range of settings with varying degrees of risk for HIV infection; street workers are more likely to be substance users than workers in massage parlors, escort services, brothels
   b. Factors affecting sex workers and HIV disease
      (1) Membership in oppressed, powerless groups (e.g., youth; women; ethnic or racial minorities; gay, lesbian, bisexual, transgender; persons with mental illness, addiction issues; economic poverty)
      (2) Psychosocial issues related to lack of power in society: Low self-esteem, depression, hopelessness, poor educational/vocational skills, poor social support combined with complex social entanglements, likelihood of lifestyle being criminalized or stigmatized
      (3) Often have history of sexual and physical abuse with medical and psychosocial sequelae
      (4) Sex workers with family/social support members with HIV are likely to have suffered multiple losses to HIV disease
      (5) May be involved in a coercive relationship with someone who requires them to continue working
      (6) Often are victims of violent crimes by patrons, employers, partners, police, vigilantes
2. Specific Issues
   a. Transmission/risk behaviors
      (1) Sex workers who use IV drugs or crack cocaine are at very high risk for infection/transmission
      (2) Low U.S. incidence of HIV transmission from women to men
      (3) Risk for workers is often higher than for patrons because workers have multiple contacts and are more likely to perform higher risk-receptive acts
      (4) Patrons will often pay 2–3 times normal rates for unprotected sex
      (5) STDs
         (a) Indicate high risk for HIV infection and transmission of new HIV infection
         (b) May increase likelihood of HIV infection in worker or patron via lesions, decreased immunity; cofactor in increasing HIV replication and viral shedding
         (c) Chronic STDs (e.g., HSV, HBV) can recur as OIs and complicate treatment of HIV disease
         (d) STDs increase in number and severity with progression of HIV disease
      (6) Women sex workers may have partners, children, and other family members who have HIV disease or are at risk for HIV
   b. Access to care/treatment or research protocols: Barriers include
      (1) Structural, related to insurance, finances; knowledge deficit related to confusing healthcare system
      (2) Substance use
      (3) Powerlessness
      (4) Fear and avoidance related to stigma of sex work
      (5) Historical indifference to women, substance users, marginalized groups by those providing health care; poor access to experimental and complementary therapies that may improve quality of life
   c. Treatment outcomes: Positive outcomes are affected by numerous factors (including barriers to care)
      (1) Late diagnosis and treatment of HIV disease and OIs
      (2) Chaotic interaction with healthcare system, lack of consistent care, incomplete treatment regimens

(3) Poor baseline health/nutritional status due to substance use, limited health care in the past

3. Specific Approaches
   a. Individual
      (1) Establish trust through open, nonjudgmental exploration of lifestyle, issues related to substance use, and health history
         (a) Allow time for relationship to develop, be patient, ask direct questions
         (b) Foster hope and independence while recognizing functional and social limitations
      (2) Assess legal history and current legal problems; be aware of current laws related to sex work and HIV
      (3) Assess connection to financial support systems such as SSI
         (a) SSI and other forms of financial assistance may allow sex worker to stop working
         (b) HIV diagnosis can increase eligibility for financial assistance
      (4) Refer to primary care provider who is able to provide sensitive, consistent care
      (5) Knowledge of working hours and substance use habits will help in making appointments that will be kept
      (6) Refer to appropriate support groups to enhance power and reduce feelings of isolation and hopelessness, and to drug treatment/detox program if desired/realistic
      (7) See also *Hopelessness*, p. 260, *Powerlessness*, p. 267
   b. Community
      (1) Use outreach teams to provide education about safer sex and safer substance use, provide connection to health care, legal services, and drug treatment
         (a) Outreach workers should include former workers and substance users who know community and culture
         (b) Multidisciplinary approach is vital

(c) Goal is to reduce risk behavior as well as provide alternatives to sex work
      (2) Work with law enforcement to provide useful interventions when sex workers are incarcerated
      (3) Direct education and outreach to "consumers" about risks related to HIV infection and transmission
      (4) Focus on overlapping strategies related to substance users (e.g., need exchanges, drug treatment/methadone maintenance programs)
      (5) Expanded use of community-based clinics and home care nursing to provide services in the areas where sex workers live

4. Specific Resources
   - COYOTE (Call Off Your Old Tired Ethics)
     [*A sex worker self-advocacy group that has chapters in several U.S. cities. There is no national clearinghouse or national office at this time.*]

L. Substance Users

1. Definition/Description of the Population
   a. People who use legal or illegal substances with the intent to alter consciousness; addiction, substance abuse, and substance misuse are terms generally applied when use becomes harmful or uncontrolled
   b. Substance use can interfere with a person's ability to access the healthcare system and manage his/her HIV disease to maximize health and quality of life
   c. Substance use exists on a continuum from minimal to maximal impact and within a social context that is value laden and tends to marginalize and criminalize users
   d. Types of substance users and their relation to HIV disease
      (1) Injecting drug users (IDUs)
         (a) Currently make up >30% of total AIDS cases; many pediatric HIV cases are related to mothers who are IDUs

(b) Active IDU negatively affects disease progression, transmission, and access to care

(c) Previous use also has implications for care (e.g., possibilities for relapse, pain control, stress management)

(d) Heroin, amphetamines, cocaine most commonly injected drugs; each has specific effects on the user and how a provider works with a patient

(e) IDUs, while often poor and marginalized, exist at all levels of society

(2) Non-IDUs

(a) Cocaine (crack smokers): Crack cocaine is highly addictive and is associated with many new infections and risk behaviors

(b) People who inhale, smoke, or ingest substances such as alcohol, prescription drugs, heroin, LSD, ecstasy

(c) Non-IDUs may have been injectors in the past and are at risk for becoming injectors again

(3) Substance use is complex and multifaceted; users often use more than one substance or route of administration depending on availability, desired high, or ability to procure

e. Other factors affecting substances users with HIV disease

(1) Mental illness, childhood sexual/physical abuse, history of familial addiction and dysfunction are highly correlated with substance use

(2) Race, ethnicity, gender, sexual preference, and class affect drug use, health, and access to health care

(3) Criminalization of lifestyle leads to marginalization, distrust of authority and institutions; access to housing, food, and healthcare is often compromised by restrictions on serving active users; the Americans with Disabilities Act prohibits withholding of health services to people who are addicts

(4) Adverse health effects of substance use

(a) Infections (e.g., abscesses; sepsis; endocarditis; CNS, hepatic, renal infections) related to unclean injection equipment, unsafe techniques, impurities in substances injected

(b) Organic syndromes related to direct effect of substances/impurities on tissues; affects skin, muscular, CNS, hepatic, renal, vascular systems

(c) Mental health: Causation or exacerbation of depression, psychosis, suicidal tendencies, isolation from social support systems, stigmatization, poor self-esteem

(d) Lifestyle-associated risks (e.g., malnutrition, TB)

2. Specific Issues

a. Transmission/risk behavior: Substance use may increase a person's risk of contracting HIV and transmitting it to others

(1) The risk increases because the person engages in risk behaviors (e.g., shared equipment, unsafe sex) while high or in exchange for substances

(2) Craving for drug may lead to unsafe practices

b. Access to care/treatment or research protocols: Barriers include

(1) Structural barriers affecting all persons relating to insurance, finances; knowledge deficit regarding confusing healthcare system

(2) Labeling substance users as immoral, noncompliant, manipulative, drug seeking, etc.

(3) Users are often disorganized due to lifestyle and altered mental status; appointments, records, medication refills may be lost, not kept, stolen

(4) Conflicts over pain medication often undermine relationship to provider

(5) Restrictions, rules, and requirements for persons to be clean and sober deter users from accessing care while using

(6) Users of illicit substances may fear

arrest, distrust institutions
- (7) Providers often refuse to treat active users who are mentally ill
- (8) Active users usually denied access to clinical trials for experimental treatments
- (9) Addiction, craving usually must be addressed by user before other needs, especially those involving stress (stress triggers craving)
- c. Treatment outcomes: Negatively affected by numerous factors (including above barriers)
  - (1) Poor underlying health related to lifestyle and substance use
  - (2) Poor nutrition, food often second to getting high
  - (3) Poor adherence to treatment plan due to disorganization, belief that "street" and prescribed drugs are not compatible
  - (4) Interactions between street drugs and prescribed drugs poorly understood
  - (5) Self-medication for pain or mental illness with substances often results in underlying problems becoming unmasked and diagnosable
  - (6) Differential diagnoses among HIV-related, substance-related, and mental health-related syndromes are often difficult or ignored
  - (7) Barriers to care often prevent diagnosis of HIV disease and related problems until too late for treatment
  - (8) Substance use, particularly rational or moderate, may provide positive coping strategies for some and improve quality of life; some substance use (e.g., marijuana, opiates) may provide symptom relief as well as have positive effects on mental status or sense of well-being
- 3. Specific Approaches
  - a. Prevention: Harm reduction—a model that attempts to reduce or eliminate risk of HIV infection/transmission by changing high-risk sex and substance-use behaviors
    - (1) Abstinence: One option in a multi-faceted approach
    - (2) Needle/syringe exchange programs
    - (3) Teaching safe injection use/techniques
    - (4) Education programs that avoid simplistic approaches (e.g., "just say no")
    - (5) Nonjudgmental approach to working with users
    - (6) Accessible, flexible, noncoercive drug treatment programs on demand
    - (7) Understanding user's relationship with substances and working to provide safer alternatives
  - b. Individual
    - (1) Establish trust through open, non-judgmental exploration of substance use
      - (a) Provider needs to have working knowledge of substance-use culture; ask questions if you do not know
      - (b) Users will often cover or minimize use until trust established; allow time for relationship to develop (can be months to years)
      - (c) Acknowledge difficulty of accessing health care; express willingness to work to overcome barriers
      - (d) User may not perceive substance use as primary problem; assess immediate needs and offer assistance
      - (e) Discuss benefits of substance use for person as well as costs; substance use is often related to primary coping mechanisms; do not attempt to remove this coping mechanism without providing a substitute
      - (f) Comprehensive substance use history may take time to complete; be patient
      - (g) Substance users are capable of making decisions concerning treatment and quality-of-life issues; respect their ability to do so
      - (h) Differentiate between the person and the effects of the drug in

order to identify with a person and his/her life

(2) Construct interventions with substance users' culture in mind

  (a) Be aware that users often do not keep appointments; drop-in schedules and rescheduling several times may be necessary

  (b) Do not schedule appointments that coincide with peak use times (beginning and mid-month when person gets "paid") as they will usually not be kept

  (c) Outreach clinics and services in areas populated by users are more easily accessed

  (d) Offer drug treatment/detox regularly after trust established; avoid making recovery a requirement for continued care

  (e) Manipulation and "scamming" are survival tools for many users; expect and acknowledge this

    i) Do not take it personally if you are scammed

    ii) Respect, trust, and negotiation are the best tools to minimize manipulation

  (f) Assess support networks, family relationships; remember that dysfunctional relationships are sometimes better than none

(3) Interventions in the acute setting

  (a) Assess substance use, most recent use

  (b) Anticipate and treat withdrawal symptoms; know that opiate and ETOH withdrawal are better understood and treated than amphetamine and cocaine withdrawal

  (c) Users expect to be judged and treated punitively; anticipate and reassure

  (d) Stress, fear, poor coping mechanisms without drugs potentiate craving

  (e) Despite best attempts, users may leave "against medical advice"

(AMA); begin discharge planning early

    i) Provide medications and referrals if possible

    ii) Attempt referral to home care agencies to complete IV therapy and provide follow-up

  (f) Primary care/community-based agency referrals are important to break cycle of using ER and hospital as only source of health care

  (g) Clear, reasonable, firm limits help patient understand expectations

  (h) Patient advocacy remains central to the nurse's role in caring for the substance user with HIV disease

  (i) Team approach with excellent communication reduces impact of attempts to split and manipulate

  (j) Assess and treat pain adequately (often the precipitating factor in users leaving AMA)

c. Community

(1) Expanded services for substance users

  (a) Legal, free access to clean injection equipment

  (b) Expanded access to drug treatment and detox, including methadone (estimated 2.8 million users of illicit drugs in U.S. with only 600,000 treatment slots available)

  (c) Design outreach and case management programs targeting substance users in a multidisciplinary approach to connect them with housing, food, health care, financial support, etc.

  (d) Develop housing options for active users

    i) Active users are usually barred from subsidized AIDS housing

    ii) Money management programs can prevent homelessness and stabilize

harm from substance use

   (e) Expanded use of community-based clinics, mobile vans, and public health and home care nursing to provide as much health care as possible in the areas users live

   (f) Rework the traditional model of hospice and palliative care to accommodate the needs of substance users with HIV disease

   (g) Expanded research into treatment of withdrawal and detoxification from cocaine and amphetamines

4. Specific Resources

- National Harm Reduction Coalition
  3223 Lakeshore Avenue
  Oakland, CA 94610
  Phone (510) 444-6969
  Fax (510) 444-6977
  [*A national coalition of needle exchange, AIDS education and outreach, and community health groups working to change perspectives on working with and providing options for substance users to reduce and eliminate the harm related to substance use.*]

- Local needle-exchange groups

- Resource guides to local drug treatment programs
  [*Always check to determine each agency's focus, approach, rules, etc. It can improve chances of success if a good match between program and patient is made first.*]

M. Women

1. Definition/Description of the Population
   a. Women with HIV acquired the infection through various mechanisms
      (1) In the U.S., most AIDS cases in women are associated directly or indirectly with IDU; however, in 1992 heterosexual transmission surpassed IDU as the leading mode of HIV acquisition in women diagnosed with AIDS
      (2) The incidence of woman-to-woman transmission of HIV is low, although 3 cases have been documented; larger studies of lesbians with HIV have found that other risk factors (e.g., injecting drug use, sex with men, transfusions) could not be ruled out as the mode of disease acquisition (Chu & Wortley, 1995; Petersen et al., 1992).
      (3) Although injecting drug use is a major source of HIV transmission; women who use non-IV drugs, particularly cocaine, may be at increased risk of acquiring HIV
         (a) May exchange sex for drugs
         (b) More likely to engage in unprotected sex
         (c) Sex partners may be current or former IDUs

   b. African-American and Hispanic women are disproportionately affected by HIV disease
      (1) Represent 76% of women with CDC-defined AIDS (CDC, 1995b)
      (2) In 1994 (*Fact sheet*, 1995), the incidence of AIDS was 15 and 7 times higher among African-American and Hispanic women, respectively, than among white women

   c. Through June 1995, 84% of women with AIDS are between the ages of 19 and 44, the primary childbearing years (CDC, 1995c)

   d. There is significant geographic variability in the prevalence of AIDS in women
      (1) Most of the women with CDC-defined AIDS live in large cities on the U.S. coasts, principally in the Northeast
      (2) The number of women with AIDS in rural areas and smaller communities is growing, particularly in the Southeast

   e. Population-based studies of childbearing women have yielded additional information about the extent of HIV in women
      (1) In 1991, 1.7/1,000 women giving birth in the U.S. were HIV infected; the significant geographic variability in rates ranged from 6/1,000 in the

Northeast to 0.5/1,000 in the Midwest (Wasser, Gwinn, & Fleming, 1993)

(2) It is estimated that in 1989, as many as 80,000 women were living with HIV in the U.S. (Gwinn, Wasser, Fleming, Karon, & Petersen, 1993)

f. In 1993, the CDC expanded its AIDS surveillance case definition for adolescents and adults

   (1) The expanded definition included invasive cervical carcinoma in addition to pulmonary TB, recurrent pneumonia, or CD4+ lymphocyte count <200/μl or percentage of CD4+ lymphocytes of total lymphocyte count

   (2) A preliminary study (Chu, Ward, & Fleming, 1993) of the impact of the expanded definition has shown a 142% increase in reported AIDS cases in men and a 182% increase in women, suggesting that the new definition may be more sensitive in identifying HIV disease manifestations in women

2. Specific Issues

  a. Transmission/risk behaviors

   (1) Why women are at risk of acquiring HIV

    (a) Power imbalances (economic, gender, cultural) make it difficult for women to negotiate safe sexual relationships

    (b) Drug dependence may increase women's exposure to unsafe situations (needle use, sex) and decrease the ability to negotiate safe ones

    (c) Lack of a sense of vulnerability or risk for HIV, particularly for women unaware of their partner's current or past risk behaviors

   (2) No single prevention strategy will work with this heterogeneous group, as different subgroups require discrete prevention efforts; women at risk through injecting drug use or sexual contact include

    (a) Women at risk through injecting drug use

    (b) Women at risk through sexual contact

     i) Adolescent girls

     ii) Heterosexual women (who may believe that monogamy means they are not at risk) may have partners with past or current hidden risks

    (c) Lesbians

     i) May believe they are not at risk because the incidence is low among women who have sex with women

     ii) Some lesbians have unprotected sex with men, which puts them at risk

     iii) Some women who have sex with women do not self-identify as lesbian and may not access information specifically targeted to lesbians

  b. Access to care/treatment or research protocols

   (1) Socioeconomic/lifestyle barriers

    (a) Lack of transportation or child care

    (b) Employment that grants no sick leave or healthcare benefits

    (c) Active drug use: Disorganized lifestyles may reduce drug users' ability to follow through with care needs; health care may be a low priority

    (d) Women with stigmatized lifestyles may shy away from contact with mainstream providers or may not fully disclose relevant information

    (e) Dependence on unsupportive or abusive partners

   (2) Psychosocial/cultural barriers

    (a) Women may have a tendency to take care of themselves last

    (b) Caregiving responsibilities as a mother or primary care provider for other ill family members may consume all available time and energy

(c) Women may not understand the language or medical vocabulary of educators and providers

(3) Healthcare environments unfriendly toward women

   (a) Long waits, no access to child care for small children

   (b) Clinic hours that conflict with school hours of older children

   (c) Complicated scheduling: Nonavailability of coordinated HIV and gynecologic care necessitate appointments at multiple clinics

(4) Insensitive or inadequate care provider(s)

   (a) Delays in proper diagnosis and treatment because providers have a lower index of suspicion for HIV disease in women, particularly if obvious risk factors are absent

   (b) Providers may not address HIV prevention issues with women as a routine part of health maintenance

   (c) Providers may assume heterosexuality and not deal appropriately with issues of lesbians/bisexual women

(5) Biases against drugs and drug users

(6) Women are underrepresented in experimental HIV/AIDS protocols

   (a) May be barred from participation in protocols by virtue of gender, presence of a uterus, or lack of surgical sterilization

   (b) Women from racial and ethnic minorities may be suspicious of experimental treatments based on past scientific abuses

   (c) As the epidemic spreads further into nonurban areas, access to trials may be reduced

c. Treatment outcomes

(1) Data on the natural history of HIV infection in women are limited to date

   (a) Most information gathered in large-scale studies of men

   (b) There are two ongoing large, multicenter cohort studies on the natural history of HIV in women (sponsored by NIH and CDC); it will be a few years before much of the data are published

   (c) Available information on the natural history of HIV in women has been compiled from small studies (DeHovitz, 1995; Melnick et al., 1994)

     i) Early manifestations center on the genital tract (e.g., *Candida vulvovaginitis*, cervical dysplasia, PID)

     ii) Anecdotal reports suggest that women with HIV experience menstrual changes (e.g., oligomenhorrea, irregular periods); however, published reports do not show significant menstrual changes in women with lower vs. higher CD4+ lymphocyte counts; see *Menstrual Irregularities*, p. 181

     iii) Esophageal candidiasis as the first OI is more common in women than in men

     iv) KS and oral hairy leukoplakia have been reported less frequently in women than in men

     v) HSV, CMV infections, bacterial pneumonia, and mycobacteremia have been reported as more frequent in women than in men

     vi) There is no documentation to show pregnancy has a significant effect on the progression of HIV disease in women

(2) Survival rates of women with HIV

   (a) Early studies found shorter survival rates in women than in men; socioeconomic status and lack of access to treatment may have been factors

   (b) More recent studies (DeHovitz, 1995; Melnick et al., 1994) have

reported contradictory findings
    (c) No evidence to suggest that women respond differently to treatments for HIV or OIs; however, definitive studies have not been done
3. Specific Approaches
    a. Individual
        (1) Prevention
            (a) Assuming heterosexuality may inhibit open communication and development of appropriate prevention plans
            (b) Individualize prevention plans; develop them in collaboration with each woman
            (c) Facilitate empowerment of women to help them make safe choices
            (d) Discuss, encourage, and refer drug users to addiction treatment services to increase their ability to make safe choices
            (e) Assess barriers to condom use and eroticize condom use with heterosexual/bisexual women
            (f) Incorporate partner whenever possible to reinforce prevention message
        (2) Treatment
            (a) Coordinate clinical care and services where possible to facilitate "one-stop shopping" for HIV care, gynecologic services, and HIV care for children
            (b) Assess a woman's social situation, particularly her family structure, as a part of the clinical history
            (c) Include psychosocial support network and empowerment in the treatment plan
            (d) Include the family (if the woman desires) and drug treatment
            (e) Don't assume heterosexuality; ask directly about relationships and sex with both men and women in order to develop an appropriate plan of care
            (f) Discuss long-term planning for minor children as early as possi-

ble; it may take women a long time to deal with this issue
            (g) Provide women with written materials to reinforce education and to provide information to family members at home
    b. Aggregate interventions
        (1) Prevention
            (a) Identify target population (e.g., women attending inner-city family planning clinic)
            (b) Conduct a needs assessment
                i) Identify the gaps between this community's needs and available resources (e.g., need for general education on how to prevent HIV infection, but providers have insufficient time)
                ii) Assess the perceived needs for an intervention (e.g., through focus groups, surveys of providers)
            (c) Develop an intervention plan
                i) Distribute information packets to every patient at her initial visit
                ii) Conduct waiting room educational sessions
            (d) Evaluate impact of the intervention
                i) Pre/postintervention questionnaires
                ii) Incidence of STD, pregnancy rates
            (e) Adjust the intervention based on the evaluation
            (f) Target prevention efforts at multiple points on healthcare continuum (e.g., school, work sites, family planning clinics)
            (g) Make prevention messages culturally sensitive and specific
        (2) Treatment
            (a) Develop outpatient clinical services that are easy for women to access
                i) Organize services with the goal of one-stop shopping where possible
                ii) Arrange clinic times to

allow for visits by women with school-age children

   iii) Make provisions for child care in clinic

  (b) Have other resources that women use frequently (e.g., drug treatment, colposcopy, support groups, family planning, case management, legal services) available for immediate referral

  (c) Discuss clinical drug trials with all women

4. Specific Resources

- National Resource Center on Women and AIDS/Center for Women's Policy Studies
  2000 P Street NW #508
  Washington, DC 20036
  (202) 872-1770
  [*Publishes written materials and videos and The Guide to Resources on Women and AIDS, a national listing of resources.*]

- National Lesbian and Gay Health Association
  1407 S Street NW
  Washington, DC 20009
  (202) 939-7880
  [*Publishes an annual directory of lesbian and gay health services, sponsors the annual Lesbian and Gay Health Conference.*]

- National Native American AIDS Prevention Center
  2100 Lake Shore Avenue #A
  Oakland, CA 94606
  (800) 283-AIDS
  [*Services include a hotline and educational information on Native American women and AIDS*]

- National Black Women's Health Project
  1211 Connecticut NW #310
  Washington, DC 20036
  (202) 835-0117
  [*Advocacy and policy organization that publishes a quarterly news magazine, Vital Signs, which includes articles on women and AIDS*]

- National Minority AIDS Council
  1931 13th Street NW
  Washington, DC 20009
  (202) 483-6622

- National Women and HIV/AIDS Project
  710 I Street SE
  Washington, DC 20003
  (202) 547-1155
  [*Advocacy organization that publishes a newsletter, Spirits, and compiled the National Women and HIV/AIDS Survey Results and Agenda*]

- National Women's Health Network
  514 10th Street NW #400
  Washington, DC 20004
  (202) 347-1140
  [*Provides educational materials on women and AIDS*]

- Sexuality Information and Education Council of the United States
  130 West 42nd Street #350
  New York, NY 10036
  (212) 819-9770
  [*National research library includes literature on women and AIDS*]

Section 7

Preventing the Transmission of HIV Infection

In the absence of an effective cure for HIV infection and AIDS, prevention is the best means of limiting the spread of infection. Preventing HIV infection and transmission requires sustained commitment to effect the process of change over the long term.

Short-term interventions are not effective. Prevention usually requires multiple interventions and strategies to change behaviors and attitudes. Healthcare professionals must critically analyze interventions before suggesting them to a given patient. Patients may need referral to sources of help with experience and broad-based resources in dealing with emotional and relationship problems (Catania et al., 1994).

The implications of the mistrust of authorities and the government on HIV-prevention programs must be considered when planning a prevention program. Paternalism and politics have figured historically in preventing HIV infection. For example, needle-exchange programs have led to heated debates, not so much about the ability of such programs to reduce the risk of transmission of HIV, but rather about fear that the program would serve to encourage illegal drug use (Des Jarlais, 1992).

Limited resources make it essential to target prevention programs precisely toward patients at highest risk. Prevention messages need to be culturally and educationally appropriate for their intended audiences or they will not be effective or even understood. For example, men of some cultures who have sex with men do not recognize the label "gay." Focus should be on the behaviors, not the labels. Messages also need to be appropriate for the patient's developmental stage and age.

For most risky behaviors prevention is aimed at abstinence or at risk reduction. Risk reduction, also called harm reduction, can help nurses design goals that are practical and can incorporate full participation from the planned participants. Harm reduction recognizes that people change gradually, not radically and has three basic principles:

- *Know that it is better to be pragmatic than idealistic.* The goal is to achieve an improvement in outcomes rather than in abstinence, which may never be achieved.
- *Establish a hierarchy of goals to reduce risk.* For example, if patients choose to continue using drugs, it is better to set a goal of them using their own needles and syringes (works) and not to share them, rather than a goal of complete abstinence.
- *Treat patients with respect and dignity.* Work with patients to problem solve how to reduce risks in ways that are acceptable to them.

Prevention messages must target general and specific populations, e.g., adolescents; gay, lesbian, and bisexual adolescents and adults; those who engage in survival sex; IDUs and needle users; the incarcerated; sex workers; women of color; men and women who have unprotected homosexual or heterosexual sex; and people who have been sexually abused or assaulted.

Risky behaviors are more important than membership in risk groups or exposure categories. There is a complex relationship in the transmission of HIV by sexual means and by blood through the use of injecting drugs. Many people engaged in risky or unprotected sexual encounters also inject drugs. Many IDUs engage in risky sex either to exchange money for drugs or foods or because of altered perceptions. This section discusses prevention of sexual transmission, transmission through injection drug use, vertical transmission (from mother to child), and prevention through vaccination.

I. PREVENTING SEXUAL TRANSMISSION

1. Definition/Description
    a. Adolescents are at high risk for acquiring HIV infection because of numerous developmental issues; need specific interventions
    b. Adolescents have sexual feelings and may have a need to act on them
    c. 75% of women and 86% of men have engaged in sexual activity by the age of 20 (CDC, 1993b)
    d. The average age of sexual debut for males and females is 15 (Sonenstein, Pleck, & Ku, 1989), but younger adolescents may be sexually active
    e. The "invisibility" of gay, lesbian, and bisexual youth may be compounded by sexual activity and risk taking
        (1) Teens may be in the process of coming out to themselves and society and engage in heterosexual activity to prove themselves straight
        (2) Those who are not acculturated in the gay community may feel that safer sex messages are not directed toward them, and therefore they are exempt from having to practice safer sex (Johnson, Bachman, & O'Malley, 1992)
        (3) The gay or bisexual adolescent male's first sexual partner is typically 7 years older than the teen, which may increase potential for exposure to HIV infection
    f. Teenage bravado makes high risk-taking activities (e.g., alcohol use, sexual activity, street drug experimentation) common
    g. One in 10 adolescent females becomes pregnant each year (Gayle et al., 1990)
    h. One in 7 adolescents aged 15–19 acquires a STD each year (Novello, 1988)
    i. About 20% of adolescents with HIV infection are hemophiliacs or recipients of blood products
    j. Seroprevalence studies do not usually include adolescents; many of the cases of AIDS in people in their 20s acquired HIV infection in adolescence
    k. Homeless teenagers are at increased risk of HIV transmission when they exchange sex for food or shelter
    l. Teenagers may not have the communication or negotiation skills necessary to ensure the use of safer sex behaviors
2. Factors increasing risk of transmission
    a. Use of alcohol and recreational drugs can impair the immune system and also break down inhibitions (Cohen & Durham, 1993); greatest risk arises from the use of drugs as an excuse for engaging in risky behaviors
    b. Lesions on genitals and mucosa, sores, or irritation can increase risk of transmission if exposed to HIV-positive body fluids
    c. Lack of self-esteem (e.g., from sexual abuse, violence) can result in decreasing the person's ability to demand safer sex behaviors
    d. Partners who are not truthful about their past history or who are not monogamous after beginning a new relationship increase potential for HIV transmission
    e. HIV is more easily transmitted from men to women than vice versa
        (1) Concentration of HIV is higher in semen than in vaginal secretions
        (2) The vagina's structure acts as a reservoir that can harbor infected semen, thus prolonging exposure
        (3) The vaginal wall is more friable and permeable than the penis
3. Primary prevention
    a. The only safe sex is no sex, or abstinence; all other sexual activity is considered *safer sex*
    b. Abstinence is a viable option for many people to be include as one aspect in the range of factual information regarding decision making and sexual activity
        (1) "Abstinence only" messages, especially if coupled with "sex is evil," are harmful and ineffective

Table 7.1   Riskiest Forms of Sexual Activity

Sexual Activity	Risk-Reduction Strategies
Unprotected anal intercourse	• Condom • Water-soluble lubricant
Unprotected vaginal intercourse	• Condom • Water-soluble lubricant • Female condom if labial lesions
Unprotected oral sex	• Condom • Rubber dam
Bondage and discipline	• Strategies for each (formerly known as S&M) specific behavior (e.g., oral sex—use of a "safe word" to signify it is not part of the sexual play when a partner says "stop")
Water sports	• Do not do if open lesions
Anal play (fisting)	• Condom • Glove/finger cot • Water-soluble lubricant • Rubber dam (short fingernails)

(2) Behavioral education to modify unsafe sexual practices is vital

c. More important than risk groups are risky behaviors and practices (see Tables 7.1 and 7.2)

d. People who choose to be sexually active need to understand their options for protection against infection

e. Protective barriers
   (1) To decrease risk of transmission of HIV
      (a) Male latex condoms: Nonlubricated condoms can be cut lengthwise and used as a barrier between two partners' mouths, anus, or vagina
      (b) Female polyurethane condoms
      (c) Latex sheets (dental dams)
   (2) Adjunctive use of spermicides and lubricants
      (a) Role of spermicides in preventing infection is uncertain
      (b) Spermicides and water-based lubricants reduce friction, may prevent condom rupture
   (3) No protective device works if the people do not know how to use it or feel uncomfortable with it; nurses need to provide suggestions on using thinner condoms and proper lubricants and suggest ways that condom use can be sensual and part of love making
   (4) Know that natural-membrane condoms do NOT consistently demonstrate prevention of HIV transmission (may have naturally occurring pores that are large enough for passage of viruses, but small enough to prevent passage of sperm [Cates & Stone, 1992])

f. Effectiveness of barrier protection
   (1) Condoms are highly effective in preventing HIV/STD transmission when used consistently and correctly as has been demonstrated by several studies of serodiscordant couples (one partner HIV positive, the other not) (Padian, Sluboski, & Jewell, 1991)
   (2) Consistent and correct condom use (see Table 7.3) results in a contraceptive failure rate as low as 2% (Trussell et al., 1991)
   (3) The female condom (Reality™) is an

Table 7.2 Safer Sexual Practices

While these are physiologically safe activities, they may not be acceptable to individual patients. Healthcare workers must be attentive to possible individual sensitivities that may to lead alienation due to the person's fear that engaging in sexual behaviors might have moral or religious implications.

- Toe-sucking
- Finger-sucking
- Body massage
- Slow dancing
- Hugging
- Dry kissing
- Computer sex
- Telephone sex
- Fantasy
- Self-pleasuring
- Abstinence
- Body-to-body rub

Table 7.3 Correct Use of Condoms

- Use a new condom with each act of oral, anal, or vaginal intercourse.
- Handle carefully to avoid damaging with sharp objects.
- Put the condom on after penis is erect and before any genital contact with the sex partner.
- Eliminate any air that may be trapped in the tip of the condom ("pinch an inch").
- Use adequate lubrication during intercourse.
- Use water-based lubricants only (e.g., K-Y jelly) with latex condoms.
- Hold the condom firmly against the base of the penis while withdrawing; withdraw while the penis is still erect to prevent slippage.

Note: From "Update: Barrier protection against HIV infection and other sexually transmitted diseases," by Centers for Disease Control and Prevention, 1993, *Morbidity and Mortality Weekly Report, 42,* p. 590.

option for women that can be controlled by the woman
  (a) Polyurethane sheath with a ring on each end for vaginal insertion
  (b) Offers protection during cunnilingus
  (c) Disadvantages: Expense and access
  (d) Insufficient study of the female condom's role in preventing pregnancy (Kurth, 1993)
g. Techniques to teach prevention: Humor, skits, playacting; brainstorming, buzz groups; new sexual scripts, role playing, participatory demonstrations (Cohen & Durham, 1993)
  h. Make evaluation part of every prevention program
4. Additional risks/considerations
  a. How will a partner react to a suggestion of safer sex?
  b. Women may be subject to abuse as a consequence of asking their partner to use a condom or may lose security of financial support (Cohen & Durham, 1993)
  c. Cultural, legal, and religious beliefs; belief systems are extremely strong.

II. PREVENTING PARENTERAL TRANSMISSION IN INJECTING DRUG USERS

1. Definition/Description
   a. IDUs are at increased risk for infection with blood-borne pathogens such as HIV-1, HBV, hepatitis C virus, HTLV-II
   b. Sharing of contaminated injection equipment is usual way HIV is transmitted (blood-borne) between those injecting drugs
   c. Cessation of drug use is possible
      (1) Review of studies of methadone programs show effectiveness in treating opioid addiction
      (2) Availability and effectiveness of treatment for cocaine abuse lags substantially behind treatment for opioid addiction; in some samples of IDUs surveyed, as many as 90% injected cocaine alone or in combination with other drugs (Normand, Vlahov, & Moses, 1995)
   d. Even with effective treatment, it is estimated that <20% of IDUs are in treatment at any given time, and as many as 50% of IDUs have no history of treatment for drug abuse (Normand et al., 1995); lack of universal coverage may result from
      (1) Insufficient treatment slots
      (2) No readiness to curtail drug use or enter treatment
      (3) Perception that treatment has intolerable side effects
      (4) Treatment options limited for certain drugs (e.g., cocaine)
2. Factors increasing risk of transmission
   a. Sharing contaminated injection equipment
      (1) Direct sharing: Passing a used needle and syringe from one person to another
      (2) Indirect sharing: Individuals might each have their own needle and syringe, but share drug-preparation equipment (e.g., "cookers" or spoons used to prepare drugs for injection; cotton used to filter out particulate matter when drawing up solution prior to injection)
      (3) Anonymous sharing: Because possession of needles and syringes may be illegal, IDUs avoid arrest risk if they do not carry injection equipment
         (a) "Shooting galleries": Clandestine locations where needles and syringes can be rented
         (b) In shooting galleries, repeated rental of needles and syringes is tantamount to sequential anonymous sharing of injection equipment
   b. Risk factors for needle sharing: The reasons why IDUs share needles are multiple and complex
      (1) Ritual embedded within the subculture
      (2) Pragmatic motivation: To avoid arrest for possession of paraphernalia
      (3) Economics: Needles and syringes cost money
3. Risk prevention
   a. Strategies to prevent parenteral transmission of blood-borne infections among IDUs
      (1) Abstinence from drug use
         (a) In theory, the most effective approach would be to never start drug use; however, evaluations of "just say no" and D.A.R.E. programs in elementary schools show modest or negligible impact
         (b) Facilitating abstinence from injecting drug use through treatment is an important strategy; alone it is insufficient
      (2) Use of sterile needles and syringes only is next best strategy for people who continue injecting drug use
         (a) Obstacles: Current U.S. paraphernalia and prescription laws prohibit possession of needles and syringes for nonmedical purposes

(b) Some community groups are concerned that unrestricted legal access to needles and syringes might encourage
  i) Nonusers to initiate drug use
  ii) Nonparenteral users to start injecting drug use
  iii) Current IDUs to increase frequency of use
  iv) Former IDUs to restart drug use
  v) Discarding contaminated needles and syringes on the street, placing the public at risk for accidental needle-stick injury
  vi) Even with access to sterile needles, levels of needle sharing might not change

(3) Needle-exchange programs
  (a) 77 programs in many U.S. cities through 1994 (Normand et al., 1995); although program characteristics vary widely, basic objectives are similar
    i) To distribute sterile syringes
    ii) To collect contaminated syringes
    iii) To establish trust and rapport with IDUs to permit education, counseling, and referrals
  (b) Evaluation: In 1993, two reports from the U.S. General Accounting Office (1993) and the University of California (Lurie et al., 1993) in conjunction with the CDC addressed questions related to needle exchange; some conclusions were
    i) "The majority of studies of needle exchange program clients demonstrated decreased rates of HIV drug risk behavior, but no decreased rates of HIV sex risk behavior" (Lurie et al., 1993, p. 18)
    ii) "Although quantitative data are difficult to obtain, those available provide no evidence that needle exchange programs increase the amount of drug use by needle exchange program clients or change overall community levels of noninjection and injection drug use" (Lurie et al., 1993, p. 15)
    iii) "Needle exchange programs in the U.S. have not been shown to increase the total number of discarded syringes and can be expected to result in fewer discarded syringes" (U.S. General Accounting Office, 1993, p. 395)
    iv) "Studies of the effect of needle exchange programs on HIV infection rates do not and, in part due to the need for large sample sizes and the multiple impediments to randomization, probably cannot provide clear evidence that needle exchange programs decrease HIV infection . . ." (Lurie et al., p. 12)

(4) See also *Substance Users*, p. 305.

III. PREVENTING VERTICAL TRANSMISSION

1. Definition/Description
   a. In the U.S., AIDS is the third leading cause of death for all women aged 25–44 years, and the leading cause of death for African-American women in this age category (CDC, 1995c)
   b. Many women in this age group have children, enhancing the potential for perinatal HIV transmission; thus HIV has become a biologic family disease
2. Pregnancy issues
   a. Estimated 80,000 women with HIV infection in United States. About 7,000 HIV-positive women deliver each year, resulting in 1,500 HIV-infected infants (CDC, 1995f).
   b. HIV-infected women who become pregnant face unique dilemmas in reproductive decision making
      (1) Determining individual risk of HIV transmission to the fetus or disease exacerbation for self is difficult (Williams, 1990)
      (2) Pregnancy decisions influenced by profound meaning of childbearing across cultures, class (Mitchell, Brown, Loftman, & Williams, 1990)
   c. Reproductive decisions of HIV-positive women are often very similar to those of HIV-negative women (Sunderland, Minkoff, Handte, Moroso, & Landesman, 1992); studies show a number of influencing factors for keeping and for terminating pregnancies in women with and without HIV (Bradley-Springer, 1994)
   d. HIV can be transmitted antepartally, intrapartally, and postpartally through breastfeeding; more than 50% of all infections thought to occur late in pregnancy or during delivery, with breastfeeding adding an additional 15%
      (1) Rates of perinatal (vertical—mother to infant) HIV transmission vary (Chin, 1994)
         (a) Lower in industrialized countries (13%–32%)
         (b) Higher in developing nations (25%–48%)
      (2) On average, 1 in 4 infants is infected (CDC, 1994e)
   e. Vertical transmission is multifactorial (Boyer et al., 1994)
      (1) Maternal and fetal viral factors (high viral load and p24 antigenemia viral type)
      (2) Immunologic (low CD4+ lymphocyte counts, antibody levels)
      (3) Clinical factors (e.g., premature rupture of membranes, premature delivery, delivery complications, mother's advanced disease state)
   f. Primary HIV infection prevention should be the fundamental goal, as it yields healthy mother and infant
   g. See also *Clinical Management of Pediatric HIV Patients*, p. 375
3. Factors increasing risk of transmission
   a. Heterosexual contact is increasing as a transmission mode: Accounts for 8% of total AIDS cases but 36% of all female cases (CDC, 1995c)
   b. Why women are at risk
      (1) Biologic vulnerability
         (a) HIV directly infects cervix or vaginal epithelium
         (b) Menses causes pH changes: Less acidic, more hospitable to HIV (Grimes, 1994)
         (c) Higher dose of HIV in sperm than in vaginal fluids (dose-response relationship)
      (2) Epidemiologic vulnerability: Seroprevalence levels in communities vary; women in these areas are more likely to encounter HIV-infected sex or drug-sharing partner
      (3) Social vulnerability
         (a) Women may be economically or otherwise reliant on partner
         (b) May not have power or skills to negotiate terms of sexual encounter
         (c) Sexual partners may lie about or be unaware of their risks and status
   c. Risk prevention

(1) Assess each client's understanding of risk behaviors
    (a) Ask whether client has sex with men, women, or both; survival sex (for drugs or money); if experienced/experiencing sexual abuse or trauma; feelings about current sexual situation
    (b) Make referrals to address identified concerns (Denenberg, 1993)
(2) Chronic vaginitis raises an index of suspicion for HIV in women
(3) Safer sex
    (a) Women are more at risk of acquiring STD from a man that men from a woman, but less able to negotiate sexual terms; thus there is a need for more female-controlled methods, such as vaginally-applied virucides (Stein, 1995)
    (b) Methods and techniques currently available provide a hierarchy of risk reduction (Hutchison & Shannon, 1993)
      i) Most effective: Abstinence, "outercourse" (mutual masturbation, frottage, etc.), use of latex male condom with spermicide containing nonoxynol-9 or other virucidal agent
      ii) Less effective/unknown effectiveness: Contraceptive sponge with spermicide, diaphragm or cervical cap with spermicide, spermicide alone, female polyurethane condom
      iii) No protection from HIV/STDs: Oral contraceptives, other hormonal methods (injections, subdermal implants) should be used in conjunction with barrier protection (condoms, spermicide)
      iv) IUDs are contraindicated due to risk of infection
(4) Substance use counseling
    (a) Many women acquire HIV through own injecting drug use or sex with IDU partner
    (b) Substance use may lead to unsafe behavior, compounding risk of sexual HIV acquisition (Berger & Vizgirda, 1993)
(5) Women need access on demand to addiction treatment but may have difficulty getting services during pregnancy or at facilities that accommodate children (Springer, 1992)

4. Enhancing perinatal health for mother and fetus/infant
  a. Antepartum: Review information for women who already are infected with HIV, and who are pregnant or considering pregnancy, on treatment options and self-care
    (1) HIV does not seem to alter pregnancy outcomes adversely, nor does pregnancy alter HIV disease course unless the woman is severely immunocompromised
    (2) Perinatal transmission rates vary, based on factors such as maternal disease state
    (3) The pregnancy decision is hers to make, with support from her health providers
      (a) If she decides to terminate the pregnancy, make appropriate referrals
      (b) If she decides to carry the pregnancy to term, assume that monitoring and care for her health and the infant's health will be provided
    (4) Weighing all the information and options may take multiple sessions
    (5) Main goal is to keep the woman as healthy as possible, avoiding coinfections and other immune system assaults that may have an adverse impact on her health status and possible perinatal transmission
    (6) Early entry into care is optimal; monitor the woman's HIV disease in additional to standard prenatal care
      (a) Draw CD4+ lymphocyte counts each trimester

(b) Offer PCP prophylaxis or anti-retroviral therapy as indicated

(c) May be cases where need for maternal treatment outweigh possible pharmacologic risk to the fetus (e.g., during a major OI)

b. Intrapartum

(1) Maintain skin integrity for infant ante/intrapartally

(2) Avoid chorionic villus sampling, percutaneous umbilical cord sampling, fetal scalp monitoring or pH sampling, vacuum extraction, etc., unless clinically indicated

(3) Some evidence of possible protective transmission effect from Cesarean section, but not conclusive and should be based on clinical indications (Kuhn, Stein, Thomas, Singh, & Tsai, 1994)

c. Postpartum

(1) Clear secretions from infant's airways (using DeLee with wall suction) from infant's eyes and other mucous membranes, and from any skin prior to parenteral contact (vitamin K, heel sticks, venipuncture)

(2) Wrap infant to avoid further ingestion of maternal secretions until bathed (Shannon, 1996)

(3) Encourage mother to bond with baby and be assured that with consistent use of universal precautions need not worry about household transmission

(4) Where safe alternatives to breast-feeding exist, encourage HIV-infected women to consider refraining from breastfeeding

5. Perinatal risk reduction

a. Prenatal testing

(1) Policy makers and others have debated ethical framework around testing of pregnant women (Faden, Geller, & Powers, 1992)

(2) CDC guidelines recommend *universal* counseling and *voluntary* HIV testing for pregnant women (CDC, 1995f)

(a) Offering counseling, testing, and referrals to care as appropriate to women and men who are sexually active or abusing substances is an important nursing intervention

(b) Approaching the test decision as a partnership builds relationships of trust between provider and patient essential for informed discussion of complex reproductive and treatment decisions

(3) Counseling and testing alone do not result in behavior change; continuing education, ongoing counseling, assurance of legal protection for reproductive choice and freedom from coercion also needed (Amaro, 1993)

(4) Counselor's attitude and approach can influence woman's acceptance of HIV testing (Meadows et al., 1990)

(5) Counseling for woman with HIV who is pregnant or considering pregnancy should be nondirective, take into account personal meanings of reproduction, and address grief work as well as clinical information for the woman herself (Holman & Kurth, 1995)

b. AZT use during and after pregnancy (see also *Clinical Management of Pediatric HIV Patients*, p. 375)

(1) Initial results from randomized, multicenter, double-blinded study (ACTG 076 clinical trial) found that AZT given after first trimester of pregnancy, during labor and delivery, then orally to newborns resulted in 67% reduction in rate of perinatal HIV transmission; of 184 infants in placebo group, 25.5% were HIV-infected vs. 8.3% of 180 children in AZT-treated group (CDC, 1994e)

(2) Another, smaller study found similar results in a group of women with lower CD4+ lymphocyte counts than ACTG 076 study (Boyer et al., 1994)

(3) Long-term effects of such AZT use in pregnancy are not yet known

(4) Women need to be provided information regarding results of these studies, and—as with the reproductive decision itself—be supported in their treatment choice.

IV. HIV-VACCINE DEVELOPMENT

A. General Information on Vaccines

1. Mechanism of action
   a. Induces immune response and immunologic memory
   b. Provides individual protection
   c. Provides protection to other members of the community (herd immunity)
2. Traditional approaches to vaccines
   a. Live attenuated vaccines
      (1) In wide use for polio (OPV), measles, mumps, and rubella
      (2) Most effective in eliciting an immune response that is similar to the response to actual antigen
      (3) Do not protect against infection but do protect against disease
      (4) Possibility of reversion to pathogenic-type virus in vivo
      (5) Adverse effects possible with all above
   b. Inactivated or killed vaccines
      (1) Formed from
         (a) Whole inactivated organisms (e.g., pertussis, cholera)
         (b) Detoxified exotoxin (e.g., diphtheria, tetanus)
         (c) Soluble capsular material (e.g., pneumococcal polysaccharide)
         (d) Components of the organism (e.g., HBV, subunit influenza)
      (2) Effective in preventing disease: Often less immunogenic than live attenuated vaccines (therefore often requiring repeated doses or boosters) and may be more reactogenic (cause more adverse side effects)
   c. Whole inactivated vaccines (e.g., first effective polio vaccine [Salk])
      (1) An effective whole inactivated vaccine has been in wide use against pertussis
      (2) A whole inactivated vaccine for cholera was in wide use until the 1970s, when it was proved to be of limited effectiveness
   d. Subunit vaccines
      (1) Use a piece of the organism or its products (e.g., exotoxin) to elicit a protective immune response (diphtheria and tetanus)
      (2) The plasma-derived hepatitis B vaccine uses purified plasma hepatitis B surface antigen to protect against hepatitis B
      (3) Recombinant hepatitis B vaccine is also a subunit vaccine
3. Newer approaches to vaccines
   a. The advent of molecular biology and the development of new techniques in genetic manipulation and recombination of DNA have greatly expanded the number of possible approaches for vaccine development
   b. Genes coding for biologically active substances have been identified and analyzed
   c. Techniques for transferring genetic material within and between organisms have been applied to vaccine development (Ellis, 1988)
      (1) Recombinant subunit vaccines (e.g., hepatitis B vaccine); made by using surface antigen produced in a recombinant expression system in yeast
      (2) Live recombinant virus vectors (hybrid viruses): Live virus (e.g., vaccinia, adenovirus) or bacteria (e.g., *Salmonella typhimurium*) carry vaccine antigens for other pathogens (Douglas, Buchbinder, Judson, & McKirnan, 1994; Ellis, 1988).
      (3) Combination vaccines: Two or more vaccines delivered in a single inoculation

B. Development, Testing, and Licensing of Vaccines

1. Vaccine development is a long and multistep process requiring integration of basic and clinical research
   a. Basic research to identify
      (1) Causative agent
      (2) Components of the organism responsible for disease

(3) Host immune response
(4) Candidate vaccines
(5) Animal-model systems for preclinical testing: Ideally, an animal model is identified in which safety, immunogenicity, and protection can be evaluated before human testing begins
b. Clinical research to demonstrate safety, efficacy in humans; usually done in three phases/trials
(1) Phase I: Evaluate short-term safety and immunogenicity at various dose levels
(2) Phase II: Evaluate safety and immunogenicity in target populations and determine optimal dose, route, and schedule
(3) Phase III: Controlled field trials to evaluate efficacy of the vaccine in preventing infection or disease (LaMontagne & Curlin, 1992)
2. Licensing (in the United States through Centers for Biologics Research and Evaluation [CBER/FDA])
3. Social acceptance and commercial interest
a. Despite the remarkable achievements of vaccine prophylaxis, the use of vaccines has always been controversial, primarily because of public concern about safety
b. Commercial interest is necessary to develop an efficient and reliable method of producing sufficient quantities of vaccine
4. Decisions about use
a. Defining populations at risk
b. Achieving wide vaccine coverage: Acceptance, access to vaccine and health care
c. Barriers to use: Cost, fear, misinformation

C. HIV Vaccines

1. HIV differs from other vaccine-preventable viral infections (Karzon, Bolognesi, & Koff, 1992)
a. Escapes immune surveillance
b. More than one route of transmission
c. Cell associated and free virus

d. Genetic diversity
e. Target is immune cell
f. Little evidence of viral elimination on recovery
2. Scientific hurdles to HIV vaccine development
a. Inadequate understanding of the correlates of immunity
(1) Role of neutralizing antibody
(2) Cell-mediated immunity
(3) Mucosal immunity
b. Lack of an adequate animal model
3. Virus variation
a. Geographic variation (9 clades identified worldwide)
b. Variation between and in individuals (FCCSET, 1993)
4. Lack of standard immunologic assays
a. Clinical studies of HIV vaccines to date have not all used standard, reproducible assays to measure immune response
b. Being able to make valid and reliable comparisons of immune responses among trials and sites is critical in evaluating the true efficacy and safety of vaccine candidates

D. State of the Science of HIV Vaccines

1. Preventive HIV-1 Vaccines
a. Preclinical testing: Studies of protection in primates (e.g., Fast, Mathieson, & Schultz, 1994; Schultz & Hu, 1993)
b. Phase I clinical trials
(1) >20 HIV-vaccine candidates have been entered into clinical trials
(2) Most are recombinant subunit vaccines (composed of envelope proteins gp160 or gp120) or recombinant poxviruses (e.g., vaccinia, canarypox) containing envelope proteins
(3) All have been well tolerated with no serious physical side effects (short-term safety)
(4) Some have been more immunogenic than others (see e.g., Fast & Walker, 1993; Walker & Fast, 1994)
(5) Problems of discrimination and other social risks have been docu-

mented (Belshe et al., 1994)
c. Phase II clinical trials: Two gp120 vaccine subunit products have been tested in Phase II clinical trials involving groups at higher risk of infection from HIV; to date, the vaccines have been well-tolerated and have induced neutralizing antibody and binding antibody in most volunteers
d. Planning for Phase III efficacy trials
    (1) Goals
        (a) To prevent infection, disease
        (b) To define and measure efficacy
    (2) Criteria/justification for beginning efficacy trials
        (a) Comparative safety/immunogenicity from clinical trials
        (b) Immunogenicity and protective efficacy from animal studies
        (c) Assessment of risks and benefits of going ahead vs. risks and benefits of waiting
        (d) Recently, WHO decided to move ahead with efficacy testing in a developing country with two gp120 vaccine candidates; in spring 1994, the NIH AIDS Advisory Council decided against proceeding in the U.S. with the same two candidates
    (3) Design of efficacy trials
        (a) Randomized, placebo controlled, double blind
        (b) Endpoints and timepoints
        (c) Length of the trial
        (d) Sample size
        (e) Behavioral counseling and assessment
    (4) Sample selection
        (a) Populations with high seroincidence
        (b) Perceive themselves to be at risk
        (c) Capable of understanding and consenting
        (d) Stable and cooperative
    (5) Ethical concerns
        (a) Protecting the rights and welfare of participants
        (b) Informed consent
        (c) Behavioral counseling
        (d) Minimizing social risks
        (e) Issues of justice
    (6) Decision making and review
        (a) National and international review (scientific and ethical)
        (b) National and regional approval
        (c) IRB approval
        (d) Data and Safety Monitoring Board
e. Planning for the use of a preventive vaccine
    (1) Target populations
    (2) Mandatory or voluntary vaccination
    (3) Cost and payment
2. Therapeutic vaccines
a. Differences between prophylactic and therapeutic vaccines
    (1) Prophylactic vaccines to prevent infection or disease in uninfected persons
    (2) Therapeutic vaccines to enhance immune response in those already infected
b. Phase I and II clinical trials
    (1) Several vaccines have been tested in Phase I or I/II trials with HIV-infected individuals
    (2) Most have been envelope subunit vaccines, but whole inactivated virus, vaccinia recombinants, and cellular antigens (soluble CD4+) have also been entered into clinical trials
    (3) All have been reassuring with respect to safety, and there is evidence of new antibody to some epitopes and increased cytotoxic activity (Karzon, 1995; Walker & Fast, 1994)
    (4) Long-term follow-up will be necessary to see if and how these vaccines affect the health and well-being of infected clients
3. International issues (Lurie et al., 1994): Complex; often both political and ethical.

Section 8

Wellness Strategies

The concept of wellness is receiving increasing attention from people who wish a direct, participatory role in their own health programs. This section reviews some of the more common strategies people living with AIDS use to enhance their quality of life, increase their capacity for healing, and strengthen their stress-management abilities. These strategies may be considered alternative, complementary, or holistic.

Holistic health care emphasizes four dimensions: nutrition, physical awareness, stress reduction, and self-responsibility (Keegan, 1988). Each patient's pattern of use of wellness and alternative strategies is personal, very private, and profound for the individual. It is in this spirit of respect and compassion that we present the following content.

Although the section is patient focused, the content is also of value to nurses, other healthcare providers, and care partners of patients to adopt for their own wellness needs.

A. Wellness and Holistic Nursing

1. Healing Paradigms: See Table 8.1
   a. Wellness nursing theories: Nightingale's Environmental Nursing; Roy's Adaptation Model; Orem's Self-Care Model
   b. Holism
      (1) Nursing theories: Rogers' Science of Human Beings/Unitary Man, Watson's Caring; Leininger's Transcultural Nursing; Newman's Systems Model
      (2) Others: Ayurvedic, traditional Chinese medicine, shamanism
2. Holistic Nursing Process
   a. Preparing the nurse: Opening yourself to possibilities, listening actively, centering (achieving a quiet, connected, calm state of being)
   b. The process
      (1) Assessment
         (a) Listen actively with the whole being
         (b) Share with the patient; open to the patient with receptivity and compassion
         (c) Identify wellness behaviors the patient uses
         (d) Identify significant health providers in patient's life (including spiritual guides)
         (e) Assess effectiveness and side effects of treatments used by patient
      (f) Focus on patient's strengths, positive behavior
      (2) Nursing diagnosis, state of being, or defining situation
      (3) Goal setting and establishing treatment plan
      (4) Intervention and implementation
      (5) Revisiting goals and treatment plan
3. Uses and Limitations
   a. Expected benefits (patient's and practitioner's) need to be explored; may include all the following and may change over time
      (1) Cure
      (2) General wellness promotion
      (3) Adjuvant restorative therapy to conventional treatment
      (4) Symptom management
      (5) Healing of emotional, physical, spiritual, and psychosocial problems
   b. Limitations and side effects
      (1) Because the intervention(s) often encompass elements of the transcendent and spiritual realms, the outcome is difficult to predict with any certainty; it is dependent on the patients needs, the skill and compassion of the practitioner, and many other factors
      (2) Interaction with other treatments
   c. The patient's intention to treat these practices as complementary (treatment used *with* standard medical therapy) vs. alternative (treatment used *instead of*

Table 8.1 Comparison of Healing Paradigms

Traditional Western View	Holistic View
"Man is the sum of his parts"	Unity of man-body-spirit
Allopathic	Healer uses whole self
Cure	Promote healing
Causality	Relativity
Human beings are center of universe	All are connected and are one with the universe
Doing	Being
"Show me"	Use of intuition
Quantitative research	Qualitative research
Illness (negative findings)	Wellness (positive findings)

standard medical therapy) needs to be explored

d. Experience, competence, and state of the healer are generally thought to affect the healing process

4. Modalities
   a. Spiritual and psychologic
      (1) Guided imagery and psychoneuroimmunology (PNI)
      (2) Music therapy, movement/dance therapy, art therapy
      (3) Humor, yoga, meditation, prayer, dreamwork
   b. Nutrition, elimination
      (1) Vegetarian
         (a) Eating low on the food chain
         (b) Macrobiotic and other balancing diets
      (2) Mega dosing of vitamins
      (3) Cleansing and detoxifying treatments (e.g., fasting, juicing, enemas)
   c. Drug and biologic: Homeopathy, herbs and teas, ozone and other oxygen therapies
   d. Energy systems: Therapeutic touch and healing touch, Reiki, acupuncture, shiatsu, reflexology, laying on of hands, chakra balancing

5. Current Areas of Research
   a. Prevalence/use of complementary modalities in specific populations
   b. Effectiveness and uses of specific complementary modalities
   c. The lived experiences of people affected by HIV

6. Resources
   a. American Holistic Nurses Association
      4101 Lake Boone Trail
      Raleigh, NC 27607
      (919) 787-5181
   b. Nurse Healers Professional Associates, Inc.
      P.O. Box 444
      Allison Park, PA 15101
      (412) 355-8476

B. Therapeutic Touch, Healing Touch, and Other Energy Modalities

1. Description
   a. Therapeutic touch (TT) is one of many modalities, both ancient and modern, used to heal by manipulating the human energy field. TT is a scientific approach similar to laying on of hands; there may be little or no physical contact between healer and patient.
   b. Healing touch (HT) is a program sponsored by the American Holistic Nursing Association (AHNA). HT uses TT and other energy modalities borrowed from ancient healing techniques such as the laying on of hands or the balancing of the chakras; both TT and HT are nurse-developed interventions from a nursing paradigm.
      (1) Scientific basis for healing touch (HT) builds on the studies using TT; however, there is a growing body of research to support HT
      (2) As with TT, HT is practiced in many settings, including independent practice
   c. Historical usage
      (1) TT was introduced into nursing practice in the early 1970s by Dr. Dolores Krieger at New York University School of Nursing
      (2) HT was introduced to nursing by Janet Mentgen, RN, in the 1980s
   d. Important concepts
      (1) Human energy field (HEF) is the life energy open system within and around each individual. HEF is a cross-cultural concept known as *chi* in Chinese, *qi* in Japanese, and *prana* in Sanskrit. Other terms could be *life force, Holy Spirit,* or *energy bodies.* This subtle nutritive energy circulates within and throughout the body. It extends beyond the corporal body, and its properties may be felt by any of the senses. To experience your own energy field by centering, hold hands 2 in. apart, slowly and consciously moving them apart

another 1–2 in., then back together without touching, then pulling apart a few inches, and repeating this inward and outward movement a few more times. You will notice an energy charge and perhaps sense the presence of a subtle substance.

(2) Universal energy field (UEF) is the collective energy from the earth

(3) Centering: Quiet, connected, calm state of being

(4) Other important components: Caring, compassion, and unconditional love; acceptance; intentionality; intuition, in addition to tactile awareness; unity of mind-body-spirit

(5) Anticipated benefits: Studies support many beneficial uses of TT and HT, such as hastening wound healing, reducing anxiety, boosting the immune system, enhancing recovery from anesthesia

(6) Application, usage, frequency: TT is probably the best known complementary independent nursing intervention; thousands of nurses are trained in TT and HT

   (a) Therapeutic touch process: Centering

     i) Assess the patient, including his/her energy field: Do a light sweep holding the healer's hands 2–4 in. above the patient

     ii) Clear, smooth, or unruffle the field

     iii) Stop when energy flow feels adequately open and even

     iv) Reassess the energy field after treatment

   (b) Healing touch process

     i) Preparing the practitioner: Be open to unconditional love, offer unconditional love, center yourself; attune to the patient and the UEF

     ii) Accessing and assessing: Use traditional and nontraditional methods, including hands, pendulum, or bells

     iii) Manipulating the energy field: Include the techniques of TT, visualization, conscious breathing, opening Chakras, gentle and conscious touch, channeling the energy from the UEF

     iv) Reassessment: Use any of the techniques described above, and nonverbal feedback from the patient

2. Relationship to People With HIV

  a. Utility: TT and HT practitioners and practice groups provide care to people with HIV in many communities and settings

  b. Level of acceptance

    (1) Both the AHNA and the Nurse Healers Professional Association (NHPA) have collected hundreds of TT and HT policies and procedures from healthcare institutions throughout the U.S.

    (2) TT and HT are consistently referred to as independent nursing interventions, but most schools of nursing do not yet teach these modalities in their curricula

    (3) Many health insurance plans reimburse nurses for TT and HT if these are included in the treatment plan

    (4) Energetic healing interventions are of interest to many patients and those patients at high risk for illness episodes

  c. Providers/facilitators of services

    (1) Attributes of skilled practitioners/healers

     (a) Compassionate; able to use intuition to guide actions

     (b) Attentive to their own physical, mental, spiritual, emotional, and psychologic health needs

     (c) Humility (awareness that the healer is the vehicle and not the source of the healing energy)

     (d) Able to be centered and grounded

(2) Types of providers: Care partners, psychotherapists, pastoral counselors, nurses, members of religious and spiritual communities, massage therapists, counselors, lay people in spiritual or religious communities

(3) Potential for harm/any regulatory oversights

  (a) It is important to note that the unity of mind-body-spirit implies that any treatment modality may have an impact on the total being; it is not surprising, therefore, that patients undergoing energy treatments for pain, for instance, may experience strong emotions associated with a repressed emotion or other phenomena

  (b) TT: NHPA has set practice standards

  (c) HT: AHNA certification of practitioners and instructors has been available since 1993

  (d) There is no licensure requirement associated with certification: Many practitioners come from other traditions beside nursing (e.g., shamanism, psychotherapy and spiritual communities) and are excellent practitioners/healers

3. Nursing Role

  a. Incorporate TT, HT, and other energetic healing activities into clinical practice, education, consultation, research, and administrative aspects of nursing

  b. Provide information about these care modalities to the general public as well as to patients and families

  c. Practice behaviors that facilitate the integration of mind-body-spirit into healthcare activities

  d. Explore personal reactions and feelings regarding these modalities and the interest or ability to engage in them

4. Future Directions

  a. Other energy modalities will join TT and HT as healing arts practiced by nurses and other practitioners/healers

in the more traditional areas of health care

(1) Reiki: An ancient Buddhist method of healing and wellness that was resurrected in Japan during the mid-1800s by Mikao Usui; Reiki practitioners channel universal energy of the earth through different positions and sequential placements of their hands

  (a) Reiki practice uses an apprentice tradition, passing knowledge from one to another directly. Training includes ritual, prayer, meditation and attunement. Levels of practice are Reiki I, Reiki II, and Reiki III (Master/Teacher).

  (b) Almost from its inception women have been accepted as Reiki practitioners, which, linked with Reiki's use of connectedness to the (mother) earth, has attracted many women who are involved in matriarchal spiritual communities

(2) Reflexology (see p. 338) and acupuncture (p. 333)

b. The currently unfamiliar concepts of energy, universal energy field, chi, and other terms will become increasingly accepted by traditional healthcare providers and nurses in particular

c. Patients' desire for compassionate, high-touch healing encounters with nurses and their other providers will become increasingly relevant to the nursing profession as a whole and, in turn, provide nursing with a renewed dedication to our art and science

C. Traditional Chinese Medicine

1. Description

  a. Traditional Chinese medicine (TCM) describes a system of medicine practiced in modern China. It derives from many medical traditions in China and has its roots in the ancient medical and spiritual practices of China and Tibet. "Traditional" reflects the fact that TCM has remained relatively unchanged over time; the techniques pass from one generation to the next.

b. In the U.S., TCM is used in professional practice by people licensed as acupuncturists; although professional standards are still emerging, a master's-degree level of education in Chinese medicine is generally required for entry into the profession, with board certification available in acupuncture and herbology

c. Diagnosis in Chinese medicine
   (1) Based on syndrome or pattern identification (*bian bing*), more than disease identification (*bian zheng*)
   (2) Pattern identification is the process of gathering and assembling a meaningful group of symptoms into a coherent clinical picture through the four examinations (*si zhen*): inspection, auscultation and olfaction, inquiring, palpation
   (3) The approach is generally holistic: It emphasizes the person (host) rather than the disease or pathogen

d. TCM encompasses several treatment modalities
   (1) Acupuncture (see p. 333): The insertion of fine, solid needles into specific sites on the body corresponding to energetic pathways in the body
   (2) Herbal medicine: Plant, mineral, and animal products taken internally or applied externally to heal the body (see *Chinese Herbal Medicine*, p. 335)
   (3) Qi gong (pronounced "chee kung"): Breathing, movement, and meditation practice (see *Qi Gong*, p. 337)
   (4) Diet and nutrition
   (5) Massage and bodywork
   (6) Cupping (glass or bamboo cups applied to the skin with a partial vacuum to cause local congestion)
   (7) Moxibustion (burning artemisia mugwort on or near acupuncture points)

e. TCM is intimately tied to the culture of China and is heavily influenced by the cosmology of that culture; however, it is being/has been successfully transplanted into other cultures

f. Important concepts: Some words do not translate clearly; others have specific meanings that differ from conventional usage
   (1) Yin and yang: Complementary principles that may be observed throughout life
       (a) Yin corresponds to elements of the feminine: Water, cold, winter, night, rest, and interior
       (b) Yang corresponds to elements of the masculine: Fire, heat, summer, day, movement, and exterior
   (2) Qi (pronounced "chee"): Vital energy, the animating force of life, it is both energy and matter; it warms, protects, and keeps all our organs in place. Blood is the nourishment that fosters the creation of every cell in the body. Qi is yang in relation to yin blood.
   (3) Essence: Carried in a woman's reproductive capacity and in a man's sperm; essence is the basis of reproduction, growth, and aging
   (4) Spirit: The intangible expression of who a person is; it includes one's personality and can be seen in the light that shines from one's eyes

g. Practitioners of TCM are licensed in 32 states, generally under the title of Licensed Acupuncturist. Status of licensure and scope of practice vary considerably from state to state; many states rely on board certification by the National Commission for the Certification of Acupuncturists (NCCA).

2. Relationship to People With HIV
   a. Utility
      (1) Immune enhancement: The concept of resistance to disease is at the heart of immunity; it is a cornerstone of TCM practice. With acupuncture the patient is not given any substance but there is a measurable outcome. The acupuncture has stimulated a healing response or restored homeostasis. The body's ability to resist or recover from a disease state has been stimulated.

(2) Symptom alleviation: Case reports and clinical case studies (Moffett & Sanders, 1995; Moffett, Sanders, Sinclair, & Ergil, 1994; Rabinowitz, 1987; Smith, 1988) have found repeatedly that TCM is useful in alleviating common, nonspecific symptoms (e.g., weight loss, diarrhea, abdominal pain, nausea, headaches, enlarged lymph glands, peripheral neuropathy, fatigue, loss of appetite, shortness of breath); it is also useful in alleviating the side effects of drugs

(3) Improvement in quality of life (QOL): Case reports and clinical studies (e.g., Medical Outcomes Study SF-36; Moffet et al., 1994) have found improvements in QOL indices such as physical functioning, role functioning (physical), general health, vitality, social functioning, role functioning (emotional), mental health

b. Level of acceptance: TCM is not widely accepted by the medical establishment

3. Nursing Role

a. Nurses can provide patient education about the appropriate use of TCM in HIV disease as adjunctive therapies

b. Nurses can be effective liaisons between physicians or other providers and the patient regarding the appropriate use of TCM for HIV-positive patients; the nurse is uniquely positioned to provide education to physicians about TCM as well as provide education about western medicine to acupuncturists

4. Future Directions

a. More states are expected to join in regulating TCM professional practice; the scope of practice for acupuncturists is being debated

b. Quality-assurance activities and practice guidelines are largely missing, although professional associations are now forming peer review bodies

c. Integration of practitioners of TCM into the healthcare system is being explored with obvious implications for issues of reimbursements

5. Resources

a. *Professional associations* (call for member state associations)

American Association of Acupuncture and Oriental Medicine
433 Front Street
Catasauqua, PA 18032
Phone (610) 433-2448
Fax (610) 433-1832

National Acupuncture and Oriental Medicine Alliance
P.O. Box 77511
Seattle, WA 98177
Phone (206) 524-3511
Fax (206) 623-4272

b. *Substance abuse*

National Acupuncture Detoxification Association
3220 N Street NW, #275
Washington, DC 20007

c. *AIDS care*

AIDS & Chinese Medicine Institute
455 Arkansas Street
San Francisco, CA 94107
Phone (415) 282-4028
Fax (415) 282-2935

d. *Education and certification of acupuncturists*

Council of Colleges of Acupuncture and Oriental Medicine
(202) 265-3370

National Commission for the Certification of Acupuncturists
P.O. BOX 97075
Washington, DC 20090
(202) 232-1404

D. Acupuncture

1. Description: The use of fine, filiform needles inserted into the body at specific sites to stimulate a healing or homeostatic response by facilitating the smooth flow of qi through the meridians (energetic pathways)

a. Historical usage

(1) Earliest use dates back 3,000 years in China

(2) First brought to the U.S. by French physicians in the 18th century, but has become established by immigrant Chinese communities

(3) Acupuncture was "discovered" by the West in 1971 following an apocryphal report by James Reston in *The New York Times*

(4) Most non-Chinese practitioners have studied in England or the U.S.

(5) Licensure began in 1973 in Nevada; currently acupuncturists are licensed in 33 states

b. Types or categories

(1) Many styles or schools of acupuncture practice (e.g., Chinese, Japanese, Korean, five-element)

(2) Auricular (ear) acupuncture is a particular application that has found widespread use in substance-abuse treatment

c. Anticipated benefits

(1) Immune enhancement, symptom alleviation, and quality-of-life benefits (see "Utility" under *Traditional Chinese Medicine*)

(2) Pain: Generally useful for painful conditions, localized or general, somatic or psychic; acupuncture triggers the release of endogenous opiates that have analgesic action, calming mind and body

(3) GI disorders: Studies (e.g., Li, Tougas, Chiverton, & Hunt, 1992) have found that acupuncture normalizes intestinal motility and gastric secretions; this normalizing function is difficult to explain, but can be understood as stimulating a homeostatic response of body functions

(4) Relaxation response obtained with most treatments

(5) Addictions have been treated with acupuncture with some very good results, in part because acupuncture releases endogenous endorphins that help alleviate cravings and withdrawal symptoms

(6) In 1996, the FDA approved the use of acupuncture needles by qualified health practitioners

d. Application, usage, frequency

(1) Acupuncture has wide application for various populations across ages and ethnicities

(2) Can be used in a variety of settings (clinics, medical offices, hospitals, drug treatment settings)

(3) Generally used on a weekly basis, but daily usage sometimes indicated

2. Relationship to People With HIV

a. Utility

(1) Useful for common, non-HIV specific complaints

(2) Helpful as an adjunctive modality in care and recovery from opportunistic infections (OIs)

b. Level of acceptance

(1) It is popular, generally not painful, and the most widely accepted part of TCM

(2) While there is some concern with acupuncture as an invasive procedure, it has a high level of safety when practiced with universal precautions

c. Providers/facilitators of services

(1) Attributes of skilled practitioners/healers

(a) State licensed, if available, or National Commission for the Certification of Acupuncturists (NCCA) board certified, including a knowledge of clean needle techniques

(b) Education or experience working with people with HIV

(c) A compassionate provider who respects the patient

(2) Types of providers

(a) Licensed acupuncturists have primary training using acupuncture as a modality of TCM

(b) Physicians may legally practice acupuncture in most states, although most do not because of lack of training

(c) Nurses may be able to provide acupuncture in some states as part of their scope of practice or under the direct supervision of a skilled physician

(d) Acupuncture detox specialists can perform acupuncture on the ear as part of a substance-abuse program in some states

(3) Potential for harm/any regulatory oversights

    (a) Possible risks with acupuncture include infection, bruising, numbness or tingling, dizziness, fainting, spontaneous miscarriage, nerve damage, or organ puncture

    (b) Most acupuncturists practice without a system for peer review or professional QA activities; many acupuncture clinics have clear standards for practice under the supervision of a clinical director

    (c) Most of the 33 states that license or certify acupuncturists use the NCCA exam as a minimum standard of competency

3. Nursing Role: This is a licensed specialty in most states, but nurses can play a valuable role as advocates for patient choice in treatments and as educators for acupuncturists and western-medicine physicians

4. Future Directions: Integration of licensed acupuncturists as healthcare providers within the system

E. Chinese Herbal Medicine

1. Description: Plant, mineral, and animal products taken internally or applied externally to heal the body; most commonly plant material ingested as a food or nutritional supplement, but sometimes in the manner of a drug or medicine

  a. Historical usage

    (1) Herbal medicine has its roots in ancient China: Herbs and foods are often indistinguishable, except in their usage; foods are medicine and vice versa

    (2) Herbs are a major part of TCM, though less well-known than acupuncture to the American public

  b. Types or categories

    (1) There are hundreds of commonly used Chinese herbs and many classical combinations for their use; some of the more than 15 categories of Chinese herbs are

    (a) Tonics: Used to strengthen and nourish the organs and address weakness of the blood, qi, essence, sinews, flesh, or bones; research in China has identified herbs that can improve nonspecific immunity, normalize various abnormal physiologic states, and increase production of lymphocytes, erythrocytes, and immunoglobulins

      i) Qi tonics (e.g., ginseng, astragalus, codonopsis, atractylodes licorice)

      ii) Blood tonics (e.g., rehmanniae, angelica, peony, lycium fruit, polygoni)

      iii) Yang tonics (e.g., deer antler, cistanches, epimedii, eucommia, cuscutae)

      iv) Yin tonics (e.g., ophiopogonis, ligustrum, tremellae, ganoderma)

    (b) Heat-clearing herbs: From a biomedical perspective these are antiinflammatory, antiviral, or antibacterial (e.g., honeysuckle, forsythia, isatidis, dandelion, viola, prunella, skullcap, coptis)

    (c) Herbs: To vitalize and move the blood to reduce capillary permeability and inflammation, activate the absorption of inflammation, and regulate the immune system (e.g., angelica, ligusticum, peony, semen persicae, salvia, curcumin, pseudoginseng)

  c. Anticipated benefits with rationale

    (1) Immune enhancement, symptom alleviation, and QOL benefits (see "Immune enhancement" under *Traditional Chinese Medicine,* p. 332)

    (2) Herbs can nourish the body and normalize digestion and assimilation, allowing the body to obtain maximum nourishment from the

diet (based on thousands of years of empirical usage)

d. Application, usage, frequency

(1) Chinese herbal medicine is a sophisticated and complex system that can be very powerful, but dangerous if misused; it is highly recommended that herbs not be self-prescribed; patients need to consult a licensed or traditional herbalist, especially for long-term use

(2) Herbs have many traditional forms

(a) Decoctions: Raw or processed herbs in bulk form are brewed as a tea or a soup

(b) Pills: Herbs may be ground up and compressed into tablets for ease of ingestion and uniformity of product

(c) Spray-dried processing: Herbs may be decocted and spray dried to create a concentrated product to be reconstituted in water or made into a tablet or capsule

(d) Tinctures and liquid extracts: Herbs may be processed with alcohol, water, or other medium to make a tincture or extraction solution

(3) Used either daily or as needed for acute conditions

2. Relationship to People With HIV

a. Utility

(1) Immune enhancement, symptom alleviation, and QOL benefits (see "Immune Enhancement" under *Traditional Chinese Medicine*)

(2) There are a number of prepared, experimental herbal formulas specifically for people with HIV (e.g., Composition A®, Enhance®)

(3) There is a category of herbs that is traditionally used to treat infections. In vitro, some of these herbs have had an inhibitory effect on HIV. No data are available from in vivo studies.

(4) Herbs have a primary utility for treating GI disorders; as a nutritional supplement, herbs can help normalize GI functions and provide nutrition

(5) Many herbs are the source of biochemically derived pharmaceutical products, so it is easy to see how the natural herbs themselves have healing properties; also, the herb in its natural form may be more or less easily absorbed and may have natural buffers

b. Level of acceptance

(1) Herbal medicines are widely used in many cultures; there is a high level of general acceptance among consumers

(2) Herbal medicines are viewed with skepticism and caution by most of the medical establishment

c. Providers/facilitators of services

(1) Attributes of skilled practitioners/healers: See *Acupuncture*, p. 333

(2) Types of providers

(a) In many states acupuncturists are trained as practitioners of Chinese herbal medicine as part of the scope of practice

(b) Physicians, nurse practitioners, and others with appropriate training may prescribe herbs

(c) Traditional herbalists who have apprenticed under a master or as a family tradition are often highly knowledgeable about herbs

(3) Potential for harm/any regulatory oversights

(a) Risks

i) Toxicities, especially in large doses or inappropriate use

ii) Individual herbs may have specific contraindications (e.g., in pregnancy)

iii) GI: Nausea, gas, vomiting, stomachache, diarrhea

iv) Other: Headache, rashes, hives, tingling of the tongue

(b) Herb/drug interactions are quite uncommon

(c) The FDA currently has few

guidelines about herbs or herbal products with respect to indications, contraindications, product manufacturing and labeling

    (d) Herb products with parts from endangered animal species, toxic ingredients, or drug constituents are unacceptable to reputable herbalists and herb distributors

3. Nursing Role: Nurses can become involved in recommending and dispensing herbal remedies and encouraging patients not to self-prescribe but instead to consult a licensed or traditional herbalist

4. Future Directions
   a. More clinical research
   b. Role of herbs as nutritional supplements to be developed

F. Qi Gong

1. Description: Qi gong means "breath exercise" or "energy work." It is also based on the movement or manipulation of the body qi (vital energy). Qi gong is variously described as exercise, movement, breathing, and meditation. Qi gong also involves focusing attention, intention, or awareness on the body and circulation of qi.
   a. Historical usage: Qi gong is the oldest modality of TCM
   b. Types or categories
      (1) Internal qi gong: Energy movement or manipulation done on oneself
      (2) External qi gong: Energy movement or manipulation done by a practitioner to a patient or student
      (3) There are countless styles of qi gong practice, of which tai chi is perhaps the most widely known
   c. Anticipated benefits with rationale
      (1) Increased body awareness and sense of balance through movement and focused awareness on the body
      (2) Increased energy through improved circulation
   d. Application, usage, frequency
      (1) Has the widest application of all TCM therapies to patients at every stage of HIV disease and can be helpful to many (more applicable generally than acupuncture or herbs)
      (2) May be practiced in almost any setting; useful for ambulatory and non-ambulatory patients
      (3) Qi gong practice should be cultivated as a part of daily hygiene and practiced regularly under the guidance of an experienced teacher

2. Relationship to People With HIV
   a. Utility
      (1) Immune enhancement, symptom alleviation, and QOL benefits (see "Utility" under *Traditional Chinese Medicine*)
      (2) Can be a powerful tool to empower people with HIV; increases body awareness, stamina, and mobility
   b. Level of acceptance: Awareness of qi gong is very limited outside Japan, China, Tibet, and India
   c. Providers/facilitators of services
      (1) Attributes of skilled practitioners/healers: Trained with a master and practiced for many years
      (2) Types of providers
         (a) Many licensed acupuncturists are not adequately trained in qi gong, nor do they maintain the kind of practice that enables them to teach others or use qi gong in their daily work
         (b) Most qi gong teachers practice qi gong as a spiritual practice or personal activity that they share with others
      (3) Potential for harm: Musculoskeletal complaints and what is known in China as "qi gong psychosis" are associated with qi gong practice without appropriate supervision, especially by those who overindulge in it

3. Nursing Role: Many of the simpler qi gong exercises can be easily and safely learned by nurses and shared with patients

4. Future Directions: Teaching qi gong to patients as part of a health maintenance or education program is a very promising area for research; patients increase their body awareness and can become involved in their own health care

G. Reflexology

1. Description
   a. An ancient healing based on the theory that there are reflex areas in the hands and feet that correspond to all parts of the body (see Figure 8.1)
   b. Stimulating the reflexes correctly can relieve tension and stress naturally
   c. There is a special dimension to reflexology for which there is no currently accepted scientific explanation; it is the direct hands-on connection between the provider and the subject, which allows a direct flow of energy between the two during the entire treatment
   d. Many subjects report that along with a reduction of stress, heightened energy levels and balance, they also feel centered and uplifted as a direct result of their involvement with the reflexologist and his/her state of being
   e. Historical usage
      (1) Reflexology is practiced in all parts of the world by different cultures
      (2) Earliest recorded documentation is a pictograph of 2,500 B.C. in the tomb of Akhmahor in Egypt that shows physicians working on a person's hands and feet
      (3) Dr. William Fitzgerald, of St. Francis Hospital, Hartford, CT, brought reflexology to the U.S. in 1916 as "zone therapy"; he taught that the body is divided into 10 vertical zones, 5 each on the left and right sides of the body
   f. Types or categories: Foot and hand reflexology
   g. Anticipated benefits
      (1) Affects all the organs and glands in the body; specific problems are altered or balanced during each session
      (2) By stimulating the reflexes in the hands or feet, reflexology leads to
         (a) Balance in the body
         (b) Stimulation of the lymphatic system
         (c) Reduction of stress
         (d) Relief of neuropathic conditions
         (e) Increased circulation
         (f) An overall sense of well-being
         (g) Reduced blood pressure
         (h) Lowered anxiety levels
         (i) Improved respiratory effort as the patient's relaxed state allows breathing to become more efficient
   h. Application, usage, frequency
      (1) Initial treatments can take ≤75 min; follow-up treatments are 45–60 min; during the initial treatment the patient is given a full, simple explanation of the principles of reflexology
      (2) Some issues to be covered during the initial meeting
         (a) Particular difficulties the patient is having; patient complaints
         (b) Duration and highlights of ailment or condition
         (c) Type of medical program patient is on, if any
         (d) Prior experience with reflexology or other alternative touch treatment
         (e) Evaluation of hands and feet and suggestions to support range of motion
         (f) Determination of the dominant hand and suggestions of ways to strengthen the nondominant side, if necessary
         (g) Assessment of walk, gait, weight distribution
         (h) Assessment of the type of shoes patient wears, checking inside and outside shoes for pressure areas
         (i) Detection of bunions, corns, calluses, unusual marks on hands and feet
      (3) After the evaluation, the reflexologist tells the patient what to expect during treatment and benefits to anticipate between treatments
2. Relationship to People With HIV
   a. Utility
      (1) Reflexology is a noninvasive, gentle modality requiring removal of nothing more than shoes and socks

Figure 8.1 Reflex Areas in the Hands and Feet

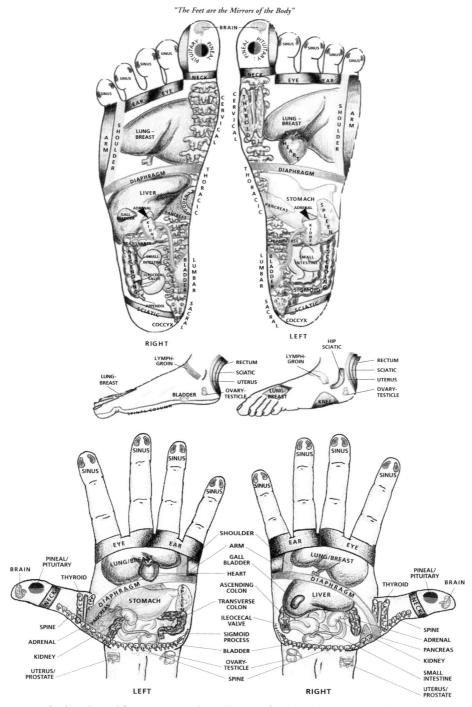

Reflex areas in the hands and feet correspond to all parts of the body; stimulating these reflexes correctly can relieve tension and stress in a natural way. (Copyright 1995 Reflexology Seminars of New York, Inc. Suite 264, 1175A 2nd Avenue, New York, NY 10021)

(2) Reflexology treatments are possible at any stage of a disease and can be given with as much gentleness or pressure that is necessary

(3) Fees vary according to location and experience of practitioner; some insurance companies will cover treatment if prescribed by a physician

b. Level of acceptance

(1) The patient's orientation to the concept of personal healing practices

   (a) In most cases, people with HIV who have been exposed to alternative methods of healing are encouraged to communicate with people with similar problems, to breathe properly, meditate, and eat nourishing food; the task for the reflexologist becomes easier because this patient is receptive to the healing process that emanates from within and is conditioned to expect the elimination of stress in the body, which helps the patient live in the present moment

   (b) For patients not yet exposed to alternatives for healing, reflexology is a wonderful introduction to balancing the body; nonverbal communication during reflexology treatments is as important as verbal because the sensitive reflexologist can guide the patient to a peaceful, balanced state of being

(2) Reflexology is well received by the HIV community: In New York City alone, three support organizations (Friends in Need, Manhattan Center for Living, the Gay Men's Health Crisis) support reflexology and encourage treatments

c. Providers/facilitators of services

(1) Attributes of skilled practitioners/healers

   (a) Compassion and empathy

   (b) Knowledge of human anatomy and physiology and a commitment to continuing self-education

   (c) Open-mindedness

   (d) Training

   (e) Dedication to their own health and well-being as demonstrated by self-care; nutritional, spiritual, mental health; and other behaviors that improve ability to engage in a therapeutic relationship with patients

   (f) People oriented

   (g) Talent for hands-on connection with people

(2) Types of providers

   (a) Trained reflexologists (may be certified)

   (b) Nurses, massage therapists, physicians; partners, friends, relatives of HIV-infected people

(3) Potential for harm/any regulatory oversight

   (a) Reflexology is safe; there are no harmful side effects

   (b) Regulatory laws are defined by each state

3. Nursing Role: Nurses caring for HIV-infected patients can implement reflexology treatments at any time during care, if they have had reflexology training

4. Future Directions

a. There is a movement in the U.S. to include reflexology in the curricula of nursing and massage therapy schools

b. The established medical community today is both more receptive to reflexology and apt to endorse its use, given the favorable experience of patients

5. Resources: Reflexology training locations

a. Reflexology Seminars of New York, Inc.
   1173a 2nd Ave #264
   New York, NY 10021
   (212) 517-5532

b. Kunz School of Reflexology
   P.O. Box 35820, Station D
   Albuquerque, NM 87176-5820
   (505) 344-9392

c. American Institute of Reflexology
   606 East Magnolia Street
   Burbank, CA 91501
   (818) 841-7741

d. The International Academy for
   Reflexology Studies
   4759 Cornell Road #D
   Cincinnati, OH 45241
   (513) 489-9328

H. Yoga

1. Description
   a. Yoga is an ancient technology from
      India incorporating asanas (physical
      postures), pranayama (breathing tech-
      niques), and mantra (sound)
   b. Yoga's technical definition is the union
      of body, mind, and spirit; also defined
      as control of the mind attained through
      specific breathing techniques
   c. Historical usage
      (1) Yoga was historically used to fine
          tune the nervous system, glandular
          system, and internal organs, and to
          open up the flow of energy along
          the spinal nerve centers (chakras) so
          the body and mind can function in
          conjunction with spirit in its purest
          form
      (2) Yoga came to the U.S. a century ago
          and has gained in popularity in the
          last decade as an alternative healing
          system
   d. Types or categories: At least 20 different
      types of yoga; they vary specifically
      from focusing on sound (Naad) to med-
      itation (Raja) to physical aspects only
      (Hatha)
      (1) Hatha: The most familiar in the U.S.,
          thus generating the false belief that
          yoga is only about physical flexibil-
          ity; with increased awareness, other
          types are being experienced as well
      (2) Kundalini (brought to the U.S. by
          Yogi Bhajan): Sound, postures, and
          breathing used or incorporated
          simultaneously with accelerated
          results
      (3) Sivenanda (brought to the U.S. from
          India by Vishnu Devananda):
          Emphasizes Hatha (physical pos-
          tures with some pranayama [breath-
          ing expansion techniques]) with an
          encompassing yogic philosophy

      (4) Iyengar (brought from India by
          Iyengar): Emphasizes perfecting
          alignment and strength in the physi-
          cal posture one is practicing; uses
          props (wood blocks, ropes) to assist
          one into the postures
      (5) Ashtanga (introduced to the West by
          Patabi Jois): Also called power yoga,
          a more gymnastic and potentially
          aerobic approach to yoga
      (6) Integral yoga: Hatha yoga as taught
          by Swami Satchidananda, with cen-
          ters throughout the U.S.; the
          approach is gentle and physical,
          though not as demanding as
          Astanga or Iyengar
      (7) There are offshoots of these types of
          yoga and contemporary adaptations
          such as yog-aerobics; however, those
          mentioned above are pure forms
          emphasizing equally the ideal con-
          nection between, and the impor-
          tance of, mind, body, and spirit
   e. Anticipated benefits
      (1) Calming of the mind (affecting both
          parasympathetic and sympathetic
          nervous systems)
      (2) Inner peace
      (3) Increased ability to face fears and
          break through them
      (4) Feelings of connectedness (not isola-
          tion)
      (5) Boosting of immune system,
          strengthening of nervous system
      (6) Strengthening and toning of muscles
          and internal organs
      (7) Increased joint flexibility and health
          resiliency
      (8) Expanded lung capacity
      (9) Increased awareness of the physical
          body
     (10) Greater connection to spirit
   f. Application, usage, frequency
      (1) Can be practiced as a disciplined
          workout routine any time of the day,
          though morning and evening are
          suggested times to practice (on a rel-
          atively empty stomach)
      (2) Daily practice is suggested any-
          where from a few minutes to 1–2
          hours

2. Relationship to People With HIV
   a. Utility
      (1) Ambulatory patients or outpatients with evident HIV-related symptoms can practice yoga daily as part of a wellness and preventive health program
      (2) For bedridden patients, certain physical postures (e.g., reclining) can be practiced as well as pranayama for breath and mind benefits
   b. Level of acceptance
      (1) Excellent in those open to alternative approaches such as meditation, relaxation, exercise, diet, and other lifestyle-changing approaches to treatment
      (2) Dr. Dean Ornish has pioneered getting integral yoga relaxation techniques covered by certain insurance companies for heart disease; 3HO (Kundalini) yoga has a center in Arizona that is covered by insurance for treatment of addictions
   c. Providers/facilitators of services
      (1) Attributes of skilled practitioners/healers
         (a) The standard for what constitutes a "good" yoga teacher is not based primarily on technical ability; less technically proficient teachers who have greater capacities for compassion and communication may be considered more skilled
         (b) Skilled practitioners in yoga are more effective if their heart is as much a part of their teaching as their head
         (c) Willingness to suggest lifestyle changes (e.g., omitting alcohol, drugs, sex) but not forcing patients or being judgmental
         (d) Practitioners see themselves as healers who facilitate the individual in self-healing (which may not mean curing) on emotional, physical, and spiritual levels
         (e) Teacher training or certification is based on weeks to a few years of training depending on the particular school of yoga; the masters are from India and are of no particular religious affiliation; no physical requirements other than proficiency at yoga
      (2) Types of providers
         (a) Practitioner: General term for a yoga therapist or instructor (teacher)
         (b) Therapists: Deal with specific mental, physical, or spiritual issues
         (c) Instructors (teachers): Teach a more generalized approach, though the yoga itself would be specific postures, breathing, mantras; a therapist also might work this way with a patient
      (3) Potential for harm
         (a) None that are specific but it is important for the individual to be sensitive to physical limits (e.g., if sitting cross-legged causes pain, the patient might sit in chair instead of on the floor); only do postures that feel acceptable
         (b) Because no standards for practice are established, it is important that the chosen yoga teacher/therapist be confident in working with this population and have resources should problems or questions arise
3. Nursing Role
   a. Nurses can take a few yoga classes to be familiar with basics of yoga to share when needed or appropriate
   b. Nurses can use yoga therapists as resources for questions and referrals to yoga centers or as teachers in the healing team (e.g., some yoga teachers have experience working with death and dying counseling)
   c. Nurses can educate other healthcare providers on the importance of yoga both physically and mentally and as a tool in helping deal with depression and mental crisis; many physicians and other healthcare professionals know

little or nothing about yoga or its beneficial properties and may view it skeptically

d. Contact local yoga centers to see if they offer classes for this population

e. Make inquiries at hospitals that might have classes taught as meditation, relaxation, or yoga

f. Inquire at local foundations or AIDS community-based organizations (e.g., Friends In Deed in New York City) as they routinely have AIDS-aware yoga teachers

4. Future Directions

a. As more yoga teachers are exposed to working with HIV/AIDS patients, more resources will become available

(1) Specialized workshops and classes will be developed and found more easily as part of curricula at yoga centers, alternative healing centers, progressive hospitals

(2) Research into the relationship between yoga and HIV/AIDS may be developed

b. Other family members, friends, or loved ones may also want to be included in yoga sessions as a way to connect and become more open and loving with each other and to resolve emotional, physical, and spiritual issues together

5. Resources

a. *Magazines*

Yoga Journal
P.O. Box 469018
Escondido, CA 92046-9018

Yoga International
Rural Route 1, Box 407
Honesdale, PA 18431
(717) 253-6241

b. *Video*

Living With AIDS Through Yoga and Meditation
388 Point McKay Gardens, N.W.
Calgary, Alberta T3B 4V8, Canada
(403) 270-9691

I. Massage

1. Description: Manipulation of soft tissue such as muscles, tendons, and ligaments by the hands

a. Historical usage

(1) Literature can be traced back to China around 2,600 B.C.

(2) The first book on massage was written by the Taoist priest-physician, Tao-Tse

(3) From China, massage was brought to Japan, India, Egypt, Assyria, Babylonia, Persia, Greece, and Rome

(4) In Europe, Henrick Ling successfully obtained state support to establish a research institute, the Royal Central Gymnastic Institute, Sweden, where he taught movement therapy, exercise, and massage during the 1840s

b. Types or categories: Among today's popular techniques are Swedish massage (effleurage, petrissage, kneading, vibration, tapotement), acupressure, amma therapy, aromatherapy, craniosacral massage, jin shin jyutsu, manual lymph drainage, myofacial release, neuromuscular therapy, ohashiatsu, on-site (seated) massage, connective tissue therapy, pre/postnatal and infant massage, reflexology, rolfing, shiatsu, sports massage, trager, triggerpoint therapy, zone therapy

c. Anticipated benefits

(1) Depending on the technique used, massage provides elasticity and mobility in muscles and tendons

(2) During injury recovery, massage

(a) Increases circulation and lymph activity

(b) Prevents formation of scar tissue

(c) Softens existing scar tissue

(d) Helps eliminate waste products

(e) Breaks down collagen resulting from inflammation

(f) Noticeably increases speed of healing

(3) Assists the nervous system in breaking the pattern of chronic pain

(4) Reduces stress and promotes feeling

of well-being and relaxation
d. Application, usage, frequency
(1) Can be used in a variety of settings (clinics, medical offices, hospitals, addiction treatment and abuse recovery settings, sports facilities, health spas, homes)
(2) Use as prescribed by physician or on maintenance level as needed; physician prescription is not required for patient self-care
(3) Generally used on a weekly or monthly basis, but sometimes indicated more frequently

2. Relationship to People With HIV
a. Utility
(1) Useful for common, non-HIV-specific complaints
(2) Helpful in decreasing HIV-related lymphedema; even though results are only temporary, they provide welcome comfort to the patient
(3) Offers caring touch to the HIV patient who is often touch deprived
(4) Provides the chronically ill with improved sense of well-being and a more positive outlook
(5) HIV/AIDS patients benefit from various techniques including lymph drainage; because the patient's condition can change frequently, appropriate treatment is at the therapist's discretion

b. Level of acceptance
(1) Only a small percentage of U.S. physicians are familiar with massage, although it is widely accepted in Europe; some nursing schools include the basics of Swedish massage in their curricula
(2) As new medical graduates are more familiar with alternative medicine, there is the potential that physicians of the future will be more likely to accept massage
(3) In general, AIDS community-based organizations recommend massage

c. Providers/facilitators of services
(1) Attributes of skilled practitioners/healers
(a) Depending on state require-

ments, licensing or certification
(b) Education or experience working with people with HIV
(c) A compassionate provider who respects the patient
(d) Knowledge of precautionary measures related to blood and body fluids

(2) Types of providers
(a) Massage therapists
(b) Nurses, physicians, chiropractors, physical therapists, although most do not because of lack of knowledge, time consumption
(c) Family and significant others can be taught some basics of massage, provided teaching includes anatomy, various systems

(3) Potential for harm/any regulatory oversights
(a) Massage is generally contraindicated during the acute stage of inflammation or injury (as may occur with cancer or acute OIs); such conditions require approval of the patient's primary care provider; all treatments need to be tailored to meet the patient's needs
(b) Possible risks with massage include lightheadedness, bruising, increased inflammation, increased lymph activity, elevated blood pressure
(c) Many massage therapists practice without a system for peer review or professional quality assurance
(d) Massage therapists are licensed in 20 states; many are certified in states where licensing is not yet required
(e) In most states where massage therapists are licensed insurance companies do not reimburse for treatment; this makes massage unaffordable for many patients and difficult to fill a physician's prescription for massage; some HIV service organizations pro-

vide referrals to volunteer massage therapists
3. Nursing Role
   a. Nurses can educate providers, patients, and families on the appropriate use of massage
   b. Nurses can incorporate massage into their practice or make referrals for massage
   c. Nurses in AIDS care can incorporate massage into their own self-care
4. Future Directions
   a. Integration of massage therapists as healthcare providers as an adjunct to other healthcare modalities and providers
   b. Increased integration of massage into stress reduction and HIV-related care

J. Individual Psychotherapy

1. Description: The goal of individual psychotherapy is to help the person accept the diagnosis, take control of their life, explore their thoughts and feelings, and in the end die peacefully
   a. Historical usage
      (1) Psychotherapy for patients with medical illness began as early as 1905 when Dr. Joseph Pratt organized a psychotherapy group for TB patients
      (2) Psychotherapy for dying patients came into its own with the publication of *On Death and Dying* by Elizabeth Kübler-Ross in 1969
      (3) Psychotherapy has been employed with HIV-infected patients since AIDS was first identified
2. Relationship to People With HIV
   a. People who are not known to be HIV positive: Before diagnosis
      (1) People who are not at risk for HIV, but nevertheless are obsessed with a fear of getting the disease
      (2) People who are at risk but have not been tested; people in this group often experience anxiety or depression (see *Anxiety*, p. 245)
         (a) Reasons for not being tested
            i) Fear their lives will be all downhill if they are HIV positive
            ii) Fear that if they are found by others to be HIV positive they will experience discrimination in housing, insurance, and the workplace
         (b) Nurses can help by encouraging testing
            i) If the person is HIV negative, the anxiety may be reduced
            ii) If the person is HIV positive, life can be prolonged by prophylactic drugs and other methods
   b. Human responses to the diagnosis with psychotherapeutic suggestions (Lego, 1994, 1996)
      (1) Early phase
         (a) Shock, anger, panic: Provide quiet, emotional connectedness
         (b) Disappointment, loss, sadness: Offer quiet reassurance, encouraging mobilization of a supportive network
         (c) Fear of incapacitation, physical and mental deterioration, deformity, pain: Encourage the patient to express all thoughts and feelings reassure the patient professional help will be available
         (d) Shame, both internal and external: Examine personal values to ensure they do not contribute to the patient's shame; help the patient talk about internal conflicts
         (e) Denial: Help the patient accept the diagnosis by reassuring that the patient will not be alone, help will be available
         (f) Suicidal thoughts: See *Potential for Violence/Harm to Self or Others*, p. 265
         (g) The "ego chill," a shudder that comes from the sudden awareness that our nonexistence is entirely possible (Erikson, 1958): Help the patient explore

thoughts and feelings about death

(2) Middle phase

(a) Loss of control: Help patients find ways to gain control of their lives by
   i) Seeking prophylactic treatment for infections
   ii) Leading a healthy lifestyle (good nutrition, exercise, meditation, communion with others); see *Meditation*, p. 355
   iii) Participating in treatment decisions

(b) Helplessness and vulnerability: Empower patients by encouraging them to reach out to others through cultural, political, or altruistic endeavors that give meaning to life; see *Powerlessness*, p. 267

(c) Passivity and victimization: Help patients replace negative thinking with positive attitudes by encouraging them to live life to its fullest and to be proactive; see *Hopelessness*, p. 260

(d) Severe reduction in self-esteem: Encourage patients to
   i) Continue work even if it must be scaled down
   ii) Spend time with supportive family and friends
   iii) Help others
   iv) Attend a support group or individual psychotherapy (see *Support Groups*, p. 348)

(e) Changes in physical appearance: Help patients reorder priorities, pointing out that relationships, work, and connections with the world at large may be more important than personal appearance; see *Body Image Disturbance*, p. 247

(f) Sense of isolation: Help patients decide who can offer the most support and who the patient wants present at death; a support group and individual psychotherapy help overcome loneliness and stigmatization see *Social Isolation*, p. 269, *Stigma*, p. 274

(g) Guilt over lifestyle when the patient is gay, bisexual, an IDU, or a female partner who has been victimized (see *Guilt*, p. 255): Help patients explore
   i) Who has caused them to feel bad or wrong
   ii) Ways to expiate guilt (e.g., by repaying money stolen for drugs)

(h) Anger and acting out: Help patients express rage verbally rather than act it out, validating the reasons for realistic anger such as problems with healthcare delivery or victimization by discrimination; help patients identify displaced anger

(i) Depression: Point out patients are turning the anger they feel toward themselves rather than expressing it openly, so encourage open expression; an advanced practice nurse with prescriptive authority may prescribe antidepressants, or refer to a provider who can evaluate patient for this need; see *Depression*, p. 248

(j) Paranoia: Help patient sort out behaviors that reflect actual anger at others, and paranoia that represents their own anger that is projected onto others

(k) Fear of violence: Discuss sources of violence at home and in the community to help patients avoid these; refer family and friends to support groups or involve social protective agencies as necessary

(l) Sense of betrayal by partners, family, or friends who may have deceived or deserted the patient: Help patients grieve the loss of belief in the other, at the same time helping them acquire new sources of comfort including the nurse, a support group, or a higher being; see *Grief and Loss,* p. 253, *Spiritual Distress,* p. 273

(m) Escape into alcohol or drugs: Help patients talk about their thoughts and feelings, rather than escape them; arrange access to prescribed pain medication as needed

(n) Somatic preoccupation: Provide health information to allay unrealistic worries; explore the anxiety that is underlying the preoccupation

(o) Projective identification: When patients unconsciously infuse the nurse with their own feelings of panic, anger, helplessness, step back, notice what is happening, and attempt to react with empathy and understanding

(3) Late phase

(a) Disinterest: Realizing the patient's need to disengage; remain emotionally available but avoid unnecessary demands

(b) Ambivalence: Recognize patient's simultaneous feelings of anger and neediness, realize they may need to be with loved ones, or may need to die alone; ask if there are friends or relatives to call or messages to be sent

(c) Life review: Realizing patients may want to review happier times or talk about regrets, be emotionally available; any and all feelings are encouraged and accepted

(d) Resolution: Recognizing death is near, help patients to accept death

(4) Special concerns: Interventions with rationale

(a) How to tell parents or children: Assess and evaluate each case individually; help patients look at all the dimensions and ramifications (*some factors such as health

status of elderly parents or life phase of the children may have a bearing on how the information is accepted; on the other hand, thinly veiled family secrets can be destructive; see p. 375 for pediatric disclosure issues*)

(b) Questions about sexuality: Help patients explore safer sex methods and nonsexual physical contact; may encourage discussion of feelings about this with partners (*most human beings need physical contact; partners may withdraw owing to fear of contagion or anticipatory grief*)

(c) Reconciliation with estranged family members: Help patients decide if reconciliation is desired even if they seem strongly defended against it; agree to be present at the reconciliation if desired and to meet with the patient afterward (*a tough exterior may cover a fear of rejection; the reconciliation is likely to arouse strong feelings that require expression and acceptance*)

(d) A "limbo" phase: When OIs are in check, encourage an enjoy-the-moment philosophy, but be alert to underlying depression (*patients can fall into a state of denial when they feel physically healthy but suffer intense depression when an infection returns*)

(e) Unfinished business: Move at the patient's pace but offer encouragement to put legal and personal affairs in order (e.g., helping plan the funeral or memorial service, leaving letters or tapes behind) (*patients may fear that to do this planning hastens the end; low self-esteem may not let them realize the importance letters or tapes may have for others after they are gone*)

(f) Resurrection fantasies as others recover from an infection: Help patient explore thoughts, feelings, wishes, and dreams, keeping reality in mind—e.g., "It's good to see John's feeling better. I guess we all wish it could last forever." (*as with all forms of denial the patient is vulnerable to "crashing" when reality sets in; resurrection fantasies represent the wish to reverse the dying process*)

(g) Talk about death: Remain alert to signs the patient is ready; when these occur, ask patients what they have been thinking about death (*thoughts and feelings about dying are always present, though often kept in abeyance. The nurse may be the only person with whom the patient can openly discuss death*)

(h) Rational suicide: Depending on ethical and moral beliefs, allow patients to discuss and explore a rational suicide plan (*many patients are reassured by knowing they have a means of controlling their own death with dignity; nurses who are in accord can help the patient accept this without guilt; nurses who believe death is in the hands of God will be unwilling and unable to enter into this discussion*)

(5) Level of acceptance

(a) Psychotherapy has become commonly accepted in our society, especially in times of crisis

(b) Acceptance by the patient depends on the fit between the patient and therapist in a psychologic or emotional, theoretical or philosophical sense

3. Providers/facilitators of services

a. Attributes of skilled practitioners/healers: A thorough knowledge of both the psychotherapeutic and HIV/AIDS disease process

b. Types of providers: Psychiatric-mental health CNSs are uniquely qualified by virtue of their knowledge of the psychotherapeutic process, AIDS, and pathophysiology; psychiatric social workers, psychiatrists, psychologists, rehabilitation counselors, other counselors

4. Nursing Role

a. Nurses caring for persons with HIV/AIDS can help by

(1) Referring to therapy patients experiencing emotional distress

(2) Encouraging them to attend their psychotherapy sessions, especially if or when they feel discouraged

(3) Supporting them through the ups and downs of psychotherapy

(4) Respecting and accepting changes in the person over time (e.g., increased anger for a period of time)

5. Future Directions: Individual psychotherapy will continue to be offered by nurses and other mental health providers

K. Support Groups

1. Description: Support groups for the HIV infected are homogenous groups led by one or two healthcare providers who are seen as equals rather than authorities over group members

a. Historical usage: Began early in the AIDS epidemic; usually sponsored by AIDS self-help groups (e.g., Gay Men's Health Crisis in New York City)

b. Types: Groups for gay men, IDUs, women

c. Properties of support groups (Rosenberg, 1984)

(1) Homogeneity of problems

(2) Victimization by a system, as opposed to psychopathology

(3) Public confession as a qualification for membership

(4) A common understanding of terms

(5) Horizontal structure, where the leader is seen as an equal rather than as an authority above the others

(6) Education and information exchanges

(7) Reality testing where members test their own perceptions on the other group members, eliciting feedback

(8) Development of coping skills

d. Application, usage, frequency

(1) Goals

(a) Acceptance of the illness

(b) Expression of otherwise "unac-

ceptable" feelings of rage, sadness, jealousy, shame, guilt
(c) Decrease in anxiety
(d) Regaining of the ability to manage their own lives
(e) Reaching out to others for practical and emotional support
(f) Acceptance of loss and death
(g) Increased self-esteem
(h) Reduction of high-risk behaviors
(i) Decisions about substance abuse
(j) Discovery of new meaning in life
(k) Reconciliation with estranged family members
(l) Discovery of ways to show concern for significant others who may be overwhelmed by the member's illness
(m) Examination of ways to leave a legacy unique to members' own lives
(2) Frequency: Groups usually meet once a week

2. Relationship to People With HIV
   a. Level of acceptance: Support groups are well accepted when members
   (1) Feel a part of the group
   (2) Find the group meaningful to them as individuals
   (3) Believe they are contributing to the group, and helping others
   b. Providers/facilitators of services
   (1) Attributes of skilled practitioners/healers
      (a) Knowledgeable of group process, AIDS, and pathophysiology
      (b) Sensitive, able to accept expressions of anger, frustration, loneliness, love, etc., without undue anxiety
      (c) Able to examine carefully own personal values and possible bias toward homosexuality or drug use
      (d) Able to discuss death and dying
      (e) Feel comfortable with persons whose death may be imminent
      (f) Able to avoid dominating the group and let natural leaders emerge

(g) Feel comfortable discussing sex
(h) Be aware of and honest about their own concerns, for example, about being at risk themselves
(i) Able to monitor concerns related to confidentiality
(2) Types of providers: Psychiatric-mental health CNSs, psychiatric social workers, psychiatrists, psychologists, rehabilitation and other counselors
(3) Potential for harm: Leaders must be alert to signs of severe depression, suicidal ideology, impending psychosis or dementia, and refer members for more intensive care when indicated

3. Nursing Role
   a. Refer newly diagnosed persons to support groups; encourage attendance
   b. Support group members during the ups and downs of group life
   c. Respect group confidentiality if members mention the names of other members
   d. Encourage members to work out conflicts in the group, rather than discussing them with the nurse or others outside the group

4. Resources
   a. American Psychiatric Association (APA)
      AIDS Steering Committee
      1400 K Street NW
      Washington, DC 20005
      (202) 682-6843
      [APA has published A Psychiatrist's Guide to AIDS and HIV Disease, a training program, computerized self-help test on the psychiatric aspects of AIDS, and training video.]
   b. American Psychological Association
      1200 17th Street NW
      Washington, DC 20036
      [The association has an office on AIDS, which has a computerized AIDS Resource Network listing those who work with HIV disease, and has published Psychology and AIDS Exchange.]

L. Dreamwork

1. Description: Dreamwork is a process
whereby a person listens to and interacts
with the unconscious, which exerts a powerful and compelling influence on their
life. The unconscious is always pushing to
be heard, either through dreams or by
leading people into life experiences that
force them to look within. By working
with our dreams—writing them down,
musing about them, telling them to receptive individuals, and dialoguing with the
figures they bring to us—people can
encounter the forgotten or discredited
parts of ourselves and better understand
our individual destinies.
   a. Historical usage
      (1) Dreams and the telling of dreams
          are probably as old as humankind
      (2) Aboriginal cultures the world over
          make a place for dreams in both reli-
          gious rituals and shamanic healing
          practices
      (3) Early Greek civilization recognized
          the healing effect of dreams; initiates
          who sought healing would "incu-
          bate" dreams by sleeping in the tem-
          ple of Asclepius
      (4) Freud and Jung pioneered the use of
          dreamwork in psychoanalytic prac-
          tice at the turn of the century
      (5) Dreamwork continues to be one
          aspect of psychoanalysis, but attend-
          ing to dreams is important in any
          practice that is concerned with psy-
          chologic health and well-being
   b. Types or categories: There are as many
      types as there are schools of psychologic
      thought—Jungian, Freudian, Kleinian,
      gestalt, etc.; each views dreams in a
      slightly different way but all involve
      some method of recording, analyzing,
      and working with the unconscious
      material presented in dreams
   c. Anticipated benefits
      (1) Wholeness: Dreams make conscious
          previously unknown aspects of the
          personality; they show us the parts
          of ourselves that were never known,
          have been forgotten, or are being
          neglected; as unconscious material
          is brought into consciousness the
          overall personality is enlarged and
          deepened
      (2) Congruence: Awareness of uncon-
          scious motivations and conflicts
          brings stability to the psyche; one
          recognizes the ebb and flow of emo-
          tion and energy as coming from
          one's inner world, rather than expe-
          riencing oneself at the mercy of out-
          side people and forces
      (3) Meaning: The unconscious is less
          concerned with day-to-day issues
          that occupy waking consciousness
          than with the overall direction of
          our lives; dreams connect us to the
          deep guiding and ordering principle
          of the psyche that determines what
          is meaningful to us as individuals
          rather than to what society tells us is
          important
      (4) Just as sleep restores the body and
          brings it back into balance, dreams
          restore and balance the psyche
   d. Application, usage, frequency
      (1) Dreamwork has universal applica-
          tion; everyone dreams, although
          some people may need help in
          remembering their dreams
      (2) Powerful dreams often come during
          serious illness or life-altering events
          when people are confronted with
          questions of mortality
      (3) Individuation—the natural process
          by which the psyche evolves—may
          be speeded up in people with AIDS;
          it is as though the unconscious, rec-
          ognizing that time may be limited,
          pushes forcefully to be heard, often
          through dreams
      (4) Looking at a single dream, sponta-
          neously offered by the patient, is like
          looking at a photograph of some-
          thing, taken from one perspective;
          working continuously with dreams
          allows the psychologic process to
          reveal itself over time; it is like look-
          ing at a series of photographs taken
          from many different perspectives
      (5) Dreamwork can be done in a variety

of settings—homes, clinics, counseling offices, hospitals, hospices
(6) Dreams should be recorded and thought about daily. Discussion with a professional can occur spontaneously following the dream or on a regular basis depending on the volume of dream material
(7) Dreamwork, as an aspect of holistic nursing, has applications in any specialty where people face serious life-altering or life-threatening illnesses
2. Relationship to People With HIV
  a. Utility: Requires commitment to remember, record, and reflect on dream images and themes
    (1) Most practical when the person is unimpaired physically and mentally
    (2) When physical limitation is present, dreams can be dictated to another person or recording machine
  b. Level of acceptance
    (1) The language of the unconscious, which is not like everyday logic, takes some getting used to
      (a) The goal of dreamwork is not interpretation, but involvement
      (b) With practice, most people can learn to engage their inner figures in a meaningful way
    (2) The deeper psyche is a never-ending source of images and stories that enrich a person's life; working with dreams becomes a lifelong habit for many who try it
  c. Providers/facilitators of services
    (1) Attributes of skilled practitioners/healers
      (a) Respect for and willingness to engage the unconscious; nurses who are interested in working with dreams may want to explore their own attitudes and experience with dreams
      (b) Education or experience working with people with HIV
    (2) Types of providers
      (a) In general, psychotherapists, counselors, and psychoanalysts
      (b) Any professional who works with people who are experiencing serious, life-altering illnesses or events
    (3) Potential for harm/any regulatory oversights
      (a) Risks: Dreams are a natural occurrence; there is no risk in listening to and recording dreams
      (b) The psyche is self-regulating; if we misunderstand what it is trying to tell us, it will try again in another way, on another occasion
      (c) Only the dreamer knows the meaning of the dream; overzealous interpretations of dreams by others are invasive to the dreamer and should be avoided
3. Nursing Role
  a. Nurses can create an environment that is conducive to dreaming itself and to sharing dreams; to tell a dream is, literally, to bare one's soul; confidentiality and privacy are of primary importance
  b. Nurses can encourage people to talk about their dreams and can learn to respond helpfully to dream material
  c. Guidelines for working with dreams
    (1) Preparing for dreamwork
      (a) A dream journal is helpful for comparing dreams and seeing overall patterns and similarities in successive dreams; keep the journal and pen at the bedside, ready for use
      (b) Whenever possible, waken naturally rather than being startled by an alarm
      (c) On waking, lie still and let the images from the night seep into awareness
      (d) If the dream has disappeared, you may be able to recall it by doing one of the following
        i) If a feeling state remains, let yourself sink into the feeling, let it wash over you; sometimes an image will come to mind that will lead back to the dream
        ii) Let your mind move slowly across the familiar

people and animals in your life to see if your memory can be jogged into remembering the dream

(2) Recording dreams: It is important to record dreams in writing or by dictation; details fade with time and dreams that are not recorded may be forgotten

    (a) All dreams are meaningful, even if fragmentary or seemingly insignificant

    (b) Include as much detail as possible about images, situations, and events in the dream

    (c) Pay special attention to how the dream opens; dreams are similar to theater—the setting or landscape when the curtain opens is important for establishing the context of the dream

    (d) Describe the sequence of events as if they were a story

(3) Amplifying dreams: What matters most is the experience of the dream itself; it is not important to interpret dreams, rather to amplify or expand on their images; you can do this by going back and walking around in the dream, reencountering the dream figures and situations from a waking standpoint, not by intellectual analysis of images and themes

    (a) After recording the dream, note down your associations to each image and situation; you might want to ask yourself: How would I describe the figures in the dream? Are the people or events known to me? What do they bring to mind? Are the dream figures acting in character? Do they remind me of anything that is happening in my life at the present?

    (b) Because dreams contain universal as well as personal images, you might want to consider whether they remind you of a myth, fairy tale, or familiar piece of art or literature

    (c) One powerful way of working with dreams is to give them physical reality in the waking world; you can do this through drawing, painting, sculpture, poetry, and movement; because dreams speak in symbolic rather than logical language, they can often be better understood by intuitive activities than by rational analysis

    (d) Active imagination is a process whereby the dreamer recalls and talks with a figure from the dream, asking what he or she wants; the dialogue allows for a relationship between the day self and the figures of the night world

(4) Understanding dreams

    (a) Dreams do not usually tell us what we already know; as a general rule, in some models of dreamwork philosophy, if we understand the dream immediately, we've probably missed the point

    (b) Think about the dream metaphorically rather than literally: For example, if the dream says you are caught in a traffic jam, it is probably not talking about a traffic jam in the outer world as much as a traffic jam in the psychologic world. The question would be: In what way are you experiencing an inner traffic jam?

    (c) Often the meaning of the dream becomes clear only with time; dreams come in series, building on each other; the pattern or story reveals itself and we begin to see how the dream relates to our condition

    (d) There are no bad dreams; dreams come to help, not to harm us; frightening dreams usually indicate the urgency with which the unconscious is trying to get our attention

d. Supervision by someone who is trained in dreamwork—psychotherapist or psychoanalyst—is very useful

M. Humor

1. Description: Humor is characterized by a
sensitivity to or appreciation of ludicrous,
absurd, incongruous, or comical events
(McGhee & Goldstein, 1983). Humor is the
creation of incongruity. Humor often
results from nonlinear reactions, from tension betweeen the expected and the unex-
pected. "The contrast between the false
comfort of fixed meanings and the shock
of new insight can generate laughter
which, in turn, may lead to new ways of
seeing" (Rico, 1991, p. 199).
   a. Historical usage
      (1) Benefits of humor noted as early as
King Solomon: "A merry heart
doeth good like a medicine"
(Proverbs 17:22)
      (2) Norman Cousins (1976) revealed
how he personally used humor therapeutically to decrease his chronic
pain; he described his belief that
humor enhances the immune system; from this sprang the therapeutic humor movement in the U.S.
   b. Types or categories
      (1) Positive humor is laughing with but
not at; humor is that which makes
you feel good and no one else feel
bad (Goodman, 1989)
      (2) Therapeutic humor: An emerging
"science" or technique used to
enhance the quality and quantity of
life of both patient and professional
caregiver
   c. Anticipated benefits
      (1) Physiologic
         (a) Stress reduction
         (b) Immune-system enhancement
         (c) Release of endorphins leading to
pain reduction, fewer pain medications used, general sense of
well-being
         (d) Laughter, especially belly laugh-
ter, massages internal organs; if
sustained for several minutes,
can have the equivalent effect on
the cardiovascular system of 10
minutes of jogging
         (e) Laughter accelerates breathing,
increases oxygen consumption,
and exercises the muscles of the
face, shoulders, diaphragm and
abdomen
         (f) Laughter as a cathartic has been
known to decrease blood pres-
sure, increase oxygenation of tissue, and decrease muscle tension
         (g) Voltaire wrote, "The art of medi-
cine consists of amusing the
patient while nature cures the
disease" (Parrott, 1992, p. 13)
      (2) Emotional
         (a) Cathartic effect in releasing grief,
anger, frustration, sorrow
         (b) Allows for new perspective and
hopefulness
         (c) Creates energy in lightening up
attitudes and focus
         (d) Assists in creating a sense of inti-
macy or social connection with
others who share mirthful experience
         (e) Provides a gracious way to cope
with many indignities of being
ill as well as witnessing individuals at their most stressed
         (f) Increases creativity and flexibil-
ity of thought
         (g) To quote Henry Ward Beecher
"A person without a sense of
humor is like a wagon without
springs—jolted by every pebble
in the road" (Parrott, 1992, p. 13)
   d. Application, usage, frequency
      (1) Clinical care
         (a) Social: May be used by patients
and staff for social bonding, creating a connection, establishing a
trusting relationship as a first
step toward greater intimacy
         (b) Embarrassment: Often used in
the helping relationship to cope
with embarrassing moments
between caregiver and patient
and to help retain dignity
         (c) Anxiety: Serves as a means of
coping with fear and anxiety until
deeper levels can be explored;
creates a safety net for emotions
that can feel overwhelming

(d) Denial: Can hide real feelings or reactions until the person is able to cope directly with the situation

(e) Complaining: Allows a safe method of complaining about care or services provided when one is in the vulnerable position of being ill and dependent

(f) Perspective: Can assist patient in reframing painful experiences by offering a fresh or different perspective, can also provide a sense of hope and joy

(g) Cathartic release: A means of releasing intense emotions (grief, joy, fear)

(h) Symptom management: May be used to control pain and decrease anxiety, thus allowing for increased oxygenation, muscle relaxation, and distraction

(2) Therapeutic humor: Individually planned approaches will allow patient to use humor to enhance healing and decrease stress; key components are

  (a) Target of humor (oneself or the situation)

  (b) Environmental conditions: Nature of the relationship, timing, circumstance where humor is shared, setting in which humor is presented

  (c) Patient receptivity

    i) Observing current uses of humor

    ii) Soliciting the role of humor in the patient's life

    iii) Observing the patient's ability to laugh at himself or herself

    iv) Observing the patient's response to the humor of others

(3) Professional caregivers

  (a) Interpersonal relationships: Humor can ease tension in the workplace and enhance working relationships

  (b) Bonding for work groups: Humor can be a means to create a sense of team, to establish intimacy between coworkers delivering very intimate care to people who are seriously ill

  (c) Stress reduction, physical health: Humor can help caregivers cope with the physiologic effects of working in high-stress environments

  (d) Cathartic: Gallows humor releases psychologically stressful feelings experienced by caregivers exposed to suffering and loss

  (e) Conflict management: Humor can be used to deal with anger and hostility and to chide group members who have violated group norms; but beware, this can be a negative use unless carefully applied

  (f) Play: Humor can serve as a source of playfulness and renewal by caregivers

2. Relationship to People With HIV

  a. Utility

    (1) Immune system enhancement

    (2) Stress reduction

    (3) Perspective shift (e.g., despair to hopefulness)

    (4) Interpersonal skill in interacting with multiple care providers

    (5) Emotional and spiritual healing

    (6) Increased quality and possible quantity of life

  b. Level of acceptance

    (1) Still an emerging therapy, scientific proof of its benefits is limited

    (2) Seen in many treatment groups as one more tool to treat the patient holistically

    (3) Growing body of resources— newsletters, national association of humor therapists, guide and resource books for establishing humor groups

  c. Providers/facilitators of services

    (1) Attributes of skilled practitioners/ healers

      (a) Training in the use of therapeutic humor

        i) Techniques

ii) Clear vision regarding own blocks to using healthy humor
iii) Ability to conduct assessment of patient and plan carefully for humor used as therapy
(b) Anyone using humor with patients needs to understand clearly the negative effects of harmful humor
(c) No national accreditation at this time
(2) Types of providers
(a) Varied professional backgrounds (nurses, chaplains, physicians, social workers, mental health therapists)
(b) Trained volunteers from non-healthcare backgrounds, professional clowns
(3) Potential for harm
(a) Used inappropriately humor can shame, increase tensions, destroy someone's self-esteem, exclude others from enjoyment, place blame, be divisive
(b) An untrained person attempting to use humor therapeutically risks psychologically harming the patient if intervention is poorly managed
3. Nursing Role
a. Educate self on the uses and principles of therapeutic humor
b. Create opportunities to use humor in practice setting
(1) Humor rooms
(2) Cartoon collections
(3) Laugh libraries (tapes, videos, books, games)
(4) Humor wagons (take the library to the patient)
(5) Comedy performances for patients and staff
(6) Bulletin boards with comics
(7) Cable TV programming with 24-hour comedy shows
c. Consider using a humor assessment form on intake
d. Evaluate humor efforts and continually attempt to improve programs

4. Future Directions
a. Increased use
(1) Train more professionals to use therapeutic humor
(2) Caregivers using programs of therapeutic humor offered at work site as stress reducer
(3) Increased numbers of HIV-infected patients creates greater need for wellness strategies that are relatively inexpensive
b. Humor may come to be recognized as an underused tool to engage the healing power of the human spirit

N. Meditation

1. Description: A practical activity in which the person focuses his or her concentration on a specific object, idea, or action for the purpose of achieve "quiet mind," i.e., going within oneself and connecting with one's higher power
a. Historical usage
(1) References to meditation as a form of or way to personal connection with a higher power and the healing benefits of meditation have been cited in most major religious traditions (e.g., Sufi, Jewish, Zen, Christian)
(2) Meditation is used frequently for stress reduction and relaxation
(3) Some cultures make a distinction between prayer and meditation; others consider the terms interchangeable
(4) Meditation has often been considered a required activity of healers in contemporary and past cultures (e.g., physician-priests, shamans)
b. Types or categories
(1) Breath counting: Complete concentration on the rhythm of one's breath
(2) Contemplation: Uninterrupted, focused concentration on ideas as they arise in one's consciousness, or concentrated focus on a chosen object, usually an object from nature (e.g., shell, stone, pine cone)

(3) Koan: A paradoxical problem or idea on which the meditator places full concentration; focusing on an issue

(4) Mantra: Repetition of a word or phrase used to focus concentration

(5) Choreographed body movements (e.g., yoga, t'ai chi, karate)

(6) Total concentration on a single, repeated action or performance of a particular type of skill (e.g., flower arranging, archery, walking, knitting, painting, weight lifting)

(7) Mysticism: Transcending physical limitations through a practiced mental/spiritual connecting to one's higher power

c. Anticipated benefits with rationale
  (1) Psychosocial
    (a) Sense of being in control on a personal level, especially in environments (such as hospitals) where patients feel depersonalized and out of control of their own bodies
    (b) Stress reduction
    (c) Pain management
  (2) Physiologic
    (a) Reduction in metabolic, heart, and respiration rates
    (b) Increased mental awareness and alertness
    (c) With much practice, more control over cardiovascular function (e.g., heart rate, blood pressure)
    (d) With expert practice, control over other organ and system functions (e.g., blood lactate level, WBC, T cells)
    (e) An increase in overall sense of well-being, connected with psychologic and emotional strengthening as outlined above
  (3) Spiritual
    (a) A consciously developed sense of having a relationship with one's higher power
    (b) A study of 100 subjects who were either HIV-positive or diagnosed with ARC or AIDS demonstrated positive relation-

ships between patient hardiness and participation in meditation or prayer (Carson, 1993)

d. Application, usage, frequency
  (1) Often used as one form of alternative healing and commonly used as part of an entire alternative healing program
  (2) One study (Nokes, Kendrew, & Longo, 1995) of complementary and alternative therapies used by HIV/AIDS patients listed meditation fifth in frequency of use; spirituality (prayer) was listed fourth

2. Relationship to People With HIV
  a. Utility
    (1) Meditation is noninvasive: It does not require financial investment or the removal of clothing and it can be done anywhere (outdoors; sitting in a chair, on the floor, on a cushion; lying on a bed)
    (2) Meditation can be part of a daily (or less frequent) self-care, stress-reduction program
    (3) Meditation can be practiced as a group activity where a prearranged group of patients and friends or family (with health professionals if desired) can have an ongoing group that meditates together; meditation can also be practiced alone, in a family, or in any other grouping
    (4) Meditation can be practiced for a 20-minute period or more, depending on the person's desire, ability, and reason for meditating
    (5) The different forms of meditation permit patients with different abilities and interests to develop their own routine; the different forms also allow for times when a patient may be more distracted (as in times of great stress or symptom distress) and find sitting quietly difficult
    (6) Meditation itself does not cost anything: Patients may want to buy a cushion to sit on, give a donation at a meditation class, or incur some other expense, but this is not necessary

b. Level of acceptance
   (1) Many formal religions practice meditation along with prayer so some patients are very familiar with meditation before they get sick
   (2) Many AIDS service organizations, community organizations, churches, and other spiritual or religious groups offer meditation sessions or special services for the public or for HIV patients in particular
   (3) Many meditation practitioners comment on how difficult it is to maintain a steady practice over time; setting time aside for meditation requires commitment and discipline
c. Providers/facilitators of services
   (1) Attributes of skilled practitioners/healers
      (a) Have their own meditation practice
      (b) Have sought formal training in meditation through master teachers, schools, or other classes; regular attendance at a meditation group that has an instructor, master, or specially-prepared (ordained) leader
      (c) Have a familiarity and comfort with the different forms of meditation
      (d) Demonstrate compassion and have the capacity to focus attention acutely; show a respect for the unconscious and for spiritual forces
   (2) Types of providers
      (a) Meditation is an integrated and formal part of Buddhism and many Buddhist groups (priests, nuns, individuals) have a wealth of experience in meditation and are very knowledgeable about related books and schools on the subject
      (b) Meditation (like prayer and contemplation) crosses all human cultures and religious categories and practitioners; people who meditate can be found in all walks of life
      (c) Nonsectarian providers who practice meditation and are not connected with any organized form of spiritual, religious or cultural group are available as teachers
   (3) Potential for harm
      (a) Meditation is a natural human activity; there is no physical harm
      (b) Beginning practitioners sometimes complain of aches and pains associated with sitting in one position for a long period of time
3. Nursing Role
   a. Conduct or support meditation sessions in inpatient units, hospices, residential facilities, etc.
   b. As a nurse, consider starting a personal meditation practice for stress reduction
   c. Include content on meditation in wellness, early intervention, or stress-management programs offered to health professionals, patients, family members, or the community at large
   d. Become familiar with different forms of mediation in order to be able to provide an overview of these forms instead of relying solely on those with which you may already be familiar
   e. Incorporate meditation period into any memorial services or times of remembrance the nursing agency staff does as part of a loss and grief event
4. Future Directionss
   a. As more interest is placed in our society and healthcare system on wellness, patient empowerment, and the connection of mind-body-spirit, meditation and similar activities will become increasingly relevant and familiar
   b. There is a growing interest in researching the effects of meditation, and a body of knowledge on the health effects of meditation is being developed
   c. As the level of acceptance increases due to the benefits and "successes" from use of meditation becoming more widely publicized, frequency of use is increasing.

Section 9

Ethical and Legal Aspects

Recognition of the AIDS epidemic highlighted ethical issues in ways both new and old. Characteristics of HIV disease, the nature of the epidemic, and the nature of the populations among whom HIV infection first became apparent were part of the reason for the emergence of ethical conflicts that appeared new. Many, in fact, were a refocus of previous ethical issues in a new frame.

I. FRAMEWORK FOR CONSIDERING ETHICAL ISSUES

1. Definition/Description
   a. Ethics is a branch of philosophy concerned with values related to human conduct, the rightness or wrongness of certain actions, and the goodness or badness of the motives or ends of such actions; ethics helps us answer questions about how we ought to behave and why, using reasoned analyses
   b. Ethical theories define what it is to act morally
      (1) They justify ethical principles to guide moral decisions and to serve as standards to evaluate actions and policies
      (2) Theories and principles of ethics guide us in searching for and appraising solutions to ethical problems
2. Approaches to ethics: There are several major approaches to ethics, which are not necessarily mutually exclusive
   a. *Consequentialism or utilitarianism:* Used to determine the rightness of an action based on consequences

   b. *Principle-based ethics:* Another approach to determine the rightness of an action
      (1) Four principles are commonly used in healthcare ethics
         (a) Nonmaleficence (avoiding harm or injury to others)
         (b) Beneficence (promoting the good or welfare of others)
         (c) Respect for autonomy (respecting the liberty, privacy, and self-determination of others)
         (d) Justice (treating others fairly)
      (2) Other relevant principles
         (a) Fidelity (keeping promises, contracts)
         (b) Veracity (telling the truth)
   c. *Ethics of care:* Emphasizes caring for others and their significant relationships, recognizing the special obligations toward and willingness to act on behalf of people with whom one has a relationship
   d. Other approaches: Rights-based approach, virtue ethics, communitarianism

358

II. SPECIFIC ETHICAL ISSUES IN HIV INFECTION AND DISEASE

Almost all the issues that have challenged bioethicists over the last several decades are those issues we are struggling with in the HIV epidemic—for example, confidentiality, discrimination, prenatal testing, abortion, privacy, individual freedom versus public compulsion, access to health care, justice in health care, informed consent and patient decision making, advance directives, end-of-life decisions, suicide and assisted suicide, the conduct of clinical trials, scientific integrity, and the education of children. Important issues are outlined below, although this is not meant to be an exhaustive list. See also Appendix G, ANA's *Code for Nurses*, p. 431.

A. Prevention and Public Health

1. HIV antibody testing of individuals and groups
   a. Basing decisions about the testing of individuals or groups on an assessment of the risks and benefits
   b. Compulsory vs. voluntary or routine testing (e.g., testing of prisoners, military recruits, applicants of insurance policies)?
   c. Counseling and informed consent for HIV antibody testing
   d. Issues related to blinded HIV seroprevalence testing: Should it be done, and if so under what circumstances?
   e. Prenatal/neonatal testing
   f. Testing of healthcare providers
   g. Paying for testing
2. Confidentiality: Does anyone beside the person being tested have a right or need to know the results?
   a. Should results be disclosed only with the consent of the person tested?
   b. What are the criteria for ethically overriding confidentiality?
   c. What are the safeguards to protect the confidentiality of patient information?
3. Discrimination
   a. Often the consequence of disclosure of information about a person's HIV status
   b. Violates the principles of justice
   c. What safeguards are in place to protect against or minimize discrimination?
4. Partner notification: Sexual partners and needle sharers are at risk of infection

   a. Do they have a right to information about a person's HIV status if that person doesn't want them to know? How is this accomplished?
   b. Duty to warn versus privilege to warn; consequences of warning others may include violence
5. Prenatal counseling
   a. What advice should an HIV-positive woman be given about pregnancy?
   b. With data that demonstrate the effectiveness of prenatal AZT in reducing the rate of transmission of HIV from mother to fetus, should all pregnant women be antibody tested?
   c. Should testing be mandatory or voluntary?
   d. If the HIV-antibody test is positive, is there an obligation to provide the patient with access to AZT?
   e. Is there an obligation for a mother to take AZT?
6. Risk-behavior counseling (children, adolescents, adults)
   a. What is the best way to teach people to reduce or avoid risky behavior while respecting their autonomy and privacy?
   b. Does providing clean needles to drug users or condoms to teenagers promote undesirable behaviors?
7. Dealing with deliberate "unsafe" behavior: How should we (as nurses, friends, fellow citizens) respond to those who deliberately practice unsafe behaviors that put others in jeopardy?

B. Providing Care to Patients

1. Obligation to care
   a. Nurses have an obligation "to provide services with respect for human dignity and the uniqueness of the client, unrestricted by considerations of social or economic status, personal attributes, or the nature of the health problem" (ANA Committee on Ethics, 1985, p. 1).
   b. What are the limits of this obligation? The risk of occupational HIV infection is very small, but other risks to the nurse include TB, CMV, hepatitis or other infections, violence, discrimination.
2. Patient advocacy: By functioning as patient advocates, nurses promote and respect patient autonomy
3. Patient decision making, informed consent
   a. Providing people with adequate and culturally appropriate information to help them make decisions about treatment and care is part of nursing care and advocacy
   b. Assessing a patient's ability to make decisions and understand information is critical because of the possibility of neuropsychiatric complications
4. End-of-life decisions, advance directives
   a. PWAs face decisions about the kind of care they want in end-stage disease; advance directives enable a patient to specify a person to make decisions in the case of incapacity (durable power of attorney) or specify interventions to be foregone (living will)
   b. PWAs have a higher incidence of suicide than those with other medical conditions; assistance with suicide is believed to be available among certain communities of gay men with AIDS (Battin, 1994)

C. Access to Care and Treatment

1. Access to care in the United States is uneven
   a. Many PWAs rely on Medicaid or have no healthcare insurance, which has a major impact on their ability to get the care and therapies they may need
   b. The growth of managed care will likely complicate the ability of PWAs and those who need complex or expensive treatment to get adequate care

D. Biomedical and Behavioral Research

1. Access to research participation and experimental therapies
   a. AIDS activists have challenged attitudes and some regulations regarding research participation and access to experimental therapies as too restrictive and discriminatory
   b. Exclusion of certain groups from research has been seen as discrimination rather than protection; access to clinical trials is seen as a benefit
   c. People with HIV infection are often willing to take the risks of unproven therapies through underground buyers' clubs and expanded access programs, instead of or in addition to clinical trials
2. Design and conduct of research
   a. Trial design, rigid exclusion criteria, the use of placebos, the need for clinical endpoints and other aspects of trial design have all been challenged by AIDS activists, researchers, and pharmaceutical companies
   b. Scientific conflicts of interest, scientific integrity, and competition in HIV research have become important areas of discussion and consciousness
3. The demand for quicker results and more efficient clinical trials, as well as issues of scientific integrity, have led to more emphasis on methods of monitoring the research participants and data through data and safety monitoring boards and other review bodies; community representatives have become involved in decisions about research through community advisory boards
4. Nurses, often in positions of monitoring patients who participate in research, are sometimes placed in the difficult position of knowing that a person is not adhering to the research protocol; disclosing this information, however, may disqualify the individual from continued participation in the research.

III. LEGAL ISSUES

While legal issues are important to people with HIV/AIDS, many legal decisions rely on state laws. Many issues are mentioned below, but the reader needs to consult other sources, including current state laws, for current details and policies.

A. Legal Issue Overview for Patients With HIV

1. Wills/powers of attorney
2. Debtor/Creditor
3. Entitlement programs
4. Guardianship
5. Insurance
6. Discrimination and AIDS in workplace policies
7. Testing of healthcare workers
8. Failure to diagnose
9. Confidentiality and duty to warn

B. Estate Planning and People with AIDS

1. Psychosocial factors and the terminal patient
2. Considerations for gay men; grounds for challenges to a will
3. Considerations for parents with children
   a. Custody provisions in the will
   b. Temporary guardianships
   c. Standby guardianships
4. The mechanics of will writing
   a. Definition of terms
   b. Laws of intestacy
   c. Disinheritance/in terrorem clause
   d. Executor appointment
   e. Beneficiary designation
   f. Conditional bequests
5. Medical decision making
   a. Living wills
   b. Directives to physicians (do-not-resuscitate [DNR] orders)
6. Forms to review (vary by institution, state)
   a. Model will form
   b. Living will form
   c. DNR form
   d. Standby guardianship form
   e. Temporary guardianship form
   f. State-by-state breakdown of living will and DNR statutes

C. Discrimination

1. AIDS as a handicap
   a. State handicap laws
   b. The Federal Rehabilitation Act of 1971: The Arline Decision—making AIDS a handicap for federal purposes
   c. State, municipal, and HIV-specific county antidiscrimination efforts
2. The Americans with Disabilities Act
   a. In the workplace
   b. Public accommodation
   c. As access to health care
3. Policy formation addressing AIDS in the workplace

D. Insurance

1. Health
   a. Insurance plans
      (1) Traditional: Fee for service
      (2) Health maintenance organizations (HMOs)
      (3) Preferred provider organizations (PPOs)
      (4) Self-insured companies
   b. Individual plan issues: Material misrepresentation
   c. Group plan issues: Preexisting conditions
   d. Special problems
      (1) Noncoverage for experimental treatments
      (2) Capping
   e. Conversion rights
      (1) To an individual policy
      (2) COBRA (group plan)
2. Life insurance
   a. HIV testing
   b. Disability and waiver of premiums
   c. Accelerated benefits
   d. Viatical settlements
      (1) "Purchases of life insurance policies from terminally ill individual. The

individual receives a lump sum of money along with insurance coverage, prior to death" (Freudenheim, 1996, p. 290).

(2) Thus the purchaser pays the life insurance premiums until the individual dies, and then the company receives the insurance benefits instead of the heirs (Freudenheim, 1996)

E. Healthcare Providers

1. Confidentiality
   a. The doctrine of HIV exceptionalism
   b. The standard
   c. The exceptions
      (1) Medical personnel
          Third-party notification
      (3) States with mandatory names reporting
   d. Testing
      (1) Informed consent and documentation
      (2) Mandatory testing situations
          (a) Ethics of the mandatory testing of newborns or pregnant women
          (b) Defendants charged with sex crimes
          (c) The incarcerated
          (d) Institutionalized minors
2. Treatment
   a. Failure to diagnose
   b. Failure to treat
3. The HIV-positive healthcare professional and the Americans with Disabilities Act

F. Family Law

1. Child custody in divorce proceedings and HIV
2. Criminalization of HIV transmission
3. Psychological factors for courts respecting HIV/AIDS, homosexuality, and lesbianism.

Section 10

Infection Control

This section addresses two aspects of infection control: preventing transmission of HIV in the patient care setting and preventing transmission of opportunistic pathogens to HIV-infected people. The content focuses on infection-control measures to prevent and reduce risks; however, information and recommendations related to preventing HIV transmission in patient care is ever evolving.

Most OIs in people with HIV are reactivated latent infections rather than new or primary ones. Information on opportunistic pathogens and prophylactic treatments is covered in Section 4, *Clinical Manifestations and Treatment of HIV Disease in Adults*.

I. PREVENTING THE TRANSMISSION OF HIV IN PATIENT CARE SETTINGS

A. Introduction

1. Transmission of HIV to healthcare workers (HCWs) has been a concern since HIV was first identified as a communicable disease
   a. In 1984, *The Lancet* reported the first case of HIV transmission as a result of an occupational exposure in Africa (Needlestick transmission, 1984)
   b. In 1987, CDC reported three cases of occupationally acquired HIV infection in the U.S. (CDC, 1987)
2. In 1990, the first incident of possible HIV transmission from a healthcare worker (HCW) to a patient was reported (CDC, 1990a)
   a. This incident created the same fear in the public that HCWs had expressed toward their infected patients
   b. The general public demanded to know
      (1) The HIV status of HCWs
      (2) What measures would be taken to maintain public safety within healthcare settings
3. 93% of U.S. AIDS cases today have resulted from human behaviors involving sexual contact or sharing needles during injecting drug use (CDC, 1995b)
4. The risk of acquiring HBV following a percutaneous exposure to blood infected with HBV can be as high as 30% in susceptible people (Hadley, 1989) (significantly greater than the risk of 0.3% for acquiring HIV infection [Gerberding, 1994])
5. Documented HIV infections: Patient to HCWs (see Table 10.1)
   a. Through December 1995, 49 HCWs with documented occupationally acquired AIDS/HIV infection have been reported; most of these infections occurred via percutaneous exposure (CDC, 1995d)
   b. An additional 102 HCWs have possible occupationally acquired HIV infection (CDC, 1995d)
      (1) Investigations have revealed no other identifiable exposure risk for HIV infection

   (2) Each HCW reported an occupational exposure; however, HIV seroconversion specifically resulting from an occupational exposure was not documented
   c. Based on 21 prospective studies reviewed by Gerberding (1995), the estimated risk of transmission of HIV following a percutaneous or needle-puncture exposure is 0.3%
   d. The estimated risk of occupational exposure to HIV following a mucocutaneous transmission is 0.1% (Gerberding, 1995)
   e. Factors associated with increased risk of HIV transmission to HCWs (CDC, 1995b)
      (1) An exposure from a terminally ill AIDS patient
      (2) An exposure with a needle that was used in a blood vessel
      (3) An exposure from a visibly bloody device
      (4) A deep puncture
   f. Some occupational infections reported among nurses have been related to
      (1) Recapping needles
      (2) Drawing blood
      (3) Administering medications
      (4) Disposing of contaminated needles
   g. Studies (Marcus et al., 1988) have suggested that almost half these occupationally related infections could have been prevented had the involved HCW (or in some instances, their co-workers) adhered to universal precautions
6. Documented HIV infections: HCW to patient
   a. The risk of HIV transmission from HCW to patient is considerably lower than that from patient to HCW (patients are less likely to come in contact with blood or body fluids of HCW in the course of care) (CDC, 1992b)
   b. To date, there has been only one documented case in the U.S., reported in 1990 (CDC, 1990a)
      (1) Transmission of HIV from a dentist to 6 patients

Table 10.1   Healthcare Workers With Documented and Possible Occupationally Acquired AIDS/HIV Infection, by Occupation, Reported Through December 1995, U.S.[1]

Occupation	Documented Occupational Transmission[2] No.	Possible Occupational Transmission[3] No.
Dental worker, including dentist	–	7
Embalmer/morgue technician	–	3
Emergency medical technician/paramedic	–	9
Health aide/attendant	1	12
Housekeeper/maintenance worker	1	7
Laboratory technical, clinical	15	15
Laboratory technical, nonclinical	3	0
Nurse	19	24
Physician, nonsurgical	6	10
Physician, surgical	–	4
Respiratory therapist	1	2
Technician, dialysis	1	2
Technician, surgical	2	1
Technician/therapist, other than those listed above	–	4
Other healthcare occupations	–	2
	49	102

[1]Healthcare workers are defined as those persons, including students and trainees, who have worked in a healthcare, clinical, or HIV laboratory setting at any time since 1978. See *MMWR, 421*, pp. 823–825.
[2]Healthcare workers who had documented HIV seroconversion after occupational exposure or had other laboratory evidence of occupational infection: 40 had percutaneous exposure, 4 had mucocutaneous exposure, 1 had both percutaneous and mucocutaneous exposures, and 1 had an unknown route of exposure. Forty-one exposures were to blood from an HIV-infected person, 1 to visibly bloody fluid, 1 to an unspecified fluid, and 3 to concentrated virus in a laboratory. Twenty of these healthcare workers developed AIDS.
[3]These healthcare workers have been investigated and are without identifiable behavioral or transfusion risks; each reported percutaneous or mucocutaneous occupational exposures to blood or body fluids, or laboratory solutions containing HIV, but HIV seroconversion specifically resulting from an occupational exposure was not documented.
Note: From "US HIV and AIDS cases reported through December 1995," by CDC, 1995, *HIV/AIDS Surveillance Report, 7*(2), p. 21.

(2) Genetic similarities of the virus found in the dentist and the subsequently infected patients was confirmed
(3) Route of transmission cannot be definitively established: Two possible explanations
   (a) Probable break in infection-control procedures
   (b) Possible intention to harm on the part of the dentist (Ciesielski et al., 1992)
c. The CDC has developed a risk model to estimate the risk of a patient acquiring HIV infection from an HIV-infected surgeon

(1) The model assumes that a surgeon will sustain a percutaneous injury during a procedure, that the sharp object causing the injury is contaminated with the surgeon's blood and subsequently comes in contact with a patient's open body cavity or wound, and that HIV will be transmitted to the patient
(2) Using this model, the CDC determined that the probability of HIV transmission from an HIV-positive surgeon to an uninfected patient is 0.0024%–0.00024% (Chamberland & Bell, 1992)

d. Look-back evaluations of the 15,000 patients treated by 32 HIV-infected HCWs showed none had acquired HIV (DiMaggio, 1993)

7. Documented HIV infections: Patient to patient
   a. In 1994, a case of patient-to-patient HIV transmission involving a healthcare provider was reported (Chant, 1993)
      (1) An HIV-negative dermatologist in Australia conducted a procedure on an HIV-positive patient; the physician then conducted a similar procedure on an HIV-negative patient
      (2) The second patient was found to have acquired the HIV virus during that dermatologic office procedure; the physician did not acquire the virus during the procedure
   b. Transmission is believed to have occurred when the physician used an instrument that acted as a vector in carrying the virus from one patient to another

8. Documented HIV infections: Patient to family caregiver in the home—8 cases of HIV transmission appear to be associated with living with or providing home care to a person with HIV disease (CDC, 1994c)
   a. Four of the cases involved nursing care; the other four resulted from living in the same household
   b. Five of the incidents were associated with documented or probable blood contact
   c. Incident/exposure causing the transmission was not determined in the three remaining cases
   d. No reported data on the degree to which universal precautions were used in these caregiving situations

B. Recommendations/Standards to Prevent Exposures

1. Centers for Disease Control and Prevention
   a. 1983
      (1) CDC recommended *blood and body fluid precautions* as an infection-control practice in order to reduce the transmission of what was later identified as HIV between HCWs and patients (Garner & Simmons, 1983)
      (2) The recommendations called for the use of precautions for blood and body fluid when a patient was known or suspected to be infected with blood-borne pathogens
   b. In 1987, the CDC recommended the adoption of *universal precautions* (see Table 10.2): All patients to be treated as if they have a blood-borne infection
      (1) All human blood and certain body fluids associated with blood-borne pathogens are treated as if known to be infectious
      (2) This approach is intended to prevent parenteral, mucous membrane, and nonintact skin exposures of HCWs to blood-borne pathogens
      (3) Universal precautions apply to
         (a) Blood and other body fluids containing visible blood, semen, and vaginal secretions
         (b) Tissues
         (c) Cerebrospinal, synovial, pleural, peritoneal, pericardial, amniotic fluids
      (4) Universal precautions do *not* apply to
         (a) Feces, nasal secretions, sputum, sweat, tears, urine, and vomitus unless they contain visible blood
         (b) Saliva, except when visibly contaminated with blood, or in the dental setting where blood contamination of saliva is predictable
   c. In 1996, the Hospital Infection Control Practices Advisory Committee published revised CDC guidelines for isolation precautions in hospitals to prevent or control nosocomial infections (Garner, 1996); the guidelines contain two tiers of precautions—standard (universal and body-substance precautions) and transmission based
      (1) Transmission-based precautions (airborne, droplet, contact) are implemented *in addition to standard precautions* when a hospitalized patient has, or is suspected to have, a highly

Table 10.2 Universal Precautions

1. All healthcare workers should routinely use appropriate barrier precautions to prevent skin and mucous-membrane exposure when contact with blood or body fluids is anticipated. Gloves should be worn for touching blood and body fluids, mucous membranes, or nonintact skin of all patients, for handling items or surfaces soiled with blood or body fluids, and for performing venipuncture and other vascular access procedures. Gloves should be changed after contact with each patient. Masks and protective eyewear or face shields should be worn during procedures that are likely to generate droplets of blood or other body fluids to prevent exposure of mucous membranes of the mouth, nose and eyes. Gowns or aprons should be worn during procedures that are likely to generate splashes of blood or other body fluids.

2. Hands and other skin surfaces should be washed immediately and thoroughly if contaminated with blood or other body fluids. Hands should be washed immediately after gloves are removed.

3. All healthcare workers should take precautions to prevent injuries caused by needles, scalpels, and other sharp instruments or devices during procedures; when cleaning used instruments; during disposal of used needles; and when handling sharp instruments after procedures. Needles should not be recapped, purposely bent or broken by hand, removed from disposable syringes, or otherwise manipulated by hand. After they are used, disposable syringes and needles, scalpel blades, and other sharp items should be placed in puncture-resistant containers for disposal; the puncture-resistant containers should be located as close as practical to the use area. Large-bore reusable needles should be placed in a puncture-resistant container for transport to the reprocessing area.

4. Although saliva has not been implicated in HIV transmission, to minimize the need for emergency mouth-to-mouth resuscitation mouthpieces, resuscitation bags, or other ventilation devices should be available for use in areas in which the need for resuscitation is predictable.

5. Healthcare workers who have exudative lesions or weeping dermatitis should refrain from all direct patient care and from handling patient-care equipment until the condition resolves.

6. Pregnant healthcare workers are not known to be at greater risk of contracting HIV infection than healthcare workers who are not pregnant; however, if a healthcare worker develops HIV infection during pregnancy, the infant is at risk of infection resulting from perinatal transmission. Because of this risk, pregnant healthcare workers should be especially familiar with and strictly adhere to precautions to minimize the risk of HIV transmission.

Note: From "Precautions to prevent transmission of HIV," by CDC, 1987, *Morbidity and Mortality Weekly Report, 36,* p. 6S.

transmissible pathogen for which additional precautions are required to interrupt transmission, for instance

  (a) For disseminated herpes zoster, additional airborne and contact precautions are recommended

  (b) For pulmonary TB, additional airborne precautions are recommended

(2) Each transmission-based precaution has specific requirements related to

  (a) Patient room assignment (e.g., private room, negative pressure room)

  (b) Personal protective equipment used (e.g., mask, gloves, gowns)

  (c) Patient transport precautions for off-unit procedures

  (d) *For contact precautions only,* patient care equipment

2. Occupational Safety and Health Administration (OSHA) blood-borne pathogen standards

  a. Specific OSHA regulations have been developed in order to protect workers against work-related hazards, including exposure to blood-borne pathogens

  b. In 1991, OSHA adopted standards (Department of Labor, 1991) that stipulate both employee and employer responsibilities to reduce the risk of blood-borne pathogen transmission in the workplace that include

    (1) The Exposure Control Plan: A written exposure control plan is necessary for the safety and health of workers and includes

(a) Identification of job classifications where there is exposure to blood or other potentially infectious materials

(b) Explanation of the protective measures currently in effect, including how hazards are communicated to employees, hepatitis B vaccination, postexposure follow-up procedures, personal protective equipment, housekeeping, record keeping

(c) Establishment of procedures to evaluate the circumstances of an exposure incident

(2) Communicating hazards to employees: All employees involved with activities with the potential of occupational exposure must receive training about the OSHA regulations as a new employee and annually thereafter

(3) Hepatitis B vaccination: All HCWs at risk for exposure to blood in the healthcare setting should be educated about the risks and benefits of HBV vaccine and offered the series

(4) Engineering and work practice controls

(a) Engineering controls isolate or remove the hazard from employees; they are used in conjunction with work practices (e.g., use of puncture-resistant, leak-proof containers to discard contaminated items like needles or other sharps that could cause a puncture)

(b) Work practice controls reduce the likelihood of exposure by altering the manner in which the task is performed, e.g.

   i) Wash hands when gloves are removed and as soon as possible after contact with blood or other infectious materials

   ii) Provide available mechanisms for immediate eye irrigation in the event of an exposure to the eye

   iii) Do not bend, recap, or remove contaminated needles unless absolutely required to do so

   iv) Do not shear or break contaminated needles

   v) Discard contaminated needles and sharp instruments in puncture-resistant biohazard-labeled containers that are accessible, maintained upright, and not overfilled

   vi) Do not eat, drink, smoke, apply cosmetics, or handle contact lenses in areas of potential occupational exposure

   vii) Use red or biohazard labels on containers to store, transport, or ship blood or other potentially infectious materials

   viii) Mouth pipetting to suction blood or other infectious materials is prohibited

(5) Personal protective equipment (PPE): Specialized clothing or equipment worn by an employee for protection against a hazard

(a) PPE must not allow blood or other potentially infectious materials to pass through to workers' clothing, skin, or mucous membranes (e.g., gloves, impervious gowns, laboratory coats, face shield, masks, eye protection)

(b) The employer is responsible for providing maintaining, disposing, and assuring the proper use of PPE

C. Management of Exposures

1. Definition of exposure
   a. The CDC defines an occupational exposure as an injury occurring during the performance of job duties that places a worker at risk of HIV infection as a result of
      (1) A percutaneous injury (needle stick or cut with a sharp object)

(2) Contact of mucous membranes or skin (especially when skin is chapped, abraded, or afflicted with dermatitis or the contact is prolonged or involving an extensive area) with blood, tissues, or other body fluids to which universal precautions apply

(3) Contact with blood, tissues, and other body fluids considered potentially infectious

  (a) Semen, vaginal secretions, and other body fluids contaminated with visible blood

  (b) Cerebrospinal, synovial, pleural, peritoneal, pericardial, and amniotic fluids

  (c) Laboratory specimens that contain HIV

2. Immediate management: Immediate first aid to the site of exposure, although of unproven benefit, is a reasonable action and not associated with any harm (Gerberding & Henderson, 1992)

a. Wash puncture wounds and other cutaneous injuries with soap and water; if the exposure breaks the skin, irrigate with sterile saline, an antiseptic, or other suitable solution

b. Decontaminate exposed oral and nasal mucous membranes by vigorous flushing with water

c. Irrigate eyes with clean water, saline, or specific sterile irrigants

3. Reporting exposures

a. Each healthcare site must have in place a mechanism to evaluate and treat an employee in the event of an exposure

b. All activities involved with the exposure, including testing, should be documented and considered confidential

4. Immediate assessment of the exposure should include relevant details

a. Site of the exposure

b. Instruments involved

c. Mechanism of exposure

d. Activity surrounding the exposure incident

e. Body fluids and volume involved, if known

f. Duration of contact

g. Type of protective barriers used

5. Evaluation of source patient

a. The source patient needs clinical and epidemiologic evaluation for HIV infection

b. Obtain informed consent from the source patient for confidential testing for HIV infection

c. Do not include the exposed HCW as part of the request and testing process of the source patient

d. Keep testing in compliance with the regulatory laws in the particular state

e. If the source patient is found to be HIV negative and has no clinical manifestations of HIV, then repeated testing and follow-up may not be necessary; if there is any evidence that the source patient may be at risk for HIV or if the exposed HCW requests it, testing and follow-up may be carried out

f. If the source patient is unknown, the decision on follow-up assessment must be on a case-by-case basis

6. Counseling and support following occupational exposure to HIV

a. HIV testing and education to prevent transmitting infection to others while testing of the HCW is ongoing

(1) Provide counseling to the HCW and offer confidential HIV testing

(2) For HCWs with reservations about being tested, offer the option of having blood obtained and stored for possible future testing (the rationale for initial baseline testing at the time of exposure is to establish the HIV status of the HCW at the time of the incident in order to document an occupational exposure to HIV)

(3) Schedule follow-up testing at 6 weeks and 3 and 6 months postexposure

(4) During the period the HCW is being tested, counsel to

  (a) Abstain from unprotected sexual intercourse, needle sharing, breastfeeding, blood/tissue/organ donation

  (b) Defer conception

  (c) Report and seek evaluation for

any signs or symptoms of viral infection such as fever, headache, lymphadenopathy, rash, pharyngitis, myalgia, fatigue

b. Emotional responses to exposures and the need for supportive counseling

   (1) A study assessing the responses has found that many HCWs have significant reactions to the exposure (e.g., anger, anxiety, denial, sadness, depression, fear, mood swings, sleep disturbances, psychosis) (Gerberding & Henderson, 1992)

   (2) The majority of HCWs experience increased anxiety as they wait for test results

   (3) HCWs may respond to the exposure with varying degrees of emotion and concern

   (4) Offer and provide supportive psychologic counseling by trained clinicians who are experienced with crisis/stress management and also knowledgeable about HIV

c. Since 1983, CDC has conducted a nationwide surveillance project to assess the risk to HCWs of acquiring HIV infection resulting from documented occupational exposure. Enrollment information may be obtained from an infection-control practitioner, state health department, or the CDC at (404) 639-1547.

7. Chemoprophylaxis

a. Research efforts to determine if and when chemoprophylaxis should be used are confounded by a number of difficult aspects (CDC, 1990b; Tokars, Marcus, Culver, et al., 1993)

   (1) The overall risk of HIV transmission is relatively low (0.3%), so enormous numbers would have to be enrolled in trials

   (2) Understanding of the factors that contribute to HIV transmission is limited

   (3) Lengthy window period from time of exposure to positive test results

   (4) Additional factors associated with HCWs' potential risky behaviors outside the workplace

b. Between January 1988 and August 1994 the CDC, in collaboration with French and British public health authorities, conducted a retrospective case-control study (CDC, 1995b)

   (1) Data were obtained from reports made to the U.S., France, and United Kingdom surveillance systems

   (2) Postexposure use of zidovudine (AZT) by HCWs was associated with a 79% lower risk for transmission of HIV compared to those HCWs who did not take AZT postexposure

   (3) As a result of these findings, the USPHS is revising their previous recommendations (CDC, 1990b) regarding postexposure use of antiretroviral agents

c. Determining chemoprophylaxis use following an exposure needs to be individualized and done by a knowledgeable clinician who is able to assess the incident and explain the appropriateness of chemoprophylaxis and the potential limitations and benefits

   (1) Experience at San Francisco General Hospital and the Clinical Center of the National Institutes of Health suggests that offering and providing AZT 500–600 mg/day within 4 hours of exposure and continuing for 4–6 weeks is safe and feasible (Gerberding, 1995)

   (2) A confounding factor is the potential limitation of AZT when the source patient has an AZT-resistant strain of the virus.

II. PREVENTING TRANSMISSION OF OPPORTUNISTIC PATHOGENS TO THE HIV INFECTED

1. See *Clinical Manifestations and Treatment of HIV Disease in Adults,* p. 46, for mode of transmission, reservoir of pathogens, and prophylactic therapies

2. Table 10.3 provides information on reducing the risk of or preventing exposure to opportunistic pathogens.

Table 10.3   Reducing the Risk of/Preventing Exposure to Opportunistic Pathogens Based on Method of Exposure: Information for Patients

Sexual Exposures

1. Patients should use male latex condoms during every act of sexual intercourse to reduce the risk of exposure to CMV, HSV, and HPV as well as to other sexually transmitted pathogens (AIII)*. Use of latex condoms will also prevent the transmission of HIV to others.
2. Patients should avoid sexual practices that may result in oral exposure to feces (e.g., oral-anal contact) to reduce the risk of intestinal infections such as cryptosporidiosis, shigellosis, campylobacteriosis, amebiasis, giardiasis, and hepatitis A and B (BIII).

Environmental and Occupational Exposures

1. Certain activities or types of employment may increase the risk of exposure to TB (BIII). These include volunteer work or employment in healthcare facilities, correctional institutions, and shelters for the homeless as well as in other settings identified as high risk by local health authorities. Decisions about whether or not to continue with such activities should be made in conjunction with the healthcare provider and should take into account such factors as the patient's specific duties in the workplace, the prevalence of TB in the community, and the degree to which precautions designed to prevent the transmission of TB are taken in the workplace (BIII). These decisions will affect the frequency with which the patient should be screened for TB.
2. Child-care providers and parents of children in child-care facilities are at increased risk of acquiring CMV infection, cryptosporidiosis, and other infections (e.g., hepatitis A, giardiasis) from children. The risk of acquiring infection can be diminished by good hygienic practices, such as hand washing after fecal contact (e.g., during diaper changing) and after contact with urine or saliva (AII). All children in child-care facilities are also at increased risk of acquiring these same infections; parents and other caretakers of HIV-infected children should be advised of this risk (BIII).
3. Occupations involving contact with animals (e.g., veterinary work and employment in pet stores, farms, or slaughterhouses) may pose a risk of crytosporidiosis, toxoplasmosis, salmonellosis, campylobacteriosis, or bartonella infection. However, the available data are insufficient to justify a recommendation against work in such settings.
4. Contact with young farm animals, especially animals with diarrhea, should be avoided to reduce the risk of cryptosporidiosis (BII).
5. Hand washing after gardening or other contact with soil may reduce the risk of cryptosporidiosis and toxoplasmosis (BIII).
6. In histoplasmosis-endemic areas, patients should avoid activities known to be associated with increased risk, including cleaning chicken coops, disturbing soil beneath bird-roosting sites, and exploring caves (CIII).
7. In coccidioidomycosis-endemic areas, when possible, patients should avoid activities associated with increased risk, including those involving extensive exposure to disturbed soil (e.g., at excavation sites, on farms, or during dust storms (CIII).

Pet-Related Exposures

Healthcare providers should advise HIV-infected persons of the potential risk posed by pet ownership. However, they should be sensitive to the possible psychologic benefits of pet ownership and should not routinely advise HIV-infected persons to part with their pets (DIII). Specifically, providers should advise HIV-infected patients of the following.

continued ▶

Table 10.3 *Continued*

General

1. Veterinary care should be sought when a pet develops diarrheal illness. If possible, HIV-infected persons should avoid contact with animals that have diarrhea (BIII). A fecal sample should be obtained from animals with diarrhea and examined for *Cryptosporidium, Salmonella,* and *Campylobacter.*
2. When obtaining a new pet, HIV-infected patients should avoid animals <6 months of age, especially those with diarrhea (BIII). Because the hygienic and sanitary conditions in pet breeding facilities, pet stores, and animal shelters are highly variable, the patient should exercise caution when obtaining a pet from these sources. Stray animals should be avoided. Animals <6 months of age, especially those with diarrhea, should be examined by a veterinarian for *Cryptosporidium, Salmonella,* and *Campylobacter* (BIII).
3. Patients should wash their hands after handling pets (especially before eating) and avoid contact with pets' feces to reduce the risk of cryptosporidiosis, salmonellosis, and campylobacteriosis (BIII). Hand washing by HIV-infected children should be supervised.

Cats

4. Patients should consider the potential risks of cat ownership such as the risk of toxoplasmosis and bartonella infection, as well as enteric infections (CIII). Those who elect to obtain a cat should adopt or purchase an animal that is >1 year of age and in good health to reduce the risk of cryptosporidiosis, bartonella infection, salmonellosis, and campylobacteriosis (BII).
5. Litter boxes should be cleaned daily, preferably by an HIV-negative, nonpregnant person; if the HIV-infected patient performs this task, he or she should wash the hands thoroughly afterward to reduce the risk of toxoplasmosis (BIII).
6. Also to reduce the risk of toxoplasmosis, cats should be kept indoors, should not be allowed to hunt, and should not be fed raw or undercooked meat (BIII).
7. Although declawing is not generally advised, patients should avoid activities that may result in cat scratches or bites to reduce the risk of bartonella infections (BII). Patients should also wash sites of cat scratches or bites promptly (CIII) and should not allow cats to lick open cuts or wounds (BIII).
8. Care of cats should include flea control to reduce the risk of bartonella infection (CIII).
9. Testing of cats for toxoplasmosis (EII) or bartonella infection (DII) is not recommended.

Birds

10. Screening of healthy birds for *Cryptococcus neoformans, Mycobacterium avium,* or *Histoplasma capsulatum* is not recommended (DIII).

Other

11. Contact with reptiles (such as snakes, lizards, turtles) should be avoided to reduce the risk of salmonellosis (BIII).
12. Gloves should be used during the cleaning of aquariums to reduce the risk of infection with *Mycobacterium marinum* (BIII).
13. Contact with exotic pets, such as nonhuman primates, should be avoided (CIII).

Food- and Water-Related Exposures

1. Raw or undercooked eggs (including foods that may contain raw eggs, such as some preparations of hollandaise sauce, Caesar and certain other salad dressings, and mayonnaise); raw or undercooked poultry, meat, or seafood; and unpasteurized dairy products may contain enteric pathogens. Poultry and meat should be cooked until no longer pink in the middle (internal temperature, >165°F). Produce should be washed thoroughly before being eaten (BIII).
2. Cross-contamination of foods should be avoided. Uncooked meats should not be allowed to come into contact with other foods; hands, cutting boards, counters, and knives and other utensils should be washed thoroughly after contact with uncooked foods (BIII).
3. Although the incidence of listeriosis is low, it is a serious disease that occurs unusually frequently among HIV-infected persons who are severely immunosuppressed. Some soft cheeses and some ready-to-eat foods

continued ▶

Table 10.3 *Continued*

Food- and Water-Related Exposures (*continued*)

(e.g., hot dogs and cold cuts from delicatessen counters) have been known to cause listeriosis. An HIV-infected person who is severely immunosuppressed and who wishes to reduce the risk of food-borne disease can prevent listeriosis by reheating these foods until they are steaming hot before eating them (CIII).

4. Patients should not drink water directly from lakes or rivers because of the risk of cryptosporidiosis and giardiasis. Even accidental ingesting of lake or river water while swimming or engaging in other types of recreational activities carries this risk (BII).

5. During outbreaks or in other situations in which a community "boil-water" advisory is issued, boiling of water for 1 minute will eliminate the risk of cryptosporidiosis (AI). Use of submicron personal-use water filters (home/office types) and/or bottled water may reduce the risk (CIII). Current data are inadequate to recommend that all HIV-infected persons boil or otherwise avoid drinking tap water in nonoutbreak settings. However, persons who wish to take independent action to reduce the risk of waterborne cryptosporidiosis may choose to take precautions similar to those recommended during outbreaks. Such decisions are best made in conjunction with the healthcare provider. Persons who opt for a personal-use filter or bottled water should be aware of the complexities involved in selecting the appropriate products, the lack of enforceable standards for the destruction or removal of oocysts, the cost of the products, and the difficulty of using these products consistently.

Travel-Related Exposures

1. Travel, particularly in developing countries, may carry significant risks for the exposure of HIV-infected persons to opportunistic pathogens, especially for patients who are severely immunosuppressed. Consultation with healthcare providers and/or with experts in travel medicine will help patients plan itineraries (BIII).

2. During travel to developing countries, HIV-infected persons are at even higher risk for food- and waterborne infections than they are in the U.S. Foods and beverages—in particular, raw fruits and vegetables, raw or undercooked seafood or meat, tap water, ice made with tap water, unpasteurized milk and dairy products, and items purchased from street vendors—may be contaminated (AII). Items that are generally safe include steaming-hot foods, fruits that are peeled by the traveler, bottled (especially carbonated) beverages, hot coffee or tea, beer, wine, and water brought to a rolling boil for 1 minute (AII). Treatment of water with iodine or chlorine may not be as effective as boiling but can be used, perhaps in conjunction with filtration, when boiling is not practical (BIII).

3. Waterborne infections may result from the swallowing of water during recreational activities. To reduce the risk of cryptosporidiosis and giardiasis, patients should avoid swallowing water during swimming and should not swim in water that may be contaminated (e.g., with sewage or animal waste) (BII).

4. Antimicrobial prophylaxis for traveler's diarrhea is not recommended routinely for HIV-infected persons traveling to developing countries (DIII). Such preventive therapy can have adverse effects and can promote the emergence of drug-resistant organisms. Nonetheless, several studies (none involving an HIV-infected population) have shown that prophylaxis can reduce the risk of diarrhea among travelers. Under selected circumstances (e.g., those in which the risk of infection is very high and the period of travel brief), the provider and patient may weigh the potential risks and benefits and decide that antibiotic prophylaxis is warranted (CIII). For those individuals to whom prophylaxis is offered, fluoroquinolones, such as ciprofloxacin (500 mg q.d.) can be considered (BIII). Trimethoprim-sulfamethoxazole (TMP-SMX) (one double-strength tablet daily) has also been shown to be effective, but resistance to this drug is now common in tropical areas. Persons already taking TMP-SMX for prophylaxis against *P. carinii* pneumonia (PCP) may gain some protection against traveler's diarrhea. For HIV-infected persons who are not already taking TMP-SMX, the provider should use caution when prescribing this agent for prophylaxis of diarrhea because of the high rates of adverse reactions and the possible need for the agent for other purposes (e.g., PCP prophylaxis) in the future.

5. All HIV-infected travelers to developing countries should carry with them a sufficient supply of an antimicrobial agent to be taken empirically should diarrhea develop (BIII). One appropriate regimen is 500 mg of ciprofloxacin bid for 3–7 days. Alternative antibiotics (e.g., TMP-SMX) should be considered

continued ▶

Table 10.3   *Continued*

Travel-Related Exposures (*continued*)

as empirical therapy for use by children and pregnant women (CIII). Travelers should consult a physician if their diarrhea is severe and does not respond to empirical therapy, if their stools contain blood, if fever is accompanied by shaking chills, or if dehydration develops. Antiperistaltic agents such as diphenoxylate and loperamide are used for the treatment of diarrhea; however, they should not be used by patients with high fever or with blood in the stool, and their use should be discontinued if symptoms persist beyond 48 hours (AII). These drugs are not recommended for children (DIII).

6. Travelers should be advised about other preventive measures appropriate for anticipated exposures, such as chemoprophylaxis for malaria, protection against arthropod vectors, treatment with immune globulin, and vaccination (AII). They should avoid direct contact of the skin with soil and sand (e.g., by wearing shoes and protective clothing and using towels on beaches) in areas where fecal contamination of soil is likely (BIII).

7. In general, live virus vaccines should be avoided (EII). An exception is measles vaccine, which is recommended for nonimmune persons. Inactivated (killed) poliovirus vaccine should be used instead of oral (live) poliovirus vaccine. Persons at risk for exposure to typhoid fever should be given inactivated parenteral typhoid vaccine instead of the live attenuated oral preparation. Yellow fever vaccine is a live virus vaccine with uncertain safety and efficacy in HIV-infected persons. Travelers with asymptomatic HIV infection who cannot avoid potential exposure to yellow fever should be offered the choice of vaccination. If travel to a zone with yellow fever is necessary and immunization is not performed, patients should be advised of the risk, instructed in methods for avoiding the bites of vector mosquitoes, and provided with a vaccination waiver letter.

8. In general, killed vaccines (e.g., diphtheria-tetanus, rabies, Japanese encephalitis) should be used for HIV-infected persons as they would be for non-HIV-infected persons anticipating travel (BIII). Preparation for travel should include a review and updating of routine vaccinations, including diphtheria-tetanus for adults and all routine immunizations for children. The currently available cholera vaccine is not recommended for persons following the usual tourist itinerary, even if travel includes countries reporting cases of cholera (DII).

9. Travelers should be told about other area-specific risks and instructed in ways to reduce those risks (BIII). Geographically focal infections that pose a high risk to HIV-infected persons include visceral leishmaniasis (a protozoan infection transmitted by the sandfly) and several fungal infections (e.g., *Penicillium marneffei* infection, coccidioidomycosis, and histoplasmosis). Many tropical and developing areas have high rates of TB.

*Letters and Roman numerals in parentheses after regimens indicate the strength of the recommendation and the quality of the evidence supporting it (adapted from Gross, P., Barrett, T., Dellinger, P., et al., 1994, "Purpose of quality standards for infectious diseases," *Clinical Infectious Diseases*, 18, 421):

A Both strong evidence and substantial clinical benefit support a recommendation for use.
B Moderate evidence—or strong evidence for only limited benefit—supports a recommendation for use.
C Poor evidence supports a recommendation for or against use.
D Moderate evidence supports a recommendation against use.
E Good evidence supports a recommendation against use.
I Evidence from at least one properly controlled randomized trial
II Evidence from at least one well-designed clinical trial without randomization, from cohort or case-controlled analytic studies (preferably from more than one center), or from multiple time-series studies or dramatic results from uncontrolled experiments
III Evidence from opinions of respected authorities based on clinical experience, descriptive studies, or reports of expert committees.

Note: From "USPHS/IDSA guidelines for the prevention of opportunistic infections in persons infected with human immunodeficiency virus" by J. Kaplan, H. Masur, K. Holmes, et al., 1995, *Clinical Infectious Diseases*, 21(Suppl. 1), pp. S19–21, reprinted by USDHHS.

Section 11

Clinical Management of Pediatric HIV Patients

his section describes the prevention, classification, diagnosis, staging, and management of HIV disease in infants and children. Guidelines for the use of antiretroviral therapies and immunomodulators, OI prophylactic regimens, and immunizations are reviewed. It focuses on nursing case issues, emphasizing the complications of HIV disease such as growth and development alterations and pain. Disclosure of the diagnosis and family-oriented care are featured as important considerations. This chapter also contains many tables that serve to organize valuable content on clinical management and diagnostic parameters.

Please see Section 2, *Pathophysiology of HIV/AIDS*, for information on pediatric epidemiology and Section 6, *Issues in Special Populations*, for information on adolescents and other related information.

I. HIV INFECTION IN INFANTS AND CHILDREN

A. Pediatric Epidemiology

See *Epidemiology of HIV Infection and AIDS*, p. 18

B. Prevention of Perinatal HIV Infection

1. Specific use of zidovudine (AZT) during pregnancy, labor and delivery, and newborn period
   a. Based on results of clinical trial ACTG 076 (see Table 11.1)
   b. Recommendations from the U.S. Public Health Service to reduce perinatal HIV transmission (CDC, 1994d)
      (1) Maximum benefit showed reduction in transmission from 25%–8% occurred when pregnant women (Connor et al., 1994)
         (a) Had CD4+ lymphocyte counts >200/µl, *and*
         (b) No previous use of AZT, *and*
         (c) Clinically well with no indications to initiate antiretroviral therapy, *and*
         (d) Interventions initiated between 14 and 36 weeks of pregnancy
      (2) Treatment regimen
         (a) During pregnancy: 100 mg AZT po 5/day
         (b) During labor and delivery: AZT IV loading dose of 2 mg/Kg/hr for 1 hour and then 1 mg/Kg until cord is clamped
         (c) Newborn infant: AZT syrup 2 mg/Kg po q6h for 6 weeks
            i) Monitor CBC q2wks
            ii) Coordination among labor and delivery, postpartum, and infant primary care is essential
            iii) Treatment adherence may be problematic
   c. Nursing concerns for implementing strategies to reduce risk of perinatal HIV transmission
      (1) Recommendations for women not meeting the original study criteria were developed by the CDC and are based on a risk-benefit discussion with numerous unknown risks (CDC, 1994d)
      (2) Knowledge regarding HIV pathogenesis and perinatal transmission is rapidly changing and may appear to conflict
      (3) Information and education of women is nondirective and should follow genetic counseling model
      (4) Risk reduction of perinatal HIV transmission must be incorporated into comprehensive prenatal care
      (5) Interventions reduce risk but do not prevent transmission

C. Diagnosis of HIV Infection in Infants and Children

1. All infants born to HIV-positive mothers will have transplacentally acquired HIV antibody
   a. Infants will test antibody positive by ELISA
   b. Maternally acquired HIV antibody can be present up to 18 months of age
2. HIV infection can be definitively diagnosed in infants >1 month of age using tests that identify the HIV antigen rather than antibody (see Figure 11.1)
   a. HIV culture: 90% sensitive at 3 months of age and nearly 100% by 6 months
   b. HIV polymerase chain reaction (PCR) has similar sensitivity
   c. Immune complex dissociated (ICD) p24 antigen capture assay can also be used to establish, but not rule out, infection
   d. Presumptive diagnosis of HIV infection can be made with one positive HIV culture or PCR and definitive diagnosis, with a confirmatory test on a different blood sample
   e. HIV can be reasonably excluded with two negative HIV cultures or PCR results on different samples if both are obtained after 1 month and the second after 4 months of age; some clinicians also use a confirmatory negative ELISA at ≥18 months of age
3. Children >18 months of age can be diag-

Table 11.1   Clinical Situations and Recommendations for Use of AZT to Reduce Perinatal Transmission

Clinical Situation	Recommendations

Pregnant HIV-infected women with CD4+ lymphocyte counts >200/μl who are at 14–34 weeks of gestation and who have
• No clinical indications for AZT, and
• No history of extensive (>6 months) prior antiretroviral therapy
	Infants who are born to HIV-infected women who have received no intrapartum AZT therapy
	• Full ACTG Protocol 076 regimen*
	  – During gestation: AZT 100 mg po 5/day
	  – During labor: Loading dose of AZT 2 mg/kg IV, then 1 mg/Kg/hr by continuous IV infusion until umbilical cord is clamped
	  – In newborn infants: AZT syrup 2 mg/Kg po q6h for 6 weeks

Pregnant HIV-infected women who are at >34 weeks of gestation, who • Have no history of extensive (>6 months) prior antiretroviral therapy, and • Do not require AZT for their own health	• Full ACTG Protocol 076 regimen
Pregnant HIV-infected women with CD4 lymphocyte counts <200/μl who are at 14–34 weeks of gestation, who have • No other clinical indications for AZT, and • No history of extensive (>6 months) prior antiretroviral therapy	• Antenatal AZT therapy to the woman for her own health benefit • Intrapartum and neonatal components of the ACTG Protocol 076 regimen
Pregnant HIV-infected women who have a history of extensive (>6 months) AZT therapy or other antiretroviral therapy before pregnancy	• Consider recommending the ACTG Protocol 076 regimen on a case-by-case basis
Pregnant HIV-infected women who have not received antepartum antiretroviral therapy and who are in labor	• Discuss the benefits and potential risks of the intrapartum and neonatal components of the ACTG Protocol 076 regimen

• Offer AZT therapy when the clinical situation permits

• Only if AZT therapy can be initiated within 24 hours of birth

*Zidovudine regimens used in the ACTG 076 study from "Reduction of maternal-infant transmission of human immunodeficiency virus type 1 with zidovudine treatment," by E. Connor, R. Sperling, T. Gelber, Kiselev, P., Scott, G., M. O'Sullivan, et al., 1994. *New England Journal of Medicine, 331*, p. 1173–1180.

Note: From "Recommendations for the use of zidovudine to reduce perinatal transmission of human immunodeficiency

nosed with a positive HIV ELISA and confirmatory Western blot
4. AIDS can be diagnosed based on clinical symptoms in conjunction with laboratory evidence of dysfunction of humoral and cellular immunity using the 1994 CDC Pediatric HIV Classification System (CDC, 1994a)

D. Natural History and Presentation of HIV in Infants and Children

1. Perinatal HIV has two patterns of presentation
   a. One third of infants present in first year of life with early onset of severe symp-

Figure 11.1   Diagnosis/Evaluation of the HIV-Exposed Infant

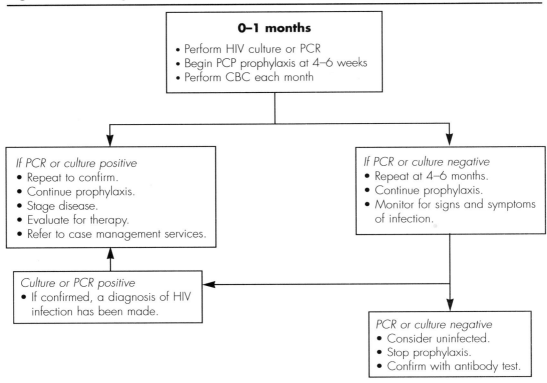

toms, rapid progression, poor prognosis (Grubman & Oleske, 1995)

(1) May represent infants infected in utero

(2) Present with severe OIs (e.g., PCP), encephalopathy, failure to thrive, and moderate to severe immune suppression within the first year of life

b. Two thirds of perinatally infected infants become symptomatic after 1 year of life with slower progression of disease, with and without immune suppression (Duliege et al., 1992; Grubman & Oleske, 1995)

(1) May be infected intrapartally

(2) Lymphoproliferative symptoms including generalized lymphadenopathy and lymphoid interstitial pneumonitis (LIP) are common

(3) Often present with general clinical manifestations of HIV, including recurrent or chronic symptoms of normal childhood illnesses (otitis media, reactive airway disease)

2. Prognosis and survival (Duliege et al., 1992; Grubman & Oleske, 1995)

a. Rapid progression

(1) Usually evidence of severe immune compromise (see Table 11.2)

(2) Frequent evidence of end organ failure (e.g., primary HIV encephalopathy, HIV cardiomyopathy, failure to thrive)

(3) May experience short stable periods in response to therapies, but disease progression is evident and life expectancy short (2–4 years)

b. Slower progression

(1) May have history of recurrent normal childhood infections (e.g., otitis media [OM], sinusitis, allergies, reactive airway disease) but no

Table 11.2   Classification System for HIV Infection in Children <13 years of Age (1994, Revised): Immunologic and Clinical Parameters

Immunologic Categories	Clinical Categories*			
1. No evidence of suppression	N1	A1	B1	C1
2. Evidence of moderate suppression	N2	A2	B2	C2
3. Severe suppression	N3	A3	B3	C3

*N: No signs or symptoms   A: Mild signs or symptoms   B: Moderate signs or symptom   C: Severe signs or symptoms (both category C and LIP in category B are reportable as AIDS to state and local health departments)

Note: From "1994 revised classification system for human immunodeficiency virus infection in children less than 13 years of age," by CDC, 1994, MMWR, 43, RR-12.

apparent symptoms of HIV infection for years

(2) Often have moderate immune suppression evidenced by CD4+ lymphocyte counts and percentage, but may have nonfunctional antibody responses (B-cell function)

E. Physiologic Impact of HIV Disease in Infants and Children

1. Immune system effects
   a. Humoral
      (1) Production of nonfunctional but elevated levels of IgG
      (2) Ineffective or variable antibody protection after acquired illness
      (3) Variable response to immunizations
   b. Cellular
      (1) Infants ages 1–6 months have normal median CD4+ lymphocyte counts of 3,200/μl (accounts for 35%–65% of all lymphocytes)
      (2) Normal CD4+ lymphocyte counts decrease with age until they reach adult range at about 6 years of age; use age-adjusted guidelines to evaluate CD4 count and percentage for infants and children
      (3) Depletion of CD4+ lymphocytes is indicative of HIV disease progression
      (4) Inverse CD4:CD8 ratio occurs as

HIV disease progresses

   c. Findings related to immunodeficiency
      (1) Recurrent bacterial/viral/fungal infections
      (2) OIs
         (a) Usually represent a primary (initial) infection (not reactivation of disease as seen in adults)
         (b) With increased survival, incidence of OIs as seen in adults may increase
         (c) Subclinical infections contracted perinatally may be expressed as immune suppression worsens (e.g., condylomata acuminata)
      (3) Neoplasms
2. Involvement of other body systems
   a. Nonspecific findings (fever, failure to thrive, lymphadenopathy, hepatosplenomegaly, diarrhea, recurrent OM, chronic nasal discharge, thrush) may occur at presentation or later in illness
   b. End organ disease and dysfunction: Neurologic (static encephalopathy, progressive encephalopathy), renal, cardiac, respiratory, GI, skin

F. CDC Classification System for Children <13 Years Old with HIV Infection

1. Principles of 1994 revised classification system (CDC, 1994a)
   a. Mutually exclusive categories

Table 11.3   Classification System for HIV Infection in Children <13 years of Age (1994, Revised): Immunologic Categories Adjusted by Age

Immunologic Category Based on CD4+ Lymphocyte Count (or Percentage)	Age of Child		
	<12 months	1–5 years	6–12 years
1. No evidence of suppression	≥ 1,500 μL (≥ 25%)	≥ 1,000 μL (≥ 25%)	≥ 500 μL (≥ 25%)
2. Evidence of moderate suppression	750–1,499 μL (15%–24%)	500–999 μL (15%–24%)	200–499 μL (15–24%)
3. Severe suppression	<750 μL (<15%)	<500 μL (<15%)	<200 μL (<15%)

Note: Adapted from "Revised classification system for human immunodeficiency virus infection in children less than 13 years of age," by CDC, 1994, *MMWR, 43,* RR-12.

b. Three parameters: Infection, clinical, and immunologic status
2. Infection status
   a. Infants whose infection status has not been definitely established are categorized with the prefix E for "perinatally exposed"
   b. Diagnosis can be established in infants (see Figure 11.1)
3. Immunologic categories (see Table 11.3)
   a. Based on CD4+ lymphocyte count or percentage adjusted for age
   b. If CD4+ lymphocyte count and percentage lead to different categories, use the more severe category
   c. Child may *not* be reclassified into a less severe category, regardless of later CD4+ lymphocyte count or percentage determinations
4. Clinical categories (see Table 11.4): Four mutually exclusive clinical categories based on signs, symptoms, or diagnoses related to HIV infection
   a. Category N (not symptomatic)
   b. Category A (mildly symptomatic)
   c. Category B (moderately symptomatic):

LIP is categorized as B because children with LIP have a better prognosis than those with other AIDS-defining conditions; but LIP is considered an AIDS-defining condition, as are category C illnesses and conditions
   d. Category C (severely symptomatic): AIDS-defining conditions in the 1987 case definition, except LIP
5. Important points in HIV classification of children
   a. Signs and symptoms related to causes other than HIV should not be used in classification (e.g., drug-induced hepatitis)
   b. HIV encephalopathy and HIV wasting syndrome are defined specifically for children
   c. Once categorized, child's category cannot improve, although clinical condition may
   d. Categories may have some usefulness for staging of disease, but data are incomplete
   e. Classification needs careful interpretation for families.

Table 11.4   Classification System for HIV Infection in Children <13 years of Age (1994, Revised): Explanation of Clinical Categories

N (No signs or symptoms)	A (Mild signs or symptoms)	B (Moderate signs or symptoms)*	C (Severe signs or symptoms)*
May have ONE from A	Two or more of the following *but none in B or C:* Lymphadenopathy Hepatomegaly Splenomegaly Dermatitis Parotitis Recurrent or persistent URI, OM, sinusitis	Anemia Neutropenia Thrombocytopenia Bacterial infections (1 episode) Oral candida (>2 months) Cardiomyopathy CMV (age <1 month) Diarrhea Hepatitis HSV (twice in 1 year) Herpes zoster Leiomyosarcoma LIP Nephropathy Nocardiosis Persistent fever Toxo (age <1 month) Varicella, disseminated	Bacterial infections (2 in 2 years) Candidiasis Cryptococcosis Cryptosporidiosis CMV (age >1 month) Encephalopathy HSV (ulcer >1 mo) Histoplasmosis Kaposi's sarcoma Lymphoma MAI MTB (disseminated) PCP PML Toxoplasmosis Wasting syndrome (failure to thrive)

*Both category C and LIP in category B are reportable as AIDS to state and local health departments

Note: Adapted from "Revised classification system for human immunodeficiency virus infection in children less than 13 years of age," by CDC, 1994, *MMWR, 43,* No. RR-12.

II. MANAGEMENT OF HIV-INFECTED INFANTS AND CHILDREN

A. Primary Interventions

1. Antiretroviral therapy
   a. Zidovudine (AZT)
      (1) Delays clinical progression
      (2) Direct antiretroviral action on CNS leads to improvements in cognitive function
      (3) Improved linear growth and weight gain, which may not be sustained
      (4) Side effects
         (a) Most common: Anemia, neutropenia
         (b) Less common: Nausea, headache, hepatic transaminase elevations, myositis
      (5) Dosage may be adjusted due to side effects or when used in combination therapy
      (6) Schedule may be modified to promote treatment adherence
      (7) Nursing implications: Family education
         (a) Negative personal family experience may affect willingness to initiate antiretroviral therapy
         (b) Treatment adherence may be complicated in families with multiple caregivers
         (c) Elixir preparation is bad tasting
   b. Didanosine (ddI)
      (1) Approved for children intolerant to AZT or who develop resistance to AZT
      (2) Leads to sustained increased in CD4+ lymphocyte counts
      (3) Some indication of improved neurodevelopmental function
      (4) Side effects (appear to be dose related): Pancreatitis, peripheral neuropathy, elevated hepatic alkaline phosphate, peripheral retinal depigmentation
      (5) Nursing implications
         (a) Suspension may be made more palatable by constituting with flavored antacid
         (b) Tablets are not palatable and families may dissolve them in acidic fluids (orange juice, lemonade)
   c. Zalcitabine (ddC)
      (1) Pilot study (Pizzo et al., 1990) showed decreased p24 antigen level and increased CD4+ lymphocyte count
      (2) Approved for use in adolescents with HIV in combination with AZT
      (3) Side effects: Skin rash, mouth sores, peripheral neuropathy not seen in low-dose trials with children
      (4) Nursing implications: Neuropathy in a child is difficult to access; removing socks and shoes, requesting foot rubs, rubbing hands on clothes or fabrics may be only clues
   d. Indications to begin antiretroviral therapy (Working Group, 1993)
      (1) Symptomatic HIV infection regardless of CD4+ lymphocyte count (see Table 11.5)
      (2) Evidence of immunosuppression (see Table 11.6)
      (3) Current information does not support the use of antiretroviral therapy in asymptomatic children with relatively intact immune systems
   e. Indications to change therapy (Working Group, 1993)
      (1) Disease progression (see Table 11.7)
      (2) Intolerance to AZT as manifested by significant and persistent toxicity
2. Combination antiretroviral therapy: Ongoing clinical trials
   a. AIDS Clinical Trial Group Study 152 (ACTG 152): Randomized double-blind clinical trial designed to compare AZT alone, ddI alone, and AZT in combination with ddI
   b. In February 1995 the Data Safety and Monitoring Board stopped the AZT monotherapy arm of the study because children in that arm had a higher rate of clinical endpoints including impaired growth, new OIs, neurologic deterioration, or death. Parents of children in that arm were told of their treatment and, based on their progress on AZT, either

Table 11.5 Initiating Antiretroviral Therapy: Clinical Criteria

Clinical Conditions that Definitively Warrant Antiretroviral Therapy

- AIDS-defining OI
- AIDS wasting syndrome
- Failure to thrive (crossing 2 percentile points or below the 5th percentile for age and falling off curve)
- HIV-related encephalopathy
- HIV-associated malignancy
- Recurrent septicemia or meningitis (2 or more episodes)
- Thrombocytopenia (platelet count <75,000/mm³ on two or more occasions)
- Hypogammaglobulinemia (total IgG/IgM/IgA <250/mm³)

Clinical Conditions that May Warrant Initiation of Antiretroviral Therapy Depending on the Overall Clinical Profile and Judgment of Healthcare Provider

- Lymphoid interstitial pneumonitis
- Parotitis
- Splenomegaly
- Recurrent oral candidiasis
- Recurrent or persistent diarrhea
- Symptomatic HIV-related cardiomyopathy
- HIV-related nephrotic syndrome
- Severe hepatic transaminitis (>5-fold normal)
- Chronic bacterial infections (sinusitis or pneumonia)
- Recurrent herpes simplex or varicella zoster
- Neutropenia (<750/mm³) or age-corrected anemia at least twice over 1 week

Note: Adapted from "Antiretroviral therapy and medical management of the human immunodeficiency virus-infected child," by Working Group on Antiretroviral Therapy, National Pediatric HIV Resource Center, 1993, *Pediatric Infectious Diseases Journal, 12*, 513–522.

Table 11.6 Initiating Antiretroviral Therapy: Immunologic Criteria

Age	CD4+ Percentage	CD4+ Lymphocyte Count
<1 year	<30	<1,750 cells/μl
1–2 years	<25	<1,000 cells/μl
2–6 years	<20	<750 cells/μl
>6 years	<20	<500 cells/μl

Note: Adapted from "Antiretroviral therapy and medical management of the human immunodeficiency virus-infected child," by Working Group on Antiretroviral Therapy, National Pediatric HIV Resource Center, 1993, *Pediatric Infectious Diseases Journal, 12*, 513–522.

a. 3TC and D4T are available only for investigational use in approved clinical trials
b. Protease inhibitors are available for use in children in 1995 in limited clinical trials
c. Therapeutic vaccine trials are ongoing
d. Ongoing clinical trials to reduce the risk of perinatal HIV transmission have newborn arms with treatment interventions dependent on mother's randomization
4. Immunomodulation: Intravenous gamma globulin (IVIG)
   a. Pooled immunoglobulin G from 3,000–6,000 donors that has been treated to destroy antigens and screened for hepatitis B surface antigen, HIV antibody, and evidence of other antigens
   b. Provides for delivery of large amounts of passive antibody protection with half-life of 21 days
   c. Offers immunomodulation for preexposure prophylaxis of bacterial and viral infections and treatment for thrombocytopenia
   d. Indications for use
      (1) Evidence of humoral immunodeficiency as defined by
         (a) Severe recurrent bacterial infections
         (b) Hypogammaglobulinemia
         (c) Poor functional antibody

continued or changed to other antiretroviral therapy.
   c. Final results of the study comparing all three arms were not available at press
   d. While AZT may remain the first choice of antiretroviral therapy, results of ACTG 152 may significantly influence providers' choice
3. Other antiretroviral chemotherapy

Table 11.7 HIV Disease Progression and Therapy-Related Decisions

Clinical Conditions that Warrant Changing Antiretroviral Therapy

- Growth failure: Crossing two percentiles or sustained deviation from a parallel curve for children who are below the 5th percentile (remediable causes should be ruled out and treated)
- Neurodevelopmental deterioration (should have at least 2 of the following)
  Impairment of brain growth (for children >2 years neuroimaging is necessary to confirm atrophy)
  Decline of cognitive function (sustained decline as defined by standardized testing)
  Clinical neurologic deterioration

Clinical Conditions that Merit Consideration of a Change in Antiretroviral Therapy

- Development of a new OI
- Symptomatic cardiomyopathy
- HIV-related nephrotic syndrome
- Severe transaminitis (>5-fold increase above normal)

Note: Adapted from "Antiretroviral therapy and medical management of the human immunodeficiency virus-infected child," by Working Group on Antiretroviral Therapy, National Pediatric HIV Resource Center, 1993, *Pediatric Infectious Diseases Journal, 12,* 513–522.

response to documented infection, or

(d) Lack of response to immunizations

 i) Children in high-prevalence measles areas who do not respond to two immunization attempts should be started on IVIG

 ii) Assess measles titers every 3–6 months to assure adequate protection due to increased morbidity and mortality related to measles (rubeola) infection in children with HIV

(2) Recurrent serious bacterial infections defined as two or more documented infections (e.g., sepsis, meningitis, pneumonia) within 1 year, or infections recalcitrant to treatment

(3) Chronic bronchiectasis: IVIG as adjunctive therapy to cyclic antibiotics and aggressive pulmonary therapy

(4) Thrombocytopenia secondary to HIV infection

e. Efficacy of IVIG

 (1) Decreased frequency of minor or serious bacterial or viral infections in children with CD4+ lymphocyte count >200/μl

 (2) Slows decline of CD4+ lymphocyte counts

f. Dosage varies for indications (immunodeficiency, bronchiectasis, thrombocytopenia)

g. Passive protection from IVIG

 (1) May need to give varicella zoster immune globulin (VZIG) if exposed to varicella

 (2) Other immunizations can be deferred if on regular IVIG

5. Modifications to routine immunizations: Children with HIV exposure/infection should receive routine childhood immunizations, except

a. Inactivated polio vaccine (IPV) should be used. Oral polio vaccine is contraindicated for children with HIV infection, exposed to HIV infection, or living in households with immunocompromised individuals as the virus may be shed.

b. Varicella vaccine is not indicated for children with HIV infection as data regarding safety and efficacy in children with immunocompromise are lacking. However, family members may receive this vaccine.

c. Children with HIV infection significantly exposed to varicella or varicella zoster would receive VZIG (see "Primary Prophylaxis," below)

d. Children with symptomatic HIV infection who are exposed to measles should receive serum immune globulin (SIG) prophylaxis (see "Primary Prophylaxis," below). Measles-susceptible children with HIV infection, particularly those <1 year old, should also receive immunoglobulin for exposure.

B. Primary Prophylaxis Against Infections (see Table 11.8)

1. *P. carinii* pneumonia (PCP)
   a. Rationale for prophylaxis
      (1) PCP is the most common serious OI in children with HIV
      (2) Peak incidence between 3 and 6 months of age, often prior to a definitive diagnosis of HIV
      (3) Most cases of PCP occur in children not identified as being at risk for HIV infection
      (4) PCP has an acute onset and carries a poor prognosis (survival is between 1 and 19 months after an acute episode)
      (5) PCP in children is the primary illness, not reactivation of previously acquired infections
   b. Indications for PCP prophylaxis in children (see Table 11.9)
      (1) All infants born to women with HIV infection should begin with prophylaxis against PCP at 4–6 weeks of age regardless of CD4+ lymphocyte count or definitive HIV infection status
      (2) All HIV-infected infants should remain on prophylaxis throughout the first year of life
      (3) Infants born exposed to HIV may discontinue PCP prophylaxis when HIV has been reasonably excluded on the basis of ≥2 negative definitive viral assays (PCR or HIV culture), both obtained at >1 month of age and one obtained after 4 months of age
      (4) Prophylaxis against PCP may be

discontinued for children with HIV infection at 1 year of age if CD4+ lymphocyte count has been monitored and has remained higher than age-adjusted parameters

(5) Children with HIV infection who have had CD4+ lymphocyte count <750/μl or CD4+ lymphocyte percentage <15% within the first year of life should continue on prophylaxis

(6) Any child started on prophylaxis because of a low CD4+ lymphocyte count should continue prophylaxis even if the CD4+ lymphocyte cell count increases

(7) All children exposed to or infected with HIV who have a CD4+ lymphocyte percentage <15% should be started on PCP prophylaxis

(8) Consider prophylaxis for children with HIV who may be at risk for PCP because of rapidly declining CD4+ lymphocytes or other evidence of severe immune compromise

(9) Children with HIV infection who have not required PCP prophylaxis should
   (a) Have their immune system monitored every 3–4 months
   (b) Begin prophylaxis if CD4+ lymphocyte counts drop below age-adjusted thresholds, indicating immune suppression

(10) All children with a prior episode of PCP should remain on lifelong prophylaxis regardless of CD4+ lymphocyte count

c. Regimens for PCP prophylaxis: TMP-SMX is first-line drug of choice
   (1) Effective in preventing PCP; improves survival
   (2) Toxicities include rash, fever, bone marrow suppression
   (3) TMP-SMX should not be started until age 4 weeks to prevent interference with bilirubin conjugation in the newborn period
   (4) For infants receiving AZT to reduce the risk of perinatal HIV transmission, TMP-SMX should not be initi-

Table 11.8   Primary Prophylaxis for HIV-Associated Infections

Infection	Indications	Prophylactic Medications	Nursing Considerations
MAC	• <12 years old with CD4+ lymphocyte <75/µl • No evidence of active disease	• 6–12 years old: Rifabutin 300 mg/day po • <6 years old: Rifabutin 5 mg/Kg/day po (max 300 mg)	• Interacts with ketoconazole and AZT • May cause GI upset or increase LFTs • Resistance develops with stopping/starting drug effectiveness • Controversial
TB	• TB infection: +PPD ≥ 5 mm induration • Significant exposure (usually household contact) in child with anergy • No evidence of active disease	• INH 10–15 mg/Kg qd (max 300 mg) for 12 months	• Treatment adherence concerns • Peripheral neuropathy (treat with vitamin B_6 q1d)
PCP	• See Table 11.9	• See Table 11.9; TMP-SMX preferred	• Neutropenia, rash
Toxoplasmosis	• Positive IgG • CD4+ lymphocytes <100/µl or severe immune suppression • CD4+ lymphocytes <15%	• TMP-SMX as indicated for PCP prophylaxis (see text)	• Neutropenia, rash
Varicella	• Exposure <48 hours preferred (96 hours maximum)	• VZIG 125 U/10 Kg (max 5 vials–625 U) • IVIG 400 mg/Kg q4wks	• Painful injection • May only ameliorate, not prevent disease • May prolong incubation
Measles	• Nonproduction of rubeola antibodies to measles immunization • Measles exposure (within 6 days)	• SIG IM 0.5 ml/Kg (max 15 ml)	• Possibility of reaction • Painful injection may ameliorate, not prevent disease

Note: Developed by M. O'Hara and D. D'Orlando for AIDS program at Children's Hospital of New Jersey, Newark, NJ.

ated until 6 weeks of age when AZT is discontinued
(5) Obtain CBCs routinely every 1–2 months to monitor for neutropenia
(6) Dosage: Divided doses 2/day, 3/week on consecutive days (M, T, W) to allow for bone marrow recovery

(7) Acceptable alternative dosing schedules
(a) A single dose 3/week on consecutive days
(b) A modified daily dose
(c) Dose divided 2/day, 3/week on alternate days (M, W, F)

Table 11.9 Recommendations for PCP Prophylaxis and CD4+ Monitoring for HIV-exposed Infants and HIV-Infected Children, by Age and HIV Infection Status

Age/HIV-Infection Status	PCP Prophylaxis	CD4+ Monitoring
Birth to 4–6 weeks, HIV exposed	No prophylaxis	1 months
4–6 weeks to 4 months, HIV exposed	Prophylaxis	3 months
4–12 months • HIV infected or indeterminate • HIV infection reasonably excluded[1]	 Prophylaxis No prophylaxis	 6, 9, and 12 months None
1–5 years, HIV infected	Prophylaxis if • CD4+ lymphocyte count <500/µL, or • CD4+ lymphocytes <15%[2,3]	Every 3–4 months[4]
6–12 years, HIV infected	Prophylaxis if • CD4+ lymphocyte count <200/µL, or • CD4+ lymphocytes <15%[3]	Every 3–4 months[4]

[1]HIV infection can be reasonably excluded among children who have had 2 negative HIV diagnostic tests (e.g., HIV culture, PCR), both performed at ≥ 1 month of age and one at ≥ 4 months of age; or ≥ 2 negative HIV IgG antibody tests performed at >6 months of age among children who have no clinical evidence of HIV disease.
[2]Children age 1–2 years receiving PCP prophylaxis and with a CD4+ lymphocyte count <750/µL or <15% at age <12 months should continue prophylaxis.
[3]Prophylaxis should be considered case by case for children who might otherwise be at risk for PCP, such as children with rapidly declining CD4+ lymphocyte counts or percentages or children with Category C conditions. Children who have had PCP should receive lifelong PCP prophylaxis.
[4]More frequent monitoring (e.g., monthly) is recommended for children whose CD4 counts or percentages are approaching the threshold at which prophylaxis is recommended.
Note: Adapted from "Revised guidelines for prophylaxis against *Pneumocystis carinii* pneumonia for children infected with or perinatally exposed to human immunodeficiency virus," by CDC, 1995, *MMWR, 44*, RR-4.

(8) Alternative regimens if TMP-SMX is not tolerated
  (a) Dapsone
    i) Side effect is mostly dose-related hemolysis
    ii) Hemolytic anemia may occur in patients with glucose-6-phosphate-dehydrogenase (G6PD) deficiency, which is more common in African Americans
    iii) Regular hematologic monitoring monthly is indicated
    iv) Available as tablets; suspension available through clinical trial only
  (b) Aerosolized pentamidine monthly (ONLY for children ≥5 years of age)
    i) Side effects include cough, bronchospasm
    ii) Not effective against extra-pulmonary PCP
  (c) IV pentamidine q2–4wks
    i) Safety and efficacy data not available
    ii) Side effects have included hyperglycemia, hypoglycemia, hypotension, cardiac dysrhythmias, renal failure, blood dyscrasias

d. Nursing considerations when initiating PCP prophylaxis
  (1) Family education
    (a) Families should be part of the decision making about treatment regimen (e.g., 3 days/week vs. daily dosing)
    (b) Families need an explanation of the purpose of prophylaxis and the indications to initiate and discontinue treatment
    (c) Prophylaxis continues regardless of other antibiotics prescribed
  (2) Treatment adherence is challenging as prevention may entail lifelong medication and child often appears well
  (3) Failure to comply with prophylaxis regimen raises medical-legal issues in some states

2. Tuberculosis
  a. Indications for prophylaxis
    (1) TB infection defined as positive PPD ≥5 mm induration in a child without anergy
    (2) Significant exposure usually involves a household contact with TB in a child with anergy
    (3) The child with significant exposure but a negative PPD may need prophylaxis and retesting in 6 months. If PPD remains negative, consider discontinuing prophylaxis.
    (4) Prophylaxis is initiated only after *active disease* has been ruled out
  b. Intervention
    (1) INH each day for 12 months
    (2) Treatment adherence is a major concern, particularly in areas of MDR-TB; consult with public health authorities (see *Mycobacterium Tuberculosis*, p. 55)
    (3) With INH use, peripheral neuropathy is possible
      (a) Neuropathy may be minimized by concomitant administration of vitamin B_6 (Cohen & Durham, 1995)
      (b) Symptoms of neuropathy (e.g., removing shoes, rubbing hands and feet on clothing or carpets) may be difficult to elicit

3. Varicella (see Table 11.8)
  a. Prophylaxis is indicated for exposure to varicella, preferably within 48 hours to maximum of 96 hours
  b. Each exposure requires prophylaxis

4. Measles
  a. Indications for prophylaxis
    (1) Measles in the immunocompromised child may be life threatening
    (2) Measles outbreaks are frequent and unpredictable
    (3) Measles is associated with severe morbidity (especially measles encephalitis and measles pneumonia) as well as mortality
    (4) Routine immunizations should begin at age 6 months in areas of epidemic measles, and again at age 12–15 months; obtain titers 6–8 weeks after vaccination to ascertain response to immunizations
  b. Prophylaxis
    (1) Children unable to mount an immune response after 2 immunization attempts as evidenced by lack of protective measles titers obtained 6–8 weeks after immunization should be considered for passive protection with IVIG
    (2) Children exposed to measles regardless of their antibody titers should receive SIG as soon as possible after exposure but within 6 days maximum
  c. Nursing considerations
    (1) IVIG is a blood product, and the child must be monitored for possible reactions
    (2) SIG is a painful injection that may ameliorate, but not prevent, disease
    (3) In the susceptible person SIG may prolong incubation

5. Toxoplasmosis (see Table 11.8)
6. *M. avium* complex (see Table 11.8): Poor treatment adherence may add to concerns regarding MDR-TB

C. Secondary Prophylaxis Against Recurrent OIs

(see Table 11.10)

1. *M. avium* complex: Lifelong prophylaxis of recurrent disease
2. Candida
   a. Indicated for severe or recurrent oral or esophageal infection
   b. Investigational therapies such as itraconazole and flucytosine have not been studied for pediatric indications
3. Herpes simplex virus: Indicated for severe recurrent infection
4. Toxoplasmosis
   a. Indicated after 1 episode of toxoplasmosis encephalitis
   b. Medication regimen is lifelong
5. Cryptococcosis
   a. Indicated after 1 episode of cryptococcal meningitis
   b. Medication regimen is lifelong
6. Cytomegalovirus (CMV)
   a. Indicated for a history of active disease
   b. Medication regimen: Two phases (induction and maintenance) using ganciclovir or foscarnet
      (1) Safety and efficacy data are limited using foscarnet in children
      (2) Oral ganciclovir in children with HIV infection is investigational
7. PCP: TMP-SMX indicated if child has had prior episode of PCP

D. Special Concerns Regarding Growth and Development

1. Failure to thrive
   a. Definition: Inability to maintain growth along a continuum appropriate for age and height
   b. Requires serial measurements of height and weight plotted on standard growth curves
   c. Assess growth in relation to height as well as age
   d. Failure to gain weight (flat) growth curve indicates need for intervention
   e. Possible etiology for failure to gain weight
      (1) Inadequate intake secondary to
         (a) Inadequate food supply at home
         (b) Anorexia
         (c) Pain related to mouth lesions, poor dental hygiene, significant caries
         (d) Difficulty swallowing related to pain from esophagitis
         (e) Nausea and vomiting possibly related to medication administration
         (f) Constipation
            i) May present as diarrhea with small frequent stools leaking around impaction
            ii) May be associated with perianal lesions, including genital warts
         (g) Fullness related to organomegaly
      (2) Poor absorption secondary to
         (a) Primary HIV infection in the gut
         (b) OIs (*Cryptosporidium;* MAC; *C. difficile; Salmonella, Shigella, Campylobacter,* and other enteric pathogens)
         (c) Diarrhea
            i) Defined as persisting >1 month with ≥2 loose stools a day
            ii) Interventions may include antidiarrheal agents only after infectious etiologies have been ruled out
      (3) Neurologic complications
         (a) May interfere with coordinated suck and swallow
         (b) Inability to chew and swallow
         (c) Time demands for feeding
      (4) Endocrine abnormalities associated with HIV
         (a) Relationship between HIV and decreased growth hormone is established
         (b) Implications for intervention with replacement growth hormone currently under study
   f. Interventions for failure to gain weight
      (1) Evaluate to rule out OIs
         (a) Obtain stool specimens for ova and parasites, C&S, C. *difficile, Cryptosporidium, Campylobacter*

Table 11.10   Secondary Prophylaxis for Recurrent Opportunistic Infections

Infection	Indications	Prophylactic Medications	Nursing Considerations
MAC	• Prior disease	• Biaxin 30 mg/kg/day, *plus* ethambutol 15–25 mg/kg/day, *or* • Clofazamine 50–100 mg/day, *or* • Ciprofloxacin 10–15 mg/kg bid (max 1.5 g), *or* rifabutin 300 mg qd	• Monitor for optic neuritis
Candida	• Severe recurrent oral infection or esophageal infection	• Fluconazole 2–8 mg/Kg/day, taper to 3/week • Ketoconazole 5–10 mg/Kg q12–24h	• Stopping medication may result in rebound infection • Use only if recurrences are severe
Toxoplasma	• Prior episode of toxoplasmosis encephalitis	• Sulfadiazine 85–120 mg/kg divided 2–4 doses, *plus* pyrimethamine 1 mg/kg (max 25 mg) qd, *plus* leukovorin 5 mg q3d	• Lifelong suppressive therapy required
Herpes simplex	• Severe recurrent infection	• Acyclovir 600–1000 mg/day (titrate to the individual) in divided doses qd	• Caution if impaired renal function • Resistance may develop with prolonged treatment
Cryptococcosis	• Documented disease	• Fluconazole 2–8 mg/Kg/day	• Lifelong suppressive therapy required
CMV	• Prior end-organ disease	*Induction* • Ganciclovir 5 mg/Kg IV q12h x 7 days, *or* • Foscarnet 60 mg/Kg IV q8h for 14 days *Maintenance* • Ganciclovir 5 mg/Kg/day, *or* • Foscarnet 60–120 mg/Kg/day	• Nephrotic toxicity • IV access concerns

Note: From "USPHS–IDSA guidelines for the prevention of opportunistic infections in persons infected with human immunodeficiency virus: A summary," by CDC, 1995, *MMWR, 7* (RR-7), p. 29.

(b) Obtain AFB culture and smear from 3 separate samples to recover MAI

(2) Evaluate to rule out malabsorption

    (a) 1 hour D-Xylose level may indicate functioning gut

    (b) D-Xylose, 0.5 g/Kg po in A.M. (NPO after midnight), and serum D-Xylose levels measured after 1 hour

    (c) Low levels (<20 mg/dl) indicates impaired absorption

        i) Maintaining use of gut is priority

        ii) Consider trying NG feeding before parenteral intervention

(3) 2-day diet recall to assess calorie intake

(4) Nutritional support with high-calorie supplements if gut functioning

(5) Appetite stimulants (e.g., megesterol acetate) have had some limited success with children if gut functioning

(6) Spicy, very sweet, or highly flavored as well as favorite foods may stimulate child's appetite

(7) NG feeding, as bolus or continuous feeds, may provide additional nutritional support or may be used as primary source of nutrition

(8) In cases of poor absorption, consider TPN for continued weight loss or during acute medical crisis

    (a) Decisions to initiate intervention should have clearly defined short- and long-term goals

    (b) Family must be involved in decision as home and caretaker must be able to support high-tech interventions

(9) All interventions should consider the social and supportive concerns of eating with family and friends and child should be encouraged to participate in regular family mealtimes

(10) Failure to gain weight is defined as wasting, meeting the CDC definition of a Class C AIDS-defining condition when the following are met

    (a) Downward crossing of two percentiles lines on standard weight-for-age growth chart in children >1 year of age, or

    (b) Persistent 10% loss of baseline body weight, or

    (c) Weight is <5% on growth chart on 2 consecutive measurements 30 days apart and is associated with chronic diarrhea or persistent (30 days) documented fever

(11) See also *Anorexia,* p. 227

2. CNS involvement

  a. Incidence likely to be higher in children than adults (true incidence unknown)

  b. Majority of all children (90%) ultimately experience some CNS involvement

  c. Severity and onset of symptoms possibly related to timing of infection during pregnancy

    (1) HIV may infect the CNS through HIV-infected macrophages in utero prior to development of blood-brain barrier

    (2) Infants with signs and symptoms of progressive encephalopathy within the first year of life have a poor prognosis

    (3) Some degree of developmental delay is common, but etiologies other than HIV must be considered

      (a) Poor or minimal prenatal care

      (b) Substance use during pregnancy

      (c) Maternal health during pregnancy

  d. Clinical spectrum of CNS symptoms

    (1) Etiology may by related to one or more of the following

      (a) Primary HIV infection of the brain (e.g., progressive encephalopathy)

      (b) Secondary neurologic complications due to OIs related to immune suppression (e.g., cryptococcosis)

      (c) CNS lesions secondary to immunodeficiency (e.g., lymphoma): AIDS-related malignancies are rare in children but need to be ruled out

      (d) HIV organ-system involvement resulting in hypoxia or stroke

(2) Progressive encephalopathy (in the absence of a concurrent condition that could explain the findings)
  (a) Defined as progressive loss of cognitive, motor or language skill, or failure to attain milestones, *or*
  (b) Impaired brain growth or acquired microcephaly (demonstrated on serial head circumferences), *or*
  (c) Brain atrophy on CT scan, *or*
  (d) Acquired symmetric motor deficits (two or more of paresis, patholigreflexes, ataxia, gait disturbances)
  (e) May be rapid, subacute with continued losses over time, or may plateau for periods of time
(3) Static encephalopathy characterized by nonprogressive cognitive or motor deficits
  (a) Over time, a static encephalopathy may begin to appear as progressive as the gap between attained and expected development widens
  (b) Evidence of hyperactivity or attention deficit may present at the preschool and school ages
  (c) Developmental delay in achieving motor or cognitive milestones is common
(4) Opportunistic infections
  (a) Less common than in adult population
  (b) More apparent as children live longer with severe immunosuppression
(5) Neuropsychiatric issues
  (a) Depression is likely to be under-recognized and underreported
  (b) Anecdotal evidence of psychosis has been reported
  (c) Changes in behavior (frustration, withdrawal, loss of interest in activities and friends) may be biologic or psychosocial in origin
  (d) Subtle changes in cognitive performance may appear before concrete neurologic signs
  (e) Strokes, seizures (see *Nervous System Complications*, p. 143),

attention deficit hyperactivity disorder (ADHD) may all have etiologies other than HIV and need careful assessment
(6) Treatment/interventions
  (a) AZT has been shown to improve neurodevelopmental function
  (b) Gains in motor function and regaining developmental milestones may be dramatic
  (c) Symptomatic interventions, including evaluations for early intervention programs, preschool handicapped placements, child study teams, as well as feeding teams are essential

E. Organ System Involvement

1. Recurrent or recalcitrant common childhood illnesses: Otitis media, sinusitis
  a. May cause significant morbidity, absence from school, ER visits
  b. Infections may be caused by unusual organisms
  c. Standard therapeutic regimens may be ineffective in eliminating infections
  d. Treatment may require more broad-spectrum antibiotics; treatment over longer periods may lead to concerns about treatment adherence and to development of resistant organisms
  e. "Failures" of therapy may erode confidence in provider or, conversely, assumptions of poor compliance on the part of the family
2. Pulmonary manifestations
  a. Lymphoid interstitial pneumonitis (LIP)
    (1) Diffuse lymphocytic infiltration of the interstitium
    (2) May be associated with co-infection of HIV and Epstein-Barr virus
    (3) Diagnosed by characteristic reticulo-nodular pattern on X ray
    (4) Symptoms of impaired gas exchange (e.g., hypoxia, clubbing) may develop over time
    (5) Treatment is symptomatic
      (a) May begin with bronchodilator, inhaled steroids similar to reactive airway disease

(b) May require systemic steroids, pulmonary tune-ups

(c) May progress to bronchiectasis, necessitating addition of cyclic antibiotics

b. Recurrent bacterial or viral pneumonia

c. PCP

  (1) Signs and symptoms: Tachypnea, hypoxia, retractions with or without cough or fever

  (2) Diagnosis may be presumptive

    (a) History of acute respiratory decomposition and interstitial infiltrates on CXR, or

    (b) Oxygen desaturation and elevated serum LD >1 U/L

  (3) Diagnosis may be definitive: Positive silver or Giemsa stain of lung tissue obtained by bronchoalveolar lavage

3. Skin/scalp lesions

a. Fungal infections, including candidiasis (mouth, diaper area, skin folds, nail beds), tinea versicolor, tinea capitis, tinea corporis

  (1) May not present with classic appearance

  (2) Treatment of infections may extend to months with limited improvements

  (3) Stopping and starting medications may lead to resistant organisms

  (4) Initial treatment usually topical but may require systemic therapy

b. Viral skin lesions

  (1) Molluscum contagiosum

    (a) May not respond to any standard therapies (liquid nitrogen or 0.1% tretinoin cream)

    (b) May spontaneously remiss, or may progressively worsen

    (c) May profoundly affect body image if located on the face

    (d) Home remedies, such as the use of tape to "pull off" the lesions, may have as much success as medical interventions

  (2) Human papillomavirus (HPV, genital warts, condylomata acuminata)

    (a) May respond to therapy and then spontaneously reoccur

    (b) Small lesions may resolve with podophyllum resin

      i) Protect surrounding skin with petroleum jelly to prevent burning on application

      ii) Treatment adherence is extremely difficult

    (c) Large lesions may require surgical excision

    (d) Treatment with interferon to shrink lesions prior to surgery has had some success

    (e) Explore possibility of sexual abuse, though children may acquire the infection in the birth canal and have no symptoms until they become immunocompromised

4. Cardiomyopathy

a. Etiology may be primary HIV infection or secondary to systemic HIV disease

b. Signs and symptoms may include onset of respiratory difficulties, feeding changes, gallop rhythm, murmur, cardiomegaly on chest x-ray

c. ECG and echocardiogram may show evidence of ventricular hypertrophy, left ventricular dysfunction, or pericardial effusion

d. Endocarditis is rare but possible in children

e. Interventions are specific to the etiology of cardiovascular disease and require consultation with pediatric cardiologist.

III. NURSING CONSIDERATIONS FOR INFANTS AND CHILDREN WITH HIV DISEASE

A. HIV as a Chronic Illness

1. Commonalities with other chronic child-hood illnesses
   a. Ongoing need for health care
   b. Psychosocial consequences of illness
      (1) Parental guilt and anxiety
      (2) Existential shock because child may predecease parents
   c. Shortened life span and decline in health over time
   d. Periods of wellness punctuated by episodes of illness
   e. Impact on the family system and its individual members
2. Rapid progressors: Nursing care balances interventions to manage treatable, life-threatening OIs with care and comfort measures associated with terminal illness
   a. Frequent assessment of families' coping strategies and resources is essential
   b. Discussion of risks and benefits of each intervention needs to be carefully woven into counseling sessions with families
   c. It is important to recognize that child's declining health, hospitalizations, invasive therapies may mimic or foretell mother's or other family member's future disease progression and may elicit powerful responses of fear, anger, sorrow, denial
3. Slower progressors: Nursing care follows chronic illness model, maximizing wellness and promoting optimal growth and development
   a. Changes in clinical condition frequently precipitate crisis as families are challenged to confront inability to cure the illness
   b. Strategies to promote family growth may be challenged by maternal illness, substance use within families, poverty, and nondisclosure of diagnosis to child
4. Special issues for schoolage children
   a. HIV infection not a contraindication to regular school attendance
   b. Body-image concerns
      (1) Short stature and poor weight gain may make child appear to be much younger than chronologic age
      (2) Delayed puberty not uncommon; prepare children and families proactively to allay anxieties
      (3) High-tech interventions (e.g., central line catheters, venous access devices) can be effectively camouflaged using strategies developed for children living with other chronic, life-threatening illness
      (4) Girls experiencing menarche should be instructed to dispose of feminine-hygiene products safely in a matter-of-fact manner to avoid perceptions of feeling unclean or contaminated

B. HIV as a Multigenerational Disease

1. Families may suffer many losses, frequent simultaneous illnesses, and multiple involvement with service agencies as well as multiple care providers
2. Infected and affected family members may have many competing needs; HIV interacts with preexisting family problems and may not be family's priority; other competing problems include
   a. Poverty, homelessness, racism
   b. Poor access to and use of medical/social services
   c. Previous/current drug use
3. Mother is usually infected and frequently is the primary caretaker
   a. Mothers frequently neglect their own care to assure appropriate services for their children
   b. Siblings are infected and affected
   c. Extended family members may be infected and are affected
   d. Caretakers for children may change frequently, requiring continuous assessment of home situation

C. Disclosure of Diagnosis to Child, Family, Community

1. Important process for families that requires ongoing discussion, review of facts and feelings, and discussion within a risk-benefit analysis; may be viewed as a continuum of total secrecy to complete openness and involves significant swings to both ends of the continuum
2. Family concerns regarding disclosing the diagnosis
   a. Fear and anxiety that the child will give up, inappropriately disclose to others, or question the etiology for the infection, thereby revealing the parent's health status, sexual activity, or drug use
   b. Limitations of family's ability to access their social-support networks
   c. Fears of ostracism or social consequences of disclosure of HIV diagnosis are often well founded
3. Issues that may encourage disclosure
   a. The burden of secrecy may be very heavy, adding to familial stresses
   b. UN Convention on the Rights of the Child states that children have the right to be involved in their own health care
   c. Child's autonomy should increase as growth occurs, and child should understand actions and consequences of medical interventions
   d. Family may explore future options for caring for one another in the event of serious or terminal illness
   e. For the school-age child, benefits include school nurse participation in medication administration, assessment of physical complaints, and information regarding presence of contagious illnesses posing a threat to immune-compromised child; risks are primarily psychosocial—discrimination, stigma, and breaches of confidentiality of HIV diagnosis
4. Balance between families' wishes and rights of the child may pose ethical dilemmas
5. Decision to "tell" should not be driven by professional concerns and needs (e.g., offering a clinical drug trial)
6. Specific nursing considerations
   a. Disagreement among healthcare team members regarding issues of disclosure are common
   b. Conflicts may interfere with the child's care and should be identified
   c. Families' statements regarding their decision not to disclose may conflict with observed behavior (e.g., discussing child's health in the child's presence, using medication names associated with HIV/AIDS), and sharing discrepancies with families may identify ambivalence
   d. As with any intervention, a decision to disclose diagnosis should be carefully planned and be developmentally appropriate. The process should be monitored and assessed continuously to assure that the child and family have a positive outcome.
   e. See *Alterations in Family Functioning*, p. 243, *Family Caregiver Burden/Strain*, p. 251, *Guilt*, p. 255, *Individual Psychotherapy*, p. 345, *Social Support*, p. 272, *Spiritual Distress*, p. 273, *Stigma*, p. 274

D. Pain

1. HIV may cause pain in all organ systems directly related to primary infection; may also result from OIs, side effects of treatments, or procedures (e.g., lumbar puncture, venipuncture)
2. Families with histories of substance abuse may be uncomfortable with certain pain-medication strategies
3. Professionals may be uncomfortable with the use of narcotics in families with substance use/misuse
4. Myths regarding pain in children (e.g., children don't remember pain, children don't perceive pain, children who play are not feeling pain, children who sleep are not in pain) apply to children living with HIV
5. Do not base strategies for relieving pain on the diagnosis, but on what the child/family reports as painful
6. Pain assessment should
   a. Occur regularly

b. Include an age- or developmentally appropriate tool (e.g., Wong-Baker Faces Scale, Poker Chips Scale, behavioral observation scale) that is used consistently

c. Be documented, including observations of behavior, physiologic signs, and verbal reports

7. Procedural pain
   a. Involve parent or support person in discussion of procedure and intervention
   b. Combine pharmacologic and nonpharmacologic interventions
   c. Use topical anesthetic (e.g., EMLA cream-lidocaine 2.5% and pilocarpine 2.5%) for venipuncture and other invasive needlestick procedures
   d. Conscious sedation should be available for all painful procedures

8. Pain associated with HIV disease
   a. May be chronic, recurrent, or intermittent
   b. May be due to primary HIV infection of end organ systems or OIs, or related to systemic disease
   c. Interventions and evaluation of therapy are based on what the child describes, not what the clinician expects
   d. World Health Organization analgesic pain ladder may be effective guide to treat pain in children
      (1) Mild pain treated with NSAIDs: When threshold of pain relief is reached, move up the ladder to
      (2) Moderate pain treated with NSAIDs, plus a weak opioid such as codeine: When threshold is reached, move up ladder to
      (3) Severe pain treated with nonopioid and add stronger opiate such as morphine, methadone, or fentanyl
   e. Pain relief should be assessed based on the child's response to treatment, regardless of dosage
   f. Narcotics may be used safely with infants, children and adolescents. Consultation with a pain management expert may be extremely beneficial.
   g. See *Pain*, p. 229.

Appendices

Appendix A

Public Health Service Revised Classification System for HIV Infection (Adolescents and Adults), 1993 Revised

The following material contains the most important aspects of the report published by CDC[1]. The complete document may be found as cited.

The classification system for HIV infection among adolescents and adults has been revised to include the CD4+ lymphocyte count as a marker for HIV-related immuno-suppression. This revision establishes mutually exclusive subgroups for which the spectrum of clinical conditions is integrated with the CD4+ lymphocyte count. The objectives of these changes are to simplify the classification of HIV infection, to reflect current standards of medical care for HIV-infected people, and to categorize more accurately HIV-related morbidity.

The revised CDC classification system for HIV-infected adolescents and adults[2] categorizes people on the basis of clinical conditions associated with HIV infection and CD4+ lymphocyte counts. The system is based on three ranges of CD4+ lymphocyte counts and three clinical categories and is represented by a matrix of nine mutually exclusive categories (Table A1). This system replaces the classification system published in 1986, which included only clinical disease criteria and which was developed before the widespread use of CD4+ T-cell testing.

---

[1]*Note:* From "1993 revised classification system for HIV infection and expanded surveillance case definition for AIDS among adolescents and adults," by CDC, 1992, *MMWR, 41*(RR-17), 1–9.

[2]Criteria for HIV infection for people ages ≥13 years: (a) repeatedly reactive screening tests for HIV antibody (e.g., enzyme immunoassay) with specific antibody identified by the use of supplemental tests (e.g., Western blot, immunofluorescence assay); (b) indirect identification of virus in host tissues by virus isolation; (c) HIV antigen detection; or (d) a positive result on any other highly specific licensed test for HIV.

Table A1   1993 Revised Classification System for HIV Infection and Expanded AIDS Surveillance Case Definition for Adolescents and Adults*

CD4+ T-cell Categories	Clinical Categories		
	(A) Asymptomatic, acute (primary) HIV or PGL[†]	(B) Symptomatic, not (A) or (C) conditions	(C) AIDS-indicator conditions
(1) ≥ 500/μl	A1	B1	C1
(2) 200–499/μl	A2	B2	C2
(3) <200/μl AIDS-indicator T-cell count	A3	B3	C3

*The shaded cells illustrate the expanded AIDS surveillance case definition. People with AIDS-indicator conditions (Category C) as well as those with CD4+ T-lymphocyte counts <200/μl
[†]PGL (persistent generalized lymphadenopathy). Clinical Category A includes acute (primary) HIV infections.

CD4+ Lymphocyte Categories

The three CD4+ lymphocyte categories are defined as follows:

- Category 1: ≥500 cells/μl
- Category 2: 200–499 cells/μl
- Category 3: <200 cells/μl

These categories correspond to CD4+ lymphocyte counts per microliter of blood and guide clinical and therapeutic actions in the management of HIV-infected adolescents and adults. The revised HIV classification system also allows for the use of the percentage of CD4+ lymphocytes.

HIV-infected people should be classified based on existing guidelines for the medical management of HIV-infected people. Thus, the lowest accurate, but not necessarily the most recent, CD4+ lymphocyte count should be used for classification purposes.

Clinical Categories

The clinical categories of HIV infection are defined as follows:

Category A

Category A consists of one or more of the conditions listed below in an adolescent or adult (≥13 years) with documented HIV infection. Conditions listed in Categories B and C must not have occurred.

- Asymptomatic HIV infection
- Persistent generalized lymphadenopathy
- Acute (primary) HIV infection with accompanying illness or history of acute HIV infection

Category B

Category B consists of symptomatic conditions in an HIV-infected adolescent or adult that are not included among conditions listed in clinical Category C and that meet at least one of the following criteria: (1) the conditions are attributed to HIV infection or are indicative of a defect in cell-mediated immunity; or (b) the conditions are considered by physi-

cians to have a clinical course or to require management that is complicated by HIV infection. Examples of conditions in clinical Category B include, but are not limited to:

- Bacillary angiomatosis
- Candidiasis, oropharyngeal (thrush)
- Candidiasis, vulvovaginal; persistent, frequent, or poorly responsive to therapy
- Cervical dysplasia (moderate or severe)/cervical carcinoma in situ
- Constitutional symptoms, such as fever (38.5°C) or diarrhea lasting >1 month
- Hairy leukoplakia, oral
- Herpes zoster (shingles), involving at least two distinct episodes or more than one dermatome
- Idiopathic thrombocytopenic purpura
- Listeriosis
- Pelvic inflammatory disease, particularly if complicated by tubo-ovarian abscess
- Peripheral neuropathy

For classification purposes, Category B conditions take precedence over those in Category A. For example, someone previously treated for oral or persistent vaginal candidiasis (and who has not developed a Category C disease) but who is now asymptomatic should be classified in clinical Category B.

Category C

Category C includes the clinical conditions listed in the AIDS surveillance case definition (Table A2). For classification purposes, once a Category C condition has occurred, the person will remain in Category C.

Equivalences for CD4+ Lymphocyte Count and Percentage of Total Lymphocytes

Compared with the absolute CD4+ lymphocyte count, the percentage of CD4+ T-cells of total lymphocytes (or CD4+ percentage) is less subject to variation on repeated measurement. However, data correlating natural his-

Table A2   Conditions Included in the 1993 AIDS Surveillance Case Definition

- Candidiasis of bronchi, trachea, or lungs
- Candidiasis, esophageal
- Cervical cancer, invasive*
- Coccidoidomycosis, disseminated or extrapulmonary
- Cryptococcosis, extrapulmonary
- Cryptosporidiosis, chronic intestinal (>1 month's duration)
- Cytomegalovirus disease (other than liver, spleen, or nodes)
- Cytomegalovirus retinitis (with loss of vision)
- Encephalopathy, HIV-related
- Herpes simplex: chronic ulcer(s) (>1 month's duration); or bronchitis pneumonitis, or esophagitis
- Histoplasmosis, disseminated or extrapulmonary
- Isosporiasis, chronic intestinal (>1 month's duration)
- Kaposi's sarcoma
- Lymphoma, Burkitt's (or equivalent term)
- Lymphoma, immunoblastic (or equivalent term)
- Lymphoma, primary, of brain
- *Mycobacterium avium* complex of *M. kansasii,* disseminated or extrapulmonary
- *Mycobacterium tuberculosis,* any site (pulmonary* or extrapulmonary)
- *Mycobacterium,* other species or unidentified species, disseminated or extrapulmonary
- *Pneumocystis carinii* pneumonia
- Pneumonia, recurrent*
- Progressive multifocal leukoencephalopathy
- *Salmonella* septicemia, recurrent
- Toxoplasmosis of brain
- Wasting syndrome due to HIV

*Added in the 1993 expansion of the AIDS surveillance case definition.

Table A3   Equivalences for Absolute Numbers of CD4+ Lymphocytes and CD4+ Percentage

CD4+ T-cell Category	CD4+ T-Cells/µl	CD4+ Percentage (%)
(1)	≥500	≥29
(2)	200–499	14–28
(3)	<200	<14

Expansion of the CDC Surveillance Case Definition for AIDS

In 1991, CDC, in collaboration with the Council of State and Territorial Epidemiologists (CSTE), proposed an expansion of the AIDS surveillance case definition. This proposal was made available for public comment in November 1991 and was discussed at an open meeting on September 2, 1992. Based on information presented and reviewed during the public comment period and at the open meeting, CDC, in collaboration with CSTE, has expanded the AIDS surveillance case definition to include all HIV-infected people with CD4+ lymphocyte counts of <200 cells/µl or a CD4+ percentage of <14. In addition to retaining the 23 clinical conditions in the previous AIDS surveillance definition, the expanded definition includes pulmonary tuberculosis, recurrent pneumonia, and invasive cervical cancer. This expanded definition requires laboratory confirmation of HIV infection in people with a CD4+ lymphocyte count of <200 cells/µl or with one of the added clinical conditions. This expanded definition for reporting cases to CDC becomes effective January 1, 1993.

In the revised HIV classification system, people in subcategories A3, B3, and C3 meet the immunologic criteria of the surveillance case definition, and those people with conditions in subcategories C1, C2, and C3 meet the clinical criteria for surveillance purposes.

tory of HIV infection with the CD4+ percentage have not been as consistently available as data on absolute CD4+ lymphocyte counts. Therefore, the revised classification system emphasizes the use of CD4+ lymphocyte counts but allows for the use of CD4+ percentages (Table A3).

Appendix B

Common Medications Used in Treating the Patient With HIV/AIDS

- Please refer to a pharmacologic text for more detailed information.
- Dosages listed reflect upper dosing ranges; patients frequently will receive lower therapeutic dosages.
- Because dosages, indications, and adverse effects may change over time, neither the author nor ANAC can be held responsible for new dosage recommendations, unforeseen adverse effects, and new indications.

Table A4 Common Medications

Generic Name (Trade Name)	Maximal Dosage	Route of Administration	Indications	Side/Adverse Effects and Interactions
Acyclovir (Zovirax)	800 mg 5/day 5–15 mg/Kg q8h	PO IV	• Herpes simplex virus (HSV) infection • Herpes zoster infection • Varicella infection	• Parenteral: Skin rash, hives, hematuria, lightheadedness, headache, diaphoresis, confusion, tremors, abdominal pain, nausea, vomiting, extreme fatigue • Oral: Skin rash, diarrhea, dizziness, headache, joint pain, nausea, vomiting, acne, anorexia, somnolence
Adenine arabinoside (Vidarabine) (Vira-A)	15 mg/Kg/day	IV, ophthalmic	• HSV infection • Herpes zoster infection • Progressive multifocal leukoencephalopathy (PML) • Varicella infection	
• Anorexia, nausea, vomiting, diarrhea,	tremors, dizziness, confusion, hallucinations	, ataxia, psychosis, leukopenia, thrombo-	• Microsporidiosis • Cryptosporidiosis	• Stomach upset, headache, dizziness, rash, fever, elevated liver function tests
All trans retinoic acid	Up to 60 mg/m²/day	PO	• Kaposi's sarcoma (KS)	• Headache, boney pain, dry mucous membranes
Amikacin (Amikin)	Up to 15 mg/Kg/day (MAC)	IV, IM	• *M. avium* complex (MAC)	• Nephrotoxicity and polyuria, any loss of hearing, ringing or buzzing, dizziness

continued ▶

Table A4   *Continued*

Generic Name (Trade Name)	Maximal Dosage	Route of Administration	Indications	Side/Adverse Effects and Interactions
Amitriptyline (Elavil)	Up to 400 mg/day	PO	• Peripheral neuropathy • Depression	• Drowsiness, dizziness, tremors, confusion, nervousness, orthostatic hypotension, hypertension, blurred vision, mydriasis, dry mouth, constipation, anorexia, paralytic ileus, urine retention, nightmares
Amphotericin-B (Fungizone)	Up to 1 mg/Kg/day	IV	• Aspergillosis • Blastomycosis • Candidiasis • Coccidioid-omycosis • Cryptococcosis • Histoplasmosis	• Fever, chills, hypokalemia, hypomagnesia, pain at site of infusion, renal failure (increased or decreased urination), paresthesias, impaired hearing, tinnitus, skin rash or itching, leukopenia, thrombocytopenia
Amphotericin-B Colloidal dispersion*	Up to 6 mg/Kg/ day	IV	• Candidiasis • Cryptococcosis • Histoplasmosis	• See amphotericin-B
Anti-B4-Blocked Ricin*		IV	• Lymphoma	• Allergic reactions, weight gain, can affect liver • Take on empty stomach.
Ampicillin (Omnipen, Omnipen-N, Polycillin, Polycillin-N, Principen, Totacillin, Totacillin-N)	Up to 150 mg/Kg/day (divided doses)	PO, IM, IV	• Salmonellosis	• Anaphylaxis, skin rash, fever, hives, itching, pseudomembranous colitis, seizures, diarrhea, nausea, vomiting, thrush, abdominal pain or cramps
Atovaquone (Mepron, formerly 566C80)	Up to 750 mg 4/day	PO	• PCP • Toxoplasmosis* • Cryptosporidium*	• Rash, nausea, diarrhea, headache, vomiting, fever, insomnia, asthenia, pruritus, thrush, abdominal pain, constipation, dizziness, anemia, neutropenia, elevated liver enzymes • Take with fatty meal.

* = Still under investigation

continued ▶

Table A4   *Continued*

Generic Name (Trade Name)	Maximal Dosage	Route of Administration	Indications	Side/Adverse Effects and Interactions
Azithromycin (Zithromax)	Up to 2,000 mg/day	PO/IV*	• Cryptosporidiosis* • MAC • Toxoplasmosis*	• Diarrhea, nausea, vomiting, abdominal pain, dyspepsia, flatulence, melena, cholestatic jaundice, dizziness, headache, somnolence, fatigue, rash, photophobia • PO: Take on empty stomach.
Bleomycin (Blenoxane)	Up to 29 U/m²	IV	• KS • Non-Hodgkin's lymphoma (NHL) • Cervical cancer	• Cough, shortness of breath (SOB), pneumonitis, fever, chills, stomatitis, confusion, syncope, diaphoresis, rashes, nausea, vomiting and anorexia
Brovavir* (BV-ARA-U)		PO	• HSV infection • Varicella zoster virus infection	• None yet reported
Carbamaze-pine (Tegretol)	Up to 1,200 mg/day	PO	• Peripheral neuropathy • Anticonvulsant	• Nausea, vomiting, drowsiness, rash, elevated LFTs, neutropenia
CD4, recombinant soluble*		IV, IM	• HIV infection	• Local reactions at injection site, fever
Ceftriaxone (Rocephin)	Up to 4 g/day (divided doses)	IM, IV	• Neurosyphilis • Salmonellosis • G+/G− infections	• Bruising, diarrhea, fever, hypotension, Stevens-Johnson syndrome, skin rash, joint pain, itching, redness, swelling, seizures, thrombophlebitis, pseudolithiasis
Chloram-phenicol (Anocol, Chloromycetin)	Up to 6 g/day (divided doses)	PO, IM, IV	• Salmonellosis	• Blood dyscrasias, abdominal distention, blue-gray skin color, low body temperature, skin rash, fever, confusion, delirium, headache, loss of vision, paresthesias, diarrhea, nausea, vomiting, sore throat, bleeding

* = Still under investigation

continued ▶

Table A4   *Continued*

Generic Name (Trade Name)	Maximal Dosage	Route of Administration	Indications	Side/Adverse Effects and Interactions
Chlorhexidine gluconate Oral Rinse (Peridex)		Oral rinse	• Prophylaxis for thrush, periodontal disease	• Change in taste; increased tartar; staining of teeth, fillings, dentures; mouth irritation
Cidofovir* (HPMPC)	5 mg/Kg/ week with progenecid	IV	• Cytomegalovirus (CMV) infection	• Nephrotoxicity, neuropathy, peripheral neuropathy
Ciprofloxacin (Cipro)	Up to 750 mg q12h	PO	• MAC	• Restlessness, tremors, seizures, crystalluria, blood in urine, dysuria, skin rash, itching, swelling of face or neck, joint pains, stiffness, visual disturbances, photosensitivity, dizziness, headache, abdominal pain, diarrhea, nausea, vomiting, insomnia, unpleasant taste in mouth • Take on empty stomach.
Clarithromycin (Biaxin)	Up to 2,000 mg/day	PO	• Cryptosporidiosis* • MAC • Toxoplasmosis*	• Nausea, vomiting, headache, rash, hearing loss, hepatotoxicity, diarrhea
Clindamycin (Cleocin)	Up to 600 mg q6h; Up to 1,800 mg q6h	PO, IM, IV	• Toxoplasmosis • Pneumocystosis	• Pseudomembranous colitis, skin rash, neutropenia, thrombocytopenia, abdominal pain, nausea and vomiting (N&V), diarrhea
Clofazimine (Lamprene)	Up to 300 mg q6h	PO	• MAC	• Colicky or burning abdominal or stomach pain, nausea, vomiting, pink or red to brownish black discoloration of skin, visual changes, GI bleeding, hepatitis or jaundice, dry rough scaly skin, anorexia, dizziness, drowsiness, dryness, burning, itching or irritation of eyes, skin rash, photosensitivity

---

* = Still under investigation

continued ▶

Table A4 *Continued*

Generic Name (Trade Name)	Maximal Dosage	Route of Administration	Indications	Side/Adverse Effects and Interactions
Clotrimazole (Mycelex Troches)	Up to 5/day	PO	• Candidiasis (oropharyngeal)	• Abdominal or stomach cramping/pain, diarrhea, nausea or vomiting
CMV immune globulin*		IV	• CMV	• Flushing, chills, muscle cramps, back pain, fever, N&V, wheezing
Colony stimulating factors (Leukine) GM-CSF (Neupogen) G-CSF (Prokine)	Up to 10 mcg/Kg/day Up to 4–8 mcg/Kg/day	IV, SC	• Neutropenia	• Fever, chills, rigors, bone pain, arthralgias, adult respiratory distress syndrome, rash, pericarditis and local erythema at site of injection, hypoxia
Cyclophospha-mide (Cytoxan) (Neosar)	Up to 1,500 mg/m²	PO, IM, IV	• NHL	• Darkening of skin and fingernails, loss of appetite, N&V, diarrhea, stomach pain, flushing and redness of face, headache, increased sweating, skin rash, loss of hair
Cycloserine (Seromycin)	Up to 1,000 mg/day	PO	• MAC • *M. tuberculosis*	• Anxiety, confusion, dizziness, drowsiness, increased irritability, increased restlessness, mental depression, hyperreflexia, speech problems
Cytarabine (Ara-C, Cytosine arabinoside, Cytosar-U)	Up to 150 mg/m²	IM, IV	• NHL • PML*	• Fever, chills, mouth or lip sores, unusual bleeding/bruising, numbness or tingling in fingers, toes or face, conjunctivitis, pain at injection site, skin rash
Dapsone (Avlosulfon, DDS)	Up to 100 mg/day	PO	• Pneumocystosis	• Hemolytic anemia, Stevens-Johnson syndrome, agranulo-cytosis (fever and sore throat) hepatic damage, methemoglobinemia • Needs acidic environment for absorption. • Take on empty stomach.

* = Still under investigation

continued ▶

Table A4   *Continued*

Generic Name (Trade Name)	Maximal Dosage	Route of Administration	Indications	Side/Adverse Effects and Interactions
Dextroam-phetamine (Dexedrine)		PO	• HIV dementia	• Restlessness, tremor, hyperactivity, insomnia, dizziness, headache, chills, dysphoria, tachycardia, palpitations, hyper/hypotension, N&V, cramps, dry mouth, diarrhea, constipation, metallic taste, anorexia, weight loss, urticaria, impotence, altered libido
Diclazuril*		PO	• Cryptosporidiosis	• N&V, fever, flulike symptoms
Didanosine (ddI, Videx)	Up to 600 mg/day	PO	• HIV infection	• Diarrhea, abdominal pain, pancreatitis, peripheral neuropathy, seizures, headaches, abnormal bone marrow function, abnormal liver function, electrolyte abnormalities, cardiac dysrhythmias, allergic reactions • Needs an alkaline environment. • Take on an empty stomach. Do not take with dapsone, intraconozole, or ketoconozole.
Doxorubicin hydrochloride (Adriamycin)	Up to 70 mg/m²	IV	• KS • NHL	• Leukopenia/infection (fever, chills, sore throat), stomatitis, esophagitis, pain at infusion site, thrombocytopenia (unusual bleeding or bruising), changes in skin color, diarrhea, nausea, vomiting, skin rash or itching, hair loss and reddish color to urine
Doxorubicin Lipsomal (Doxil)	20 mg/m² q3wks	IV	• KS • NHL	• See Doxorubicin

* = Still under investigation

continued ▶

Table A4 *Continued*

Generic Name (Trade Name)	Maximal Dosage	Route of Administration	Indications	Side/Adverse Effects and Interactions
Dronabinol (Marinol)	Up to 15 mg/m²/dose	PO	• HIV wasting • Antiemetic	• Irritability, insomnia, restlessness, hot flashes, sweating, mood changes, confusion, personality changes, hallucinations, depression, nervousness, anxiety, vision changes, hypotension
Epoetin alfa, recombinant (Epogen, Eprex, Procrit)	Initial dose: Up to 100 U/Kg/week Maintenance: 100 U Kg/week	IV, SC	• Anemia associated with HIV infection or AZT therapy	• Chest pain, edema, tachycardia, headache, hypertension, polycythemia, seizures, SOB, skin rash, arthralgias, asthenia, diarrhea, nausea, fatigue, flulike syndrome after each dose • *Note:* Should be temporarily discontinued if hematocrit reaches or exceeds 36%.
Ethambutol (Myambutol)	15–25 mg/Kg/day	PO	• MAC • *M. tuberculosis*	• Skin rash, fever, arthralgias, numbness, blurred vision, eye pain, red-green color blindness, any loss of vision, abdominal pain, anorexia, nausea, vomiting, headache, mental confusion, increased serum uric acid levels
Ethionamide (Trecator-SC)	Up to 100 mg/day	PO	• *M. tuberculosis*	• Yellow skin/eyes, tingling, burning or pain in hands or feet, mental depression, confusion, mood or mental changes, coldness, decreased sexual ability, dry and puffy skin, weight gain, hyperglycemia, blurred/lost vision, skin rash
Etoposide (VePesid)	Up to 200 mg/m²	IV, PO	• KS • NHL	• Leukopenia, thrombocyto-penia, stomatitis, ataxia paresthesias, tachycardia, SOB or wheezing, pain at site of injection, N&V and loss of appetite, diarrhea, fatigue, loss of hair

continued ▶

Table A4   *Continued*

Generic Name (Trade Name)	Maximal Dosage	Route of Administration	Indications	Side/Adverse Effects and Interactions
Famciclovir (Famvir)	Up to 1,500 mg/day	PO	• Herpes simplex varicella zoster • Herpes zoster infection	• N&V, diarrhea, headache, fatigue, dizziness
Fluconazole (Diflucan)	Up to 1,200 mg/day	PO, IV	• Candidiasis • Coccidioido-mycosis • Cryptococcosis	• Abnormal liver function, Stevens-Johnson syndrome, nausea, headache, skin rash, vomiting, abdominal pain, diarrhea • Amphoterecin: Do not administer together; antagonistic. • Coumarin anticoagulants: Increased protime (PT). • Astemizole and terfenadine: Inhibits metabolism therefore increases cardiovascular toxicity (e.g., dysrhythmias, palpitations, syncope). • Phenytoin: Increased phenytoin plasma levels. • Rifampin: Increased metabolism of fluconazole, may decrease fluconazole plasma concentration by as much as 20%. • Sulfonyurea antidiabetic agents: Fluconazole may inhibit sulfonyurea metabolism; the resulting drug levels lead to hypoglycemia.
Flucytosine (Ancobon, 5-Fluorocytosine, 5FC)	Up to 150 mg/Kg/day (divided in 4 equal doses)	PO	• Candidiasis • Cryptococcosis	• Anemia, sore throat, fever, unusual bleeding/ bruising, confusion, sensitivity to sunlight, abdominal pain, diarrhea, loss of appetite, N&V, dizziness, lightheaded-ness, drowsiness, headache
Fluoxetine (Prozac)	Up to 80 mg/day	PO	• Depression	• Anxiety, agitation, N&V, anorexia • Liver enzymes (P_{450}) inhibition

continued ▶

Table A4 *Continued*

Generic Name (Trade Name)	Maximal Dosage	Route of Administration	Indications	Side/Adverse Effects and Interactions
Foscarnet sodium (Foscavir)	Up to 120 mg/Kg/dose	IV	• CMV infection • HSV infection • HIV infection • Varicella infection	• Headaches, nausea, anorexia, hypomagnesia, elevated creatinine, mild proteinuria, renal failure, decrease in calcium hyperphos-phatemia, fatigue, irritability, tremors, seizures, genital ulcers
Ganciclovir (Cytovene, formerly known as DHPG)	3,000 mg/day Up to 5 mg/Kg/dose	PO IV Intravitreal implants*	• CMV infection • HSV infection	• Granulocytopenia, thrombocytopenia, anemia, mood changes, fever, skin rash, abnormal liver function, phlebitis, loss of appetite
Gentamicin liposome injection*		IV	• MAC	• Urinary frequency, increased thirst, anorexia, N&V, muscle twitching, paresthesias, seizures, impaired hearing, itching, skin rash, impaired vision
gp120 vaccines* gp160 vaccines*		IM	• Preventive, therapeutic, and perinatal vaccines	• Malaise, myalgia, headache, fever, tenderness and induration at injection site
Granisetron (Kytril)	Up to 40 mcg/Kg/day	IV, PO	• Antiemetic	• Headache, somnolescence, diarrhea, constipation
Guaifenesin (Humabid)	Up to 2,400 mg/day	PO	• Decongestant	• N&V, GI upset
Haloperidol (Haldol)	Up to 100 mg/day	PO, IV, IM	• Psychosis • Antiemetic	• Extrapyramidal effects, agitation, sedation, hallucination
Human growth hormone* (Humatrope) (Protropin)		SC	• Immunomodu-lation • Wasting syndrome	• Sodium and water retention, edema, carpal tunnel syndrome, increased intracranial pressure
Hypericin*		IV	• HIV infection	• Elevated liver function tests, photosensitivity, paresthesias

* = Still under investigation

continued ▶

Table A4   *Continued*

Generic Name (Trade Name)	Maximal Dosage	Route of Administration	Indications	Side/Adverse Effects and Interactions
Indinavir (Crixivan)	Up to 2,400 mg/day	PO	• HIV infection	• Elevated liver enzymes and bilirubin, N&V, diarrhea, headache, malaise, nephrolithiasis • Need to take on empty stomach. Recommend 6–8 glasses of water/day. • Take 1 hr before or after ddl. • Inhibits metabolism of rifampin. • Ketoconozole reduces indinavir metabolism.
Interferon-alfa recombinant (Intron-A, Roferon-A, Kemron) (Alferon)	Up to 100 MU/week	IM, SC	• HIV infection • KS	• Parenteral: Flulike syndrome (fever, myalgias, malaise), leukopenia, elevated liver enzymes, weight loss, hair loss, fatigue, proteinuria, reversible congestive cardiomyopathy (weight gain and signs of right- or left-sided congestive heart failure) • Oral: No side effects have been reported with low-dose oral interferon-alpha
Interleukin-2 recombinant*	Up to 10 MU/m^2	IV, SC	• HIV infection • KS	• Fluid retention, hypotension, fever, chills, elevated creatinine, elevated BUN, oliguria, anuria, azotemia, fatigue, weight gain, tachycardia, N&V, transient changes in liver function studies, headache, lightheaded-ness, dizziness, mental changes, pulmonary symptoms, anemia, leukocytosis, skin rash, mylagia, arthralgia
Isoniazid (INH, Izonid, Laniazid, Nydrazid, Tubizid)	Up to 300 mg/day	PO, IM, IV	• *M. tuberculosis*	• Loss of appetite, N&V, diarrhea, numbness, tingling, burning/pain in hands or feet, fever, sore throat, unusual bleeding/ bruising, skin rash, pain at injection site, arthralgia, seizures, depression, psychosis, blurred vision with or without eye pain

* = Still under investigation

continued ▶

Table A4 *Continued*

Generic Name (Trade Name)	Maximal Dosage	Route of Administration	Indications	Side/Adverse Effects and Interactions
Itraconazole (Sporanox)	Up to 600 mg/day	PO	• Aspergillosis • Candididiasis • Cryptococcosis • Histoplasmosis	• N&V, headaches, rash, diarrhea, anorexia, fever, headache, dizziness, pruritus, hypotension, hypokalemia, elevated liver enzymes, impotence • Take on empty stomach.
Ketoconazole (Nizoral)	Up to 600 mg/day	PO	• Candidiasis	• Hepatitis, N&V, diarrhea, dizziness, drowsiness, gynecomastia, headache, skin rash, itching, impotence, insomnia, photophobia • Needs acidic environment for absorption; take on empty stomach. • Rifampin: Decreases ketoconazole plasma levels. • Coumarin anticoagulants: May increase protime. • Phenytoin: May alter metabolism of both drugs. • Terfenadine and astemizole: Ketoconazole may inhibit terfenadine and astemizole metabolism and may increase cardiac toxicity.
Lamivudine (3-TC, Epivir)	Up to 600 mg/day	PO	• HIV infection	• Neutropenia, rash, insomnia, fever, headache, fatigue, diarrhea, vasculitis, photophobia, paresthesias
Letrazuril*		PO	• Cryptospo-ridiosis	• N&V rash
Leucovorin (Citrovorum, Folinic Acid, Wellcovorin)	Up to 100 mg/m²/dose	PO, IM, .IV	• Prophylaxis and treatment of toxicity related to methotrexate, pyrimethamine, trimethoprim, trimetrexate	• Skin rash, hives, itching, wheezing

* = Still under investigation

continued ▶

Table A4   *Continued*

Generic Name (Trade Name)	Maximal Dosage	Route of Administration	Indications	Side/Adverse Effects and Interactions
Megestrol-acetate (Megace oral suspension)	Up to 1,200 mg/day	PO	• HIV wasting	• Impotence, diarrhea • Alteration of menstrual pattern with unpredictable bleeding, visual disturbances, headache, insomnia, pain in abdomen, depression, skin rashes, peripheral edema, acne, increased body hair, increased breast tenderness, loss of scalp hair
Methylene blue	1–2 mg/Kg/day	IV, PO	• Methemoglobi-nemia	• N&V, diarrhea, dizziness, mental confusion
Methotrexate (Folex, Folex PFS, Mexate, Mexate-AQ)	Up to 250 mg/m²	PO, IM, IV	• NHL	• GI ulceration or bleeding, enteritis, intestinal perforation, leukopenia, bacterial infections, septicemia, thrombocy-topenia, stomatitis, renal failure, hyperuricemia, cutaneous vasculitis, hepatotoxicity, anorexia, N&V, boils
Methylpheni-date (Petalin, Ritalin)		PO	• HIV dementia	• Tachycardia, hypertension, chest pain, tremors, allergic reactions, anemia, convulsions, leukopenia, agitation, confusion, anorexia, nervousness, insomnia, headache, N&V
Mexiletine (Mexitril)	Up to 2,000 mg/day	PO	• HIV peripheral neuropathy	• Chest pain, rapid or irregular heart beats (PVCs), leukopenia, thrombocy-topenia, dizziness, lightheaded-ness, tremors, ataxia, N&V, confusion, impaired vision, headache, diarrhea, constipation, tinnitis, rash, insomnia, slurred speech
Mitoguazone (MGBG, M-GAG)	Up to 600 mg/m²	IV	• NHL	• N&V, myopathy, mucositis, anorexia

continued ▶

Table A4 *Continued*

Generic Name (Trade Name)	Maximal Dosage	Route of Administration	Indications	Side/Adverse Effects and Interactions
Nevirapine* (BI-RG-587)		PO	• HIV infection	• Rash, thrombocytopenia, fever
Nimodipine* (Nimotop)	Up to 90 mg q4h	PO	• HIV dementia	• Decreased blood pressure
Nystatin (Mycostatin, Nilstat, Nystex)		PO	• Candidiasis (oropharyng-eal)	• Diarrhea, N&V, stomach pain
Octreotide (Sandostatin)	Up to 1,500 mcg q8h	SC	• HIV-related diarrhea	• Hyperglycemia, hypoglycemia, abdominal pain, diarrhea, N&V, pain at injection site, headache, fatigue, dizziness, edema, hepatic dysfunction
Ondansetron (Zofran)	0.15 mg/Kg/dose	PO, IV	• Antiemetic	• Diarrhea, headaches
Oxadralone*	Up to 20 mg/day	PO	• HIV wasting	• Anabolic steroid side effects: Masculinizing effects in women (facial hair growth, deepened voice), feminizing effects in men (breast development) • Edema, jaundice, hepatic carcinoma, N&V
Paclitaxel (Taxol)	Up to 250 mg/m^2	IV (Use nonpolyvinyl chloride tubing)	• KS	• Neutropenia, thrombocy-topenia, headache, fatigue, peripheral neuropathy, bradycardia, N&V, diarrhea, mucositis, hair loss, arthralgia, fever, taste alterations, urticaria, rashes
Paromomycin sulfate (Humatin, Aminosidin)	Up to 150 mg/Kg/day (4 divided doses)	PO	• Cryptosporidiosis	• N&V, diarrhea, renal damage
Paroxetine (Paxil)	Up to 50 mg/day	PO	• Depression	• Anxiety, agitation, N&V, anorexia

* = Still under investigation

continued ◗

Table A4   *Continued*

Generic Name (Trade Name)	Maximal Dosage	Route of Administration	Indications	Side/Adverse Effects and Interactions
Pentamidine isethionate (Nebupent, inhalation; Pentam parenteral)	IV: 3–4 mg/ Kg/day Inhalation: 300–600 mg	IV, inhalation	• Pneumocystosis	• Parenteral: Skin rash, hyperglycemia, hypotension, pain/tenderness at injection site, redness/flushing of face, metallic taste in mouth • Inhalation: Chest pain, congestion, coughing, dyspnea, pharyngitis, wheezing, skin rash, metallic taste in mouth, pneumothorax
Peptide T*		SC, intranasal	• Immunomodu-lation • HIV dementia • Neuropathy	• None yet reported
PMEA*		IV	• HIV infection	• None yet reported
Prednisone (Deltasone, Meticortin, Orasone, Prednicen-M, Strerepred)		PO	• HIV myopathy • PCP (as adjunctive therapy)	• Rectal irritation, bleeding, impaired vision, diabetes mellitus, psychic disturbances, delayed wound healing, infection
Primaquine	Up to 60 mg/day	PO	• PCP • *Microsporidium*	• Methemoglobinemia, hemolytic anemia, agranulocytosis
Pyrazina-mide (PZA)	20–35 mg/Kg/day	PO	• *M. tuberculosis*	• Joint pain, loss of appetite, unusual tiredness or weakness, swelling of joints, itching rash, nausea
Pyrimethamine (Daraprim)	Up to 100 mg/day (need to add folinic acid to regimen)	PO	• Pneumocystosis • Toxoplasmosis	• Folic acid deficiency (loss of taste, glossitis, diarrhea, sore throat, dysphagia, ulcerative, stomatitis), fever, bleeding, bruising, fatigue, skin rash, seizures, anorexia, vomiting
Rifabutin (Ansamycin)	Up to 600 mg/day	PO	• MAC infection (for prophylaxis and treatment of disease)	• Increase in both liver enzymes and creatinine, uveitis, rash, fever, leukopenia, GI distress, hemolysis, arthralgias

* = Still under investigation

continued ▶

Table A4   *Continued*

Generic Name (Trade Name)	Maximal Dosage	Route of Administration	Indications	Side/Adverse Effects and Interactions
Rifampin (Rifadin, Rifadin IV, Rimactane)	Up to 600 mg/day	PO, IV	• M. tuberculosis	• Dizziness, fever, headache, muscle and bone pain, rash, itching, skin redness, sore throat, loss of appetite, N&V, bloody or cloudy urine, diarrhea, sore mouth or tongue • Discoloration of urine, feces, sputum, sweat or tears • Rifampin induces liver enzymes responsible for the inactivation of a number of drugs including verapamil, digitalis derivatives, quinoine, dapsone, cyclosporine, chloramphen- icol, oral anticoagulants, estrogens, oral contraceptives, benzodiazepine, narcotics, and fluconazole.
Ritonavir (Norvir)	1,200 mg/day	PO (store in refrigerator)	• HIV infection	• Taste perversions, asthenia, headache, anorexia, dizziness, circumoral paresthesia, increased liver enzymes • Drugs may increase serum levels of the following and are, therefore, contraindicated: Benzadiazepines, opiates, terfenadine, astemizole, antidysrhythmics, calcium channel blockers, fluoxetine, sertraline, paroxetine
Saquinavir (Invirase)	Up to 1,500 mg/day	PO	• HIV infection	• N&V, increased CPK, neutropenia, AST elevation
Sertraline (Zoloft)	Up to 200 mg/day	PO	• Antidepressant	• Anxiety, agitation, N&V, anorexia • Liver enzynes (P_{450}) inhibition
SP303T*		Topical	• HSV infection	• None yet reported
Stavudine (Zerit, d4T)	40 mg q12h (>60 Kg) 30 mg q12h (<60 Kg)	PO	• HIV infection	• Peripheral neuropathy, hepatotoxicity, anemia, headache, nausea

* = Still under investigation

continued ▶

Table A4   *Continued*

Generic Name (Trade Name)	Maximal Dosage	Route of Administration	Indications	Side/Adverse Effects and Interactions
Sulfadiazine	Up to 8 g/day	PO	• Toxoplasmosis	• Fever, itching, skin rash, hepatitis, photosensitiv-ity, blood dyscrasias, blistering, peeling of skin, hematuria, crystalluria, dizziness, headache, anorexia, N&V, diarrhea
Sulfadoxine and pyrimethamine (Fansidar)	Sulfadoxine: 500 mg Pyrimethamine: 25 mg	PO	• Pneumocystosis	• Stevens-Johnson syndrome, toxic epidermal necrolysis, fulminant hepatic necrosis, photosensitivity, bleeding/bruising, folic acid deficiency (loss of taste, glossitis, diarrhea, sore throat, dysphagia, ulcerative stomatitis), skin rash, fatigue, aching in joints or muscles, hematuria, dysuria, goiter, tremors, seizures, headache, dizziness, N&V
Sulfame-thoxazole and trimethoprim (SMX) (Bactrim, Bethaprim, Cheragan W/TMP, Cotrim, Septra, Sulfamethoprim, Sulfaprim, Sulfatrim, Sulfoxaprim, Triazole, Uroplus)	Up to 20 mg/Kg/day	PO, IV	• Isosporiasis • Pneumocystosis • Salmonellosis • Toxoplasmosis	• Skin rash, itching, Stevens-Johnson syndrome (myalgia, arthralgia, redness, blistering, peeling/ loosening of the skin, extreme fatigue), lysphagia, fever, leukopenia (sore throat), thrombocy-topenia, hepatitis (dark urine pale stools, yellow skin/ sclera), cystalluria, hematuria, diarrhea, dizziness, headache, anorexia, N&V
Testosterone	200 mg q2wks q2–3wks	IM	• Depression • Muscle wasting	• In females: Menstrual irregularities, deepened voice, excessive hair growth • In males: Bladder irritability, breast soreness, frequent or continuing erections • Both sexes: Edema, dizziness, headaches, fatigue, bleeding, N&V, diarrhea, redness or pain at injection site

continued ▶

Table A4   *Continued*

Generic Name (Trade Name)	Maximal Dosage	Route of Administration	Indications	Side/Adverse Effects and Interactions
Thalidomide*	Up to 25 mg/Kg/day	PO	• Immunomodulation • Wasting syndrome	• Sedation, severe congenital abnormalities in developing fetuses, neurotoxicity
Thymopentin*		SC	• Immunodulation	• Respiratory congestion, pain at injection site, headache, pain at injection site, sleep disorders, fatigue, GI side effects, pruritus, elevated liver enzymes
Tricosanthin* (Compound Q)		IV	• Antiviral	• CNS toxicity
Trimethoprim* (Proloprim, Trimpex)	Up to 20 mg/Kg/day	PO	• Salmonellosis • Pneumocystosis	• Headache, methemoglobinemia, skin rash, itching, alteration in taste, sore mouth or tongue, anorexia, diarrhea, N&V, abdominal pain, cramping
Trimetrexate glucuronate (Neutrexim)	45 mg/m²/day	IV	• Pneumocystosis • Toxoplasmosis*	• Decrease in neutrophil and platelet counts, diarrhea, reversible liver function abnormalities, nephrotoxicity, skin rash, fever, mucositis
Valacyclovir (Valtrex)	1 g q8h° 3/day	PO	• CMV infection* • HSV infection • Herpes zoster infection • Varicella infection	• *See Acyclovir*
Vinblastine (Velban, Velsar)	Up to 10 mg/m²	IV, Intralesional	• KS	• Fever, chills, cough, hoarseness, painful/difficult urination, pain/redness at site of injection, mouth and lip sores, rectal bleeding, dizziness, difficulty in walking, double vision, drooping eyelids, headache, jaw pain, mental depression, numbness/tingling in fingers and toes, pain in fingers or toes, pain in testicles, weakness, N&V, loss of hair

* = Still under investigation

continued ▶

Table A4   *Continued*

Generic Name (Trade Name)	Maximal Dosage	Route of Administration	Indications	Side/Adverse Effects and Interactions
Vincristine (Oncovin, Vincasar PES, Vincrex)	Up to 1.4 mg/m²/day	IV, Intralesional	• KS • NHL • Cervical cancer	• Constipation, dizziness, dysuria, joint pain, flank pain, visual changes, ataxia, drooping eyelids, headache, jaw pain, numbness or tingling in fingers or toes, pain in testicles, weakness, hyponatremia, leukopenia, thrombocy-topenia, stomatitis • Syndrome of inappropriate antidiuretic hormone (SIADH) evidenced by agitation, confusion, dizziness, hallucinations, anorexia, mental depression, seizures, insomnia, loss of consciousness
Zalcitabine (HIVID, ddC)	0.75 mg q8h	PO	• HIV infection	• Pancreatitis, peripheral neuropathy, oral aphthous ulcers, fever, rash, stomatitis • Take on empty stomach.
Zidovudine (Retrovir, formerly known as AZT)	Up to 1,200 mg/day	PO, IV	• HIV infection	• Anemia, leukopenia, neutropenia, platelet count changes (increased or decreased), anorexia, asthenia, diarrhea, dizziness, fever, headache, nausea, insomnia, malaise, myalgia, pain in abdomen, rash, somnolence, taste alteration • Take on empty stomach.

Bibliography

AHFS Drug Information. (1995). Bethesda, MD: American Society of Hospital Pharmacists.

Gilman, A., Goodman, L., & Gilman, A. (1994). *The pharmacological basis of therapeutics.* New York: Macmillan.

Olin, B., Hebel, S., Connel, S., & Dombek, C. (1995). *Facts and comparisons.* St. Louis, MO: Lippincott.

Sande, M., & Volberding, P. (1995). *The medical management of AIDS* (4th ed.). Philadelphia: Saunders.

Appendix C

The FDA Drug-Approval Process

Experimental treatments play a significant role in the care of people infected with HIV. Interpretation of the drug-approval process and how the AIDS epidemic has influenced this field is integral to the development and maintenance of state-of-the-art care.

It is of historic importance to note that "as a result of widely perceived abuses on the part of drug manufacturers and biomedical researchers" (Edgar & Rothman, 1990, p. 112) as recently as 1962, the U.S. drug-approval system (administered by the Food and Drug Administration [FDA]) was transformed into the highly regulated process that exists today. This process may err on the side of caution. To delay approval of a drug for safety reasons may preclude its being available to those who desperately need it. This thoroughness, which appears as lethargy in the eyes of the AIDS community, has spurred both the FDA and AIDS activists to action to modify the system.

The drug-approval process set up in the early 1960s and still in use today consists of two stages: premarketing and postmarketing. The premarketing stage, where the initial investigation occurs, is the focus of this appendix.

Phase 1 trials, intended to test for safety only, form the riskiest part of the process as the drug is administered to human participants for the first time. These trials typically involve fewer than 100 people and last only several weeks. If the drug passes this test, the process then moves to *Phase II* to determine efficacy. Finally, the drug moves to *Phase III* trials, which test for long-term side effects. There are hundreds of participants in this phase and the trials could last several years.

Once a drug successfully completes *Phase III* it moves into premarketing evaluation. It is at this point that the FDA performs further analysis for safety and efficacy. In order for a sponsor's *new drug application* (NDA) to be approved, it is imperative that the analysis yield a significant amount of evidence to confirm that the study design, measures, and outcomes were appropriate for the drug's labeling, or intended use. The FDA would then approve the drug for use, based on the indication (Edgar & Rothman, 1990).

The AIDS epidemic has abbreviated this process in several ways. First, Phases I, II, and III often overlap. Second, "the FDA has enacted a special 1-AA internal agency designation for AIDS-related drugs to ensure that they receive the highest priority in all stages of the drug review process" (Young, Norris, Levitt, & Nightingale, 1988, p. 2267). Lastly, the trials are *randomized* (computer assigns research regimen to the participant) and *double blinded* (neither the researchers nor the participants know for sure which regimen they have been assigned). *Placebo-controlled* trials (comparing one therapy to a sugar pill) are mostly obsolete, following questions raised from the concerned community about the ethics of offering a placebo in the face of terminal disease.

There is also a lexicon of new regulatory language. It is important to note that terms may overlap, depending on the source, and some clarification of these terms follows.

A drug receives *treatment IND* (investigational new drug) status if

1. The drug is intended to treat a serious or life-threatening disease.
2. There is no comparable or satisfactory alternative or therapy to treat that stage of the disease in the target population.
3. The drug is under investigation in a controlled clinical trial under an IND in effect for the trial, or all clinical trials have been completed.
4. The sponsor for the controlled clinical trial is actively pursuing marketing approval of the investigational drug with due diligence (Young et al., 1988).

The status can be applied to a drug as early as Phase II during the clinical trials process. In the case of serious (but not life-threatening) disease, a drug may be made available during

Phase III. *Compassionate use IND* status indicates that an experimental drug has been made available on a compassionate basis to individuals who cannot tolerate or are failing standard therapy. "These protocols are designed to serve a limited number of people on a case-by-case basis. Entry requirements are often strict. Paperwork may be considerable, sometimes as much as for a clinical trial, but newer programs are reducing the amount required" (AIDS Institute, 1992, p. 2).

Compassionate-use IND is not to be confused with *parallel track.* The parallel track program permits a broader distribution of the experimental drugs that have completed safety testing. Not only is this described in the literature for those who cannot tolerate or who are failing standard therapy (as with compassionate use), but it also goes one step further and makes the drug available to those unable to participate in a clinical trial (Phase I/II/III study) or who live too far from a clinical trial site (AIDS Institute, 1992). Treatment IND, compassionate use, and parallel track may be referred to collectively as *expanded access* and are often used interchangeably.

The term *orphan drug program* predates AIDS and is rarely used today. It describes a drug that has been abandoned due to the costs of the traditional clinical trials process. Labeling a drug with orphan drug status creates "special incentives to produce drugs for small markets" (Edgar & Rothman, 1990, p. 120).

Finally, *accelerated approval* resolutions, available since December 1992, enable the pharmaceutical industry to use a speedier approval mechanism for new drugs that which may be indicated for serious or life-threatening illnesses "if the FDA finds that early data on a candidate agent are reasonably likely to predict clinical benefit. This shortcut to licensing, based on surrogate markers of efficacy rather than the hard endpoints such as disease progression and death, can cut years off the standard trial- and review-calendar" (Mascolini & Chang, 1994, p. 6). For example, ddI was approved in 6 months using this accelerated process.

Buyers' clubs or *underground* may provide additional avenues to obtaining treatments. The buyers' clubs provide access to experimental or alternative therapies for HIV and opportunistic infections. They are generally operated by the HIV community. "Typically, buyers' clubs help individuals take advantage of the FDA's long standing policy of permitting personal use imports of non-approved medications, generally by importing multiple supplies at once" (Hodel & Franke-Ruta, 1991, p. 1).

In general, the FDA's position is that these clubs are inappropriately taking advantage of the system. The FDA allows any individual to import drugs if the product (1) is intended for personal use, (2) is not for commercial distribution, (3) is not in excessive amounts (a 3-month supply), (4) is appropriately identified for the intended use, and (5) is supervised by a licensed U.S. physician. A person who meets the stated criteria is permitted to cross the U.S. border in possession of the drugs, or use the mail system as well (Edgar & Rothman, 1990). Thus, the FDA policy is not in direct correlation with the operational motives of the buyers' club circuit. The FDA is apparently monitoring the activity of such clubs.

The drug-approval process presents challenges to the clinician to provide cost-effective, state-of-the-art care while, in many cases, holding the ethical bottom line as well.

Appendix D

Selected Adult Laboratory Values

Table A5

Type of Test	Normal Value/Range	Comments
ELISA (enzyme-linked immunosorbent assay)	Negative (no HIV infection)	• HIV-antibody screening test; if positive, must be confirmed with Western blot. • Antibody assays do not detect HIV-antibody in the earliest stages of infection; the interval between HIV infection and appearance of antibody in the blood varies (<6 months after infection in most people this period [Wilber, 1994]) • Positive test: 98% sensitivity; 99.8% specificity
Western Blot (WB)	Negative (no HIV infection)	• HIV-antibody test used to confirm a positive ELISA; a positive WB shows antibody bands against any 2 of 3 potential antigens. • An "indeterminate" pattern is nondiagnostic, reacting against only one antigen (Wilber, 1994). • "False" positive WB and ELISA may be seen in newborns in the presence of maternal HIV antibodies.
p24 antigen assays	Negative (no HIV infection or asymptomatic HIV infection)	• Qualitative measure of free HIV viral antigen in serum or plasma. • Current test only measures positive with higher viral load. • Low sensitivity in asymptomatic, HIV+ people with CD4+ lymphocyte counts >200/μl. • Often measures positive with acute antiretroviral syndrome (Saag, Crain, & Decker, 1991)
Qualitative DNA-PCR (polymerase chain reaction)	Negative (no HIV infection)	• Qualitative measure of cell-associated proviral DNA. In HIV+ people with CD4+ lymphocytes <1000/μl, 100% positive (100% sensitivity). • Useful in documenting neonatal infection (Sanford, Sande, & Gilbert, 1995).
Qualitative RNA-PCR	Negative (no HIV infection)	• Qualitative measure of cell-free or cell-associated viral RNA. • 100% sensitivity (100% positive) in HIV+ people with CD4+ lymphocytes <1000/μl. • Technique in development (Sanford et al., 1995)
PBMC (peripheral blood mononuclear cell co-culture)	Negative (no HIV infection)	• Measures infectious, cell-associated virus. • Expensive, labor-intensive culture process. • In HIV+ people with CD4 <500, 95%–100% sensitivity (Sanford et al., 1995).

continued ▶

Table A5 *Continued*

Type of Test	Normal Value/Range	Comments
CD4+ cells T-helper T4 lymphocyte "T-cells"	Normal values a mean of 800–1,050/µl, with a range representing two standard deviations of about 450–1,400/µl	• CD4+ cells are a primary target of HIV infection. As HIV infection advances, the number of CD4+ cells declines progressively. • Test is used to stage the disease, provide guidelines for differential diagnosis of patient complaints, and dictate therapeutic decisions about antiviral treatment and prophylaxis of opportunistic disease (Laurence, 1993). • Individual variability in results up to 15% can be seen in the course of 1 day. Small variations in the number of WBCs, or in the percentage of lymphocytes greatly influences CD4+ counts (Hughes et al., 1993).
CD4+ lymphocyte percentage	HIV negative: >30%.	• Measures the percentage of total lymphocytes with the CD4+ marker. • Test shows less diurnal variation than measurement of CD4+ lymphocyte count (Laurence, 1993).
bDNA (Branched Chain DNA Signal Amplification Assay)	Negative (no HIV infection)	• Quantitative measure of HIV RNA in plasma. Emerging technique to measure viral load and potentially to follow the activity of antiviral drug treatment. • Detection limit is 5,000 virions/ml. Can detect and quantitate HIV RNA in 80%–90% of HIV+ people with CD4+ lymphocytes <500/µl (Elbeik & Feinberg, 1994).
QC-PCR (Quantitative Competitive Polymerase Chain Reaction)	Negative (no HIV infection)	• Quantitative measure of HIV viral load. Copies HIV RNA in plasma into a DNA form, which is then amplified and measured. • Can detect HIV RNA in plasma of *all* infected people, with as few as 50 virions/ml. Emerging technique (Elbeik & Feinberg, 1994).
Quantitative Cell Culture/Plasma Culture	Negative (no HIV infection)	• Labor-intensive technique for measuring viral load. • Cells of HIV+ people are diluted in 10-fold increments, and the endpoint is the reciprocal of the highest dilution that is positive for the p24 antigen (Elbeik & Feinberg, 1994).
Beta-2 Microglobulin	103 ± 24 mmol/L	• A nonspecific marker of CD4+ lymphocyte activation. A surrogate marker sometimes used to predict HIV disease progression. • Higher levels (>3.5) correlate with disease progression, but the test is a less specific surrogate than CD4+ lymphocyte count (Sanford et al., 1995).
Neoptrin	Mean 3.7 ± 1.8 mmol/L	• A marker of monocyte-macrophage activation. • Higher levels (>15 ng/ml) correlate HIV disease progression (Sanford et al., 1995).

continued ▶

Table A5   *Continued*

Type of Test	Normal Value/Range	Comments
Toxoplasmosis serology (IgG antibody)	Negative = no latent infection Positive = latent infection	• HIV+ people with evidence of latent toxoplasmosis infection may be candidates for prophylactic therapy; in those with CNS symptoms, evidence of latent infection assists in the development of differential diagnoses. HIV+ people without evidence of latent infection may be counseled to avoid unnecessary exposure. • 15% of HIV+ patients with toxoplasmosis may have "false" negative serology (Lawlor, Fischer, & Adelman, 1995).
CMV serology	Negative = no latent infection Positive = latent infection	• Very high prevalence of anti-CMV antibody in the blood and urine in the general population make this test of little value in predicting or diagnosing CMV disease in HIV+ people.

Appendix E

Central Venous Access Devices

1. Central venous access devices (CVADs) are commonly used in clinical management of HIV disease for
   a. Intravenous therapies for OIs/malignancies
   b. Parenteral nutrition
2. Types most frequently used (design characteristics make each unique): Hickman, Broviac, Groshong, implanted port, PICC
3. Great deal of concern about potential morbidity associated with AIDS patients using a CVAD
   a. Particularly concerned when receiving concomitant myelosuppressive agents (e.g., ganciclovir, AZT) on long-term basis (Stanley, Charlebois, Harb, & Jacobson, 1993)
   b. No clear evidence that risk factors for AIDS patients differ from other patients when using a CVAD (van der Pijl & Frissen, 1992; Vannucci, 1993)
4. Appropriate care of device appears to be single most important factor in reducing potential for infections (see Table A6 for various characteristics and issues related to care and maintenance)
   a. Use strict aseptic technique when accessing device
   b. Minimize catheter manipulation and entry into the system
   c. Change gauze dressings every 48–72 hours or when wet, loose, or soiled; change transparent dressing q7d
5. Potential complications
   a. Infection
      (1) Systemic, local, or in port pocket
      (2) Risk increased with multilumens and increased catheter manipulation
      (3) Treat with antibiotics; may need to remove catheter
   b. Thrombosis of vein, diagnosed via venogram
      (1) May result in superior vena cava syndrome
      (2) Symptoms include dyspnea, edema of face, neck, shoulder, arm
      (3) Treat with heparin or coumadin therapy; may need to remove catheter
   c. Catheter occlusion, partial or complete
      (1) Catheter tip may be abutting vessel wall; change in patient's position will relieve occlusion
      (2) Fibrin sheath at tip of catheter may be able to infuse but cannot aspirate blood; treat with Urokinase or hydrochloric acid installation
   d. Catheter tip migration, particularly with PICC
      (1) Most commonly into internal jugular vein
      (2) Frequent vomiting or bouts of severe coughing increase risk
      (3) Symptoms include gurgling sound in ear, referred pain in jaw, ear, teeth
   e. Pinch-off syndrome
      (1) Documented uncommon occurrence, may cause catheter fracture
      (2) Catheter is compressed between rib and clavicle with patient movement
      (3) Once fracture occurs, distal segment of catheter may embolize to pulmonary artery or right ventricle
      (4) Treat by removal of catheter and retrieval of embolized catheter
   f. Damage to catheter (most frequent cause is accidental cut in catheter)
      (1) Clamp with smooth-edged clamp or latex or plastic covered clamp proximal to catheter
      (2) Follow manufacture's recommendations for repair of line
   g. PICC
      (1) Phlebitis within first 10 days of insertion
      (2) Tenderness and erythema occur anywhere from puncture site to several inches above
      (3) Treat with rest and elevation of extremity, apply heat.

Table A6   Characteristics, Care, and Maintenance of CVADs

Type	Characteristics	Indications	Care/Maintenance Issues
Hickman	• Inserted in central vein • Tip terminates in superior vena cava • Made of silicone • Tunneled • Dacron cuff distal to exit site • Single or multilumens • Length determined by site of insertion • Internal diameter 0.5–1.6 mm; may differ in double/triple lumens	Long-term venous access (>30 days)	• Tape securely, especially during first 2 weeks of insertion until tissue adheres to cuff. • Keep catheter clamped at all times when not in use. • Avoid use of scissors near catheter. • Change injection cap at least weekly or prn. • Flush with 10 ml normal saline after blood sampling and infusions. • Flush with anticoagulant following intermittent infusion and routinely per policy/procedure. • Repair according to manufacturer's guidelines.
Broviac	• Inserted in central vein • Tip terminates in superior vena cava • Made of silicone • Tunneled • Dacron cuff distal to exit site • Single or multilumens • Length determined by site of insertion • Interior lumen smaller than Hickman • Frequently used in children	Long-term venous access (>30 days)	• Tape securely, especially during first 2 weeks of insertion until tissue adheres to cuff. • Keep catheter clamped at all times when not in use. • Avoid use of scissors near catheter. • Change injection cap at least weekly or prn. • Flush with 10 ml normal saline after blood sampling and infusions. • Flush with anticoagulant following intermittent infusion and routinely per policy/procedure. • Repair according to manufacturer's guidelines.
Groshong	• Inserted in central vein • Tip terminates in superior vena cava • Made of silicone • Tunneled • Dacron cuff distal to exit site • Catheter tip is closed with 2-way valve • Single or multilumens • Does not require heparin lock because of valve	Long-term venous access (>30 days)	• Tape securely, especially during first 2 weeks of insertion until tissue adheres to cuff. • Avoid use of scissors near catheter. • Change injection cap at least weekly or when needed. • Flush with 10 cc normal saline after blood sampling and infusions.

continued ▸

Table A6   *Continued*

Type	Characteristics	Indications	Care/Maintenance Issues
Groshing (continued)	• Has blue stripe and transparent covering as distinguishing characteristics • These unique design features are also used for PICC made by this manufacturer		• Valve design eliminates need to flush with anticoagulant. • Repair according to manufacturer's guidelines.
Implanted Port	• Inserted in central vein • Tip terminates in superior vena cava • Usually made of silicone rubber • Port with self-sealing septum encased in titanium or plastic housing—usually implanted in infraclavicular fossa • Totally implanted beneath the skin • Accessed percutaneously with noncoring needle • Tunneled • Single or double lumen • Internal diameter ranges from 0.6–2.7 mm • Catheter may be preconnected to port, or attached at time of insertion • Catheter may be inserted via a peripheral vein before entering a central vein and the port would be found on the forearm; when catheter directly inserted into a chest vein port may be found on the chest	Long-term venous access (>30 days) may be most acceptable to patients concerned with body image	• Change noncoring needle weekly. • May use xylocaine spray or ice as anesthetic agent to reduce discomfort from port puncture. • Insert needle until it hits needle stop at back of port; do not rock needle from side to side in port. • Anchor needle carefully to prevent displacement. • Confirm needle placement before infusions by aspirating after slowly injecting 5 ml saline; have patient change position if there is no blood return as tip may be abutting vessel wall. • Flush after blood sampling and infusion with at least 10 ml saline. • Never forcibly flush port if resistance is felt (may dislodge thrombus or rupture catheter). • Flush with anticoagulant once a month when not in use. • Pump pressure not to exceed 40 psi. • Clamp tubing when solution is not infusing to prevent blood from occluding catheter. • Flow rates through port dependent on internal diameter and noncoring needle gauge.
PICC	• Inserted in the antecubital fossa, through the cephalic or basilic vein • Tip terminates in axillary vein, subclavian vein, or superior vena cava • Made of silicone, elastomeric hydrogel, or polymer • Nontunneled	Therapies lasting at least 10 days to 6 weeks, for patients who would be compromised by surgical central line placement.	• To prevent potential phlebitis, wash powdered gloves with saline or use forceps to handle catheter during insertion. • X-ray before use if tip terminates in superior vena cava. • Apply antimicrobial ointment to insertion site for first 24 hours. • Change dressing after first 24 hours.

continued ▶

Table A6 *Continued*

Type	Characteristics	Indications	Care/Maintenance Issues
PICC (*continued*)	• Catheter tip may have Groshong tip with closed 2-way valve • Single or double lumens • Length is dependent on anatomical measurement of patient, 33.5–60 cm • Internal diameter is 18–23 gauge • Introducer needle 15–22 gauge	Usual life of catheter is about 6 weeks, but catheters have remained in place for several months.	• Warm moist compresses 20 minutes 4 times daily in first 48 hours may prevent phlebitis. • Flush with at least 5 ml saline after blood sampling and infusions. • Use Luer-lock connections to prevent tubing disconnection. • Repair according to manufacturer's guidelines.

Appendix F

HIV Assessment Tool (HAT)

This questionnaire lists many symptoms, some of which are associated with HIV infection. Not every HIV-positive person experiences these symptoms, and the presence of these symptoms is not necessarily indicative of HIV infection. Please describe your current condition by answering each of the following questions.

Mark a vertical line through each of the lines below the question at the point that best shows what is happening to you at present (within the past week)—see the following example:

How do you feel?

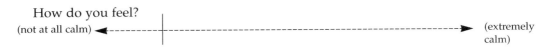

(not at all calm) ◄-------- | --► (extremely calm)

Now make your mark on the line following each question in order to answer the question.

General Symptoms

1. Have you lost any weight in the past 3 months?

   (No) ◄--► (≥20 lb)

2. Do you have white patches in your mouth?

   (No) ◄--► (All over my mouth)

3. Do you have pain in your mouth?

   (No) ◄--► (All the time)

4. Do you have diarrhea?

   (No) ◄--► (Many times a day)

5. Do you have headaches?

   (Constantly) ◄--► (No)

6. Are you dizzy?

   (No) ◄--► (All the time)

7. Do you have trouble remembering things?

   (Very forgetful) ◄--► (No)

8. Do you have difficulty sleeping?

   (No) ◄--► (Unable to sleep)

428

9. Do you have trouble with your vision?

(No) ◄--► (All the time)

10. Is your speech slurred?

(Always) ◄--► (No)

11. Do you have difficulty walking?

(No) ◄--► (Unable to walk)

12. Do you have weakness in your extremities?

(No) ◄--► (Very weak)

13. Do you have pains, numbness, or tingling?

(Severe pains) ◄--► (No)

14. Do you have any unusual bleeding, such as bruises?

(No) ◄--► (Every day)

15. Do you sweat at night?

(Every night) ◄--► (No)

16. Do you have fever(s)?

(Daily) ◄--► (No)

17. Do you have difficulty breathing?

(No) ◄--► (Unable to breathe)

18. Do you have a cough?

(Constant cough) ◄--► (No)

19. Do you feel tired?

(No) ◄--► (Always)

20. Do you have sores on your skin?

(No) ◄--► (All over my body)

21. Do you have a skin rash?

(No) ◄--► (All over my body)

22. Do you have lumps under your skin?

(In many places) ◄--► (No)

General Well-Being

23. Are you able to work at your usual tasks (job, housework)?

(No) ◀--▶ (Normal for me)

24. Is your appetite good?

(Normal for me) ◀--▶ (No)

25. Do you worry more?

(Normal for me) ◀--▶ (A great deal)

26. Do you go out socially?

(No) ◀--▶ (Normal for me)

27. Are you sexually satisfied?

(Normal for me) ◀--▶ (No)

28. Is your life satisfying?

(Normal for me) ◀--▶ (No)

29. Do you feel useful?

(Normal for me) ◀--▶ (No)

30. Is your family supportive of you?

(No) ◀--▶ (Normal for me)

31. Are your significant others supportive?

(Normal for me) ◀--▶ (No)

32. Are you lonely?

(Yes) ◀--▶ (Normal for me)

33. Do you feel hopeful about the future?

(Normal for me) ◀--▶ (No)

34. Have you noticed any changes in your private area?

(No) ◀--▶ (Many changes)

Note: From "Development of an HIV assessment tool," by K. Nokes, K. Wheeler, & J. Kendrew, 1994, *Image, 26,* 133–138. Used by permission.

Appendix G

Code for Nurses

1. The nurse provides services with respect for human dignity and the uniqueness of the client, unrestricted by considerations of social or economic status, personal attributes, or the nature of health problems.

2. The nurse safeguards the client's right to privacy by judiciously protecting information of a confidential nature.

3. The nurse acts to safeguard the client and the public when health care and safety are affected by the incompetent, unethical, or illegal practice of any person.

4. The nurse assumes responsibility and accountability for individual nursing judgments and actions.

5. The nurse maintains competence in nursing.

6. The nurse exercises informed judgment and uses individual competence and qualifications as criteria in seeking consultation, accepting responsibilities, and delegating nursing activities to others.

7. The nurse participates in activities that contribute to the ongoing development of the profession's body of knowledge.

8. The nurse participates in the profession's efforts to implement and improve standards of nursing.

9. The nurse participates in the profession's efforts to establish and maintain conditions of employment conducive to high quality nursing care.

10. The nurse participates in the profession's effort to protect the public from misinformation and misrepresentation and to maintain the integrity of nursing.

11. The nurse collaborates with members of the health professions and other citizens in promoting community and national efforts to meet the health needs of the public.

Note: From "Code for Nurses with Interpretive Statements," by American Nurses Association, 1985, Kansas City, MO. Reprinted with permission.

References

Adams, R., & Victor, M. (1993). Epilepsy and other seizure disorders. In *Principles of neurology* (5th ed., pp. 273–279). New York: McGraw-Hill.

AHCPR. (1994). *Evaluation and management of early HIV infection: Clinical practice guideline* (publication no. 94-0572). Rockville, MD: US Department of Health and Human Services.

AIDS 89 Summary: A practical synopsis of the fifth international conference. (1990). Philadelphia: Philadelphia Sciences Group.

AIDS Institute, NY State Department of Health. (1992). *Experimental treatments for HIV and AIDS.* New York: Author.

Amaro, H. (1993). Reproductive choice in the age of AIDS: Policy and counselling issues. In C. Squire (Ed.), *Women and AIDS — Psychological perspectives* (pp. 20–41). London: Sage.

American Nurses Association Committee on Ethics. (1985). *Code for nurses with interpretive statements.* Kansas City, MO: Author.

American Public Health Association. (1996, April). White House report points to need for more AIDS awareness among nation's youth. *The Nation's Health,* p. 5.

Anand, A., Carmosino, L., & Glatt, A. (1994). Evaluation of recalcitrant pain in HIV-infected hospitalized patients. *Journal of Acquired Immune Deficiency, 7,* 52–56.

Anderson, R., Grady, C., & Ropka, M. (1994). A comparison of calculated energy requirements to measured resting energy expenditure in HIV-1-infected subjects. *JANAC, 5*(6), 30–34.

Armstrong, D. (1995). Listeria monocytogenes. In G. Mandell, J. Bennett, & R. Dolin (Eds.), *Principles and practice of infectious diseases* (4th ed., pp. 1880–1885). New York: Churchill-Livingston.

Augustyniak, L., et al. (1990). *Regional seropositivity rates for HIV infection in patients with hemophilia.* Abstract presented at the Sixth International Conference on AIDS, San Francisco.

Balzer, J. (1992). The nursing process applied to family health promotion. In M. Stanhope & J. Lancaster (Eds.), *Community health nursing* (pp. 453–469). St. Louis, MO: Mosby Year Book.

Bartlett, J. (1994a). *Medical management of HIV infection.* Glenview, IL: Physicians & Scientists Publishing.

Bartlett, J. (l994b). *The Johns Hopkins Hospital guide to medical care of patients with HIV infection.* Baltimore: Williams & Wilkins.

Battin, M. (1994). Going early, going late: The rationality of decisions about suicide in AIDS. *Journal of Medicine and Philosophy, 19,* 571–594.

Bayer, S., & DeCherney, A. (1993). Clinical manifestations and treatment of dysfunctional uterine bleeding. *JAMA, 269,* 1823–1828.

Belshe, R., Clements, M., Dolin, R., Graham, B., Corey, L., Gorse, G., Schwartz, D., Keefer, M., Wagner, L., McElrath, J., et al. (1994). Interpretation of serodiagnostic tests for HIV in the 1990s: Impact of HIV vaccine studies in uninfected volunteers. *Annals of Internal Medicine, 272,* 475–480.

Bennett, M. (1990). Stigmatization: Experiences of persons with acquired immune deficiency syndrome. *Issues in Mental Health Nursing, 11,* 141–154.

Berger, B., & Vizgirda, V. (1993). Prevention of HIV infection in women and children. In F. Cohen & J. Durham (Eds.), *Women, children, and HIV/AIDS* (pp. 60–82). New York: Springer.

Berger, T. (1990). Dermatologic manifestations of HIV infection. In P. Cohen, M. Sande, and P. Volberding (Eds.), *The AIDS knowledge base* (5.3.1–25). Waltham, MA: Medical Publishing Group.

Berger, T. (1995). Dermatologic care in the AIDS patient. In M. Sande & P. Volberding (Eds.), *The medical management of AIDS* (4th ed., pp. 208–223). Philadelphia: Saunders.

Bernard, S. (1993). *HIV infection: A clinical manual* (2d ed., pp. 109–124). Boston: Little, Brown.

Berry, D. (1993). The emerging epidemiology of rural AIDS. *Journal of Rural Health, 9,* 293–304.

Bidlack, W., & Smith, C. (1984). The effect of nutritional factors on hepatic drug and toxicant metabolism. *Journal of the American Dietary Association, 84,* 892–898.

Bondmass, M. (1994). Cardiac manifestations of acquired immune deficiency syndrome and nursing implication. *Medical-Surgical Nursing, 3,* 42–48.

Borcich, A., & Kotler, D. (1991). Biology of HIV infection. In T. Allen-Mersh and L. Gottesman (Eds.), *Anorectal diseases in AIDS* (p. 313). London: Hodder and Stoughton.

Bouchard, P., Sui, P., Reach, G., et al. (1982). Diabetes mellitus following pentamidine-induced hypoglycemia in humans. *Diabetes, 31,* 40–45.

Boyer, P., Dillon, M., Navaie, M., et al. (1994). Factors predictive of maternal-fetal transmission of HIV-1. *JAMA, 271,* 1923–1930.

Bradley-Springer, L. (1994). Reproductive decision-making in the age of AIDS. *Image, 26,* 241–247.

Bramble, K. (1991). Body image. In I. Lubkin (Ed.), *Chronic illness: Impact and interventions* (2d ed., pp. 218–231). Boston: Jones and Bartlett.

Brown, M., & Powell-Cope, G. (1993). Times of loss and dying: Experiences of AIDS family caregivers. *Research in Nursing and Health, 16,* 179–191.

Buehler, J., Petersen, L., & Jaffe, H. (1995). Current trends in the epidemiology of HIV/AIDS. In M. Sande & P. Volberding (Eds.), *The medical management of AIDS* (4th ed., pp. 3–21). Philadelphia: Saunders.

Bureau of Justice Statistics. (1995a). *Prisoners in 1994* (NCJ-151654). Annapolis Junction, MD: Bureau of Justice Statistics Clearing House.

Bureau of Justice Statistics. (1995b). *HIV in prisons and jails, 1993* (NCJ-152765). Annapolis Junction, MD: Bureau of Justice Statistics Clearing House.

Calabrese, J., Kling, M., & Gold, P. (1987). Alterations in immunocompetence during stress, bereavement, and depression: Focus on neuroendocrine regulation. *American Journal of Psychiatry, 144,* 1123–1134.

Campbell, J. (1992). Violence against women. *Nursing and Health Care, 13,* 464–470.

Carpenito, L. (1993). *Nursing diagnosis: Application to clinical practice* (5th ed.). Philadelphia: Lippincott.

Carson, V. (1993). Prayer, meditation, exercise and special diets: Behaviors of the hardy person with HIV/AIDS. *JANAC, 4*(3), 18–28.

Catania, J., Coates, T., Golden, E., Dolcinic, M., Peterson, J., Kegeles, S., Siegel, D., & Fullilove, M. (1994). Correlates of condom use among black, Hispanic, and white heterosexuals in San Francisco: The AMEN longitudinal survey. *AIDS Education and Prevention, 6*(1), 12–26.

Cates, W., & Stone, K. (1992). Family planning, sexually transmitted diseases, and contraceptive choice: A literature update. *Family Planning Perspective, 24*(6), 75–84.

CDC. (1981). Kaposi's sarcoma and pneumocystis pneumonia among homosexual men—New York and California. *MMWR, 31,* 507–515.

CDC. (1982). Update on acquired immunodeficiency syndrome (AIDS) among patients with hemophilia. *MMWR, 31,* 48.

CDC. (1987). Update: Human immunodeficiency virus infections in health care workers exposed to blood of infected patients. *MMWR, 36,* 285–289.

CDC. (1990a). Possible transmission of HIV to a patient during an invasive dental procedure. *MMWR, 39,* 489–493.

CDC. (1990b). Public health service statement on management of occupational exposure to human immunodeficiency virus, including considerations regarding zidovudine post exposure use. *MMWR, 39*(RR-1), 1–14.

CDC. (1991a). The HIV epidemic: The first 10 years. *MMWR, 40,* 357–368.

CDC. (1991b). Premarital sexual experiences among adolescent women, United States, 1970–1988. *MMWR, 39,* 929–932.

CDC. (1992a). HIV infection in two brothers receiving intravenous therapy for hemophilia. *MMWR, 41,* RR-14.

CDC. (1992b). Update: Investigations of patients who have been treated by HIV infected health care workers. *MMWR, 41,* 344–346.

CDC. (1993a). HIV transmission between two adolescent brothers with hemophilia. *MMWR, 42,* RR-49.

CDC. (1993b). Update: Mortality attributable to HIV infection among persons aged 25–44 years, United States, 1991 and 1992. *MMWR, 42,* 870–872.

CDC. (1994a). 1994 Revised classification system for human immunodeficiency virus infection in children less than 13 years of age. *MMWR, 43,* No. RR-12.

CDC. (1994b). AIDS among racial/ethnic minorities—United States, 1993. *MMWR, 43,* 653–655.

CDC. (1994c). *HIV/AIDS Surveillance Report, 6*(2), 21.

CDC. (1994d). Recommendations of the US Public Health Service Task Force on the use of zidovudine to reduce perinatal transmission of HIV. *MMWR, 43,* RR-11.

CDC. (1994e). Zidovudine for the prevention of HIV transmission from mother to infant. *MMWR, 43,* 285–287.

CDC. (1995a). *AIDS information: Reported cases of AIDS and HIV infection in health care workers* (Document #320230). Atlanta, GA: Author.

CDC. (1995b). Case control study of HIV seroconversion in health-care workers after percutaneous exposure to HIV-infected blood—France, United Kingdom, and United States, January 1988–August 1994. *MMWR, 44,* 929–933.

CDC. (1995c). US HIV and AIDS cases reported through June 1995. *HIV/AIDS Surveillance Report, 7*(1), 15–16.

CDC. (1995d). *HIV/AIDS Surveillance Report, Year-end edition, 7*(2), 1–39.

CDC. (1995e). USPHS/IDSA guidelines for the prevention of opportunistic infections in persons infected with human immunodeficiency virus: A summary. *MMWR, 44*(RR-8), 1–33.

CDC. (1995f). USPHS recommendations for human immunodeficiency virus counseling and voluntary testing for pregnant women. *MMWR, 7*(RR-7), 7–15.

CDC. (1996). Update: Mortality attributable to HIV infection among persons aged 25–44 years—United States, 1994. *MMWR, 45*(6), 121–125.

Chamberland, M., & Bell, D. (1992). HIV transmission from HCW to patient. What is the risk? *Annals of Internal Medicine, 116,* 871–873.

Chang, R., Wong, G., Gold, J., & Armstrong, D. (1993). HIV-related emergencies: Frequency, diagnoses, and outcome. *Journal of General Internal Medicine, 6,* 465–469.

Chant, K., et al. (1993). Patient to patient transmission of HIV in private surgical consulting rooms. *Lancet, 342,* 1548–1549.

Cheitlin, M. (1994). Cardiac involvement in HIV disease. In P. Cohen, M. Sande, & P. Volberding (Eds.), *The AIDS knowledge base* (2d ed., pp. 5.14.1–14). Boston: Little, Brown.

Chernow, B., Schooley, R., Dracup, K., et al. (1990). Serum prolactin concentrations in patients with acquired immune deficiency syndrome. *Critical Care Medicine, 18,* 440–441.

Chiasson, R., Keraly, J., & Moore, R. (1995). Race, sex, drug use, and progression of human immunodeficiency virus disease. *New England Journal of Medicine, 333,* 751–756.

Chiasson, M., & Wright, T. (1995). HIV infection in women. In G. Mandel and D. Micovan (Eds.), *Atlas of infectious diseases (Vol. 1: AIDS)* (pp. 19.2–18). Philadelphia: Current Medicine, Inc.

Chin, J. (1994). The growing impact of the HIV/AIDS pandemic on children born to HIV-infected women. *Clinical Perinatology, 21,* 1–14.

Chlebowski, R., Grosvenor, M., Kruger, S., Tai, V., & Beall, G. (1993). Dietary intake, nutritional status, and immunologic function in patients with HIV infection [abstract Th.B.202]. *International Conference on AIDS 1990, 6,* 168.

Chu, Q., Medeiros, L., Fisher, A., Chaquette, R., & Crowley, J. (1995). Thrombotic thrombocytopenic purpura and HIV infection. *Southern Medical Journal, 88*(1), 82–86.

Chu, S., Ward, J., & Fleming, P. (1993, October). *Impact of the expanded AIDS surveillance definition on the ascertainment of HIV morbidity in women.* Abstract presented at the American Public Health Association 121st Annual Meeting, San Francisco.

Chu, S., & Wortley, P. (1995). Epidemiology of HIV/AIDS in women. In H. Minkoff, J. DeHovitz, & A. Duerr (Eds.), *HIV infection in women* (pp. 2 – 12). New York: Raven Press.

Chung, J., & Magraw, M. (1992). A group approach to psychosocial issues faced by HIV-positive women. *Hospital and Community Psychiatry, 43,* 891 – 894.

Ciesielski, C., Marianos, D., Ou, C., Dumbaugh, R., Witte, J., Berkelman, R., et al. (1992). Transmission of HIV in a dental practice. *Annals of Internal Medicine, 116,* 795 – 805.

Cohen, F., & Durham, J. (1993). *Women, children, and HIV/AIDS.* New York: Springer.

Cohen, F., & Durham, J. (Eds.). (1995). *Tuberculosis: A sourcebook for nursing practice.* New York: Springer.

Coker, R., Vivani, M., Gazzard, B., et al. (1993). Treatment of cryptococcis with liposomal amphotericin B (AmBisome) in 23 patients with AIDS. *AIDS, 7,* 829 – 835.

Colon, H., Sahai, H., Robles, R., & Matos, T. (1995). Effects of a community outreach program in HIV risk behaviors among injection drug users in San Juan, Puerto Rico: An analysis of trends. *AIDS Education and Prevention, 7,* 195 – 209.

Connor, E., Sperling, R., Gelber, R., Kiselev, P., Scott, G., O'Sullivan, M., et al. (1994). Reduction of maternal-infant transmission of human immunodeficiency virus type 1 with zidovudine treatment. *New England Journal of Medicine, 331,* 1173 – 1180.

Connor, R., & Ho, D. (1992). Etiology of AIDS: Biology of human retroviruses. In V. DeVita, S. Hellman, & S. Rosenberg (Eds.), *AIDS etiology, diagnosis, treatment and prevention* (pp. 13 – 38). Philadelphia: Lippincott.

COSSMHO (National Coalition of Hispanic and Human Services Organizations). (1991). *HIV/AIDS: The impact on Hispanics in selected states.* Washington, DC: Author.

Cousins, N. (1976). *Anatomy of an illness.* New York: Dutton.

Crandall, C., & Coleman, R. (1992). AIDS-related stigmatization and the disruption of social relationships. *Journal of Social and Personal Relationships, 9,* 163 – 177.

Cullen, B. (1993). An introduction to human retrovirus. In B. Cullen (Ed.), *Human retroviruses* (pp. 1 – 15). Oxford, England: Oxford University Press.

Curran, J., Jaffe, H., Hardy, A., Morgan, W., Selick, R., & Donders, T. (1988). Epidemiology of HIV Infection and AIDS in the United States. *Science, 239,* 610 – 616.

Curran, J., Jaffe, H., Hardy, A., Morgan, W., Selik, R., & Donders, T. (1988). Epidemiology of HIV infection and AIDS in the United States. *Science, 239,* 610 – 616.

Cu-Uvin, S., Warren, D., Mayer, K., Peipert, J., Anderson, J., Klein, R., Schoenbaum, E., Holmberg, S., Schuman, P., Vlahov, D., for HER Study Group. (1995, February 24). *Prevalence of genital tract infections in HIV seropositive women.* Presentation FC1-178 at HIV Infection in Women: Setting a New Agenda, Washington, DC.

Danielson, C., Hamel-Bissell, B., & Winstead-Fry, P. (1993). *Families, health & illness.* St. Louis, MO: Mosby Year Book.

De Cock, K. (1984). AIDS: An old disease from Africa? *British Medical Journal, 289,* 306 – 308.

DeHovitz, J. (1995). Natural history of HIV infection in women. In H. Minkoff, J. DeHovitz, & A. Duerr (Eds.), *HIV infection in women* (pp. 57 – 71). New York: Raven Press.

Denenberg, R. (1993). Gynecological considerations in the primary care setting. In A. Kurth (Ed.), *Until the cure: Caring for women with HIV* (pp. 34 – 46). New Haven: Yale University Press.

Department of Labor, Occupational Safety and Health Administration. (1991). Occupational exposure to bloodborne pathogens: Final rule. *Federal Register, 56,* 64004 – 182.

Des Jarlais, D. (1992). The harm reduction approach. *PAACNOTES, 4*(3), 149 – 150.

DiClemente, R. (1992). *Adolescents and AIDS: A generation in jeopardy.* Newbury Park, CA: Sage.

DiMaggio, S. (1993). State regulations and the HIV positive health care professional: A response to a problem that does not exist. *American Journal of Law and Medicine, 19,* 497 – 522.

Dimming the lights, carrying the flame. (1994, December 7). *Deaf Life.*

Dobs, A., Dempsey, M., Landeson, P., & Polk, B. (1988). Endocrine disorders in men infected with human immunodeficiency virus. *American Journal of Medicine, 84,* 611 – 616.

Dolnick, E. (1993). Deafness as culture. *Atlantic Monthly, 272*(3), 37 – 53.

Douglas, J., Buchbinder, S., Judson, F., & McKirnan, D. (1994). Participation of gay/bisexual men in preventive HIV vaccine trials: Baseline attitudes and concerns. *AIDS Research and Human Retroviruses, 10*(Suppl.2), S257 – S260.

Drew, W., Buhles, W., & Erlich, K. (1995). Management of herpes virus infections (CMV, HSV, VZV). In M. Sande & P. Volberding (Eds.), *The medical management of AIDS* (4th ed., pp. 512 – 536). Philadelphia: Saunders.

Dubler, N., & Sidel, V. (1991). AIDS and the prison system. In D. Nelkin, P. Willis, & S. Parris (Eds.), *A disease of society: Cultural and institutional responses to AIDS.* New York: Cambridge University Press.

Duesberg, P. (1991). AIDS epidemiology: Inconsistencies with human immunodeficiency virus and with infectious disease. *Proceedings of the National Academy of Science, 88,* 1575 – 1579.

Duliege, A., Messiah, A., Blanch, S., Tardieu, M., Griscelli, C., & Spira A. (1992). Natural history of human immunodeficiency virus type 1 infection in children: Prognostic value of laboratory tests on the bimodal progression of the disease. *Pediatric Infectious Diseases Journal, 11*, 630–635.

Durkheim, E. (1951). *Suicide*. Glencoe, IL: Free Press. Originally published in 1897.

Dworkin, B., Wormser, G., & Rosenthal, W. (1985). Gastrointestinal manifestations of the acquired immune deficiency syndrome: A review of 22 cases. *American Journal of Gastroenterology, 80*, 774–778.

Easterbrook, P., Chmiel, J., Hoover, D., Saah, A., Kaslow, R., Kinglsey, L., & Detels, R. (1993). Racial and ethnic differences in human immunodeficiency virus Type I (HIV-1) seroprevalence among homosexual and bisexual men. *American Journal of Epidemiology, 138*, 415–429.

Edgar, H., & Rothman, D. (1990). New rules for new drugs: The challenge of AIDS to regulatory process. *Millbank Quarterly, 68*(Suppl.1), 111–142.

Eeftinck-Schattenkerk, J., van Gool, T., van Ketel, R., et al. (1991). Clinical significance of small intestinal microsporidiosis in HIV-infected individuals. *Lancet, 337*, 859–868.

Eichold, S. (1995). HIV care in correctional facilities *Journal of Correctional Health Care, 2*, 111–112.

Elbeik, T., & Feinberg, M. (1994). HIV isolation and quantitation methods. In P. Cohen, M. Sande, & P. Volberding (Eds.), *The AIDS* knowledge base (2d ed., pp. 2.4.1–19). Boston: Little, Brown.

Ellerbrock, T., Wright, T., Bush, T., Dole, P., Brudney, &., & Chiasson, M. (1996). Characteristics of menstruation in women infected with human immunodeficiency virus. *Obstetrics and Gynecology*.

Ellerbrock, T., Wright, T., Rice, R., & Chiasson, M. (1995, February 24). *Genital tract infections in HIV-infected women.* Presentation FC1-180 at HIV Infection in Women: Setting a New Agenda. Washington, DC.

Ellis, R. (1988). New technologies for making vaccines. In S. Plotkin & E. Mortimer (Eds.), *Vaccines* (pp. 568–575). Philadelphia: Saunders.

Engstrom, J., Lowenstein, D., & Bredesen, D. (1989). Cerebral infarctions and transient neurologic deficits associated with acquired immune deficiency syndrome. *American Journal of Medicine, 86*, 528–532.

Erikson, E. (1958). *Young man Luther: A study in psychoanalysis and history.* New York: Norton.

Erikson, E. (1978). *Childhood and society* (2d ed.). New York: Norton.

Erlich, K., Safrin, S., & Mills, J. (1994). Herpes simplex virus. In P. Cohen, M. Sande, & P. Volberding (Eds.), *The AIDS knowledge base* (2d ed., pp. 6.12.1–19). Boston: Little, Brown.

Essex, M. (1992). Origin of AIDS. In D. DeVita, S. Hellman, & S. Rosenberg (Eds.), *AIDS etiology, diagnosis, treatment and prevention* (pp. 3–11). Philadelphia: Lippincott.

Essex, M., & Kanki, P. (1988). The origins of the AIDS virus. *Scientific American, 259*, 64–71.

European Collaborative Study. (1992). Risk factors for mother-to-child transmission of HIV-I infection. *Lancet, 339*, 1007–1012.

Fact sheet on HIV/AIDS and the deaf community (brochure). (1995). Los Angeles: AIDS Education/Services for the Deaf (AESD).

Faden, R., Geller, G., & Powers, M. (1992). *AIDS, women and the next generation.* New York: Oxford University Press.

Fast, P., Mathieson, B., & Schultz, A. (1994). Efficacy trials of AIDS vaccines: How science can inform ethics. *Current Opinion in Immunology, 6*, 691–697.

Fast, P., & Walker, M. (1993). Human trials of experimental AIDS vaccines. *AIDS, 7*(Suppl.1), S147–S159.

Fauci, A. (1984). Acquired immune deficiency syndrome: Epidemiologic, clinical, immunologic and therapeutic considerations. *Annals of Internal Medicine, 100*, 92–106.

Fauci, A. (1988). The human immunodeficiency virus: Infectivity and mechanisms of pathogenesis. *Science, 239*, 617–622.

FCCSET (Federal Coordinating Committee on Science, Engineering, and Technology). (1993). *Report of the working group on HIV vaccine development and international field trials.* Washington, DC: Author.

Feigal, E., Murphy, E., Vraniza, K., Bacchetti, P., Chiasson, R., Drummond, J., Blattner, W., McGrath, M., Greenspan, J., & Moss, A. (1991). Human T cell lymphotropic virus types I and II in intravenous drug users in San Francisco: Risk factors associated with seropositivity. *Journal of Infectious Diseases, 164*, 36–42.

Fischl, M., Fayne, T., & Flanagan, S. (1988). *Seroprevalence and risks of HIV infections in spouses of persons infected with HIV.* Abstract 4060 presented at the Fourth International Conference on AIDS, Stockholm, Sweden.

Fish, D., Ampel, N., Galgiani, M., et al. (1990). Coccidioidomycosis during human immunodeficiency virus infection: A review of 77 patients. *Medicine, 69*, 384–391.

Flaskerud, J. (1995). Psychosocial and psychiatric aspects. In J. Flaskerud & P. Ungvarski (Eds.), *HIV/AIDS: A guide to nursing care* (3d ed., pp. 308–338). Philadelphia: Saunders.

Fleisher, G. (1991). Epstein-Barr virus. In R. Belshe (Ed.), *Textbook of human virology* (2d ed., pp. 862–888). St. Louis, MO: Mosby Year Book.

Fletcher, R., Fletcher, S., & Wagner, E. (1988). *Clinical epidemiology: The essentials* (2d ed.). Baltimore: Williams & Wilkins.

Folkman, S., Chesney, M., Pollack, L., & Coates, T. (1993). Stress, control, coping, and depressive mood in human immunodeficiency virus-positive and -negative gay men in San Francisco. *Journal of Nervous and Mental Disease, 181*, 409–416.

Formenti, S., Gill, P., & Rarick, M. (1989). Primary central nervous system lymphoma in AIDS: Results of radiation therapy. *Cancer, 63*, 1101–1107.

Forthal, D., Gordon, R., Larsen, R., et al. (1992). Cigarette smoking increases the risk of developing crytococcal meningitis (abstract #Po B 3173). *International Conference on AIDS, 8:* B.115.

Frater, R. (1990). Surgical management of endocarditis in drug addicts and long-term results. *Journal of Cardiovascular Surgery, 5,* 63–67.

Frater, R., Sisto, D., & Condit, D. (1989). Cardiac surgery in human immunodeficiency virus (HIV) carriers. *European Journal of Cardio-Thoracic Surgery, 3,* 146–150.

Freidson, E. (1970). *Profession of medicine: A study of the sociology of applied knowledge.* New York: Dodd, Mead.

Freudenheim, E. (1996). *Healthspeak: A complete dictionary of America's health care system.* New York: Facts on File, Inc.

Fricke, W., et al. (1992). Human immunodeficiency virus infection due to clotting factor concentrates: Results of the Seroconversion Surveillance Project. *Transfusion, 32,* 8.

Fried, J., LoPresti, J., Micon, M., et al. (1980). Serum triiodythronine values: Prognostic indicators of acute mortality due to Pneumocystis carinii pneumonia associated with AIDS. *Annals of Internal Medicine, 110,* 970–975.

Friedman, M. (1992). *Family nursing: Theory and practice* (3d ed.). Norwalk, CT: Appleton & Lang.

Gallin, J. (1994). Quantitative and qualitative disorders of phagocytes. In K. Isselbacher, E. Braunwald, J. Wilson et al. (Eds.), *Harrison's principles of internal medicine* (13th ed., pp. 329–337). New York: McGraw-Hill.

Garner, J. (1996). Special report: Guideline for isolation precautions in hospitals. *Infection Control and Hospital Epidemiology, 17,* 53–80.

Garner, J., & Simmons, B. (1983). Guidelines for isolation precautions in hospitals. *Infection Control, 4*(Suppl.), 245–325.

Gayle, H., Keeling, R., Garica-Tunon, M., et al. (1990). Prevalence of the human immunodeficiency virus among university students. *New England Journal of Medicine, 323,* 1538–1541.

Gerberding, J. (1994). Incidence and prevalence of human immunodeficiency virus, hepatitis B virus, hepatitis C virus, and cytomegalovirus among health care personnel at risk for blood exposure: Final report from a longitudinal study. *Journal of Infectious Diseases, 170,* 1410–1417.

Gerberding, J. (1995). Management of occupational exposures to bloodborne viruses. *New England Journal of Medicine, 333,* 444–451.

Gerberding, J., & Henderson, D. (1992). Management of occupational exposures to bloodborne pathogens: Hepatitis B virus, hepatitis C virus and human immunodeficiency virus. *Clinical Infectious Diseases, 14,* 1179–1185.

Gift, A. (1989). Clinical measurement of dyspnea. *Dimensions of Critical Care Nursing, 8,* 210–216.

Ginzberg, H., Weiss, S., MacDonald, M., et al. (1985). HTLV-III exposure among drug users. *Cancer Research, 45*(Suppl.), 4605s–4608s.

Glick, M. (1994). Intraoral manifestations associated with HIV disease. In M. Glick (Ed.), *Dental management of patients with HIV disease* (pp. 153–182, 247–255). Chicago: Quintessence.

Goffman, E. (1963). *Stigma: Notes on the management of spoiled identity.* Englewood Cliffs, NJ: Prentice-Hall.

Goodman, D., Teplitz, E., & Wishner, A. (1987). Prevalence of cutaneous disease in patients with acquired immune deficiency syndrome (AIDS) or AIDS-related complex. *Journal of the American Academy of Dermatology, 17,* 210–220.

Goodman, J. (1989). Laughing matters: Taking your job seriously and yourself lightly. *Orthopedic Nursing, 8*(3), 11–13.

Graham, R., Forrester, M., Wysong, J., Rosenthal, T., & James, P. (1995). *HIV/AIDS in the rural United States: Epidemiology and health services delivery.* Rural Health Working Paper Series (No. 6). Buffalo, NY: New York Rural Health Research Center.

Greenberger, N. (1986). *Gastrointestinal disorders: A pathophysiological approach* (3d ed.). Chicago: Year Book Medical Publishers.

Greenblatt, R., Hilton, J., Palacio, H., Landers, D., Clanton, K., Cohen, J., Brosgart, C., Ameli, N., Wofsky, C., & Padian, N. (1995, February 24). *Prevalence of genital tract infections in HIV seropositive women.* Presentation FC1-177 at HIV Infection in Women: Setting a New Agenda, Washington, DC.

Grimes, D. (1994, Fall). Contraception, STDs, and risk-taking behavior: Highlights from a recent ARHP conference. *The Contraception Report,* pp. 4–7.

Grubman, S., & Oleske, J. (1995). HIV in infants, children and adolescents. In G. Wornser (Ed.), *A clinical guide to AIDS and HIV.* New York: Raven Press.

Guenter, P., Muurahainen, N., Simons, G., Kosok, A., Cohan, G., Rudenstein, R., & Turner, J. (1993). Relationships among nutritional status, disease progression, and survival in HIV infection. *Journal of AIDS, 6,* 1130–1138.

Gwinn, M., Wasser, S., Fleming, P., Karon, J., & Petersen, L. (1993, June). *Increasing prevalence of HIV infection among childbearing women, United States, 1989–1991.* Abstract presented at the Ninth International Conference on AIDS, Berlin.

Hadley, W. (1989). Infection of the health-care worker by HIV and other blood-borne viruses: Risk, protection and education. *American Journal of Hospital Pharmacy, 46*(Suppl. 3), S4–S7.

Hambleton, J. (1995). Hematologic manifestations of HIV infection. In M. Sande & P. Volberding (Eds.), *The medical management of AIDS* (4th ed., pp. 318–331). Philadelphia: Saunders.

Haseltine, W. (1992). The molecular biology of HIV-1. In V. DeVita, S. Hellman, & S. Rosenberg (Eds.), *AIDS etiology, diagnosis, treatment and prevention* (pp. 39–59). Philadelphia: Lippincott.

Havlir, D., & Ellner, J. (1995). Mycobacterium avium complex. In G. Mandell, J. Bennett, & R. Dolin (Eds.), *Principles and practice of infectious diseases* (4th ed., pp. 2250–2264). New York: Churchill-Livingstone.

Heidenreich, P., Eisenberg, M., Kee, L., Somelofski, C., Hollander, H., Schuller, M., & Cheitlin, M. (1993, June). *Pericardial effusion in HIV-positive patients: Incidence and survival.* Paper presented at Scientific Meeting of The American Society of Echocardiography, Orlando, FL.

Hellerstein, M. (1992). Pathophysiology of lean body wasting and nutrient unresponsiveness in HIV/AIDS: Therapeutic implications. *Nutrition in HIV/AIDS, 1,* 17–25.

Hellerstein, M. (1994). HIV-associated metabolic disturbances and body composition abnormalities: Therapeutic implications. *AIDSFILE, 8*(1), 1–4.

Herek, G., & Capitanio, J. (1993). Public reaction to AIDS in the United States: A second decade of stigma. *American Journal of Public Health, 83,* 574–577.

Hirschtick, R., Glassroth, J., Jordan, M., Wilcosky, T., Wallace, J., Kvale, P., Markowitz, N., Rosen, M., Mangura, B., Hopewell, P., & the Pulmonary Complications of HIV Infection Study Group. (1995). Bacterial pneumonia in persons infected with the human immunodeficiency virus. *New England Journal of Medicine, 333,* 845–851.

Hodel, D., & Franke-Ruta, G. (1991, Nov/Dec). Notes from the underground-crackup crackdown! *PWA Health Group Newsletter,* pp. 1–7.

Hollander, H. (1991). Neurologic and psychiatric manifestations of HIV disease. *Journal of General Internal Medicine, 6*(Suppl.), S24–S31.

Holman, S., & Kurth, A. (1995). HIV counseling and testing for women. In P. Kelly, S. Holman, R. Rothenberg, & S. Holzemer (Eds.), *Primary care of women and children with HIV infection* (pp. 149–173). Boston: Jones & Bartlett.

Hoyt, M., Nokes, K., Newshan, G., Staats, J., & Thorn, M. (1994). The effect of chemical dependency on pain perception in persons with AIDS. *JANAC, 4*(3), 33–38.

Hughes, M., Stein, D., Gundacker, H., Valentine, F., Phair, J., & Volberding, P. (1993). Within-subject variation in CD4 lymphocyte count in asymptomatic human immunodeficiency virus infection: Implications for patient monitoring. *Journal of Infectious Diseases, 169,* 28–36.

Hutchison, M., & Shannon, M. (1993). Reproductive health and counseling. In A. Kurth (Ed.), *Until the cure: Caring for women with HIV* (pp. 47–65). New Haven: Yale University Press.

International Association for the Study of Pain. (1979). Subcommittee on taxonomy of pain: A list of definitions and notes on usage. *Pain, 6,* 248–252.

Itescu, S. (1991). Diffuse infiltrate lymphocytosis syndrome in human immunodeficiency virus infection of Sjogren's-like disease. *Rheumatic Disease Clinics of North America, 17,* 99–115.

Janis, I. (1983). *Short-term counseling.* New Haven, CT: Yale University Press.

Johnson, L., Bachman, J., & O'Malley, P. (1992). *Data from the 1991 monitoring the future survey, Ann Arbor, University of Michigan.* Rockville, MD: National Institute on Drug Abuse.

Johnson, R. (1992). Family development. In M. Stanhope & J. Lancaster (Eds.), *Community health nursing* (pp. 431-449). St. Louis, MO: Mosby Year Book.

Johnston, F., Alistair, R., Bird, G., & Bjornsson, C. (1995). Immunohistochemical characterization of endometrial lymphoid cell populations in women with human immunodeficiency virus. *Obstetrics and Gynecology, 83,* 586–593.

Jones, E., Farina, A., Hastorf, A., Markus, H., Miller, D., Scott, R., with French, R. (1984). *Social stigma: The psychology of marked relationships.* New York: Freeman.

Jones, W., & Curran, J. (1994). Epidemiology of AIDS and HIV infection in industrialized countries. In S. Broder, T. Merigan, & D. Bolognesi (Eds.), *Textbook of AIDS medicine* (pp. 91–109). Baltimore: Williams & Wilkins.

Jonsen, A., & Stryker, J. (Eds.). Correction systems. In *The social impact of AIDS in the United States* (pp. 176–197). Chicago, IL: National Commission on Correctional Health Care.

Kapembwa, M., Fleming, S., Wells, C., Fiddian, P., Orr, M., & Griffin, G. (1991). Azidothymidine (AZT) absorption in AIDS-related small intestinal disease (SID) [abstract M.B. 2264]. *International Conference on AIDS, 7,* 248.

Kaplan, J., Masur, H., Holmes, K., McNeil, M., Schonberger, L., Navin, R., Hanson, D., Gross, P., & Jaffe, H. (1995). USPHS/IDSA guidelines for the prevention of opportunistic infections in persons infected with human immunodeficiency virus: Introduction and overview. *Clinical Infectious Diseases, 21*(Suppl. 1), S1–S31.

Kaplan, L., & Northfelt, D. (1995). Malignancies associated with AIDS. In M. Sande & P. Volberding (Eds.), *The medical management of AIDS* (4th ed., p. 561, table 28.3). Philadelphia: Saunders.

Kaplan, M. (1989). Human retroviruses: A common virology. *Transfusion Medicine Reviews, 3*(Suppl.1), 4–8.

Karzon, D. (1995). Potential for adverse reactions from HIV vaccines. In Office of Technology Assessment (Ed.), *Adverse reactions to HIV vaccines: Medical, ethical, legal issues* (pp. 27–63). Washington, DC: US Congress.

Karzon, D., Bolognesi, D., & Koff, W. (1992). Development of a vaccine for the prevention of AIDS, a critical appraisal. *Vaccine, 10,* 1039–1052.

Keat, A., & Rowe, I. (1991). Reiter's syndrome and associated arthritides. *Rheumatic Disease Clinics of North America, 17,* 25–42.

Keegan, L. (1988). The history and future of healing. In B. Dossey, L. Keegan, C. Guzzetta, & L. Kolkmeier (Eds.), *Holistic nursing: A handbook for practice* (pp. 56–76). Rockville, MD: Aspen.

Klein, R., Quart, A., & Small, C. (1991). Periodontal disease in heterosexuals with acquired immune deficiency syndrome. *Journal of Periodontology, 62,* 535–540.

Korn, A., Landers, D., Green, J., & Sweet, R. (1993). Pelvic inflammatory disease in immunodeficiency virus-infected women. *Obstetrics and Gynecology, 82,* 765–768.

Kotler, D., Tierney, A., Wang, J., & Pierson, R. (1989). Magnitude of body-cell-mass depletion and the timing of death from wasting in AIDS. *American Journal of Clinical Nutrition, 50,* 444–447.

Kramer, A., et al. (1990). *ACTU without walls.* Abstract presented at the Sixth International Conference on AIDS, San Francisco.

Kübler-Ross, E. (1969). *On death and dying.* New York: Macmillan.

Kuhn, L., Stein, Z., Thomas, P., Singh, T., & Tsai, W-Y. (1994). Maternal-infant HIV transmission and circumstances of delivery. *American Journal of Public Health, 84,* 1110–1115.

Kurth, A. (1993). *Until the cure: Caring for women with HIV.* New Haven, CT: Yale University Press.

LaMontagne, J., & Curlin, G. (1992). Vaccine clinical trials. In W. Koff & H. Six (Eds.), *Vaccine research and developments* (pp. 197–222). New York: Marcel Dekker.

Laryea, M., & Gien, L. (1993). The impact of HIV-positive diagnosis on the individual, Part 1. *Clinical Nursing Research, 2,* 245–263.

Last, J. (Ed.). (1988). *A dictionary of epidemiology.* New York: Oxford University Press.

Laurence, J. (1993). T-cell subsets in health, infectious disease, and idiopathic CD4+ T lymphocytopenia. *Annals of Internal Medicine, 119,* 55–62.

Lawlor, G., Fischer, T., & Adelman, D. (1995). *Manual of allergy and immmunology* (3d ed.). Boston: Little, Brown.

Lee, B. (1995). Drug interactions and toxicities in patients with AIDS. In M. Sande & P. Volberding (Eds.), *The medical management of AIDS* (4th ed., pp. 161–182). Philadelphia: Saunders.

Lee, B., & Täuber, M. (1994). Histoplasmosis. In P. Cohen, M. Sande, & P. Volberding (Eds.), *The AIDS knowledge base* (2d ed., pp. 6.9.1–7). Boston: Little, Brown.

Lego, S. (1994). *Fear and AIDS/HIV: Empathy and communication.* Albany, NY: Delmar Publications.

Lego, S. (1996). The client with HIV-infection. In S. Lego (Ed.), *Psychiatric nursing: A comprehensive reference* (pp. 338–344). Philadelphia: Lippincott.

Lerner, P. (1995). Nocardia species. In G. Mandell, J. Bennett, & R. Dolin (Eds.), *Principles and practice of infectious diseases* (4th ed., pp. 2273–2280). New York: Churchill-Livingston.

Lew, E., Dieterich, D., Poles, M., et al. (1995). Gastrointestinal emergencies in the patient with AIDS. *Critical Care Clnics, 11,* 531–560.

Li, Y., Tougas, G., Chiverton, S., & Hunt, R. (1992). The effect of acupuncture on gastrointestinal function and disorders. *American Journal of Gastroenterology, 87,* 1372–1381.

Lilienfeld, D., & Stolley, P. (1994). *Foundations of epidemiology* (3d ed.). New York: Oxford University Press.

Lindegren, M., Hanson, C., Miller, K., Bryers, R., & Onorata, T. (1994). Epidemiology of immunodeficiency virus infection in adolescents, United States. *Pediatric Infectious Disease Journal, 13,* 525–535.

Lindenmann, J. (1994). Duesberg on AIDS—Stretching our benevolence beyond its limits. *International Archives of Allergy and Applied Immunology, 103,* 128–130.

Loveland-Cherry, C. (1992). Issues in family health promotion. In M. Stanhope & J. Lancaster (Eds.), *Community health nursing* (pp. 470–483). St. Louis, MO: Mosby Year Book.

Loveless, M., Bell, L., & Coodley, G. (1993, June). *Pain associated with HIV disease and its complications.* Abstract WS-831-6 presented at the Ninth International Conference on AIDS, Berlin.

Lubeck, D., Bennett, C., Mazonson, P., et al. (1993). Quality of life and health service use among HIV-infected patients with chronic diarrhea. *Journal of AIDS, 6,* 478–484.

Lurie, P., Reingold, A., Bowser, B., et al. (1993). *The public health impact of needle exchange programs in the United States and abroad.* San Francisco: University of California Press.

Lurie, P., Bishaw, M., Chesney, M., Cooke, M., Fernandes, M., & Hearst, N. (1994). Ethical, behavioral, and social aspects of HIV vaccine trials in developing countries. *JAMA, 271,* 295–301.

Lyons, S., Jupp, P., & Schoub, B. (1986). Survival of HIV in the common bedbug (letter). *Lancet, 2*(8497), 45.

MacMahon, B., & Pugh, T. (1970). *Epidemiology: Principles and methods.* Boston: Little, Brown.

Mann, J., Tarantola, D., & Better, T. (1992). *AIDS in the world/The Global AIDS Policy Coalition.* Cambridge, MA: Harvard University Press.

Marcus, R., & the CDC Cooperative Needlestick Surveillance Group. (1988). Surveillance of health care workers exposed to blood from patients infected with HIV. *New England Journal of Medicine, 319,* 1118–1123.

Mascolini, M., & Chang, H. (1994). Tougher requirements ahead for accelerated drug approval? *Journal of the Physicians Association for AIDS Care, 1*(10), 6–9.

McCaffery, M. (1979). *Nursing management of the patient with pain.* Philadelphia: Lippincott.

McCain, N., & Gramling, L. (1992). Living with dying: Coping with HIV disease. *Issues in Mental Health Nursing, 13,* 271–284.

McGhee, P., & Goldstein, J. (Eds.) (1983). *Handbook of humor research.* New York: Springer.

McKay, E., & De Palma, F. (1991). *AIDS in the Hispanic community: An update.* Washington, DC: National Council of La Raza.

Meadows, J., et al. (1990). Voluntary HIV testing in the antenatal clinic: Differing uptake rates for individual counseling midwives. *AIDS Care, 2,* 229–233.

Melnick, S., Sherer, R., Louis, T., Hillman, D., Rodriguez, E., Lackman, C., Capps, L., Brown, L., Carlyn, M., Korvick, J., & Deyton, L. (1994). Survival and disease progression according to gender of patients with HIV infection. *JAMA, 272,* 1915–1921.

Membreno, Irany, I., Dere, W., et al. (1987). Adrenocortical function in acquired immune deficiency syndrome. *Journal of Clinical Endocrinal Metabolism, 65,* 482–487.

Miller, G. (1991). Molecular approaches to epidemiologic evaluation of viruses as risk factors for patients who have chronic fatigue syndrome. *Reviews of Infectious Diseases, 13*(Suppl.1), S119–S122.

Miller, S., Hohmann, E., & Pegues, D. (1995). Salmonella (including salmonella typhi). In G. Mandell, J. Bennett, & R. Dolin (Eds.), *Principles and practice of infectious diseases* (4th ed., pp. 2013–2032). New York: Churchill-Livingston.

Mitchell, J., Brown, G., Loftman, P., & Williams, S. (1990). HIV infection in pregnancy: Detection, counseling, and care. *Pediatric AIDS and HIV Infection: Fetus to Adolescent, 1,* 78–82.

Mofenson, L., & Wolinsky, S. (1992). Current insights regarding vertical transmission. In P. Pizzo & C. Wilfert (Eds.), *Pediatric AIDS: The challenge of HIV infection in infants, children, and adolescents* (2d ed., pp. 179–203). Baltimore: Williams & Wilkins.

Moffett, H., & Sanders, P. (1995). Identification of symptoms most responsive to Chinese medicine in AIDS care according to patient surveys. (Monograph). San Francisco: American College of Traditional Chinese Medicine Press.

Moffett, H., Sanders, P., Sinclair, T., & Ergil, K. (1994). Using acupuncture and herbs for the treatment of HIV infection: The American College of Traditional Chinese Medicine experience. *AIDS Patient Care, 8,* 194–199.

Moinpour, C., McCorkle, R., & Saunders, P. (1988). Measuring functional status. In M. Frank-Stromborg (Ed.), *Instruments for clinical nursing research* (pp. 23–46). Norwalk, CT: Appleton & Lange.

Moxon, E. (1995). Haemophilus influenzae. In G. Mandell, J. Bennett, & R. Dolin (Eds.), *Principles and practice of infectious diseases* (4th ed., pp. 2039–2045). New York: Churchill-Livingston.

Musher, D. (1995). Streptococcus pneumoniae. In G. Mandell, J. Bennett, & R. Dolin (Eds.), *Principles and practice of infectious diseases* (4th ed., pp. 1811–1826). New York: Churchill-Livingston.

Nabel, G. (1993). The role of cellular transcription factors in the regulation of human immunodeficiency virus gene expression. In B. Cullen (Ed.), *Human retroviruses* (pp. 49–73). Oxford, England: Oxford University Press.

Nahmias, A., Weiss, J., Yan, X., Lee, F., Kousi, R., Shanfield, M., Matthew, T., Bolognesi, D., Durack, D., Mofulsky, A., et al. (1986). Evidence for human infection with an HTLV III/LAV-like virus in Central Africa. *Lancet, 1,* 1279–1280.

National AIDS Clearinghouse. (1995). *Facts about HIV/AIDS and race/ethnicity* (Doc. # 293). Rockville, MD: CDC.

National Council of La Raza. (1992). *State of Hispanic America 1991: An overview.* Washington DC: Author.

Needlestick transmission of HTLV-III from a patient infected in Africa. (1984). *Lancet, 2,* 1376–1377.

Newshan, G., & Wainapel, S. (1993). Pain characteristics and their management in persons with AIDS. *JANAC, 4*(2), 53–59.

Nokes, K., Kendrew, J., & Longo, M. (1995). Alternative/complementary therapies used by persons with HIV disease. *JANAC, 6*(4), 19–24.

Nokes, K., Wheeler, K., & Kendrew, J. (1994). Development of an HIV assessment tool. *Image, 26,* 133–138.

Norman, C. (1985). AIDS virology: A battle on many fronts. *Science, 230,* 518–521.

Normand, J., Vlahov, D., & Moses, L. (Eds.). (1995). *Preventing HIV transmission: The role of sterile needles and bleach.* Washington, DC: National Academy Press.

North American Nursing Diagnosis Association. (1994). *Nursing diagnosis: Definitions and classifications.* Philadelphia: Author.

Novello, A. (1988). *Report of the secretary's work group on pediatric HIV infection and disease.* Washington, DC: US Department of Health and Human Services.

Obuch, M., Maurer, T., Bewcher, B., et al. (1992). Psoriasis and human immunodeficiency virus infection. *Journal of the American Academy of Dermatology, 27,* 667–673.

Olshevsky, M., Schlomo, N., Zwang, M., & Burger, R. (1989). *The manual of natural therapy: A practical guide to alternative medicine.* New York: Citadel Press.

Osei, K., Falk, J., Nelson, K., et al. (1984). Diabetogenic effect of pentamidine. *American Journal of Medicine, 77,* 41–46.

Otto, H. (1973). A framework for assessing family strengths. In A. Reinhardt & M. Quinn (Eds.). *Family-centered community nursing.* St. Louis, MO: Mosby.

Padian, N., Sluboski, S., & Jewell, N. (1991). The effect of number of exposures on the risk of heterosexual HIV transmission. *Journal of Infectious Diseases, 161,* 883–887.

Parrott, L. (1992). The psychology of humor. *Humanities Today, 12*(1), 12–13.

Pavlakis, G. (1992). Structure and function of the human immunodeficiency virus type 1. *Seminars in Liver Disease, 12,* 103–107.

Perry, S. (1990). Organic mental disorders caused by HIV: Update on early diagnosis and treatment. *American Journal of Psychiatry, 147,* 254–263.

Petersen, L., Doll, L., White, C., Chus, S., & the HIV Blood Donor Study Group. (1992). No evidence for female to female transmission among 96,000 female blood donors. *Journal of Acquired Immune Deficiency Syndromes, 5,* 853–855.

Pizzo, P., Butler, K., Balis, F., et al. (1990). Dideoxycytidine alone and in an alternating schedule with zidovudine in children with symptomatic human immunodeficiency virus infection. *Journal of Pediatrics, 117,* 799–808.

Planelles, V., Li, Q., & Chen, I. (1993). The biological and molecular basis for cell tropism in HIV. In B. Cullen (Ed.), *Human retroviruses* (pp. 17–48). Oxford, England: Oxford University Press.

Powell-Cope, G. (1995). The experiences of gay couples affected by HIV infection. *Qualitative Health Research, 5*(1), 36–62.

Powell-Cope, G., & Brown, M. (1992). Going public as an AIDS family caregiver. *Social Science & Medicine, 34,* 571–580.

Pursell, K., Telzak, E., & Armstrong, D. (1992). Aspergillus species colonization and invasive disease in patients with AIDS. *Clinical Infectious Diseases, 14,* 141–148.

Rabinowitz, N. (1987). Acupuncture and other adjunctive therapy in the treatment of the acquired immune deficiency syndrome. *American Journal of Acupuncture, 15,* 35–42.

Ragni, M., et al. (1991). The natural history of HIV infection in hemophilia. *Hemophilia and von Willebrand Disease in the 1990s* (p. 383). Amsterdam: Excerpta Medica.

Reed, P. (1992). An emerging paradigm for the investigation of spirituality in nursing. *Research in Nursing and Health, 15,* 349–357.

Reillo, M. (1993). Hyperbaric oxygen therapy for the treatment of debilitating fatigue associated with HIV/AIDS. *JANAC, 4*(3), 33–38.

Rico, G. (1991). *Pain and possibility.* New York: Perigree Books.

Rogers, M. (1988). Pediatric HIV transmission. *Pediatric Annals, 17,* 324–331.

Rold, J. (1995). Inmates participation in research: The regulatory framework. *Correct Care, 9*(2), 7–10.

Rosenberg, P. (1984). Support groups: A special therapeutic entity. *Small Group Behavior, 15,* 173–186.

Rosenberg, Z., & Fauci, A. (1991). Immunopathogenesis of HIV infection. *FASEB Journal, 5,* 2382–2387.

Sadick, N., McNutt, N., & Kaplan, M. (1990). Papulosquamous dermatoses of AIDS. *Journal of the American Academy of Dermatology, 22,* 1270–1277.

Saag, M., Crain, M., & Decker, W. (1991). High-level viremia in adults and children infected with human immunodeficiency virus: Relation to disease stage and CD4+ lymphocyte levels. *Journal of Infectious Diseases, 164,* 72–80.

Sande, M., & Volberding, P. (1995). *The medical management of AIDS* (4th ed.). Philadelphia: Saunders.

Sanford, J., Sande, M., & Gilbert, D. (1995). *The Sanford guide to HIV/AIDS therapy.* Vienna, VA: Antimicrobial Therapy, Inc.

Schambelan, M., & Grunfeld, C. (1995). Endocrinologic manifestations of HIV infection. In M. Sande & P. Volberding (Eds.), *The medical management of AIDS* (4th ed., pp. 343–357). Philadelphia: Saunders.

Schecter, G. (1994). *Mycobacterium tuberculosis* infection. In P. Cohen, M. Sande, & P. Volberding (Eds.), *The AIDS knowledge base* (2d ed., pp. 6.5.1–6). Boston: Little, Brown.

Schecter, W. (1991). Examination of the anus and rectum in the HIV infected patient. In T. Allen-Mersh & L. Gottesman (Eds.), *Anorectal diseases in AIDS* (pp. 75–87). London: Hodder and Stoughton.

Scherer, Y., Haughey, B., Wu, Y., & Kuhn, M. (1992, October). AIDS: What are critical care nurses' concerns? *Critical Care Nurse,* 23–29.

Schneider, J., & Conrad, P. (1980). In the closet with illness: Epilepsy, stigma potential and information control. *Social Problems, 28,* 32–44.

Schoenfeld, P., & Feduska, N. (1990). Acquired immunodeficiency syndrome and renal disease: Report of the National Kidney Foundation—National Institutes of Health Task Force on AIDS and Kidney Disease. *American Journal of Kidney Disease, 16,* 14–25.

Schofferman, J. (1988). Pain: Diagnosis and management in the palliative care of AIDS. *Journal of Palliative Care, 4,* 46–49.

Schram, N. (1990). Refining safer sex. *Focus, 5,* 3–4.

Schultz, A., & Hu, S. (1993). Primate models for HIV vaccines. *AIDS, 7*(Suppl.1), S161–S170.

Selik, R., Castro, K., & Pappaioanou, M. (1988). Racial/ethnic differences in the risk of AIDS in the United States. *American Journal of Public Health, 78,* 1539–1545.

Selik, R., Castro, K., & Pappaioanou, M. (1989). Birthplace and the risk of AIDS among Hispanics in the United States. *American Journal of Public Health, 79,* 836–839.

Shah, P., Smith, J., Wells, C., Barton, S., Kitchen, V., & Steer, P. (1994). Menstrual symptoms in women infected by the human immunodeficiency virus. *Obstetrics and Gynecology, 83,* 397–400.

Shannon, M. (1994, May). *Presentation on HIV in women.* American College of Nurse-Midwives Annual Meeting. Nashville, TN.

Shepp, D., Tang, L., Raumando, M., & Kaplan, M. (1994). Serious *Pseudomonas aeruginosa* infection in AIDS. *Journal of AIDS, 7,* 823–831.

Siegel, K., & Krauss, B. (1991). Living with HIV infection: Adaptive tasks of seropositive gay men. *Journal of Health and Social Behavior, 32,* 17–32.

Singer, E., Zorilla, C., Fahy-Chandon, B., Chi, S., Syndulko, K., & Tourtellotte, W. (1993). Painful symptoms reported by HIV-infected men in a longitudinal study. *Pain, 54,* 15–19.

Singh, S., Fermie, O., & Peters, W. (1992, July). *Symptom control for individuals with advanced HIV in a suacute residential unit: Which symptoms need palliation?* Abstract PoB5248 presented at the Eighth International Conference on AIDS, Amsterdam.

Smith, M. (1988). AIDS: Results of Chinese medical treatment show frequent symptom relief and some apparent long-term remissions. *American Journal of Acupuncture, 16,* 105–112.

Sonenstein, F., Pleck, J., & Ku, L. (1989). Sexual activity, condom use, and AIDS awareness among adolescent males. *Family Practice Perspective, 21,* 152–158.

Springer, E. (1992). Effective AIDS prevention with active drug users: The harm reduction model. In M. Shernoff (Ed.), *Counseling chemically dependent people with HIV illness.* New York: Haworth Press.

Stahl-Bayliss, C., Kalman, C., & Laskin, O. (1986). Pentamidine-induced hypoglycemia in patients with AIDS. *Clinical Pharmacologic Therapy, 34,* 271–275.

Stanley, H., Charlebois, E., Harb, G., & Jacobson, M. (1993). Central venous catheter infections in AIDS patients receiving treatment for cytomegalovirus disease. *Journal of AIDS, 7,* 272–278.

Stansell, J., & Murray, J. (1994). Pulmonary complications of human immunodeficiency virus infection. In J. Murray & J. Nadel (Eds.), *Textbook on respiratory medicine* (2d ed., pp. 2333–2367). Philadelphia: Saunders.

Steffe, E., King, J., Inciardi, J., Flynn, N., Goldstein, E., Tonjes, T., & Benet, L. (1990). The effects of acetaminophen on zidovudine metabolism in HIV-infected patients. *Journal of Acquired Immune Deficiency Syndrome, 3,* 691–694.

Stein, D. (1992). *The natural remedy book for women.* Freedom, CA: Crossing Press.

Stein, Z. (1995). More on women and the prevention of HIV infection. *American Journal of Public Health, 83,* 1485–1487.

Steinhart, R., Reingold, A., Taylor, F., Anderson, G., & Wenger, J. (1992). Invasive *Haemophilus influenzas* infection in men with HIV infection. *JAMA, 268,* 3350–3352.

Stevens, J., Zierler, S., Dean, D., Goodman, A., Chalfern, B., & DeGroot, A. (1995). Prevalence of prior sexual abuse and HIV risk-taking behaviors in incarcerated women in Massachusetts. *Journal of Correctional Health Care, 2,* 137–149.

Stine, G. (1993). *Acquired immune deficiency syndrome: Biological, medical, social, and legal issues.* Englewood Cliffs, NJ: Prentice-Hall.

St. Mary's Medical Center. (1993). *HIV review.* San Francisco: Author.

Stoeckle, M. (1995). Human herpesvirus 6 and human herpesvirus 7. In G. Mandell, J. Bennett, & R. Dolin (Eds.), *Principles and practice of infectious diseases* (4th ed., pp. 1317–1379). New York: Churchill Livingstone)

Stricker, R. (1991). Hemostatic abnormalities in HIV disease. *Hematology/Oncology Clinics of North America, 5,* 249–265.

Sunderland, A., Minkoff, H., Handte, J., Moroso, G., & Landesman, S. (1992). The impact of serostatus on women's reproductive decisions. *Obstetrics & Gynecology, 79,* 1027–1031.

Tami, T., & Lee, K. (1994). Otolaryngologic manifestations of HIV disease. In P. Cohen, M. Sande, & P. Volberding (Eds.), *The AIDS knowledge base* (2d ed., pp. 5.29.1–25). Boston: Little, Brown.

Tang, W., & Kaplan, E. (1989). Thyroid hormone levels in the acquired immune deficiency syndrome (AIDS) or AIDS-related complex. *Western Journal of Medicine, 151,* 627–631.

Task Force on Nutrition Support in AIDS. (1989). Guidelines for nutrition support in AIDS. *Nutrition, 5*(1), 39–46.

Tokars, J., Marcus, R., Culver, D., Schable, C., McKibben, P., Bandea, C., & Bell, D. (1993). Surveillance of HIV infection and zidovudine use among health care workers after occupational exposure to HIV infected blood. *Annals of Internal Medicine, 118,* 913–918.

Trussell, J., Jatcher, R., Cates, W., Stewart, F., & Kost, K. (1991). Contraceptive failure rates in the United States: An update. *Study of Family Planning, 21*(4), 51–54.

Van Biema, D. (1994, April 4). Silence really does equal death: AIDS. *Time,* pp. 76–77.

van der Pijl, H., & Frissen, P. (1992). Experience with a totally implantable venous access device (port-a-cath) in patients with AIDS. *AIDS, 6,* 709–713.

Vannucci, A., Nardi, G., Cargnel, A., Tocalli, L., Rech, R., & Rapati, D. (1993). Prevalence rate of infective pathogen agents on cultured central venous catheters in AIDS patients. *International Conference on Aids, 9,* 313.

Vilaliano, P., Russo, J., Young, H., Becker, J., & Maiuro, R. (1991). The screen for caregiver burden. *Gerontologist, 31*(1), 76–83.

Vilaliano, P., Young, H., Russo, J. (1991). Burden: A review of measures used among caregivers of individuals with dementia. *Gerontologist, 31*(1), 67–75.

Vitting, K., Gardenswartz, M., Zabetakis, P., Trapper, M., Gleim, G., Agawal, M., & Michelis, M. (1990). Frequency of hyponatremia and nonosmolar vasopressin release in the acquired immunodeficiency syndrome. *JAMA, 263,* 973–978.

Walker, M., & Fast, P. (1994). Clinical trials of candidate AIDS vaccines. *AIDS, 8*(Suppl.1), S213–S236.

Wallace, J., Rao, A., Glassroth, J., et al. (1993). Respiratory illness in persons with human immunodeficiency virus infection. *American Review of Respiratory Disease, 148,* 1523–1529.

Waskin, H., Stohr-Green, J., Helmick, C., & Sattler, F. (1988). Risk factor for hypoglycemia associated with pentamidine therapy for pneumocystis pneumonia. *JAMA, 260,* 345–347.

Wasser, S., Gwinn, M., & Fleming, P. (1993). Urban-non urban distribution of HIV infection in childbearing women in the United States. *Journal of Acquired Immune Deficiency Syndromes, 6,* 1035–1042.

Weber, J. (1984). Is AIDS an epidemic form of African Kaposi's sarcoma? Discussion paper. *Journal of the Royal Society of Medicine, 77,* 575–576.

Weiner, D. (1992). Insights into HIV infection and pathogenesis. *Pathobiology, 60,* 177–180.

Weitz, R. (1990). Living with the stigma of AIDS. *Qualitative Sociology, 13*(1), 23–38.

Wexner, S., Smithy, W., Milsom, J., & Dailey, T. (1986). The surgical management of anorectal disease in AIDS and pre-AIDS patients. *Diseases of the Colon and Rectum, 29,* 719–723.

Wilber, J. (1994). HIV-antibody testing: Methodology. In P. Cohen, M. Sande, & P. Volberding (Eds.), *The AIDS knowledge base* (2d ed., pp. 2.2.1–9). Boston: Little, Brown.

Wilkes, G. (1995). *Cancer and HIV: Clinical nutrition pocket guide.* Boston: Jones & Bartlett.

Williams, A. (1990). Reproductive concerns of women at risk for HIV infection. *Journal of Nurse-Midwifery, 35,* 292–298.

Wilson, H., & Kneisl, C. (1996). *Psychiatric nursing* (5th ed.). Menlo Park, CA: Addison-Wesley.

Witkin, S. (1990). Sensitization to sperm as a risk factor for the heterosexual transmission of HIV. In N. Alexander, H. Gabelnick, & J. Spieler (Eds.), *Heterosexual transmission of AIDS* (pp. 205–212). New York: Wiley-Liss.

Wolkimor, A., Barone, J., Hardy, H., & Cotton, J. (1990). Abdominal and anorectal surgery and the acquired immune deficiency syndrome in heterosexual drug users. *Diseases of the Colon and Rectum, 33,* 267–270.

Working Group on Antiretroviral Therapy, National Pediatric HIV Resource Center. (1993). Antiretroviral therapy and medical management of the human immunodeficiency virus infected child. *Pediatric Infectious Disease Journal, 12,* 513–522.

Wright, D., Lennox, J., James, W., et al. (1991). Generalized chronic dermatophytosis in patients with human immunodeficiency virus type 1 infection and CD4 depletion. *Archives of Dermatology, 127,* 265–266.

Wright, T., Ellerbrock, T., Chiasson, M., Van deVanter, N., Sun, X., & The New York Cervical Disease Study. (1994). Cervical intraepithelial neoplasia in women infected with human immunodeficiency virus: Prevalence, risk factors, and validity of Papanicolaou smears. *Obstetrics and Gynecology, 84,* 586–593.

Young, F., Norris, J., Levitt, J., & Nightingale, S. (1988). The FDA's new procedures for the use of investigational drugs in treatment. *JAMA, 259,* 2267–2270.

Bibliography

Abbey, J., & Close, L. (1979). A study of control of shivering during hypothermia. *Communicating Nursing Research, 12,* 2–3.

Aboulafia, D., & Mitsuyasu, R. (1991). Hematologic abnormalities in AIDS. *Hematology/Oncology Clinics of North America, 5,* 195–214.

Ada, G., Blanden, B., & Milbacher, A. (1992). HIV: To vaccinate or not to vaccinate? *Nature, 359,* 572.

Adall, K., Cockerell, C., & Petrie, W. (1994). Cat scratch disease, bacillary angiomatosis, and other infections due to rochalimaea. *New England Journal of Medicine, 330,* 1509–1515.

AHCPR. (1992). *Acute pain management: Operative or medical procedures and trauma* (publication no. 92-0043). Rockville, MD: U.S. Department of Health and Human Services.

AHFS Drug Information. (1995). Bethesda, MD: American Society of Hospital Pharmacists.

AIDS Action Foundation Working Group. (1994, April). *HIV preventive vaccines: Social, ethical, and political considerations for domestic efficacy trials.* Washington, DC: Author.

Airhihenbuwa, C., DiClemente, R., Wingood, G., & Lowe, A. (1992). HIV/AIDS Education and Prevention among African Americans: A focus on culture. *AIDS Education and Prevention, 4,* 267–273.

Albrecht, H., & Stellbrink, H. (1994). Hiccups in people with AIDS. *Journal of AIDS, 7,* 735.

Albrecht, G., Walker, V., & Levy, J. (1982). Social distance from the stigmatized: A test of two theories. *Social Science and Medicine, 16,* 1319–1327.

American College of Physicians. (1994). Position Paper: Human immunodeficiency virus (HIV) infection. *Annals of Internal Medicine, 120,* 310–319.

American Nurses Association. (1993). *Peer support for the HIV positive nurse.* Washington, DC: Author.

American Nurses Association. (1994). *Nursing and HIV/AIDS.* Washington, DC: Author.

American Psychiatric Association. (1994). *Diagnostic and statistical manual* (4th ed. rev.). Washington, DC: Author.

Annas, G. (1990). Faith (healing), hope, and charity at the FDA: The politics of AIDS drug trials. In L. Gostin (Ed.), *AIDS and the health care system* (pp. 183–196). New Haven: Yale University Press.

Arno, P., & Feiden, K. (1992). *Against the odds: The story of AIDS drug development.* New York: HarperCollins.

Barrett, E. (1983). *An empirical investigation of Martha E. Rogers principle of helicy: The relationship of human field motion and power.* Unpublished Doctoral Dissertation. New York University.

Barrick, B., Berkebile, C., Cuda, S., Govoni, L., Grady, C., Hahn, B., Rosenthal, Y., Sears, N., & Megill, M. (1988, April). *Motivations of persons volunteering for an AIDS vaccine trial.* Abstract 6575 presented at the Fourth International Conference on AIDS, Stockholm, Sweden.

Bartlett, J. (1990). *Pocketbook of infectious disease therapy.* Baltimore: Williams & Wilkins.

Bartlett, J., & Finkbeiner, A. (1991). *The guide to living with HIV infection.* Baltimore: Johns Hopkins University Press.

Baumann, S. (1993). Problems in the mental health assessment of persons with HIV. *JANAC, 4*(4), 36–43.

Bayer, R. (1993). The ethics of blinded HIV surveillance testing. *American Journal of Public Health, 83,* 496–497.

Bayer, R. (1994). Ethical challenges posed by zidovudine treatment to reduce vertical transmission of HIV. *New England Journal of Medicine, 331,* 1223–1225.

Bayer, R. (1995). AIDS, ethics, and activism. In R. Bluger, E. Bobby, & Fineberg, H. (Eds.), *Society's choices: Social and ethical decision making in biomedicine* (pp. 458–476). Washington, DC: National Academy Press.

Bayer, R., Levine, C., & Wolf, S. (1986). HIV antibody screening: An ethical framework for evaluating proposed programs. *JAMA, 256,* 1768–1774.

Beach, R. (1993). Appetite and anorexia. *PAACNOTES,* 413–416,434.

Beauchamp, T., & Childress, J. (1994). *Principles of biomedical ethics* (4th ed.) New York: Oxford University Press.

Beck, A., Rush, A., Shaw, B., & Emery, G. (1979). *Cognitive therapy of depression.* New York: Guilford Press.

Beckett, A., & Rutan, J. (1990). Treating people with ARC and AIDS in group psychotherapy. *International Journal of Group Psychotherapy, 40,* 19–28.

Belkin, G., Fleishman, J., Stein, M., Piette, J., & Mor, V. (1992). Physical symptoms and depressive symptoms among individuals with HIV infection. *Psychosomatics, 33,* 416–427.

Bellanti, J., Kadlec, J., & Escobar-Gutiérrez, A. (1994). Cytokines and the immune response. *Clinical Immunology, 41*(4), 597–621.

Benditt, J. (1995). Conduct in science. *Science, 268,* 1705–1718.

Biegel, D., Sales, E., & Schulz, R. (1991). *Family caregiving in chronic illness.* Newbury Park, CA: Sage.

Biwas, P., Poli, G., Orenstein, J., & Fauci, A. (1994). Cytokine-mediated induction of human immunodeficiency virus (HIV) expression and cell death in chronically infected U1 cells: Do tumor necrosis factor alpha and gamma interferon selectively kill HIV-infected cells? *Journal of Virology, 68*(4), 2598–2604.

Bjune, G., & Gedde-Dahl, T. (1993). Some problems related to risk-benefit assessments in clinical trials of new vaccines. *IRB: A Review of Human Subjects Research, 15*(1), 1–5.

Blaser, M. (1995). Campylobacter species. In G. Mandell, J. Bennett, & R. Dolin (Eds.), *Principles and practice of infectious diseases* (4th ed., pp. 1947–1956). New York: Churchill-Livingston.

Block's ethnic/cultural assessment guide. (1991). In C. Helvie (Ed.), *Community health nursing: Theory and practice* (pp. 332–340). New York: Springer.

Bolognesi, D. (1991). AIDS vaccines: Progress and unmet challenges. *Annals of Internal Medicine, 114,* 161 – 162.

Borkowski, W., Krasinski, K., Pollack, H., Hoover, W., Karl, A., & Ilmet-Moore, T. (1992). Early diagnosis of HIV infection in children under 6 months of age: A comparison of polymerase chain reaction, culture, and plasma antigen capture techniques. *Journal of Infectious Diseases, 166,* 616 – 619.

Borrow, P., Lewicki, H., Hahn, B., Shaw, G., & Oldstone, M. (1994). Virus-specific CD8+ cytotoxic T-lymphocyte activity associated with control of viremia in primary human immunodeficiency virus type 1 infection. *Journal of Virology, 68,* 6103 – 6110.

Breda, S., Gigliotti, F., Hammerschlag, P., & Schiella, R. (1988). Pneumocystis carinii in the temporal bone as a primary manifestation of the acquired immune deficiency syndrome. *Annals of Otology Rhinology Laryngology, 97,* 427 – 431.

Brennan, B. (1988). *Hands of light.* New York: Bantam.

Brensilver, J., & Goldberger, E. (1996). *A primer of water, electrolyte, and acid-base syndromes* (8th ed.). Philadelphia: F. A. Davis.

Brinson, R. (1985). Hypoalbuminemia, diarrhea, and the acquired immune deficiency syndrome. *Annals of Internal Medicine, 102,* 413.

Brown, M., & Powell-Cope, G. (1991). AIDS family caregiving: Transitions through uncertainty. *Nursing Research, 40,* 338 – 345.

Bryant, R. (1992). Acute and chronic wounds. *Nursing management.* St. Louis, MO: Mosby.

Cabaj, R. (1994). Assessing suicidality in the primary care setting. *AIDS File, 8*(4), 7 – 9.

Cain, R. (1991). Relational contexts and information management among gay men. *Families in Society, 72,* 344 – 352.

Cain, J., & Amend, W. (1993). Esophagitis causing intractable hiccups. *Annals of Internal Medicine, 119,* 249.

Callery, M., Culhane, B., Francis, C., Harrington, P., Pavel, J., & Snyder, E. (1990). *Transfusion therapy guidelines for nurses.* National Blood Resource Education Program, National Heart Lung and Blood Institute, NIH Publication No. 90-2668.

Cameron, D., Simonsen, J., & D'Costa, L. (1989). Female-to-male transmission of the human immunodeficiency virus type I: Risk factors for seroconversion in men. *Lancet, 36,* 593.

Cameron, M. (1993). *Living with AIDS: Experiencing ethical problems.* Newbury Park, CA: Sage.

Cameron, M., Crisham, P., & Lewis, D. (1993). The nature of ethical problems experienced by persons with acquired immune deficiency syndrome: Implications for nursing ethics education and practice. *Journal of Professional Nursing, 9,* 327 – 330.

Carlson, R., & Shield, B. (Eds.). (1989). *Healers on healing.* New York: Perigree.

Carson, V., Soeken, K., Shanty, T., & Terry, L. (1990). Hope and spiritual well-being: Essentials for living with AIDS. *Perspectives in Psychiatric Care, 26*(2), 28 – 34.

Carter, L. (1993). Influences of nutrition and stress on people at risk for neutropenia: Nursing implications. *Oncology Nursing Forum, 20,* 1241 – 1250.

Carwein, V., & Berry, D. (1992). HIV issues for rural hospitals in U.S. frontier areas. *Journal of Rural Health, 8,* 221 – 226.

Caruso, C., Hadley, B., Shukla, R., Frame, P., & Khoury, J. (1992). Cooling effects and comfort of four cooling blanket temperatures in humans with fever. *Nursing Research, 41,* 68 – 72.

Catania, A., Airaghi, L., Manfredi, M., Vivirito, M., Milazzo, F., Lipton, J., & Zanussi, C. (1993). Proopiomelanocortin-derived peptides and cytokines: Relations in patients with acquired immunodeficiency syndrome. *Clinical Immunology and Immunopathology, 66*(1), 73 – 79.

CDC. (1987a). Recommendations for the prevention of HIV transmission in health-care settings. *MMWR, 38*(2S), 1S – 17S.

CDC. (1987b). Revision of the CDC surveillance case definition for acquired immunodeficiency syndrome. *MMWR, 36*(1S).

CDC. (1992a). 1993 revised classification system for HIV infection and expanded surveillance case definition for AIDS among adolescents and adults. *MMWR, 41,* RR-17.

CDC. (1992b). Childbearing and contraception: Women at risk for HIV infection. Selected sites. *MMWR, 41,* 135 – 144.

CDC. (1994). Update: Trends in AIDS diagnosis and reporting under the expanded surveillance definition for adolescents and adults, 1993. *MMWR, 43,* 826 – 831.

CDC. (1995a). 1995 revised guidelines for prophylaxis against *P. carinii* pneumonia for children infected with or perinatally exposed to HIV. *MMWR, 44,* RR-4.

CDC. (1995b). Update: AIDS among women—United States, 1994. *MMWR, 44,* 81 – 84.

Center for Population Options. (1991). *National school condom availability campaign and clearinghouse.* Washington, DC: Author.

Chantilly Report. (1994). *Alternative medicine: Expanding medical horizons.* A report to the National Institutes of Health on alternative medical systems and practices in the United States (Pub. No. 94-066). Washington, DC: US Government Printing Office.

Chenitz, W. (1992). Living with AIDS. In J. Flaskerud & P. Ungvarski (Eds.), *HIV/AIDS: A guide to nursing care* (2d ed., pp. 440 – 459). Philadelphia: Saunders.

Cherry, B., & Giger, J. (1995). African-Americans. In J. Giger & R. Davidhizar (Eds.), *Transcultural nursing: Assessment and intervention* (pp. 165 – 203). St. Louis, MO: Mosby.

Chopra, D. (1989). *Quantum healing: Exploring the frontiers of mind/body medicine.* New York: Bantam.

Chu, S., Buehler, P., Flemming, L., & Berkelman, R. (1990). Epidemiology of reported cases of AIDS in lesbians, United States, 1989 – 90. *American Journal of Public Health, 11,* 1380 – 1381.

Cimoch, P. (1992). Current agents for the management of wasting and malnutrition in HIV/AIDS. *Nutrition and HIV/AIDS, 1,* 27 – 32.

Clark, J., McGee, R., & Preston, R. (1992). Nursing management of responses to the cancer experience. In J. Clark & R. McGee (Eds.), *Oncology Nursing Society core curriculum for oncology nursing* (2d ed., pp. 67–155). Philadelphia: Saunders.

Clatts, M., & Mutchler, K. (1989). AIDS and the dangerous other: Metaphors of sex and deviance in the representation of disease. *Medical Anthropology, 10,* 105–114.

Coale, M., & Robson, J. (1980). Dietary management of intractable diarrhea in malnourished patients. *Journal of the American Dietetic Association, 76,* 444–450.

Coldiron, B., & Bergstrasser, P. (1989). Prevalence and clinical spectrum of skin disease in humans infected with the human immunodeficiency virus. *Archives of Dermatology, 125,* 551–527.

Cole, R., & Cooper, S. (1991, December–January). *Lesbian exclusion from HIV/AIDS education: Ten years of low-risk identify and high-risk behavior.* SIECUS Report.

Colletti, M., German, M., McDonnell-Keenan, A., Zeller, J., & Balkstra, C. (1989). Immunologic system. In M. Thompson et al. (Eds.), *Clinical nursing* (2d ed., pp. 1302–1399). St. Louis, MO: Mosby.

Cooke, M. (1994). Patient rights and physician responsibility: four problems in AIDS care. In P. Volberding & M. Jacobson (Eds.), *AIDS clinical reviews 1993/4* (pp. 253–266). New York: Marcel Dekker.

Cooper, E. (1989). Controlled clinical trials of AIDS drugs: The best hope. *JAMA, 261,* 2444–2445.

Corea, G. (1992). *The invisible epidemic: The story of women and AIDS.* New York: HarperCollins.

Comroe, J, (1966). Some theories of the mechanism of dyspnea. In J. Howell & E. Campbell (Eds), *Breathlessness* (pp. 1–7). Boston: Blackwell Scientific.

Cunningham, R. (l992). *Prevention of infection in patients receiving myelosuppressive chemotherapy.* New York: Triclinical Communications.

Cunningham, R., & Bonam-Crawford, D. (1993) The role of fibrinolytic agents in the management of thrombotic complications associated with vascular access devices. *Nursing Clinics of North America, 28,* 900.

Dalpan, G., & McArthur, J. (1994). Diagnosis and management of sensory neuropathies in HIV infection. *AIDS Clinical Care, 6*(2), 9–12.

Dalton, H. (1989). Living with AIDS, Part 2: AIDS in blackface. *Daedalus, Journal of the American Academy of Arts and Sciences, 181,* 205–228.

Daniel, D., Kirchkoff, F., Czajak, S., Sehgal, P., & Desrosiers, R. (1992). Protective effects of a live attenuated HIV vaccine with a deletion in the nef gene. *Science, 258,* 1938–1941.

Dascombe, M. (1985). The pharmacology of fever. *Progress in Neurobiology, 25,* 327–373.

Deliacorte, F., & Alexander, P. (Eds.). (1987). *Sex work: Writings by women in the sex industry.* Pittsburgh: Cleis Press.

Demi, A. (1986). Grief as a growth process. In R. McCorkle & G. Hongladarum (Eds.), *Issues and topics in cancer nursing* (pp. 171–184). Norwalk, CT: Appleton-Century-Crofts.

Demi, A. (1996). Loss and grief. In R. Craven & C. Hinkle (Eds.), *Fundamentals of nursing: A functional approach* (2d ed., pp. 1466–1493). Philadelphia: Lippincott.

Demi, A., & Miles, M. (1987). Parameters of normal grief: A Delphi study. *Death Studies, 11,* 397–412.

Denker, A. (1989). *Nursing care of children with acquired immunodeficiency syndrome: A grounded theory approach.* Doctoral dissertation, University of Miami, FL.

Dewar, R., Highbarger, H., Sarmiento, M., et al. (1994). Application of branched DNA signal amplification to monitor Human Immunodeficiency Virus Type 1 burden in human plasma. *Journal of Infectious Diseases, 170,* 1172–1179.

Diaz, T., Buehler, J., Castro, K., & Ward, J. (1993). AIDS trends among Hispanics in the United States. *American Journal of Public Health, 83,* 504–509.

Dierich, M., Ebenbichler, C., Marschang, P., Fürst, G., Thielens, N., & Arlaud, G. (1994). HIV and human complement: Mechanisms of interaction and biological implication. *Immunology Today, 14,* 435–440.

Dilley, J. (1992). Management of neuropsychiatric disorders in HIV-spectrum patients. In M. Sande & P. Volberding (Eds.), *The medical management of AIDS* (pp. 218–233). Philadelphia: Saunders.

Dinarello, C. (1984). Interleukin-1. *Review of Infectious Diseases, 6*(1), 51–95.

Dixon, D., Rida, W., Fast, P., & Hoth, D. (1993). HIV vaccine trials: Some design issues including sample size calculations. *Journal of AIDS, 6,* 485–496.

Doka, K. (1989). *Disenfranchised grief.* Lexington, MA: Lexington.

Donohue, M. (1991). *The lived experience of stigma in individuals with AIDS: A phenomonological investigation.* Unpublished dissertation, Adelphi University, New York.

Dorn, N., Henderson, S., & South, N. (Eds.). (1992). *AIDS: Women, drugs and social care.* London: Falmer Press.

Dosey, B., Keegan, L., Guzzetta, C., & Kolkmeier, L. (1988). *Holistic nursing: A handbook for practice.* Rockville, MD: Aspen.

Drancourt, M., Mainardi, J., Brouqui, P. Vandenesch, F., Carta, A., Lehnert, F., Etienne, J., Goldstein, F., Acar, J., & Raoult, D. (1995). *Bartonella (Rochalimae) quintana* endocarditis in three homeless men. *New England Journal of Medicine, 332,* 419–428.

DuPont, H. (1995). Shigella species (bacillary dysentery. In G. Mandell, J. Bennett, & R. Dolin (Eds.), *Principles and practice of infectious diseases* (4th ed., pp. 2033–2039). New York: Churchill-Livingston.

Durham, J. (1991). The HIV epidemic: Ethical and legal dimensions. In J. Durham & F. Cohen (Eds.), *The person with AIDS: Nursing perspectives* (2d ed., pp. 361–387). New York: Springer.

Durham, J. (1994). The changing HIV/AIDS epidemic. Emerging psychosocial challenges for nurses. *Nursing Clinics of North America, 29*(1), 9–18.

Dwyer, J., Salvato-Schille, A., Coulston, A., Casey, V., Cooper, W., & Selles, W. (1995). The use of unconventional remedies among HIV-positive men living in California. *JANAC, 6*(1), 17–28.

Eisenberg, D. (1985), *Encounters with Qi: Exploring Chinese medicine.* New York: Penguin.

El-Sadr, W., Oleske, J., & Agins, B. (1994). *Evaluation and management of early HIV infection.* Clinical practice guideline No. 7. (AHCPR Publication No. 94-0572). Rockville, MD: AHCPR, Public Health Service, U.S. Department of Health and Human Services.

Enel, P., Charrel, J., Larher, M., Reviron, D., Manuel, C., & San Marco, J. (1991). Ethical problems raised by anti-HIV vaccination. *European Journal of Epidemiology, 7,* 147–153.

English, A. (1990). Treating adolescents: Legal and ethical considerations. *Medical Clinics of North America, 74,* 1097–1112.

Erickson, R. (1980). Oral temperature differences in relation to thermometer and technique. *Nursing Research, 29,* 157–164.

Esparza, J. (1993). WHO-GPA vaccine endeavors: Progress and expectations. *AIDS Research and Human Retroviruses, 9*(Suppl.1), S133–S135.

Esparza, J., Osmanov, S., Kallings, L., & Wigzell, H. (1991). Planning for HIV vaccine trials: The WHO perspective. *AIDS, 5*(Suppl.2), S159–S163.

Fabry, J. (1988). *Guideposts to meaning: Discovering what really matters.* Oakland, CA: New Harbinger.

Faden, R., Geller, G., & Powers, M. (Eds.). (1991). *AIDS, women and the next generation.* New York: Oxford University Press.

Farran, C., Herth, K., & Popovich, J. (1994). *Hope and hopelessness: Critical clinical constructs.* Newbury Park, CA: Sage.

Fauci, A. (1993a). Multifactorial and multiphasic components of the immunopathogenic mechanisms of HIV disease. *Huitième Colloque des Cent Gardes,* 81–85.

Fauci, A. (1993b). Multifactorial nature of human immunodeficiency virus disease: Implications for therapy. *Science, 262,* 1011–1018.

Fauci, A., & Lane, H. (1994). Human immunodeficiency virus (HIV) disease: AIDS and related disorders. In K. Isselbacher et al. (Eds.), *Harrison's principles of internal medicine* (pp. 1566–1618). New York: McGraw-Hill.

Fine, M., & Asch, A. (1988). Disability beyond stigma: Social interaction, discrimination, and activism. *Journal of Social Issues, 44*(1), 3–21.

Finn, A., & Plotkin, S. (1991). Immunization. In G. Wilson, E. Braunwald, K. Isselbacher, R. Petersdorf, J. Martin, A. Fauci, & R. Root (Eds.), *Harrison's principles of internal medicine* (12th ed., pp. 472–478). New York: McGraw-Hill.

Fitch, F., Lancki, D., & Gajewski, T. (1993). T-cell-mediated immune regulation. In W. Paul (Ed.), *Fundamental immunology* (pp. 733–800). New York: Raven Press.

Flaskerud, J. (1989). *AIDS/HIV infection: A reference guide for nursing professionals.* Philadelphia: Saunders.

Flaskerud, J., & Ungvarski, P. (1995). *HIV/AIDS: A guide to nursing care* (3d ed.). Philadelphia: Saunders.

Flaws, B. (1990). *Nine ounces: A nine part program for the prevention of AIDS in HIV positive persons.* Boulder, CO: Blue Poppy Press.

Fleischman, A., Post, L., & Dubler, N. (1994). Commentary: Mandatory newborn screening for human immunodeficiency virus. *Bulletin of the New York Academy of Medicine, 71,* 4–17.

Fletcher, J., & Wispelwey, B. (1994). AIDS and ethics: Clinical, social, and global. In S. Broder, T. Merrigan, & D. Bolognesi (Eds.), *Textbook of AIDS medicine* (pp. 855–170). Baltimore: Williams & Wilkins.

Friedland, R., & McCracken, G. (1995). Management of infections caused by antibiotic-resistant *Streptococcus pneumoniae. New England Journal of Medicine, 331,* 377–382.

Folkman, S., Chesney, M., & Christopher-Richards, A. (1994). Stress and coping in caregiver partners of men with AIDS. *Psychiatric Clinics of North America, 17*(1), 35–53.

Fox, A. (1994). Confronting the use of placebos for pain. *American Journal of Nursing, 94,* 42–45.

Fulton, J., & Johnson, G. (1993). Using high-dose morphine to relieve cancer pain. *Nursing93, 23*(2), 34–39.

Galle, P., & McRae, M. (1992). Amenorrhea and chronic anovulation. *Postgraduate Medicine, 92,* 255–260.

Galvin, T. (1992). Micronutrients: Implications in human immunodeficiency virus disease. *Topics in Clinical Nutrition, 7*(3), 63–73.

Gamble, R., & Getzel, G. (1989). Group work with gay men with AIDS. *Social Casework, 70,* 172–179.

Garrison, J., & Shepherd, S. (1989). *Cancer and hope: Charting a survival course.* Minneapolis: CompCare.

Gautier, E. (1993). *The legal rights and obligations of HIV-infected health care workers.* San Francisco: American Association of Physicians for Human Rights and the National Lawyers Guild AIDS Network.

Gee, G., & Moran, T. (Eds.) (1988). *AIDS: Concepts in nursing practice.* Baltimore, MD: Williams & Wilkins.

Gelberg, L., Linn, L., Usatine, R., & Smith, M. (1990). Health, homelessness, and poverty. *Archives of Internal Medicine, 150,* 2325–2330.

George, J. (1990). *Nursing theories: The base for professional nursing.* East Norwalk, CT: Appleton & Lange.

Gerber, R. (1988). *Vibrational medicine.* Santa Fe, NM: Bear.

Gerberding, J. (1991). Reducing occupational risk of HIV infection. *Hospital Practice, 26,* 103–108.

Gillon, R. (1994). *Principles of health care ethics.* New York: Wiley.

Gilman, A., Goodman, L., & Gilman, A. (1994). *The pharmacological basis of therapeutics.* New York: Macmillan.

Girard, M. (1994). Human immunodeficiency virus. In S. Plotkin & E. Mortimer (Eds.), *Vaccines* (2d ed., pp. 823–866). Philadelphia: Saunders.

Global Programme on AIDS. (1992). *Potential vaccine strategies using HIV vaccines in developing countries.* Geneva: WHO/GPA.

Goldberger, E. (1986). *A primer of water, electrolyte, and acid-base syndromes* (7th ed., p. 34). Philadelphia: Lea & Febiger.

Goldstein, J., & Kornfield, J. (1987). *Seeking the heart of wisdom.* Boston: Shambala.

Gorter, R. (1991). Management of anorexia-cachexia with cancer and HIV infection, *Oncology, 5*(Suppl.9), 13–17.

Grady, C. (1989a). Acquired immunodeficiency syndrome: The impact on professional nursing practice. *Cancer Nursing, 12*(1), 1–9.

Grady, C. (1989b). Ethical issues in providing nursing care to human immunodeficiency virus-infected populations. *Nursing Clinics of North America, 24,* 523–534.

Grady, C. (1992). Ethical aspects. In J. Flaskerud & P. Ungvarski (Eds.), *HIV/AIDS: A guide to nursing care* (2d ed., pp. 424–439). Philadelphia: Saunders.

Grady, C. (1995). *In search of an AIDS vaccine: Ethical issues in development and testing.* Bloomington: Indiana University Press.

Grady, C., & Kelly, G. (1996). State of the science: HIV vaccine development. *Nursing Clinics of North America, 31,* 25–39.

Graham, B., & Wright, P. (1995). Candidate AIDS vaccines. *New England Journal of Medicine, 333,* 1331–1339.

Graziosi, C., Pantaleo, G., Butini, L., et al. (1993). Kinetics of human immunodeficiency virus type 1 (HIV-1) DNA and RNA synthesis during primary HIV-1 infection. *Proceedings of the National Academy of Science, 90,* 6405–6409.

Greipp, M. (1992). Undermedication for pain: An ethical model. *Advances in Nursing Science, 15*(1), 44–53.

Grossman, A. (1991). Gay men and HIV/AIDS: Understanding the double stigma. *JANAC, 2*(4), 28–32.

Grossman, A. (1994). Homophobia: A cofactor of HIV disease in gay and lesbian youth. *JANAC, 5*(1), 39–43.

Grossman, M., & Cohen, S. (1991). Immunization. In D. Stites & A. Terr (Eds.), *Basic and clinical immunology* (7th ed., pp. 723–741). Norwalk: Lange Medical Books.

Grunfield, C., & Feingold, K. (1992). Metabolic disturbances and wasting in the acquired immuno-deficiency syndrome. *New England Journal of Medicine, 327,* 329–337.

Hackney, A. (1990). Women's health section. *American Journal of Nursing, 90*(9), 17.

Hagerty, B., Lynch-Sauer, J., Patusky, K., & Bouwsema, M. (1993). An emerging theory of human relatedness. *Image, 25,* 291–296.

Hall, B. (1991). The struggle of the diagnosed terminally ill person to maintain hope. *Nursing Science Quarterly, 3,* 177–184.

Hall, B. (1994). Ways of maintaining hope in HIV disease. *Research in Nursing and Health, 17,* 283–293.

Hall, J., & Stevens, P. (1988). AIDS: A guide to suicide assessment. *Archives of Psychiatric Nursing, 1,* 115–120.

Hanley, E., & Lincoln, P. (1992). HIV infection in women: Implications for nursing practice. *Nursing Clinics of North America, 27,* 925–936.

Hardy, L. (Ed). (1991). *HIV screening of pregnant women and newborns.* Committee on prenatal and newborn screening for HIV infection, Institute of Medicine. Washington, DC: National Academy Press.

Hay, L. (1987). *You can heal yourself.* Carson, CA: Hay House.

Haybach, P. (1993). Tuning in to ototoxicity. *Nursing83, 23*(6), 34–41.

Haynes, B. (1993). Scientific and social issues of human immunodeficiency virus vaccine development. *Science, 260,* 1279–1286.

Hays, R., McKusick, L., Pollack, L., Hilliard, R., Hoff, C., & Coates, T. (1993). Disclosing HIV seropositivity to significant others. *AIDS, 7,* 425–431.

Hedge, B. (1990). The psychological impact of AIDS. *AIDS Care, 2,* 381–383.

Hellon, R. (1981). Neurophysiology of temperature regulation: Problems and perspectives. *Federation Proceedings, 40,* 2804–2807.

Heurta, S., & Oddi, L. (1992). Refusal to care for patients with human immunodeficiency virus: Issues and responses. *Journal of Professional Nursing, 8,* 221–230.

Hibbard, P., Rubin, R., (1991). Fever in the immunocompromised host. In P. Macowiak (Ed.), *Fever: Basic mechanisms and management* (pp. 197–218). New York: Raven Press.

Hilleman, M. (1992a). Impediments, imponderables and alternatives in the attempt to develop an effective vaccine against AIDS. *Vaccine, 10,* 1053–1058.

Hilleman, M. (1992b). The dilemma of AIDS vaccines and therapy: Possible clues from comparative pathogenesis with measles. *AIDS research and human retroviruses, 8,* 1743–1748.

Ho, A., & Dole, V. (1979). Pain perception in drug-free alnd methadone-maintained human ex-addicts. *Proceedings of the Society for Experimental Psychology and Medicine, 162,* 392–395.

Hoffman, J., Cetron, M., Farley, M., Baughman, W., Facklam, R., Elliott, J., Deaver, K., & Breiman, R. (1995). The prevalence of drug-resistant *Streptococcus pneumoniae* in Atlanta. *New England Journal of Medicine, 324,* 481–486.

Holtzclaw, B. (1990). Control of febrile shivering during amphotericin B therapy. *Oncology Nursing Forum, 17,* 521–524.

Holtzclaw, B. (1992). The febrile response in critical care: State of the science. *Heart & Lung, 21,* 482–501.

Holtzclaw, B. (1993a). Monitoring body temperature. *AACN Clinical Issues, 4*(1), 44–55.

Holtzclaw, B. (1993b). Thermal balance. In M. Kinney, D. Packa, & S. Dunbar (Eds.), *AACN's clinical reference for critical care nursing* (3d ed., pp. 365–378). St. Louis: Mosby Year Book.

Hopps, H., Meyer, B., & Parkman, P. (1988). Regulation and testing of vaccines. In S. Plotkin & E. Mortimer (Eds.), *Vaccines* (pp. 576–586). Philadelphia: Saunders.

Horburgh, C. (1991). *Mycobacterium avium* complex infection in the acquired immunodeficiency syndrome. *New England Journal of Medicine, 324,* 1332–1338.

Hori, T., Nakashima, T., Take, S., Kaizuka Y., Mori T., & Katafuchi, T. (1991). Immune cytokines and regulation of body temperature, food intake and cellular immunity. *Brain Research Bulletin, 27,* 309–311.

Hoyt, M., & Staats, J. (1991). Wasting and malnutrition in patients with HIV/AIDS. *JANAC, 2*(3), 16–28.

Hughes, A., Jones, D., & Walent, R. (1994). Nursing management of the adult with advanced HIV disease: Inpatient care. In P. Cohen, M. Sande, & P. Volberding (Eds.), *The AIDS knowledge base* (2d ed., pp. 4.14.1–19). Boston: Little, Brown.

Hutchison, C. (1995). Healing touch research update. *Healing Touch Newsletter, 5*(2), 2.

Insler, M. (1987). *AIDS and the other sexually transmitted diseases and the eye.* Orlando: Grune and Stratton.

Isaacman, S. (1993). HIV surveillance testing: Taking advantage of the disadvantaged. *American Journal of Public Health, 83,* 597–598.

Israel, D., & Plaisance, K. (1991). Neutropenia in patients infected with human immunodeficiency virus. *Clinical Pharmacology, 10,* 268–279.

Jackson, M., & McSwane, D. (1992). Homelessness as a determinant of health. *Public Health Nursing, 9,* 185–192.

Jaffe, H. (1993). Value of non-vaccine prevention research in trials. *AIDS Research and Human Retroviruses, 9*(Suppl.1), S151–S152.

Jawetz, E., Melnick, J., & Adelberg, E. (1991). *Medical microbiology* (19th ed., pp. 419–440). Norwalk, CT: Appleton & Lange.

Johanson, G., & Kurtz, R. (1989). *Grace unfolding.* New York: Bell Tower.

Joy, W. (1979). *Joy's way: A map for the transformational journey.* New York: Putnam.

Kahn, J. (1992). Anti-human immunodeficiency virus therapeutics: Now and the future. *Seminars in Liver Disease, 12,* 121–127.

Kaptchuk, T. (1983). *The web that has no weaver: Understanding Chinese medicine.* New York: Congdon and Weed.

Katz, I. (1981). *Stigma: A social psychological analysis.* Hillsdale, NJ: Lawrence Erlbaum.

Kelly, J., St. Lawrence, J., Smith, S., Hood, H., & Cook, D. (1987). Stigmatization of AIDS patients by physicians. *American Journal of Public Health, 77,* 789–791.

Kelly, P., Holman, S., Rothenberg, R., & Holzemer, S. (Eds.). (1995). *Primary care of women and children with HIV: A multidisciplinary approach to care.* Boston: Jones & Bartlett.

Kemp, C. (1994). Spiritual care in terminal illness: Practical applications for nurses. *American Journal of Hospice and Palliative Care, 11*(5), 31–36.

Keusch, G., & Thea, T. (1993). Malnutrition in AIDS. *Medical Clinics of North America, 77,* 795–814.

Klaassen, R., Mulder, J., Vlekke, A., et al. (1990). Autoantibodies against peripheral blood cells appear early in HIV infection and their prevalence increases with disease progression. *Clinical and Experimental Immunology, 81*(1), 11–17.

Kluger, M. (1991). Fever: Role of pyrogens and cryogens. *Physiology Review, 71*(1), 93–127.

Koenig, S., Conley, A., Brewah, Y., et al. (1995). Transfer of HIV-1-specific cytotoxic T lymphocytes to an AIDS patient leads to selection for mutant HIV variants and subsequent disease progression. *Nature Medicine, 1,* 330–336.

Koff, W., & Glass, M. (1992). Future directions in HIV vaccine developments. *AIDS Research and Human Retroviruses, 8*(8), 1313–1315.

Koff, W., Wescott, S., & Hoth, D. (1990). Clinical trials of AIDS vaccines. In S. Putney & D. Bolognesi (Eds.), *AIDS vaccine research and clinical trials* (pp. 425–438). New York: Marcel Dekker.

Kotler, D., Culpepper-Morgan, J., Tierney, A., & Klein, E. (1986). Treatment of disseminated cytomegalovirus infection with 9-(1,3-dehydroxy-2-propoxymethyl) guanine: Evidence of prolonged survival in patients with the acquired immunodeficiency syndrome. *AIDS Research, 2,* 299–308.

Kugler, K., & Jones, W. (1992). On conceptualizing and assessing guilt. *Journal of Personality and Social Psychology, 62,* 317–327.

Kurth, A. (Ed.). (1993b). *Until the cure: Caring for women with HIV.* New Haven, CT: Yale University Press.

Lamendola, F. (1993). HIV+ nurses: Caring for our own. *American Nurse, 25*(3), 5.

Lamendola, F., & Newman, M. (1994). The paradox of HIV/AIDS as expanding consciousness. *Advances in Nursing Science, 16*(3), 13–21.

Lang, N. (1991). Stigma, self-esteem, and depression: Psycho-social responses to risk of AIDS. *Human Organization, 50*(1), 66–72.

Leaf, A., Laubenstein, L., Raphael, B., et al. (1988). Thrombotic thrombocytopenic purpura associated with Human Immunodeficiency virus type 1 infection. *Annals of Internal Medicine, 109,* 194–197.

Lebovits, A., Lefkowitz, M., McCarthy, D., Simon, R., Wilpon, H., Jung, R., & Fried, E. (1989). The prevalence and management of pain in patients with AIDS: A review of 134 cases. *Clinical Journal of Pain, 5,* 245–248.

LeShan, L. (1975). *How to meditate.* New York: Bantam.

Letvin, N. (1993). Vaccines against human immunodeficiency virus-progress and prospects. *New England Journal of Medicine, 329,* 1400–1405.

Levin, M. (1993). The day after an AIDS vaccine is discovered: Management matters. *Journal of Policy Analysis and Management, 12,* 438–455.

Levine, C., Dubler, N., & Levine, R. (1991). Building a new consensus: Ethical principles and policies for clinical research on HIV/AIDS. *IRB: A review of human subjects research, 13*(1–2), 1–17.

Levine, S. (1982). *Who dies?* Garden City, NY: Anchor Books.

Levy, R., Bredesen, D., & Rosenbaum, M. (1988). Neurological complications of HIV infection. *AIDS, 1,* 41–64.

Limandri, B. (1989). Disclosure of stigmatizing conditions: The discloser's perspective. *Archives of Psychiatric Nursing, 3*(2), 69–78.

Lindley, C., Dalton, J., & Fields, S. (1990). Narcotic analgesia: Clinical pharmacology and therapeutics. *Cancer Nursing, 13*(1), 28–38.

Lipscomb, J., & Love, C. (1992). Violence toward health care workers–An emerging occupational hazard. *American Association of Occupational Health Nurses Journal, 40,* 219–228.

Lisson, E. (1989). Ethical issues in pain management. *Seminars in Oncology Nursing, 5,* 114–119.

Lo, B. (1990b). Ethical dilemmas in HIV infection. *Journal of the American Podiatric Medicine Association, 80,* 26–30.

Lo, B. (1992). Ethical dilemmas in HIV infection: What have we learned? *Law, Medicine, & Health Care, 20*(1–2), 92–103.

Lo, B., Steinbrook, R., Cooke, M., Coates, T., Walters, E., & Hulley, S. (1989). Voluntary screening for HIV infection: Weighing the benefits and harms. *Annals of Internal Medicine, 110,* 727–733.

Longo, M., Spross, J., & Locke, A. (1990). Identifying major concerns of persons with acquired immunodeficiency syndrome: A replication. *Clinical Nurse Specialist, 4*(1), 21–26.

Lyons, C., & Fahrner, R. (1990). HIV in women in the sex industry and/or injection drug users. *NAACOG's Clinical Issues in Perinatal Health Nursing: AIDS in Women, 1*(1), 33–40.

Mackey, R. (1995). Discover the healing power of therapeutic touch. *AJN, 95*(4), 27–32.

Macrae, J. (1988). *Therapeutic touch: A practical guide.* New York: Knopf.

Marcusen, D., & Sooy, C. (1985). Otolaryngologic and head and neck manifestations of acquired immunodeficiency syndrome (AIDS). *Laryngoscope, 95,* 401–405.

Marin, G., & Marin, B. (1990). Perceived credibility of channels and sources of AIDS information among Hispanics. *AIDS Education and Prevention, 2,* 154–161.

Martin, J. (1987). Sustaining care of persons with AIDS. In J. Durham & F. Cohen (Eds.), *The Person with AIDS Nursing perspectives* (pp. 161–177). New York: Springer.

Martin, J., & Dean, L. (1993). Bereavement following a death from AIDS: Unique problems, reactions, and special needs. In M. Stroebe, W. Stroebe, & R. Hanson (Eds.), *Handbook of bereavement: Theory, research, and intervention* (pp. 317–330). New York: Cambridge University Press.

Mattson, S. (1987). The need for cultural concepts in nursing curricula. *Journal of Nursing Education, 26*(5), 206–207.

Mazbar, S., Schoenfeld, P., Humphreys, M. (1990). Renal involvement in patients infected with HIV: Experience at San Francisco General Hospital. *Kidney Int., 37,* 1325–1332.

McCaffery, M., & Beebe, A. (1989). *Pain : A clinical manual for nursing practice.* St. Louis, MO: Mosby.

McCaffery, M., & Vourakis, C. (1992). Assessment and relief of pain in chemically dependent patients. *Orthopedic Nursing, 11*(2), 13–27.

McCance-Katz, E., Hoecker, J., & Vitale, N. (l987). Severe neutropenia ssociated with anti-neutrophil antibody in a patient with acquired immuno-deficiency virus infection. *British Journal of Haematology, 66,* 337–340.

McDougal, J., Kennedy, M., Nicholson, J., et al. (1987). Antibody response to human immunodeficiency virus in homosexual men. *Journal of Clinical Investigation, 80,* 316–324.

McDowell, B. (1995). The National Institutes of Health Office of Alternative Medicine: Evaluating research outcomes. *Alternative and Complementary Therapies 1*(1), 17–25.

McWirter, D., & Mattison, A. (1984). *The male couple: How relationships develop.* Englewood Cliffs, NJ: Prentice-Hall.

Mentgen, J., Bulbrook, M. (1994). *Healing touch: Level I notebook.* Carrboro, NC: North Carolina Center for Healing Touch.

Mezzenzana, M., Orlando, G., Rapati, D., Quirino, T., Vigevani, G., & Cargnel, A. (1992). Permanent vascular catheter complications in AIDS patients. *International Conference on AIDS, 8,* 109.

Miles, A., Mellor, C., & Gazzard, B. (1990). Surgical management of anorectal disease in HIV positive homosexuals. *British Journal of Surgery, 77,* 869–871.

Miller, F., & Brody, H. (1995). Professional integrity and physician-assisted death. *Hastings Center Report, 25*(5), 8–12.

Miller, H., Turner, C., & Moses, L. (1990). *AIDS: The second decade.* Washington, DC: National Academy Press National Commission on AIDS. (1993).

Minkoff, H., DeHovitz, J., & Duerr, A. (Eds.). (1995). *HIV infection in women.* New York: Raven Press.

Mintz, M. (1992). Neurologic abnormalities. In R. Yogen & E. Connor (Eds.), *Management of HIV infection in infants and children.* St. Louis, MO: Mosby Year Book.

Mofenson, L., Moye, J., Bethel, J., Hirschhorn, R., Jordan, C., & Nugent, R. (1992). Prophylactic intravenous immunoglobulin in HIV-Infected Children With CD4+ counts of 0.20 x 10⁹/L or more. *JAMA, 268,* 483–488.

Monagle, J., & Thomasma, D. (Eds.). (1994). *Health care ethics: Critical issues.* Rockville, MD: Aspen.

Mondragon, D., Kirkman-Liff, B., & Schneller, E. (1991). Hostility to people with AIDS: Risk perception and demographic factors. *Social Science and Medicine, 32,* 1137–1142.

Montbriand, M. (1993). Freedom of choice. *Oncology Nursing Forum, 20,* 1195–1207.

Montbriand, M. (1994). An overview of alternative therapies chosen by patients with cancer. *Oncology Nursing Forum, 21,* 1547–1554.

Morgan, S. (1990). A comparison of three methods of managing fever in the neurologic patient. *Journal of Neuroscience Nursing, 22*(1), 19–24.

Morrison, C. (1987). Establishing a therapeutic environment: Institutional resources. In J. Durham & F. Cohen (Eds.), *The person with AIDS: Nursing perspectives* (pp. 110–125). New York: Springer.

Morrison, C. (1992). The HIV epidemic: Ethical issues for the next decade. *Critical Care Nursing Clinics of North America, 4,* 421–428.

Mount, B. (1993). Whole person care: Beyond psychosocial and physical needs. *American Journal of Hospice and Palliative Care, 10*(1), 28–37.

Mukau, L., Talamini, M., Sitzmann, J., Burns, C., & McGuire, M. (1992). Long-term central venous access vs. other home therapies: Complications in patients with acquired immunodeficiency syndrome. *Journal of Parenteral and Enteral Nutrition, 16,* 455–459.

Munson, R. (1992). *Intervention and reflection: Basic issues in medical ethics* (4th ed.). Belmont, CA: Wadsworth.

Murphy, M., Metcalfe, P., Waters, A., et al. (1987). Incidence and mechanism of neutropenia and thrombocytopenia in patients with Human Immunodeficiency Virus infection. *British Journal of Haematology, 66,* 337–340.

Murphy, T., & Walters. L. (1994). The moral significance of AIDS. *Journal of Medicine and Philosophy, 19,* 519–523.

Murray, J., Garay, S., Hopewell, P., Mills, J., Snider, G., & Stover, D. (1987). Pulmonary complications of the acquired immune deficiency syndrome: An update. *American Review of Respiratory Diseases, 135,* 504–509.

National Center for Nursing Research. (1990). *HIV infection: Prevention and care.* Bethesda, MD: U.S. Department of Health and Human Services.

National Commission on AIDS. (1993). *AIDS: An expanding tragedy.* Washington, DC: Author.

National Research Council. (1993). *The social impact of AIDS in the United States.* Washington, DC: National Academy of Sciences Press.

NCDHappenings. (1994–5, Winter). Newsletter of the National Coalition on Deaf Community and HIV, Inc.

Niu, M., Stein, D., & Schnittman, S. (1994). Primary human immunodeficiency virus type 1 infection: Review of pathogenesis and early treatment intervention in humans and animal retrovirus infections. *Journal of Infectious Diseases, 168,* 1490–1501.

Noddings, N. (1984). *Caring: A feminine approach to ethics and moral education.* Berkeley, CA: University of California Press.

Nokes, K. (1995). Nursing care of women. In J. Flaskerud & P. Ungvarski (Eds.), *AIDS/HIV infection: A guide to nursing care* (3d ed., pp. 243–259). Philadelphia: Saunders.

Novick, A. (1988). Some ethical issues associated with HIV vaccine trials. *AIDS Public Policy Journal, 3*(3), 46–48.

Nunes, J., Raymond, S., Nichols, P., Leuner, J., & Webster, A. (1995). Social support, quality of life, immune function, and health in persons living with HIV. *Journal of Holistic Nursing, 13,* 174–198.

O'Brien, M., & Pheifer, W. (1993). Physical and psychosocial nursing care for patients with HIV infection. *Nursing Clinics of North America, 28,* 303–316.

O'Connell, P. (1990). AIDS: A medical rehabilitation perspective. *Occupational Therapy in Health Care, 7*(2/3/4), 19–43.

O'Dowd, M. (1993). Suicidal behaviors and AIDS. *HIV/AIDS and Mental Hygiene, 3*(1), 1–4.

O'Dowd, M., Biderman, D., & McKegney, F. (1993). Incidence of suicidality in AIDS and HIV positive patients attending a psychiatry outpatient program. *Psychosomatics, 34*(1), 33–40.

O'Hara, M. (1995). Care of children with HIV infection. In P. Kelly, S. Holman, R. Rothenberg, & S. Holzemer (Eds.), *Primary care of women and children with HIV infection.* Boston: Jones and Bartlett.

Oldstone, M. (1994). HIV neurons and cytotoxic T lymphocytes. In R. Price & S. Perry (Eds.), *HIV, AIDS and the brain* (pp. 89–97). New York: Raven Press.

Olin, B., Hebel, S., Connell, S., & Dombek, C. (1995). *Facts and comparisons.* St. Louis, MO: Lippincott.

O'Neill, W., & Sherrard, J. (1993). Pain in human immunodeficiency virus disease: A review. *Pain, 54,* 3–14.

OrthoBiotech. (1992). *Understanding and managing anemia in the HIV-infected patient.* OrthoBiotech, Inc., PCT-186AA.

Overby, K., Lo, B., & Litt, F. (1988) Knowledge and concerns about acquired immune-deficiency syndrome with hemophilia. *Pediatrics, 83,* 204–210.

Padian, N. (1990). Heterosexual transmission: Infectivity and risks. In N. Alexander, H. Gabelnick, & J. Spieler (Eds.), *Heterosexual transmission of AIDS* (pp. 25–34). New York: Wiley-Liss.

Pallares, R., Linares, J., Vadillo, M., Cabellos, C., Manresa, F., Viladrich, P., Martin, R., & Gudiol, F. (1995). Resistance to penicillin and cephalosporin and mortality from severe pneumococcal pneumonia in Barcelona, Spain. *New England Journal of Medicine, 333,* 474–480.

Patton, J., Manning, K., Case, D., & Owen, J. (1994). Serum lactic dehydrogenase and platelet count predict survival in thrombotic thrombocytopenic purpura. *American Journal of Hematology, 47,* 94–99.

Payne, R. (1989). Pain in the drug abuser. In R. Payne & K. Foley (Eds.), *Current therapy of pain* (pp. 47–53). Philadelphia: Decker.

Petricciani, J., Gracher, V., Sizaret, A., & Regan, P. (1989). Vaccines: Obstacles and opportunities from discovery to use. *Review of Infectious Diseases, 11,* S524–S529.

PHS proposes "parallel track" for new AIDS drugs. (1990). *Public Health Reports, 105,* 541–542.

Pinching, A. (1994). AIDS: Health care ethics and society. In R. Gillon (Ed.), *Principles of health care ethics* (pp. 903–915). New York: Wiley.

Pinsky, L., & Douglas, P. (1992). *The essential HIV treatment fact book.* New York: Pocket Books.

Pizzo, P., & Wilfert, C. (Eds.). (1994). *Pediatric AIDS: The challenge of HIV infection in infants, children, and adolescents* (2d ed.). Baltimore: Williams & Wilkins.

Plowmen, V., & Ringering, L. (1994). CMV retinitis: A silent disabler. *Pacific Center Journal, 6*(3), 2–4.

Pluda, J., Mitsuya, H., & Yarchoan, R. (1991). Hematologic effects of AIDS therapies, Hematologic abnormalities in AIDS. *Hematology/Oncology Clinics of North America, 5,* 229–245.

Pollack, M. (1995). Pseudomonas aeruginosa. In G. Mandell, J. Bennett, & R. Dolin (Eds.), *Principles and practice of infectious diseases* (4th ed., pp. 1980–2003). New York: Churchill-Livingston.

Porter, J., Glass, M., & Koff, W. (1989). Ethical considerations in AIDS vaccine testing. *IRB: A Review of Human Subjects Research, 11*(3), 1–4.

Posey, E. (1988). Confidentiality in an AIDS support group. *Journal of Counseling and Development, 66,* 226–227.

Powell-Cope, G. (1994). Family caregivers of persons with AIDS: Negotiating partnerships with professional health care providers. *Nursing Research, 43,* 324–330.

Price, R., & Worley, J. (1995). Management of neurologic complications of HIV-1 infection and AIDS. In M. Sande & P. Volberding (Eds.), *The medical management of AIDS* (pp. 261–288). Philadelphia: Saunders.

Principi, N., Marchisio, P., Tornaghi, R., Onorato, J., Massironi, E., & Picco, P. (1991). Acute otitis media in human immunodeficiency virus-infected children. *Pediatrics, 88,* 566–571.

Pugh, K., O'Donnell, I., & Catalan, J. (1993). Suicide and HIV disease. *AIDS CARE, 5,* 391–400.

Ragsdale, D., & Morrow, J. (1990). Quality of life as a function of HIV classification. *Nursing Research, 39,* 355–359.

Rando, T. (1986). *Loss and anticipatory grief.* Lexington, MA: Lexington.

Raufman, J. (1988). Odynophagia/dysphagia in AIDS. In S. Friedman (Ed.), *Gastroenterology clinics of North America* (pp. 599–614). Philadelphia: Saunders.

Relman, D. (1995). Has trench fever returned? *New England Journal of Medicine, 332,* 463–464.

Rhodes, V., & Watson, P. (1987). Symptom distress—The concept: Past and present. *Seminars in Oncology Nursing, 3,* 242–247.

Rhoten, D. (1982). Fatigue and the postsurgical patient. In C. Norris (Ed.), *Concept clarification in nursing.* Rockville, MD: Aspen.

Richman, D. (1987). The toxicity of azidothymidine in the treatment of patients with AIDS and AIDS-related complex. *New England Journal of Medicine, 317,* 192–197.

Robb, V. (1994). The Hotel Project: A community approach to persons with AIDS. *Nursing Clinics of North America, 29,* 521–531.

Robb, V. (1995). Working on the edge: Palliative care for substance users with AIDS. *Journal of Palliative Care, 11*(2), 50–53.

Rose, M. (1993). The human faces of women with HIV/AIDS. *Florida Journal of Public Health, 5*(1), 8–10.

Roth, D., & LeVier, E. (Eds.). (1990). *Being human in the face of death.* Santa Monica, CA: IBS Press.

Rothman, D., & Edgar, H. (1991). AIDS activism and ethics. *Hospital Practice, 26*(7), 135–142.

Rothstein, S., Kohan, D., & Cohen, N. (1988). Otologic disease in patients with acquired immunodeficiency syndrome. *Annals of Otology Rhinology Laryngology, 97,* 636–640.

Rudd, A., & Taylor, D. (Eds.). (1992). *Positive women: Voices of women living with AIDS.* Toronto: Second Story Press.

Ryan, L. (1984). AIDS: A threat to physical and psychological integrity. *Topics in Clinical Nursing, 6*(2), 19–25.

Ryan, M., & Shattuck, A. (1994). *Treating AIDS with Chinese medicine.* Berkeley, CA: Pacific View Press.

Sabin, A. (1992). Improbability of effective vaccination against HIV because of its intracellular transmission and rectal portal of entry. *Proceedings of the National Academy of Sciences, 89,* 8852–8855.

Saunders, J. (1990). Gay and lesbian widowhood. In R. Kus (Ed.), *Keys to caring* (pp. 224–243). Boston: Alyson Publications.

Saunders, J. (1995). Ethical issues related to the care of persons with HIV. In J. Flaskerud & P. Ungvarski (Eds.). *HIV/AIDS: A guide to nursing care* (3d ed., pp. 364–388). Philadelphia: Saunders.

Saunders, J., & Buckingham, S. (1988). When depression turns deadly. *Nursing, 18*(7), 59–64.

Saunders, J., & Underwood, P. (1991). HIV infection: Helping adolescents choose safer behaviors. *Journal of Child and Adolescent Psychiatric and Mental Health Nursing, 4,* 132–136.

Saunders, J., & Valente, S. (1994). Nurses' grief. *Cancer Nursing, 17,* 318–325.

Savage, S. (1993). Addiction in the treatment of pain: significance, recognition and management. *Journal of Pain and Symptom Management, 8,* 265–278.

Scadden, D., Zon, L., & Groopman, J. (1989). Pathophysiology and management of HIV-associated hematologic disorders. *Blood, 74,* 1455–1463.

Scambler, G. (1984). Perceiving and coping with stigmatizing illness. In R. Fitzpatrick, J. Hinton, S. Newman, G. Scambler, & J. Thompson (Eds.), *The experience of illness* (pp. 203–226). New York: Tavistock.

Scambler, G., & Hopkins, A. (1990). Generating a model of epileptic stigma: The role of qualitative analysis. *Social Science and Medicine, 30,* 1187–1194.

Schmidt, C. (1995). The basics of therapeutic touch. *RN, 58*(6), 50–54.

Schneider, S., Taylor, S., Kemeny, M., & Hammen, C. (1991). AIDS-related factors predictive of suicidal ideation of low and high intent among gay and bisexual men. *Suicide and Life-Threatening Behavior, 21,* 313–328.

Schutt, R., & Garrett, G. (1992). *Responding to the homeless: Policy and practice.* New York/London: Plenum Press.

Scott, R. (1974). The construction of conceptions of stigma by professional experts. In D. Boswell & J. Wingrove (Eds.), *The handicapped person in the community* (pp. 108–121). New York: Tavistock.

Segal, J. (1987). *Living beyond fear: A course for coping with the emotional aspects of life-threatening illness.* North Hollywood, CA: Newcastle.

Semple, S., Patterson, T., Temoshok, L., McCutchan, J., Straits-Tröster, Chandler, J., & Grant, I. (1993). Identification of psychobiological stressors among HIV-positive women, *Women & Health, 20*(4), 15–36.

Seney, F., Burns, D., Silva, F. (1990). Acquired immunodeficiency syndrome and the kidney. *American Journal of Kidney Disease, 16,* 1–13.

Sepkowitz, K., Telzak, E., Carrow, M., & Armstrong, D. (1993). Fever among outpatients with advanced human immunodeficiency virus infection. *Archives of Internal Medicine, 153,* 1909–1912.

Shacknai, D. (1992). Wealth = Health: The public financing of AIDS care. In N. Hunter & W. Rubinstein (Eds.), *AIDS agenda: Emerging issues in civil rights* (pp. 181–201). New York: New Press.

Shernoff, M., & Springer, E. (1992). Substance use and AIDS: Report from the front lines. *Journal of Chemical Dependency Treatment, 5,* 35–48.

Shilts, R. (1988). *And the band played on.* New York: Viking Penguin.

Siegal, B. *Love, medicine and miracles.* New York: Harper & Row.

Siminoff, L., Erlen, J., & Lidz, C. (1991). Stigma, AIDS and quality of nursing care: State of the science. *Journal of Advanced Nursing, 16,* 262–269.

Simpson, D. (1995). Neurologic manifestations of HIV disease. *Improving the Management of HIV Disease, 3*(4), 12–16.

Singer, E., & Germaniskis, L. (1995). HIV and peripheral neuropathy. *Journal of the International Association of Physicians in AIDS Care, 1*(6), 30–33.

Slater, L., & Welch, D. (1995). Rochalimaea species (recently renamed Bartonella). In G. Mandell, J. Bennett, & R. Dolin (Eds.), *Principles and practice of infectious diseases* (4th ed., pp. 1741–1747). New York: Churchill-Livingston.

Smith, P., Hayes, R., & Mulder, D. (1991). Epidemiological and public health considerations in the design of HIV vaccine trials. *AIDS, 5*(Suppl.2), S105–S111.

Snow, W. (1993). Efficacy trials, design and implementation: Working with the community. *AIDS Research and Human Retroviruses, 9*(Suppl.1), S153–S154.

Sontag, S. (1988). *AIDS and its metaphors.* New York: Farrar, Straus and Giroux.

Sowell, R., Bramlett, M., Guildner, S., Gritzmacher, D., & Martin, G. (1991). The lived experience of survival and bereavement following the death of a lover from AIDS. *Image, 23,* 89–94.

Spector, R. (1991). *Cultural diversity in health and illness* (3d ed.). East Norwalk, CT: Appleton and Lange.

Springer, E. (1991). Effective AIDS prevention with active drug users: The harm reduction model. *Journal of Chemical Dependency Treatment, 4,* 141–157.

Squire, C. (Ed.). (1993). *Women and AIDS: Psychological perspectives.* Newbury Park, CA: Sage.

Starace, F. (1993). Suicidal behavior in people infected with human immunodeficiency virus: A literature review. *International Journal of Social Psychiatry, 39*(1), 64–70.

Stein, D. (1995). *Essential Reiki: A complete guide to an ancient healing art.* Freedom, CA: Crossing Press.

Stein, R. (1992). The development of an HIV vaccine. In W. Koff & H. Six (Eds.), *Vaccine research and developments* (pp. 223–244). New York: Marcel Dekker.

Stevens, P., & Hall, J. (1988). Stigma, health beliefs and experiences with health care in lesbian women. *Image, 20*(2), 69–73.

Stimmel, B. (1983). *Pain, analgesia and addiction: The pharmacological treatment of pain.* New York: Raven Press.

Strang, J. (1992). Harm reduction for drug users: Exploring the dimensions of harm, their measurement, and strategies for reductions. *AIDS & Public Policy Journal, 7,* 145–152.

Swanson, J. (1992). Genital herpes and prevention of HIV infection: The report of a study in progress. *JANAC, 3*(3), 30–36.

Swiss Group for Clinical Studies on AIDS. (1988). Zidovudine for the treatment of thrombocytopenia associated with human immunodeficiency virus. *Annals of Internal Medicine, 109,* 718–721.

Tagney, J. (1990). Assessing individual differences in proneness to shame and guilt: Development of the self-conscious affect and attribution inventory. *Journal of Personality and Social Psychology, 59*(1), 102–111.

Tagney, H., Wagner, P., & Gramzow, R. (1992). Proneness to shame, proneness to guilt and psychopathology. *Journal of Abnormal Psychology, 101,* 469–478.

Takigiku, S., Brubaker, T., & Hennon, C. (1993). A contextual model of stress among parent caregivers of gay sons with AIDS. *AIDS Education and Prevention, 5*(1), 25–42.

Taylor, E., Amenta, M., & Highfield, M. (1995). Spiritual Care Practices of Oncology Nurses. *Oncology Nursing Forum, 22*(1), 31–39.

Thomas, C. (Ed.). (1989). *Taber's cyclopedic medical dictionary* (16th ed.). Philadelphia: Davis.

Thomas, D. (1994). The racial divide: The effect of race on treating HIV. In *Positively aware* (p. 30). Chicago: Chicago's Test Positive Aware Network.

Tinette, M., Baker, D., McAvay, G., Claus, E., Garrett, P., Gottschalk, M., Koch, M., Trainor, K., & Horwitz, R. (1994). A multifactorial intervention to reduce the risk of falling among elderly people living in the community. *New England Journal of Medicine, 331,* 821–827.

Travin, S., Lee, H., & Bluestone, H. (1990). Prevalence and characteristics of violent patients in a general hospital. *New York State Journal of Medicine, 90,* 591–595.

Treisman, G. (1994). Mental health care of HIV patients (Part I). *AIDS Clinical Care, 6*(8), 63–66.

Triemstra, M., et al. (1995). Mortality in patients with hemophilia. *Annals of Internal Medicine, 123,* 823–827.

Tripp-Reimer, T., Brink, P., & Saunders, J. (1991). Cultural assessment: Content and process. In B. Spradley (Ed.), *Readings in Community Health Nursing* (4th ed., pp. 503–511). New York: Lippincott.

Tunnell, G. (1991). Complications in group psychotherapy with AIDS patients. *International Journal of Group Psychotherapy, 41,* 481–497.

Twiname, B. (1993). The relationship between HIV classification and depression and suicidal intent. *JANAC, 4*(4), 28–35.

Ungvarski, P. (1992). Nursing care of the adult client with AIDS and cytomegalovirus infection. *JANAC, 3*(1), 13–14.

Ungvarski, P., & Schmidt, J. (1995). Nursing managements of the adult client. In J. Flaskerud & P. Ungvarski (Eds.), *AIDS/HIV infection: A guide to nursing care* (3d ed., pp. 134–184). Philadelphia: Saunders.

Ungvarski, P., & Staats, J. (1995). Clinical manifestations of AIDS in adults. In J. Flaskerud & P. Ungvarski (Eds.), *AIDS/HIV infection: A guide to nursing care* (3d ed., pp. 81–133). Philadelphia: Saunders.

USDHHS. (1993, September 7). *Progress report: HIV infection.* Washington, DC: Author.

U.S. General Accounting Office. (1993). *Needle exchange programs: Research suggests promise as an AIDS prevention strategy* (GAO/HRD-93-60). Washington, DC: US Government Printing Office.

Valente, S., Saunders, J., & Uman, G. (1993). Self-care, psychological distress and HIV disease. *JANAC, 4*(4), 15–25.

Valentine, P. (1993). *HIV and minority populations* (HIV training manual). Washington, DC: Howard University National AIDS Minority Information & Training Program.

Valeri, A., & Nevsy, A. (1991). Acte and chronic renal disease in hospitalized AIDS patients. *Clinical Nephrology, 35,* 110–118.

Vallerand, A. (1994). Street addicts and patients with pain: Similarities and differences. *Clinical Nurse Specialist, 8*(1), 11–15.

Van Servellen, G., Lewis, C., & Leake, B. (1990). The stresses of hospitalization among AIDS patients on integrated and special care units. *International Journal of Nursing Studies, 27,* 235–247.

Veenstra, J., vanDer Lelie, J., Murder, J., & Reiss, P. (1993). Low-grade thrombotic thrombocytopenic purpura with HIV-1 infection: Case report. *British Journal of Haematology, 83,* 346–347.

Vermund, S. (1994). The efficacy of human immuno-deficiency virus vaccines: Methodological issues in preparing for clinical trials. In A. Nicolosi (Ed.), *Models and methods of epidemiologic research on HIV infection* (pp. 1–21). New York: Raven Press.

Vermund, S., Fischer, R., Hoff, R., Rida, W., Sheon, A., Lawrence, D., Hoth, D., & Barker, L. (1993). Preparing for HIV vaccine efficacy trials: Partnerships and challenges. *AIDS Research and Human Retroviruses, 9*(Suppl.1): S127–S132.

VonRoen, J. (1993). Pharmacologic interventions for HIV-related anorexia and cachexia. *Oncology, 7*(11), 95–99.

Wadland, W., & Gleeson, C. (1991). A model for psychosocial issues in HIV disease. *Journal of Family Practice, 33*(1), 82–86.

Wagner, K., & Cohen, J. (1993). Programs and policies for prevention. In A. Kurth (Ed.), *Until the cure: Caring for women with HIV* (pp. 228–238). New Haven, CT: Yale University Press.

Waldevogel, F. (1995). Staphylococcus aureus (including toxic shock syndrome). In G. Mandell, J. Bennett, & R. Dolin (Eds.), *Principles and practice of infectious diseases* (4th ed., pp. 1754–1784). New York: Churchill-Livingston.

Walkey, F., Taylor, A., & Green, D. (1990). Attitudes to AIDS: A comparative analysis of a new and negative stereotype. *Social Science and Medicine, 30,* 549–552.

Walters, L. (1988). Ethical issues in the prevention and treatment of HIV infection and AIDS. *Science, 239,* 597–602.

Weiner, B., Perry, R., & Magnusson, J. (1988). An attributional analysis of reactions to stigmas. *Journal of Personality and Social Psychology, 55,* 738–748.

Weiner, M., & Epstein, F. (1970). Signs and symptoms of electrolyte disorders. *Yale Journal of Biological Medicine, 43,* 76.

Weiss, R. (1973). *Loneliness: The experience of emotional and social isolation.* Cambridge, MA: MIT Press.

Weiss, R. (1992). The management of abnormal uterine bleeding. *Hospital Practice, 27*(10A), 55–78.

Weller, S. (1993). A meta-analysis of condom effectiveness in reducing sexually transmitted HIV. *Social Science Medicine, 12,* 1635–1644.

Wesson, D., Ling, W., & Smith, D. (1993). Prescription of opioids for the treatment of pain in patients with addictive disease. *Journal of Pain and Symptom Management, 8,* 289–297.

Whedon, M., & Shedd, P. (1989). Prediction and prevention of patient falls. *Image, 21,* 108–114.

Whitley, D. (1991). *STDs: Sexually transmitted diseases.* Arlington, Texas: Fairview Publications.

Williams, J. (1987). *Psychology of women. Behavior in a biosocial context* (3d ed.). New York: Norton.

Wolff, P., & Yetter Lunt, J. (1990). Nursing in the nineties: The nurse caring process. *Journal of Holistic Nursing, 8,* 3–21.

World Health Organization guidelines for cholera control. (1986). Geneva, Switzerland: WHO.

Wormser, G. (Ed.). (1992). *AIDS and other manifestations of HIV infection* (2d ed.). NY: Raven Press.

Wuthnow, R. (1994). *Sharing the journey. Support groups and America's new quest for community.* New York: Free Press.

Young, F. (1988). The role of the FDA in the effort against AIDS. *Public Health Reports, 103,* 242–245.

Zepp, S. (1993, October). The "potential for injury" and the risk for falls in patients with HIV disease. *AIDS Patient Care,* 249–252.

Zuger, A. (1991). AIDS and the obligations of health care professionals. In F. Reamer (Ed.), *AIDS and ethics* (pp. 215–239). New York: Columbia University Press.

Zurlo, J., et al. (1992). Sinusitis in HIV-1 infection. American Journal of Medicine, 93, 157–162.

Index

DATE DUE

NOV - 9 1999		
OCT 2 6 '00		